Stedman's

OPHTHALMOLOGY
WORDS

THIRD EDITION

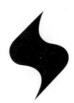

Stedman's
OPHTHALMOLOGY
WORDS

THIRD EDITION

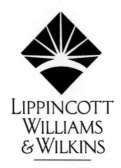

LIPPINCOTT
WILLIAMS
& WILKINS

Publisher: Julie K. Stegman
Series Managing Editor: Trista A. DiPaula
Associate Managing Editor: Steve Lichtenstein
Typesetter: Peirce Graphic Services, LLC.
Printer & Binder: Malloy Litho, Inc.

Printed in the United States of America

2004

Library of Congress Cataloging-in-Publication Data

Stedman, Thomas Lathrop, 1853–1938.
  Stedman's ophthalmology words.—3rd ed.
    p. ; cm. — (Stedman's word books)
  Includes bibliographical references.
  ISBN 0-7817-4420-2 (alk. paper)
  1. Ophthalmology—Terminology.
  [DNLM: 1. Ophthalmology—Terminology—English.   WV 15 S812s 2004]
  I. Title: Ophthalmology words.   II. Title.   III. Series.

RE20.S7 2004
617.7'001'4—dc22
                                                                2003018926
                                                                        01
                                            1 2 3 4 5 6 7 8 9 10

Contents

ACKNOWLEDGMENTS vii

EDITOR'S PREFACE ix

PUBLISHER'S PREFACE.. xi

EXPLANATORY NOTES xiii

A-Z WORD LIST.. 1

APPENDICES A1

   1.   Anatomical Illustrations................................. A1

   2.   Cranial Nerves A21

   3.   Sample Reports and Dictation A29

   4.   Common Terms by Procedure A42

   5.   Drugs by Indication A47

Acknowledgments

An important part of our editorial process is the involvement of medical transcriptionists—as advisors, reviewers, and/or editors.

We extend special thanks to Sandy Kovacs, CMT, FAAMT, and Amy Stummer, for editing the manuscript, helping resolve many difficult questions, and contributing material for the appendix sections. We are grateful to our Editorial Advisory Board members, including Pat Forbis, CMT; Robin Koza; Nicole Peck, CMT; Lauri Rebar; Tina Whitecotton, MT; and Sandra Wideburg, CMT, who were instrumental in the development of this reference. They recommended sources and shared their valuable judgment, insight, and perspective.

We also extend thanks to Darcy Johnson for working on the appendix. Additional thanks to Helen Littrell for performing the final prepublication review. Other important contributors to this edition include Marty Cantu, CMT; Janice Deal, RN, BSN; Dr. Howard Greene; Shemah Fletcher; Darcy Johnson; Cheryl A. Letner, CMT; Wendy Ryan, RHIT; Kathy Rockel, CMT; and Mary Chiara Zaratakiewicz.

And, as always, Barb Ferretti played an integral role in the process by reviewing the content files for format, updating the content, and providing a final quality check. Special thanks also goes to Lisa Fahnestock for her assistance with this work.

As with all our *Stedman's* word references, this resource incorporates the suggestions and expertise of our many contacts in the medical transcriptionist community. Thanks to all of our advisory board participants, reviewers, and editors; AAMT meeting attendees; and others who have written us with requests and comments—keep talking, and we'll keep listening.

Editor's Preface

What are tools of the trade? Well, it depends on your "trade." If you are a carpenter, a hammer might be a useful tool, but if you are a cab driver, a hammer would not work as well as a finely-tuned car. If you are an MT, a computer, headset, transcriber, and foot pedal comes to mind. What transcriptionist can do without reference books? I know I sure can't!

When I first began transcribing back in the late 70s, I had three medical reference books: a medical dictionary, PDR, and *Surgeon's Syllabus*. Lucky for me, I worked in an Air Force medical center in Germany, and the doctors were available to talk to whenever we had a question. They were more than willing to help us with the spelling of new instruments or new procedures, but as we all know, doctors are not very reliable when it comes to spelling. Thank goodness for the development of the *Stedman's Word Book* series. These books provide printed documentation of the many uncertain terms and spellings we had been trying to find for years.

This Third Edition of *Stedman's Ophthalmology Words* is another addition in the fine collection of reference materials published by Lippincott Williams & Wilkins. We have added many new terms that relate to LASIK and the new procedure, LASEK. More words are included pertaining to the subspecialty, neuroophthalmology and to some of the diseases which affect eyes including diabetes and thyroid disease. The appendix has detailed photographs of the anatomy of the eye plus drugs by indication, sample reports, tables of nerves and more.

I'd like to thank Amy Stummer for working with me on this book. She provided a second pair of eyes and solved many of our research questions. We worked very diligently to produce an end product that MTs and other medical language professionals will find useful. Many thanks to Trista DiPaula for her continued confidence in my editing skills and Barb Ferretti for her expert online editing skills. Finally, thank you, LWW for continuing to provide excellent reference books that MTs can use with confidence.

Sandy Kovacs, CMT, FAAMT

Publisher's Preface

Stedman's Ophthalmology Words, Third Edition, offers an authoritative assurance of quality and exactness to the wordsmiths of the healthcare professions—medical transcriptionists, medical editors and copyeditors, health information management personnel, court reporters, and the many other users and producers of medical documentation.

In *Stedman's Ophthalmology Words, Third Edition,* users will find protocols, diagnoses, and therapeutic procedures, new techniques, lab tests, clinical research terms, as well as abbreviations with their expansions pertinent to ophthalmology. The appendix sections, substantially enhanced over the previous edition, provide anatomical illustrations with useful captions and labels; a table of nerves; sample reports; common terms by procedure; and drugs by indication.

This new edition, including more than 60,000 entries, includes the *Stedman's Word Book Series* trademarks: terms fully cross-indexed by first and last word, an A-Z format with main entries and subentries, and appendix material for additional comprehension and application of the terminology.

We at Lippincott Williams & Wilkins strive to provide you with the most up-to-date and accurate word references available. Your use of this Word Book will prompt new editions, which we will publish as often as updates and revisions justify. We welcome your suggestions for improvements, changes, corrections, and additions—whatever will make this *Stedman's* product more useful to you. Please complete the postage-paid card in this book for future suggestions and recommendations, or visit us online at www.stedmans.com.

Explanatory Notes

Medical transcription is an art as well as a science. Both approaches are needed to correctly interpret the dictation of a physician, whose language is a product of education, training, and experience. This variety in medical language means that there are several acceptable ways to express certain terms, including jargon. *Stedman's Ophthalmology Words, Third Edition,* provides variant spellings and phrasings for many terms. These elements, in addition to complete cross-indexing, make *Stedman's Ophthalmology Words, Third Edition,* a valuable resource for determining the validity of terms as they are encountered.

Alphabetical Organization
Alphabetization of main entries is letter by letter as spelled, ignoring punctuation, spaces, prefixed numbers, or other characters. For example:

VSG 2/3F graphic card
V-slit lamp
VSR

Terms beginning or ending with Greek letters show the Greek letters spelled out and listed alphabetically. For example:

alpha, α
    a. angle
    a. crystallin

In subentry alphabetization, the abbreviated singular form or the spelled-out plural form of the noun main entry word is ignored.

Format and Style
All main entries are in **boldface** to expedite locating a sought-after term, to enhance distinction between main entries and subentries, and to relieve the textual density of the pages.

Irregular plurals and variant spellings are shown on the same line as the singular or preferred form of the word. For example:

ampulla, pl. ampullae
disk, disc

Hyphenation

As a rule of style, multiple eponyms (e.g., Mears-Rubash approach) are hyphenated. Also, hyphens have been added between a manufacturer and one or more eponyms (e.g., Vital-Metzenbaum dissecting scissors). Please note that in many cases, hyphenation is a question of style, not of accuracy, and thus is a matter of choice.

Possessives

Possessive forms have been dropped in this reference for the sake of consistency and conformance with the guidelines of the American Association for Medical Transcription (AAMT) and other groups. Please note, however, that in many cases, retaining the possessive, like hyphenating, is a question of style, not of accuracy, and thus is a matter of choice. To form the possessive of a word, simply add the apostrophe or apostrophe "s" to the end of the word.

Cross-indexing

The word list is in an index-like main entry-subentry format that contains two combined alphabetical listings:

(1) A *noun* main entry-subentry organization, which is typical of the A-Z section of medical dictionaries like *Stedman's:*

guard
    cataract knife g.
    ether g.
    eye knife g.

bed
    capillary b.
    corneal stromal b.
    recipient b.

(2) An *adjective* main entry-subentry organization, which lists words and phrases as you hear them. The main entries are the adjectives or modifiers in a multiword term. The subentries are the nouns around which the terms are constructed and to which the adjectives or modifiers pertain:

cystoid
  c. body
  c. cicatrix
  c. cicatrix of limbus

pigmentary
  p. deposits on lens
  p. dilution
  p. dispersion glaucoma

This format provides the user with more than one way to locate and identify a multiword term. For example:

hemorrhagic
  h. glaucoma

glaucoma
  hemorrhagic g.

epithelial
  e. inclusion cyst

cyst
  epithelial inclusion c.

It also allows the user to see together all terms that contain a particular descriptor, as well as all types, kinds, or variations of a noun entity. For example:

ocular
  o. adnexa
  o. adnexal tumor
  o. albinism

multifocal
  m. chorioretinal disease
  m. choroiditis
  m. choroiditis with panuveitis

Wherever possible, abbreviations are separately defined and cross-referenced. For example:

FOZR
  front optic zone radius

front
  f. optic zone radius (FOZR)

radius
  front optic zone r. (FOZR)

References

In addition to the manufacturers' literature we gather at various medical meetings, scientific reports from hospitals, and the lists of our MT Editorial Advisory Board members (from their daily transcription work), we used the following sources for new terms in *Stedman's Ophthalmology Words, Third Edition.*

Books

The AAMT Book of Style, 2ⁿᵈ Edition. Modesto, CA: AAMT, 2002.

Bartlett JD, Bennett ES, Fiscella RG, Jeanus SD, Rowsey JJ, Zimmerman TJ. *2003 Ophthalmic Drug Facts.* Philadelphia: Lippincott Williams & Wilkins, 2002.

Drake E. *Sloane's Medical Word Book, 4ᵗʰ Edition.* Philadelphia: Saunders, 2001.

Hoffman J, Ledford JK. *Quick Reference Dictionary of Eyecare Terminology, 3ʳᵈ Edition.* Thorofare, NJ: Slack, 2002.

Lance LL. *Quick Look Drug Book.* Baltimore: Lippincott Williams & Wilkins, 2003.

Pavan-Langston D. *Manual of Ocular Diagnosis and Therapy, 5ᵗʰ Edition.* Philadelphia: Lippincott Williams & Wilkins, 2002.

Rhee DJ, Deramo VA. *Wills Eye Drug Guide: Diagnostic and Therapeutic Medications, 2ⁿᵈ Edition.* Philadelphia: Lippincott Williams & Wilkins, 2001.

Rhee DJ, Pyfer MF. *Wills Eye Manual: Office and Emergency Room Diagnosis and Treatment of Eye Disease, 3ʳᵈ Edition.* Philadelphia: Lippincott Williams & Wilkins, 1999.

Stedman's Medical Dictionary, 27ᵗʰ Edition. Baltimore: Lippincott Williams & Wilkins, 2000.

Trobe JD, Hackel RE. *Field Guide to the Eyes.* Philadelphia: Lippincott Williams & Wilkins, 2002.

Vander JF, Gault JA. *Ophthalmology Secrets, 2ⁿᵈ Edition.* Philadelphia: Hanley & Belfus, 2002.

Images

Agur AMR, Lee MJ. *Grant's Atlas of Anatomy, 10th Edition.* Baltimore: Lippincott Williams & Wilkins, 1999.

Battista K, Baltimore, MD. From Oatis C. *Kinesiology: The Mechanics and Pathomechanics of Human Movement.* Baltimore: Lippincott Williams & Wilkins, 2003.

Caldwell S, Pikesville, MD. From *Stedman's Medical Dictionary, 27th Edition.* Baltimore: Lippincott Williams & Wilkins, 2000.

Hardy NO, Westport, CT. From *Stedman's Medical Dictionary, 27th Edition.* Baltimore: Lippincott Williams & Wilkins, 2000.

LifeART Nursing Collection 3, CD-ROM. Baltimore: Lippincott Williams & Wilkins.

LifeART Pediatrics Collection 1, CD-ROM. Baltimore: Lippincott Williams & Wilkins.

LifeART Super Anatomy Collection 2, CD-ROM. Baltimore: Lippincott Williams & Wilkins.

LifeART Super Anatomy Collection 4, CD-ROM. Baltimore: Lippincott Williams & Wilkins.

LifeART Super Anatomy Collection 7, CD-ROM. Baltimore: Lippincott Williams & Wilkins.

LifeART Super Anatomy Collection 9, CD-ROM. Baltimore: Lippincott Williams & Wilkins.

Ward L, Salt Lake City, UT. From Fuller J, RN, PhD & Schaller-Ayers J, RN, MNSc, PhD. *A Nursing Approach, 2nd Edition.* Philadelphia: J.B. Lippincott Company, 1994.

Journals

American Journal of Ophthalmology. New York: Elsevier Science, 2000–2003.

Cornea. New York: Raven Press, 1999–2002.

Current Opinion in Ophthalmology. Philadelphia: Lippincott Williams & Wilkins, 2002.

Journal of Neuro-Ophthalmology. Philadelphia: Lippincott Williams & Wilkins, 1999–2002.

Latest Word. Philadelphia: Saunders, 1999–2003.

Ophthalmology. Philadelphia: Elsevier Science, 1999–2003.

Ophthalmology Times. Duluth, MN: Advanstar Communications, Inc., 1999–2003.

Optometry and Vision Science. Philadelphia: Lippincott Williams & Wilkins, 1999–2003.

Retina. Philadelphia: Lippincott Williams & Wilkins, 1999–2002.

Websites

http://cns-web.bu.edu/pub/

http://med-aapos.bu.edu/

http://ods.od.nih.gov/databases/ibids.html

http://www.aao.org/

http://www.arvo.org/

http://www.ascrs.org/

http://www.djo.harvard.edu

http://www.emedicine.com/oph/

http://www.eyecancer.com/

http://www.eyecarecontacts.com/eyecare_connection_home.html

http://www.eyemdlink.com/

http://www.hsls.pitt.edu/intres/health/ophth.htm

http://www.lensmart.com

http://www.medscape.com/ophthalmologyhome

http://www.meei.harvard.edu/

http://www.mic.ki.se/Diseases/c11.html

http://www.mt-advisor.com/

http://www.nei.nih.gov

http://www.noah-health.org/english/illness/eye/eye.html

http://www.ophthal.org/

http://www.ophthalmologyresource.com/

http://www.revophth.com/

http://www.rpbusa.org/hc2/index.asp

http://www.wilmer.jhu.edu/

α (*var. of* alpha)
A
    accommodation
    A band
    crofilcon A
    cyclofilcon A
    cyclosporin A
    dimefilcon A
    droxifilcon A
    focofilcon A
    hefilcon A
    Intron A
    A Maddox line
    A measurement
    Muro Opcon A
    A pattern
    pentafilcon A
    perfilcon A
    phemfilcon A
    silafocon A
    A syndrome
    tetrafilcon A
    ultraviolet A (UVA)
AA
    accommodative amplitude
    amplitude of accommodation
AACG
    acute angle-closure glaucoma
AAMD
    atrophic age-related macular degeneration
AAO
    American Academy of Ophthalmology
    American Academy of Optometry
AAP
    achromatic automated perimetry
AAPOS
    American Association of Pediatric
    Ophthalmology and Strabismus
Aarskog syndrome
Aase syndrome
ab
    ab externo
    ab externo filtering operation
    ab externo trabeculectomy
    ab interno approach
Abadie sign
abaissement
Abbe
    A. refractometer
    A. value
abducens
    a. facial paralysis
    a. internuclear neuron
    a. nerve (CN VI)
    a. nerve fascicle

a. nerve palsy
a. nerve paralysis
a. paresis
abducent nerve (N.VI, CN VI)
abduct
abduction
    absence of a.
    congenital absence of a.
    a. deficit
abductor muscle
aberrant
    a. degeneration
    a. regeneration
    a. regeneration of nerve
    a. reinnervation of the oculomotor
    nerve
aberrated
    a. acuity chart
    a. eye
aberration
    angle of a.
    anterior-surface a.
    chromatic lens a.
    color a.
    coma a.
    corneal lens a.
    coupling of a.
    crystalline lens a.
    curvature a.
    dioptric a.
    distantial a.
    distortion a.
    lateral a.
    lens a.
    longitudinal a.
    low total spherical a.
    meridional a.
    monochromatic a.
    newtonian a.
    oblique a.
    ocular total higher-order a.
    (OTHA)
    optical a.
    positive spherical a.
    postoperative laser in situ
    keratomileusis visual a.
    postoperative LASIK visual a.
    reduction of a.
    regeneration a.
    spatially resolved wavefront a.
    spherical lens a.
    visual a.
aberrometer
    Hartmann-Shack wavefront a.

aberrometer *(continued)*
    Shack-Hartmann a.
    state-of-the-art a.
aberrometry
    clinical applications of a.
aberroscope
    objective cross-cylinder a.
ABES
    American Board of Eye Surgeons
abetalipoproteinemia
Abex-Turner incision
ability vergence
Abiotrophia defectiva
abiotrophy
    retinal a.
ABK
    aphakic bullous keratopathy
ablation
    broad-beam a.
    eccentric a.
    excimer laser a.
    hyperopic a.
    panretinal a.
    peripheral retinal a.
    pituitary a.
    toric a.
    treatment zone laser a.
    wavefront-guided a.
    a. zone
ablatio retinae
ablepharia
ablepharon
ablephary
ablepsia, ablepsy
ABMD
    anterior basement membrane dystrophy
Abney effect
abnormal
    a. harmonious retinal
      correspondence
    a. nearwork-induced transient
      myopia
    a. staining pattern
    a. unharmonious retinal
      correspondence
abnormality
    angle of a.
    congenital a.
    eyelid a.
    facial movement a.
    intraretinal microvascular a. (IRMA)
    microvascular a.
    retinal a.
    saccadic a.
    skeletal a.
    vascular a.
    vertebrobasilar vascular a.
ABO
    American Board of Ophthalmology

abrade
abrader
    cornea a.
    Howard a.
Abraham
    A. iridectomy laser lens
    A. iridotomy
    A. peripheral button iridotomy lens
    A. YAG laser lens
abrasio corneae
abrasion
    central a.
    conjunctival a.
    a. of cornea
    corneal a. (CA)
    traumatic corneal a.
abrin
abscess, pl. abscesses
    cerebral a.
    corneal a.
    fulminant a.
    lacrimal a.
    orbital subperiosteal a.
    psoriatic corneal a.
    retrobulbar a.
    a. ring
    ring a.
    scleral tunnel a.
    subperiosteal a.
    vitreous a.
abscessus siccus corneae
abscission
    corneal a.
absence of abduction
absent guttata
Absidia corymbifera
absinthe
absolute
    a. accommodation
    a. glaucoma
    a. hemianopsia
    a. hyperopia
    a. intensity threshold acuity
    near point a.
    a. scotoma
    a. strabismus
absolutum
    glaucoma a.
absorbable
    a. gelatin film
    a. suture
Absorbonac ophthalmic
absorptance
    radiant a.
absorption
    fluorescent treponemal antibody a.
    a. line
abtorsion

AC
    accommodative convergence
    anterior chamber
        Eye Drops AC
        AC eye drops
        AC tube inserter
        Visine AC
a.c.
    before meals
AC/A
    accommodative
        convergence/accommodation ratio
acanthamebiasis
Acanthamoeba
    A. *castellanii*
    A. cyst
    A. endophthalmitis
    A. keratitis
    A. keratitis pseudodendrites
    A. *mauritaniensis*
    A. *polyphaga*
acanthocytosis
acantholysis
acanthoma fissuratum
acanthosis nigricans
acarica
    blepharitis a.
ACC
    anterior central curve
Acc
    accommodation
accelerometer
accessoriae
    glandulae lacrimales a.
accessory
    a. fiber
    a. lacrimal gland
    a. nucleus
    a. organ of eye
accidental
    a. image
    a. mydriasis
accommodation (A, Acc)
    absolute a.
    amplitude of a. (AA)
    binocular a.
    breadth of a.
    bright-field a.
    convergence a. (CA/C)
    a. of crystalline lens
    dark-field a.
    defective a.

a. disorder
esodeviation a.
esotropia a.
excessive a.
far point of a. (FPA)
fusion with a.
Helmholtz theory of a.
a. insufficiency
iridoplegia a.
light and a. (L&A)
near point of a. (NPA)
near-point a.
negative a.
open-loop a.
paralysis of a.
a. paresis
a. phosphene
a. phosphene of Czermak
pinhole a.
position a.
positive a.
punctum proximum of a.
pupils equal, reactive to light
    and a. (PERLA)
pupils equal, round, reactive to
    light and a. (PERRLA)
range of a.
reflex a.
a. reflex
relative a.
residual a.
a. response
reticule a.
a. rule
a. spasm
spasm of a.
steady-state a.
subnormal a.
tonic a.
accommodation-convergence ratio
accommodative
    a. adaptation
    a. amplitude (AA)
    a. asthenopia
    a. convergence (AC)
    a. convergence/accommodation ratio
        (AC/A)
    a. cyclophoria
    a. effort syndrome
    a. esodeviation
    a. esophoria
    a. esotropia

NOTES

accommodative *(continued)*
- a. insufficiency (AI)
- a. IOL
- a. palsy
- a. pupillary reflex
- a. response
- a. spasm
- a. squint
- a. stimulus
- a. strabismus
- a. target

accommodometer

accreta
- cataracta membranacea a.

Accugel lens
Accu-Line surgical marking pen
AccuMap multifocal objective perimeter
accumulation
- lipid a.

Accurate Surgical and Scientific Instruments (ASSI)

Accurus
- A. peeler-cutter (APC)
- A. 2500 probe
- A. vitreoretinal surgical system

Accuscan Transducer 400
Accutane
Accutome
- A. black diamond blade
- A. black diamond clear cornea keratome
- A. LRI diamond knife
- A. side-port diamond knife

Accuvac smoke evacuation attachment
aceclidine
acellular
- a. dermis
- a. diurnal allograft
- a. matrix

ACES
- American College of Eye Surgeons

acetaldehyde
acetaminophen with codeine
acetanilid
acetate
- Anecortave a.
- aqueous uranyl a.
- cellulose a.
- cortisone a.
- Cortone A.
- dexamethasone a.
- fluorometholone a.
- glatiramer a.
- hydrocortisone a.
- medroxyprogesterone a.
- paramethasone a.
- phenylmercuric a.
- potassium a.
- prednisolone a.
- sodium a.
- zinc a.

acetazolamide
acetohexamide
acetonide
- triamcinolone a.

acetoxycyclohexamide (AXM)
acetoxyphenylmercury
aceturate
- diminazene a.

acetylcholine
- a. chloride
- a. receptor deficiency

acetylcholinesterase deficiency
acetylcysteine
N-acetyl-beta-D-glucosamidase
ACG
- angle-closure glaucoma

achiasma
achloropsia
achromat
achromate
achromatic
- a. automated perimetry (AAP)
- a. axis
- a. doublet
- a. objective
- a. spectacle lens
- a. threshold
- a. vision

achromatism
achromatopia
achromatopic
achromatopsia, achromatopsy
- atypical a.
- central a.
- cerebral a.
- complete a.
- cone a.
- incomplete a.
- rod a.
- typical a.
- X-linked a.

achromia
achromocytosis
Achromycin Ophthalmic
Achroplan nonapplanating 40x immersion objective lens
acid
- aminocaproic a.
- boric a.
- a. burn
- folinic a.
- hyaluronic a.
- a. maltase deficiency
- meibum oleic a.
- tranexamic a.

acid-fast
    a.-f. bacillus
    a.-f. stain
acidophilic adenoma
acid-resistant penicillin
acid-Schiff
    periodic a.-S. (PAS)
acinar
    a. dropout
    a. lacrimal gland
Acinetobacter calcoaceticus
acinus, pl. **acini**
    lacrimal gland a.
ACIOL
    anterior chamber intraocular lens
        ACIOL implant
ACL
    acromegaloid features, cutis verticis
        gyrata, corneal leukoma
aCL
    anticardiolipin
aclastic
ACM
    anterior chamber maintainer
acne
    a. ciliaris
    a. rosacea
    a. rosacea blepharoconjunctivitis
    a. rosacea conjunctivitis
    a. rosacea corneal ulcer
    a. rosacea keratitis
    a. rosacea meibomianitis
acnes
    Propionibacterium a.
A-constant
acorea
acorn-shaped eye implant
acoustic
    a. nerve
    a. neuroma
    a. spot
acoustical
    a. shadowing
    a. sonolucent
acquired
    a. abducens nerve lesion
    a. alexia
    a. astigmatism
    a. color defect
    a. distichia
    a. dyschromatopsia
    a. entropion
    a. esotropia
    a. gustolacrimal reflex
    a. Horner syndrome
    a. III nerve lesion
    a. immune response
    a. immunodeficiency syndrome
        (AIDS)
    a. jerk nystagmus
    a. melanosis
    a. myopathic ptosis
    a. ocular motor apraxia
    a. pendular nystagmus
    a. retinoschisis
    a. syphilis
    a. toxoplasmosis retinitis
acquisita
    epidermolysis bullosa a.
ACR
    Clear Eyes ACR
Acremonium
acritochromacy
acrocephalosyndactyly of Apert
acrodermatitis enteropathica
acromegaloid features, cutis verticis
    gyrata, corneal leukoma (ACL)
acrylate
    silicone a.
acrylic
    a. hydroxyapatite implant
    a. intraocular lens
    a. lens implant
AcrySof
    A. foldable intraocular lens
    A. MA60 lens
    A. Natural intraocular lens
    A. Natural IOL
    A. single-piece IOL
a-crystallin/small heat-shock gene
ACS
    Alcon Closure System
    Automated Corneal Shaper
    ACS needle
ACT
    alternate cover test
actinic
    a. conjunctivitis
    a. hyperplasia
    a. keratitis
    a. keratosis
    a. prurigo
    a. ray ophthalmia
    a. retinitis

NOTES

Actinobacillus actinomycetemcomitans
Actinomadura madurae
Actinomyces
    A. israelii
    A. nevi
Actinomycetales
actinomycetemcomitans
    Actinobacillus a.
actinomycin D
action
    mechanism of a.
    mode of a.
    primary a.
    secondary a.
Activase
activator
    tissue plasminogen a. (TPA, tPA)
    urokinase-type plasminogen a.
    (UPA)
active pterygium
activity
    A.'s of Daily Vision Scale
    (ADVS)
    intrinsic sympathomimetic a.
    laser a.
actomyosin ATPase
actual degree of independence
Acuiometer
acuity
    absolute intensity threshold a.
    Bailey-Lovie distance visual a.
    best-corrected visual a. (BCVA)
    best-uncorrected visual a. (BUVA)
    binocular visual a.
    a. card procedure
    central visual a.
    a. of color vision (VC)
    corrected visual a. (Va_{cc})
    detection a.
    distance visual a. (DVA)
    dynamic visual a.
    grating a.
    high-contrast distance visual a.
    (HCDVA)
    identification a.
    Jaeger a.
    line of visual a.
    low-contrast distance visual a.
    (LCDVA)
    mean a.
    minimum perceptible a.
    minimum separable a.
    near visual a. (NVA)
    numerical visual a.
    perceptible a.
    potential visual a.
    resolution a.
    separable a.
    Snellen visual a.

    spatial a.
    stereoscopic a.
    Teller visual a.
    true visual a. (TVA)
    uncorrected visual a. (UCVA)
    Vernier visual a.
    visibility a.
    visual discriminatory a. (VDA)
    a. visual projector
Acular
    A. drops
    A. Ophthalmic
    A. PF
aculeiform cataract
Acuson
    A. 128 apparatus
    A. ultrasound
acute
    a. angle-closure glaucoma (AACG)
    a. anular outer retinopathy
    a. atopic conjunctivitis
    a. catarrhal conjunctivitis
    a. catarrhal rhinitis
    a. chalazion
    a. chronic glaucoma
    a. congestive conjunctivitis
    a. congestive glaucoma
    a. contagious conjunctivitis
    a. dacryocystitis
    a. diffuse serous choroiditis
    a. epidemic conjunctivitis
    a. follicular conjunctivitis
    a. hemorrhagic conjunctivitis
    a. idiopathic blind spot enlargement
    syndrome
    a. idiopathic demyelinating optic
    neuritis
    a. intermittent primary angle-closure
    glaucoma (A/I-PACG)
    a. macular neuroretinopathy
    a. multifocal placoid pigment
    epitheliopathy (AMPPE)
    a. posterior multifocal placoid
    pigment epitheliopathy (APMPPE)
    a. primary angle-closure glaucoma
    (APACG)
    a. red eye (ARE)
    a. retinal necrosis (ARN)
    a. retinal necrosis syndrome
    a. spastic entropion
    a. sterile inflammation
    a. zonal occult outer retinopathy
    (AZOOR)
Acuvue
    A. Bifocal contact lens
    A. brand toric contact lens
    A. 1-Day disposable lens
    A. disposable contact lens
    A. Etafilcon A lens

A. Toric contact lens
A. 2-week UV-blocking disposable lens
acyclic nucleoside analogue
acyclovir
Adams
A. operation
A. operation for ectropion
Adapettes
Adaprolol
adaptation
accommodative a.
color a.
dark a.
light a.
photopic a.
retinal a.
scotopic a.
adapter
Sheehy-Urban sliding lens a.
Volk Minus noncontact a.
Volk retinal scale a.
Volk ultra field aspherical lens a.
Volk yellow filter a.
Zeiss cine a.
adaptive immunity
adaptometer
Collin 140 color a.
color a.
Feldman a.
Goldmann-Weekers dark a.
adaptometry
dark a.
AdatoSil
add
near a.
a. power
adduct
adduction
a. impairment
a. lag
adductor muscle
A-dellen
adenine arabinoside
adenoid cystic carcinoma
adenologaditis
adenoma
acidophilic a.
basophilic a.
chromophobe a.
endocrine-inactive a.

Fuchs a.
invasive a.
parathyroid a.
pituitary a.
pleomorphic a.
prolactin-secreting a.
sebaceous a.
a. sebaceum
adenomectomy
medical a.
adenophthalmia
adenosine monophosphate (AMP)
adenoviral
a. conjunctivitis
a. keratoconjunctivitis
adenovirus (ADV)
a. 3, 7, 8, 19
a. conjunctivitis
a. monoclonal antibody
a. type 34
adequacy
blink a.
adherence syndrome
adherens
leukoma a.
macula a.
zonula a.
adherent
a. cataract
a. lens
a. leukoma
adhesion
cell a.
chorioretinal a.
cicatricial a.
thermal a.
vitreoretinal a.
adhesive
Brown sterile a.
cyanoacrylate tissue a.
Nexacryl tissue a.
a. syndrome
tissue a.
Adie
A. syndrome
A. tonic pupil
adiposa
blepharoptosis a.
cataracta a.
pseudophakia a.
ptosis a.

NOTES

adipose
    a. body
    a. tissue
adiposus
    arcus a.
aditus orbitae
adjunct anesthetic agent
adjunctive
    a. mitomycin C
    a. MMC
adjustable suture
adjuster
    Seibel paracentesis valve a.
    Serdarevic suture a.
adjustment
    early postoperative suture a.
    (EPSA)
    intraoperative suture a. (ISA)
    late postoperative suture a. (LPSA)
    postoperative a.
    suture a.
adjuvant microwave thermotherapy
Adler operation
administration
    intraocular a.
adnatum
    ankyloblepharon filiforme a.
adnexa
    ocular a.
    a. oculi
adnexal
adolescent cataract
adrenal
    a. disorder
    a. hypertension
adrenaline
adrenergic drug
adrenochrome deposit
adrenoleukodystrophy
adrenomedullin
Adson forceps
Adsorbate
Adsorbocarpine Ophthalmic
Adsorbonac
Adsorbotear Ophthalmic Solution
adtorsion
adult
    a. inclusion conjunctivitis
    a. medulloepithelioma
adult-onset
    a.-o. cataract
    a.-o. diabetes mellitus (AODM)
    a.-o. foveomacular dystrophy
    (AOFMD)
adultorum
    blennorrhea a.
adumbration
ADV
    adenovirus

advanced
    A. Glaucoma Intervention Study
    (AGIS)
    a. pellucid marginal degeneration
    A. Relief Visine
    A. Shape Technology Refractive
    Algorithm (ASTRA)
advancement
    capsular a.
    a. flap
    a. procedure
    tendon a.
advancing wave-like epitheliopathy
    (AWE)
Advent pachymeter
ADVS
    Activities of Daily Vision Scale
AE-2910 Carones LASEK pump
AE-2920 Carones LASEK spatula
AE-7277 Rubenstein LASIK Cannula
AE-7618 Tsuneoka irrigating chopper
Aebli corneal section scissors
aegypticus
    Haemophilus a.
AEO
    apraxia of eyelid opening
aerial
    a. haze
    a. image
aerogenes
    Enterobacter a.
Aeromonas hydrophila
aerosol keratitis
Aerosporin
aeruginosa
    Pseudomonas a.
AES
    antielevation syndrome
Aesculap
    A. argon ophthalmic laser
    A. excimer laser
Aesculap-Meditec
    A.-M. excimer laser
    A.-M. MEL60 system
A-esotropia
aesthesiometer (*var. of* esthesiometer)
A-exotropia
afferent
    a. nerve
    a. pupillary defect (APD)
    a. visual pathway
    a. visual symptom
afferentiation
AFI
    amaurotic familial idiocy
afocal
    a. optical system
    a. telescope

A

africanum
  Mycobacterium a.
aftercataract bur
aftereffect
afterimage
  complementary a.
  negative a.
  positive a.
  a. test
afterimagery
afternystagmus
afterperception
aftervision
AG
  Amsler grid
against-the-rule (ATR)
  a.-t.-r. astigmatism
agar
  chocolate a.
  nonnutrient a.
  Sabouraud dextrose a.
Agarwal irrigating phaco chopper
age
  postconceptual a.
agenesis
  colossal a.
agent
  adjunct anesthetic a.
  alternate coupling a.
  coupling a.
  intraocular anesthetic a.
  reversal a.
  systemic hyperosmolar a.
  topical hyperosmolar a.
ageotropic nystagmus
age-related
  a.-r. cataract
  a.-r. degenerative retinoschisis
  a.-r. disciform macular degeneration
  A.-r. Eye Disease Study (AREDS)
  a.-r. macular degeneration (AMD, ARMD)
  a.-r. maculopathy (ARM)
  a.-r. ptosis
agglutination
  lid a.
  plasmoid a.
agglutinin
  Arachis hypogea a.
  Ricinus communis a.
  Ulex europaeus a. 1 (UEA-1)

aggregate
  cellular a.
aggregation
aging
  Canadian Study of Health and A.
AGIS
  Advanced Glaucoma Intervention Study
AGL-400
  Mira AGL-400
aglaucopsia
AGN 192024
Agnew
  A. canaliculus knife
  A. canthoplasty
  A. keratome
  A. operation
  A. tattooing needle
Agnew-Verhoeff incision
agnosia
  apperceptive a.
  color a.
  optic a.
  topographic a.
  visual a.
  visual-spatial a.
agonist-antagonist relationship
agonist muscle
Agrikola
  A. lacrimal sac retractor
  A. operation
  A. refractor
  A. tattooing needle
AGV
  Ahmed glaucoma valve
  AGV pars plana clip
Ahlström syndrome
AHM
  anterior hyaloid membrane
Ahmed
  A. device
  A. drainage seton
  A. glaucoma biplate
  A. glaucoma biplate valve
  A. glaucoma drainage tube
  A. glaucoma valve (AGV)
  A. glaucoma valve implantation
  A. shunt tube
  A. tube extender
  A. valve implant
AI
  accommodative insufficiency

NOTES

AICA
anterior inferior cerebellar artery
AICA syndrome
Aicardi syndrome
aid
low-vision a.
AIDS
acquired immunodeficiency syndrome
Longitudinal Study of Ocular
Complications of AIDS (LSOCA)
Studies of the Ocular
Complications in AIDS (SOCA)
AIDS-related
AIDS-r. complex (ARC)
AIDS-r. retinitis
aileron
Aimark perimetry
aiming beam
AION
anterior ischemic optic neuropathy
A/I-PACG
acute intermittent primary angle-closure
glaucoma
air
a. bag-associated trauma
a. bubble
a. cell
a. chamber
a. cystitome
A. Force test grid target
a. injection cannula
intraocular a.
intraorbital a.
a. rifle
air-block glaucoma
air-fluid exchange
AIRLens contact lens
air-puff
a.-p. contact tonometer
a.-p. noncontact tonometer
Airy
A. cylindric lens
A. disk
AK
astigmatic keratotomy
Akahoshi
A. acrylic intraocular lens forceps
A. acrylic IOL loading forceps
A. Combo PreChopper
A. hydrodissection cannula
A. implantation forceps
A. nucleus manipulator
A. nucleus sustainer
A. Phaco PreChopper
A. Universal PreChopper
Akarpine Ophthalmic
AK-Beta
AK-Chlor Ophthalmic

AK-Cide
AK-C. Ophthalmic
AK-C. Suspension
AK-Con-A
AK-Con ophthalmic
AK-Dex Ophthalmic
AK-Dilate Ophthalmic Solution
Aker lens pusher
AK-Fluor
AK-Homatropine Ophthalmic
akinesia
Nadbath a.
O'Brien a.
orbital a.
retrobulbar a.
Scheie a.
supraorbital a.
Van Lint a.
akinesis
pupillary sphincter a.
akinetic
akinetopsia
cerebral a.
AK-Lor
AK-Mycin
AK-NaCl
AK-Nefrin Ophthalmic Solution
AK-Neo-Cort
AK-Neo-Dex Ophthalmic
aknephascopia
Akorn OcuCaps
AK-Pentolate
AK-Poly-Bac Ophthalmic
AK-Pred Ophthalmic
AKPro Ophthalmic
AK-Rinse
AK-Spore
AK-S. H.C. Ophthalmic Ointment
AK-S. H.C. Ophthalmic Suspension
AK-S. Solution
AK-Sulf
AK-S. Forte
AK-S. Ophthalmic
AK-Taine
AK-Tate
AK-T-Caine
AK-Tetra
AKTob Ophthalmic
AK-Tracin Ophthalmic
AK-Trol Suspension
Akura PDAK marker
AK-Vernacon
Akwa
A. Tears
A. Tears lubricant eye drops
A. Tears lubricant ophthalmic
ointment
A. Tears solution
AK-Zol

AL
  axial length
al
  Vizor al
Alabama
  A. tying forceps
  A. University utility forceps
Alabama-Green
  A.-G. clamp
  A.-G. needle holder
alacrima
Alamar blue redox reaction
Alamast
ala minor ossis sphenoidalis
Aland eye disease
Alan-Thorpe lens
Albalon
  A. Liquifilm
  A. Liquifilm Ophthalmic
Albalon-A
  A.-A Liquifilm
  A.-A Ophthalmic
Albamycin
albedo retinae
albendazole
Albenza
Albers-Schönberg disease
albescens
  retinitis punctata a.
albicans
  Candida a.
albinism
  autosomal-dominant
  oculocutaneous a.
  autosomal-recessive ocular a.
  (AROA)
  Bergsma-Kaiser-Kupfer
  oculocutaneous a.
  Donaldson-Fitzpatrick
  oculocutaneous a.
  localized a.
  minimal pigment oculocutaneous a.
  Nettleship-Falls X-linked ocular a.
  ocular a.
  oculocutaneous a.
  partial a.
  punctate oculocutaneous a.
  tyrosinase-negative type
  oculocutaneous a.
  tyrosinase-positive type
  oculocutaneous a.
  yellow-mutant oculocutaneous a.

albinoidism
  oculocutaneous a.
  punctate oculocutaneous a.
albinotic fundus
albipunctate fundus
albipunctatus
  fundus a.
Albright disease
albuginea oculi
albugo
albuminuric
  a. amaurosis
  a. retinitis
Alcaine Drop-Tainers
Alcaligenes xylosoxidans
Alclear
alcohol
  benzyl a.
  polyvinyl a. (PVA)
  a. well
alcoholic amblyopia
Alcon
  A. Accurus vitrectomy cutter
  A. AcrySof SA30AL single-piece
  lens
  A. A-OK crescent knife
  A. A-OK ShortCut knife
  A. A-OK slit knife
  A. applanation pneumatonograph
  A. aspiration
  A. aspirator
  A. Closure System (ACS)
  A. cryoextractor
  A. cryophake
  A. cryosurgical unit
  A. CU-15 4-mil needle
  A. Digital B 2000 ultrasound
  A. disposable drape
  A. EyeMap EH-290 corneal
  topography system
  A. hand cautery
  A. I-knife
  A. indirect ophthalmoscope
  A. irrigating/aspirating unit
  A. irrigating needle
  A. 20,000 Legacy unit
  A. MA30BA optic Acrysof lens
  A. 10,000 Master unit
  A. microsponge
  A. phacoemulsification unit
  A. reverse cutting needle

NOTES

Alcon *(continued)*
    A. Saline Especially for Sensitive Eyes Solution
    A. spatula needle
    A. Surgical instrument
    A. suture
    A. taper cut needle
    A. taper point needle
    A. tonometer
    A. ultrasound pachometer
    A. vitrectomy probe
    A. vitrector
Alcon-Biophysic Ophthascan S
Alconefrin
AL:CR
    axial length/corneal radius
    AL/CR ratio
ALD
    average lens density
Alder anomaly
Alder-Reilly phenomenon
aldose reductase
Alexander-Ballen retractor
Alexander law
alexia
    acquired a.
    literal a.
    optical a.
    pure a.
    subcortical a.
alexic
Alezzandrini syndrome
alfa-2a
    interferon a.
Alfonso
    A. cutting platform
    A. diamond corneal transplant blade
    A. guarded bur
    A. nucleus forceps
    A. nucleus trisector
    A. pediatric eyelid speculum
Alfonso-McIntyre nucleus spoon
Alger
    A. brush
    A. brush rust ring remover
algera
    dysopia a.
    dysopsia a.
Alges bifocal contact lens
algorithm
    Advanced Shape Technology Refractive A. (ASTRA)
    FastPac a.
    Lindstrom-Casebeer a.
    Swedish interactive thresholding a. (SITA)
Alhazen theory
Alidase

Alien WildEyes lens
alignment
    ocular a.
    primary gaze a.
aliquot
Alizarin Red S dye
ALK
    automated laser keratomileusis
alkali
    a. burn
    a. burn of cornea
    a. burn to eye
alkaline burn
alkaloid
    belladonna a.
    dissociated a.
    ergot a.
    miotic a.
    undissociated a.
alkaptonuria
ALK-E
    automated lamellar keratoplasty-Excimer
Alkeran
alkyl ether sulfate
All
    A. Clear
    A. Clear AR
    A. Pupil II indirect ophthalmoscope
allachesthesia
    optical a.
Allegra
allele
Allen
    A. cyclodialysis
    A. figure
    A. operation
    A. orbital implant
    A. preschool card
    A. stereo separator
Allen-Braley
    A.-B. forceps
    A.-B. implant
Allen-Burian trabeculotome
Allen-ePTFE ocular implant
Allen-Schiötz tonometer
Allen-Thorpe
    A.-T. goniolens
    A.-T. gonioscopic prism
    A.-T. lens
Aller-Chlor
Allerest eye drops
Allergan
    A. AMO Array S155 lens
    A. Enzymatic Cleaner
    A. Humphrey laser
    A. Humphrey lensometer
    A. Humphrey perimeter
    A. Humphrey photokeratoscope
    A. Humphrey refractor

A. Medical Optics (AMO)
A. Medical Optics photokeratoscope
allergen
allergic
a. blepharitis
a. blepharoconjunctivitis
a. conjunctivitis
a. eye disease
a. keratoconjunctivitis
a. pannus
a. phlyctenulosis
a. response
a. rhinitis
allergica
iritis recidivans staphylococcal a.
Allergy Drops
AllerMax Oral
Allescheria boydii
allesthesia
visual a.
alligator scissors
Allis forceps
Alloderm
allograft
acellular diurnal a.
application of acellular diurnal a.
a. corneal rejection
epithelium-deprived orthotopic
corneal a.
keratolimbal a. (KLA)
limbal a.
living-related conjunctival limbal a.
(lr-CLAL)
allografting
limbal cell a.
allokeratoplasty
allopathic keratoplasty
allophthalmia
alloplastic donor material
allopurinol
alloxan diabetes
all-Perspex
a.-P. CQ lens
a.-P. Kelman Omnifit lens
all-PMMA intraocular lens
Allport
A. cutting bur
A. operation
all-*trans*-retinal
Almocarpine
Almocetamide
Alocril ophthalmic solution

Aloe reading unit
Alomide
A. drops
A. ophthalmic solution
alone
lens a.
alopecia orbicularis
Alpar implant
Alpern cortex aspirator/hydrodissector
alpha, α
a. angle
A. Chymar
a. crystallin
a. herpes virus
alpha-2a
alpha-2-adrenergic agonist agent,
ophthalmic
alpha-agonist
alpha-antagonist
alpha₁-antitrypsin
alphabet keratitis
alpha-chymotrypsin cannula
alpha-chymotrypsin-induced glaucoma
AlphaCor hydrogel synthetic cornea
Alphadrol
Alphagan P
alpha-methyldopa
alpha-methyl-*p*-tyrosine
ALPI
argon laser peripheral iridoplasty
Alpidine
Alport syndrome
Alred
Alrest
Alrex ophthalmic suspension
Alström
A. disease
A. syndrome
Alström-Hallgren syndrome
Alström-Olsen syndrome
Alsus-Knapp operation
Alsus operation
ALT
argon laser trabeculopexy
alteplase
Alternaria alternata
alternata
Alternaria a.
alternate
a. coupling agent
a. cover test (ACT)
a. cover-uncover test

NOTES

alternate *(continued)*
    a. day esotropia
    a. day strabismus
    a. hyperdeviation
alternating
    a. amblyopia
    a. esotropia
    a. exophoria
    a. exotropia
    a. Horner syndrome
    a. hypertropia
    a. hypotropia
    a. light test
    a. mydriasis
    a. oculomotor hemiplegia
    a. strabismus
    a. sursumduction
    a. tropia
alternation
alternative
    photoreceptor transplantation
    ineffective a.
    Soft Mate Enzyme A.
alternocular
altitudinal
    a. field
    a. hemianopsia
    a. scotoma
    a. visual field defect
ALTK
    automated lamellar therapeutic
    keratoplasty
    ALTK system microkeratome
ALTP
    argon laser trabeculoplasty
Alumina implant
aluminum
    a. chloride
    a. eye shield
    a. oxide implant
Alvis
    A. curette
    A. fixation forceps
    A. foreign body spud
    A. operation
Alvis-Lancaster sclerotome
AM
    myopic astigmatism
AMA
    American Medical Association
amacrine
    a. cell
    a. cell somata
Amadeus microkeratome
amaurosis
    albuminuric a.
    Burns a.
    cat's eye a.
    central a.

    a. centralis
    cerebral a.
    congenital a.
    a. congenita of Leber
    diabetic a.
    gaze-evoked a.
    gutta a.
    hysteric a.
    intoxication a.
    Leber congenital a.
    a. nystagmus
    a. partialis fugax
    pressure a.
    reflex a.
    saburral a.
    sympathetic a.
    toxic a.
    uremic a.
amaurotic
    a. cat's eye
    a. familial idiocy (AFI)
    a. mydriasis
    a. nystagmus
    a. pupil
    a. pupillary paralysis
ambient
ambiopia
amblyope
amblyopia
    alcoholic a.
    alternating a.
    ametropic a.
    anisometric a.
    anisometropic a.
    A Randomized Trial Comparing
    Part-Time Versus Full-Time
    Patching for A.
    A Randomized Trial Comparing
    Part-Time Versus Minimal-Time
    Patching for Moderate A.
    arsenic a.
    astigmatic a.
    axial a.
    color a.
    a. crapulosa
    crossed a.
    a. cruciata
    deprivation a.
    eclipse a.
    esotropic a.
    ethyl alcohol a.
    ex a.
    a. ex anopsia
    exertional a.
    functional a.
    hysteric a.
    hysterical a.
    index a.
    irreversible a.

meridional a.
microstrabismic a.
moderate a.
nocturnal a.
nutritional a.
occlusion a.
organic a.
postmarital a.
postoperative a.
quinine a.
receptor a.
reflex a.
refractive a.
relative a.
reverse a.
reversible a.
sensory a.
strabismal a.
strabismic a.
superimposed a.
suppressed a.
suppression a.
tobacco a.
tobacco/alcohol a.
toxic a.
traumatic a.
A. Treatment Study
uremic a.
West Indian a.
amblyopiatrics
amblyopic
amblyoscope
major a.
Worth a.
Ambrose suture forceps
ambulatory vision
AMD
age-related macular degeneration
exudative AMD
amebiasis
amebic keratitis
ameboid
a. keratitis
a. ulcer
amelanotic
a. choroidal melanoma
a. lesion
ameliorate
ameloblastic neurilemoma
Amenabar
A. capsule forceps
A. counterpressor

A. discission hook
A. iris retractor
A. lens
A. lens loupe
America
Eye Bank Association of A.
(EBAA)
American
A. Academy of Ophthalmology
(AAO)
A. Academy of Optometry (AAO)
A. Association of Pediatric
Ophthalmology and Strabismus
(AAPOS)
A. Board of Eye Surgeons
(ABES)
A. Board of Ophthalmology (ABO)
A. College of Eye Surgeons
(ACES)
A. Hydron
A. Hydron instrument
A. leishmaniasis
A. Medical Association (AMA)
A. Medical Optics
A. Medical Optics Baron lens
A. National Standards Institute
(ANSI)
A. National Standards Institute
standard
A. Optical (AO)
A. Optical Hardy-Rand-Rittler color
plate
A. Optometric Association (AOA)
A. Society of Cataract and
Refractive Surgery (ASCRS)
A. Society of Contemporary
Ophthalmology (ASCO)
A. Society of Ophthalmic Plastic
and Reconstruction Surgery
A. Surgical Instrument Company
(ASICO)
Ames test
ametrometer
ametropia
axial a.
curvature a.
defocus-induced a.
index a.
position a.
refractive a.
transient a.
ametropic amblyopia

NOTES

Amicar
amifloxacin
amikacin
Amikin
amine
    vasoactive a.
aminoaciduria cataract
aminocaproic acid
aminoglutethimide
aminoglycoside
aminophylline
aminopyridine
4-aminoquinoline
aminosteroid
amiodarone
amitriptyline
Ammon
    A. blepharoplasty
    A. canthoplasty
    A. dacryocystotomy
    A. filament
    A. fissure
    A. operation
    A. scleral prominence
ammonia alkali burn
ammonium
    a. hydroxide alkali burn
    a. lactate
amnesic color blindness
amnifocal lens
amniotic
    a. band syndrome
    a. membrane
    a. membrane transplantation
AMO
    Allergan Medical Optics
    AMO Array foldable intraocular lens
    AMO Array multifocal ultraviolet-absorbing silicone posterior chamber intraocular lens
    AMO Endosol Extra
    AMO HPF 500 pump
    AMO Ioptex Model ACR 360 foldable acrylic lens
    AMO Phacoflex II foldable intraocular lens
    AMO PhacoFlex lens and inserter
    AMO Prestige advanced cataract extraction system
    AMO Prestige Phaco System
    AMO Series 4 phaco handpiece
    AMO Set-Up
    AMO Vitrax viscoelastic solution
    AMO YAG 100 laser
amobarbital
amodiaquine
Amoils
    A. cryoextractor

    A. cryopencil
    A. cryophake
    A. cryoprobe
    A. cryosurgical unit
    A. epithelial scrubber
    A. refractor
    A. retractor
amorphic lens
amorphous
    a. corneal deposit
    a. corneal dystrophy
amotio retinae
amoxicillin
amoxicillin/clavulanate
AMP
    adenosine monophosphate
amphetamine
amphiphilic drug
amphodiplopia
amphotericin B
amphoterodiplopia
amplitude
    a. of accommodation (AA)
    accommodative a. (AA)
    artificial eye a.
    binocular a.
    b-wave a.
    cone b-wave a.
    convergence a.
    divergence a.
    flicker a.
    a. of fusion
    fusional convergence a.
    fusional divergence a.
    fusion with a.
    increased vertical fusional a.
    rod b-wave a.
    rod-cone a.
    vertical fusional vergence a.
AMPPE
    acute multifocal placoid pigment epitheliopathy
ampulla, pl. ampullae
    a. canaliculi lacrimalis
    a. ductus lacrimalis
    a. of lacrimal canal
    a. of lacrimal duct
amputator
    Smith intraocular capsular a.
Amsler
    A. aqueous transplant needle
    A. chart
    A. corneal graft
    A. grid (AG)
    A. grid test
    A. operation
    A. scleral marker
Amsoft lens

Amvisc
A. Plus
A. Plus solution
amyloid
a. body
a. cellulitis
a. corneal degeneration
a. deposit
a. P component
subcutaneous a.
amyloidosis
conjunctival a.
localized a.
orbital a.
primary familial a.
secondary a.
systemic a.
Amytal
ANA
antinuclear antibody
Anacel
anaclasis
anaerobic
a. medium
a. ocular infection
anaglyph test
anagnosasthenia
Anagnostakis operation
analgesia
surface a.
analgesic
opiate a.
analmoscope
Pickford-Nicholson a.
analog
prostaglandin a.
thymidine a.
analogue
acyclic nucleoside a.
analphalipoproteinemia
analysis, pl. **analyses**
astigmatic vector a.
bivariate a.
Cochran-Mantel-Haenszel a.
corneal topographic a.
digital-imaging a.
endothelial cell a.
Fourier harmonic a.
image a.
immunochromatography a.
infrared image a.
linkage a.

logistic discriminant a.
morphometric a.
Neale Reading A.
pedigree a.
photograph reading a.
A. of Radial Keratotomy (ARK)
retinal thickness a. (RTA)
Topcon noncontact morphometric a.
a. of variance (ANOVA)
vector a.
Western immunoblotting a.
Analytical Instruments image analyzer
analyzer
Analytical Instruments image a.
Dicon ocular blood flow a.
Eye Scan corneal a.
Friedmann visual field a.
GDx nerve fiber a.
Humphrey Field A. 750 (HFA)
Humphrey Instruments vision a.
Humphrey lens a.
Humphrey visual field a.
nerve fiber layer a.
Ocular blood flow a.
Paradigm ocular blood flow a.
P55 Pachymetric A.
profile a.
retinal thickness a. (RTA)
Tomey retinal function a.
Vision a.
ViVa binocular infrared vision a.
anamorphosis
anangioid disk
anaphoria
anaphylactic
a. conjunctivitis
a. reaction
a. shock
anaphylaxis
anastigmatic lens
anastomosis, pl. **anastomoses**
chorioretinal venous a.
retinal-choroidal a.
anatomic
a. equator
a. strabismus
a. success
anatomy
intracanalicular a.
intracranial a.
intraocular a.

NOTES

17

anatomy *(continued)*
    intraorbital a.
    topographic a.
anatropia
anatropic
ANCA
    antineutrophil cytoplasmic antibody
Ancef
anchor
    a. hook
    a. suture
anchor/fixation
    Searcy a.
anchoring suture
Ancobon
Andersen syndrome
Anderson-Kestenbaum procedure
Androgen Tear
Anecortave acetate
Anectine
Anel
    A. operation
    A. probe
    A. syringe
anemia
    aplastic a.
    macrocytic a.
    Mediterranean a.
    normocytic hypochromic a.
    pernicious a.
    sickle cell a.
anemone cell tumor
anencephaly
Anergan
anergy
anesthesia
    cornea a.
    endotracheal a.
    exam under a. (EUA)
    general a.
    infraorbital a.
    intracameral a.
    intraorbital a.
    modified Van Lint a.
    needleless regional a.
    O'Brien a.
    orbital a.
    peribulbar a.
    retrobulbar a.
    sub-Tenon parabulbar a.
    topical a.
    Van Lint a.
anesthetic
    general a.
    inhalation a.
    local a.
    a. ointment
    topical a.

anetoderma
    Jadassohn-type a.
aneurysm
    arteriovenous a.
    basilar artery a.
    berry a.
    carotid a.
    cavernous sinus a.
    cerebral artery a.
    cirsoid a.
    communicating artery a.
    fusiform a.
    giant a.
    IC-PC a.
    IC-PC artery a.
    internal carotid-posterior
      communicating artery a.
    intracranial a.
    Leber miliary a.
    miliary a.
    ophthalmic artery a.
    a. of orbit
    orbital a.
    racemose a.
    a. of retinal arteriole
    retinal artery a.
    saccular a.
    suprasellar a.
aneurysmal bone cyst
Angelman syndrome
Angelucci
    A. operation
    A. syndrome
angiitis
    frosted branch a.
angio-Behçet disease
angioblastic meningioma
angiodiathermy
angioedema
angioendotheliomatosis
    neoplastic a.
Angiofluor Lite
angiogenesis
angiogram
    fluorescein a.
    Heidelberg retina a. (HRA)
angiography
    anterior segment fluorescein a.
      (ASFA)
    carotid a.
    cerebral radionuclide a.
    computed tomographic a.
    digital subtraction indocyanine
      green a. (DS-ICGA)
    fluorescein a. (FA)
    fluorescein angiography/indocyanine
      green a. (FA/ICGA)
    Heidelberg retinal a.
    ICG a.

A

indocyanine green a. (ICGA)
intravenous fluorescein a. (IVFA)
IV retinal fluorescein a.
magnetic resonance a. (MRA)
orbital a.
retinal a.
vertebral a.

angioid retinal streak

angiokeratoma
a. corporis diffusum
a. corporis diffusum universale
diffuse a.

angioma
cavernous a.
conjunctival a.
episcleral a.
nerve head a.
orbital a.
racemose a.
retinal a.
spider a.
von Hippel a.

angiomatosis
cerebroretinal a.
encephalofacial a.
encephalotrigeminal a.
meningocutaneous a.
a. of retina
a. retinae
retinal a.
retinocerebellar a.
Sturge-Weber encephalotrigeminal a.

angiopathia retinae juvenilis
angiopathic retinopathy
angiopathy
cerebral amyloid a.

angiophakomatosis
angiosarcoma
orbital a.

angioscopy
fluorescein fundus a.

angioscotoma
angioscotomata
angioscotometry
angiosis streak
angiospasm
angiospastic retinopathy
angiotensin
angle
a. of aberration
a. of abnormality
alpha a.

anomaly a.
a. of anomaly
a. of anterior chamber
anterior chamber a.
a. of aperture
apical a.
ASSI Phaco Chopper 90-degree a.
biorbital a.
cerebellopontine a. (CPA)
chamber a.
contact a.
convergence a.
critical a.
deformity a.
a. of deviation
a. of direction
disparity a.
divergent cut a.
drainage a.
a. of eccentricity
elevation a.
a. of emergence
filtration a.
a. of Fuchs
gamma a.
a. of incidence
incident a.
iridial a.
iridocorneal a.
a. of iris
Jacquart a.
kappa a.
lambda a.
large kappa a.
lateral a.
limiting a.
medial a.
meter a.
minimum separable a.
minimum visible a.
minimum visual a.
ocular a.
optic a.
pantoscopic a.
a. of polarization
posterior a.
prism a.
a. recession
a. of reflection
a. of refraction
refraction a.
space of iridocorneal a.

NOTES

19

angle *(continued)*
    a. of squint
    squint a.
    a. structure
    tarsal a.
    visual a.
    water-contact a.
    wetting a.
    a. width
    zipped a.
angle-closure glaucoma (ACG)
angled
    a. capsule forceps
    a. counterpressor
    a. discission hook
    a. iris hook and IOL dialer
    a. iris retractor
    a. iris spatula
    a. left/right cannula
    a. lens loupe
    a. manipulator
    a. nucleus removal loupe
    a. probe
    a. suction tube
angle-fixated lens
angle-recession glaucoma
angle-supported lens
angling
    pantoscopic a.
angor ocularis
Angosky syndrome
Angström
    A. law
    A. unit
angular
    a. aqueous sinus plexus
    a. blepharitis
    a. blepharoconjunctivitis
    a. conjunctivitis
    a. distance
    a. gyrus
    a. iridocornealis
    a. junction of eyelid
    a. line
    a. vein
angularis
    blepharitis a.
    vena a.
angulated iris spatula
angulation
    haptic a.
angulus
    a. iridis
    a. iridocornealis
    a. oculi lateralis
    a. oculi medialis
anhydrase
    carbonic a. (CA)
    a. glycerol

anicteric
aniridia
    a. in the newborn
    sporadic a.
    traumatic a.
Anis
    A. irrigating vectis
    A. lens-holding forceps
    A. microforceps model 2-848
    A. radial marker
    A. staple lens
    A. suture placement marker
aniseikonia
    spectacle-induced a.
aniseikonic lens
anisoaccommodation
anisochromatic
anisochromia
anisocoria
    benign a.
    central a.
    a. contraction
    essential a.
    physiologic a.
    see-saw a.
    simple a.
anisometric amblyopia
anisometrope
anisometropia
    axial a.
    myopic a.
    refractive a.
anisometropic amblyopia
anisophoria
    induced a.
anisopia
anisotropal
anisotropy
ankyloblepharon
    external a.
    a. filiforme adnatum
    a. totale
ankylosing spondylitis
anlage
    lacrimal duct a.
annual replacement
annular *(var. of* anular)
annulus *(var. of* anulus)
anomalopia
anomaloscope
    Kamppeter a.
    Nagel a.
    a. plate test (APT)
    Spectrum color vision meter
    712 a.
anomalous
    a. disk
    a. fixation
    a. projection protan

a. retinal correspondence (ARC)
a. trichromatism
a. trichromatopsia
a. vessel
anomaly
Alder a.
angle of a.
a. angle
Axenfeld a.
Axenfeld-Reiger a. (ARA)
Chédiak-Higashi a.
Chédiak-Steinbrinck-Higashi a.
coloboma a.
coloboma, heart defects, atresia
choanae, retarded growth, genital
hypoplasia, and ear a.'s
(CHARGE)
congenital a.
craniofacial a.
developmental a.
excavated optic disk a.
facial a.
Klippel-Feil a.
lacrimal angle duct a.
location a.
morning glory optic disk a.
oculocephalic vascular a.
optical disk a.
optic disk a.
osseous a.
Peters a.
Rieger a.
Steinbrinck a.
anomia
color a.
anophoria
anophthalmanopia
anophthalmia
consecutive a.
primary a.
secondary a.
anophthalmic socket
anophthalmos
congenital a.
anopsia
amblyopia ex a.
ex a.
anorthopia
anorthoscope
anotropia
ANOVA
analysis of variance

anoxia
ANSI
American National Standards Institute
ANSI standard
antagonist
contralateral a.
folic acid a.
inhibitional palsy of contralateral a.
ipsilateral a.
thromboxane receptor a.
$_H$1-antagonist
antazoline
naphazoline and a.
a. phosphate and naphazoline HCl
Antazoline-V Ophthalmic
anteflexion of iris
antenatal testing
anterior
a. axial developmental cataract
a. axial embryonal cataract
a. axonal embryonal cataract
a. basal membrane
a. basement membrane dystrophy
(ABMD)
camera bulbi a.
camera oculi a.
a. capsulectomy
a. capsule shagreen
a. capsulotomy
a. central curve (ACC)
a. cerebral artery
a. chamber (AC)
a. chamber angle
a. chamber angle width
a. chamber cleavage syndrome
a. chamber inflammation
a. chamber intraocular lens
(ACIOL)
a. chamber intraocular lens implant
a. chamber IOL
a. chamber irrigating vectis
a. chamber irrigator
a. chamber lymphoma
a. chamber maintainer (ACM)
a. chamber paracentesis
a. chamber reaction
a. chamber shallowing
a. chamber sinus
a. chamber synechia scissors
a. chamber tap
a. chamber trabecula
a. chamber tube

NOTES

anterior *(continued)*
  a. chamber washout
  a. chamber washout cannula
  a. choroiditis
  a. ciliary artery
  a. ciliary vein
  a. compressive optic neuropathy
  a. conjunctival artery
  a. conjunctival vein
  a. corneal curvature
  a. corneal staphyloma
  a. corneal surface
  a. cylinder
  a. embryotoxon
  a. epithelium corneae
  A. Eye Segment Analysis System
  a. focal point
  a. hyaloidal fibrovascular proliferation
  a. hyaloid membrane (AHM)
  a. hydrophthalmia
  a. inferior cerebellar artery (AICA)
  a. ischemic optic neuritis
  a. ischemic optic neuropathy (AION)
  a. keratoconus
  a. knee of von Wilbrand
  lamina elastica a.
  a. lens capsule
  a. lenticonus
  a. limiting lamina
  limiting lamina a.
  a. limiting ring
  a. lip
  a. loop traction
  a. megalophthalmus
  a. mosaic crocodile shagreen
  a. ocular segment
  a. optic chiasmal syndrome
  a. optic zone
  a. optic zone diameter
  a. peripheral curve
  a. polar cataract
  a. pole
  a. pole of the eye
  a. pole of the lens
  a. proliferative vitreoretinopathy (APVR)
  a. puncture
  a. pyramidal cataract
  a. scleritis
  a. sclerochoroiditis
  a. sclerotomy
  a. segment examination
  a. segment of eye
  a. segment fluorescein angiography (ASFA)
  a. segment inflammation
  a. segment necrosis
  a. segment sleeve
  a. stromal micropuncture
  a. subcapsular cataract (ASC)
  a. symblepharon
  a. synechia
  a. uveitis
  a. visual pathway
  a. visual pathway dysfunction
  a. visual pathway glioma
  a. vitrectomy

anteriores
  limbus palpebrales a.
  vena ciliares a.

anterior-surface aberration

anterius
  foramen lacerum a.

anterograde degeneration

anteroposterior
  a. axis
  a. axis of Fick

Anthony orbital compressor

anthracis
  Bacillus a.

antiacetylcholine
  a. receptor antibody
  a. receptor antibody assay

anti-ACh receptor antibody

antiadrenergic drug

antiangiogenesis injection

antibiotic
  bacteriocidal a.
  bacteriostatic a.
  broad-spectrum a.
  fluoroquinolone a.
  fortified a.
  intravitreal a.
  prophylactic a.
  subconjunctival a.
  Triple A.

antibody, pl. **antibodies**
  adenovirus monoclonal a.
  antiacetylcholine receptor a.
  anti-ACh receptor a.
  anticardiolipin a.
  anti-CD 154 monoclonal a.
  antilens protein a.
  antilipoarabinomannan-B a.
  antineutrophil cytoplasmic a. (ANCA)
  antinuclear a. (ANA)
  antiphospholipid a.
  antirecoverin a.
  antiretina a.
  apolipoprotein E a.
  chromogranin a.
  complement-fixing a.
  cytokeratin 7, 20 a.
  cytotoxic a.
  diolipin a.

ELISA a.
glial fibrillary acidic protein a.
HIV-specific a.
homotropic a.
humanized anti-Tac monoclonal a.
immunodominant a.
indirect fluorescent a.
Kermix a.
monoclonal a.
neurofilament triplets a.
neuron-specific endolase a.
pancytokeratin a.
perinuclear antineutrophil
  cytoplasmic a. (pANCA)
S-100 protein a.
stimulatory a.
synaptophysin a.
treponemal a.
anticalbindin cell
anticardiolipin (aCL)
a. antibody
anticataract drug
anti-CD 154 monoclonal antibody
anticholinergic drug
anticomplement immunofluorescence
antielevation syndrome (AES)
antigen
Australia a.
early a.
EBV-associated a.
EBV nuclear a.
epithelial membrane a. (EMA)
extractable nuclear a.
fluorescent-antibody-to-membrane a.
  (FAMA)
HLA-A29 a.
HLA-B5 a.
HLA-B7 a.
HLA-B15 a.
HLA-B27 a.
HLA-DR4 a.
human leukocyte a. (HLA)
ICAM-1 a.
Kveim a.
major histocompatibility a.
nuclear a.
rheumatoid-associated nuclear a.
transplantation a.
viral capsid a.
antigen-1
leukocyte function associated a.-1
  (LFA-1)

antigen-presenting cell
antiglaucoma surgery
antiglial fibrillary acidic protein
Antihist-1
anti-Hu syndrome
antilens protein antibody
antilipoarabinomannan-B antibody
Antilirium
antimetropia
antimicrobial treatment
antimonate
meglumine a.
antimongoloid slant
**antineutrophil cytoplasmic antibody
  (ANCA)**
antinuclear antibody (ANA)
antiophthalmic
antioxidant
a. enzyme
a. supplement
antipericyte autoantibody
antiphospholipid (aPL)
a. antibody
a. syndrome
antirecoverin antibody
antireflection coating
antiretina antibody
antisuppression exercise
antitonic
antitorque suture
anti-VEGF injection
antiviral
antixerophthalmic
Antley-Bixler syndrome
Anton
A. symptom
A. syndrome
Anton-Babinski syndrome
antonina
facies a.
Antoni pattern
antrophose
anular, annular
a. bifocal contact lens
a. cataract
a. corneal graft
a. corneal graft operation
a. infiltrate
a. keratitis
a. macular dystrophy
a. plexus
a. ring

NOTES

anular *(continued)*
- a. scleritis
- a. scotoma
- a. staphyloma
- a. synechia
- a. ulcer

anulus, annulus
- a. ciliaris
- a. of conjunctiva
- a. iridis major
- a. iridis minor
- a. tendineus communis
- a. of Zinn
- a. zinnii

Anxanil

AO
American Optical
- AO Ful-Vue diagnostic unit
- AO lens
- AO Reichert Instruments applanation tonometer
- AO Reichert Instruments binocular indirect ophthalmoscope
- AO Reichert Instruments Ful-Vue diagnostic unit
- AO Reichert Instruments lensometer
- AO Reichert Instruments Project-O-Chart
- AO rotary prism
- AO Vectographic Project-O-Chart slide

AOA
American Optometric Association

AoDisc Neutralizer

AODM
adult-onset diabetes mellitus

AOFMD
adult-onset foveomacular dystrophy

AoSept
- A. Clear Care
- A. Disinfectant
- A. Lens Holder and Cup

AO-XT 166 lens

AO2
anterior optic zone
- AO2 diameter (AO2D)

APACG
acute primary angle-closure glaucoma

A-pattern
- A-p. esotropia
- A-p. exotropia
- A-p. strabismus

APC
Accurus peeler-cutter

APD
afferent pupillary defect

Apert
- acrocephalosyndactyly of A.
- A. syndrome

aperture
- angle of a.
- a. disk
- numerical a. (NA)
- orbital a.
- palpebral a.
- pupillary a.
- a. ratio

apex, pl. **apices**
- corneal a.
- a. fracture
- orbital a.
- petrous a.
- A. Plus excimer laser
- prism a.
- a. of prism
- tumor a.

aphacic (*var. of* aphakic)

aphake

aphakia, aphacia
- binocular a.
- extracapsular a.
- monocular a.

aphakic, aphacic
- a. bullous keratopathy (ABK)
- a. contact lens
- a. correction
- a. cystoid macular edema
- a. detachment
- a. eye
- a. glaucoma
- a. lens
- a. pupillary block
- a. spectacles

aphasia
- Broca a.
- optic a.
- visual a.

aphose

aphotesthesia

aphotic

aphrophilus
- *Haemophilus par a.*

apical
- a. angle
- a. clearance
- a. cone
- a. radius
- a. tumor
- a. zone
- a. zone of cornea

apices (*pl. of* apex)

apicitis

apiospermum
- *Scedosporium a.*

aPL
antiphospholipid

aplanatic
    a. focus
    a. lens
aplanatism
aplasia
    chiasmal a.
    lacrimal nucleus a.
    macular a.
    a. of optic nerve
    optic nerve a.
    punctum a.
    retinal a.
aplastic anemia
APMPPE
    acute posterior multifocal placoid
    pigment epitheliopathy
apochromatic
    a. lens
    a. objective
apocrine gland
apolipoprotein
    a. E
    a. E antibody
Apollo
    A. conjunctivitis
    A. disease
aponeurosis
aponeurotic ptosis
apoplectic
    a. glaucoma
    a. retinitis
apoplexy
    occipital a.
    pituitary a.
    a. of pituitary
    retinal a.
ApopTag modification
apoptosis
apotripsis
apparatus
    Acuson 128 a.
    ciliary a.
    dioptric a.
    experimental a.
    Frigitronics nitrous oxide
      cryosurgery a.
    Golgi a.
    Howard-Dolman a.
    lacrimal a.
    a. lacrimalis
    a. suspensorius lentis
    Vactro perilimbal suction a.

appearance
    beaten-bronze a.
    beaten-copper a.
    beaten-metal a.
    cobblestone a.
    cushingoid a.
    dendritiform a.
    dropped-socket a.
    feathery a.
    fluffy a.
    granular a.
    leonine a.
    mottled a.
    optic nerve head a.
    salt-and-pepper a.
    snake-like a.
    spongy a.
    squashed-tomato a.
appendage of eye
apperceptive
    a. agnosia
    a. prosopagnosia
applanation
    a. pressure
    tension by a. (TAP)
    a. tension (AT)
    a. tonometer
    a. tonometry (AT)
applanator
    Johnston LASIK Flap A.
applanometer
applanometry
application
    a. of acellular diurnal allograft
    autologous serum a.
    diathermy a.
    pilot a.
applicator
    beta therapy eye a.
    cotton-tipped a.
    Gass dye a.
    Gifford a.
Appolonio lens
apposition
    central choroidal a. (CCA)
approach
    ab interno a.
    Berke a.
    Caldwell-Luc a.
    fornix a.
    Iliff a.
    limbal a.

NOTES

approach *(continued)*
> Lynch a.
> pars plana a.
> transcaruncular-transconjunctival a.
> transpunctal endocanalicular a.

apraclonidine
> a. HCl
> a. hydrochloride
> a. ophthalmic solution

apraxia
> acquired ocular motor a.
> Cogan congenital oculomotor a.
> congenital ocular motor a.
> (COMA)
> constructional a.
> eyelid a.
> a. of eyelid opening (AEO)
> a. of gaze
> ocular motor a.
> oculomotor a.

Apresoline
A-Probe
> Soft-Touch A-P.

APT
> anomaloscope plate test
> APT-5 Color Vision Tester

APVR
> anterior proliferative vitreoretinopathy

Aquaflex contact lens
Aqua-Flow
AquaLase cataract removal system
aqua oculi
Aquasight lens
AquaSite
> A. Ophthalmic Solution
> A. PF

Aquasonic 100 gel
Aqua-Tears
aqueductal stenosis
aqueous
> a. chamber
> a. crystalline penicillin G
> fibrinous a.
> a. flare
> a. fluid
> a. humor
> a. humor drainage
> a. humor eye
> a. humor flow
> a. inflow
> a. layer of tear film
> a. misdirected glaucoma
> a. misdirection
> a. misdirection syndrome
> a. outflow
> a. paracentesis
> plasmoid a.
> a. suppressant
> a. tap

> a. tear deficiency (ATD)
> a. tear layer
> a. transplant needle
> a. tube shunt
> a. uranyl acetate
> a. vein

aqueous-influx phenomenon
aquocapsulitis
aquosus
> humor a.

AR
> autorefraction
> All Clear AR
> AR 1000 refractor

ARA
> Axenfeld-Reiger anomaly

Ara-A
Arabic eye test
arabinoside
> adenine a.

Arachis hypogea agglutinin
arachnoid
> a. hemorrhage
> a. sheath

arachnoidal cyst
arachnoiditis
> chiasma a.
> chiasmal a.
> opticochiasmatic a.
> optochiasmatic a.

Aralen Phosphate
Arbelaez LASIK spatula/protector
arborescent
> a. cataract
> a. keratitis

arborization
> pattern a.
> a. pattern

ARC
> AIDS-related complex
> anomalous retinal correspondence
> unharmonious ARC

arc
> a. and bowl perimeter
> a. of contact
> nuclear a.
> a. perimetry
> a. scotoma
> a. staining
> xenon a.

arcade
> inferior retinal a.
> inferior temporal a.
> inferotemporal a.
> limbal a.
> major a.
> superior vascular a.
> temporal vascular a.
> vascular a.

arc-flash conjunctivitis
arch
  orbital a.
  Salus a.
  superciliary a.
  supraorbital a.
Archer lesion
architecture
  iris a.
  nasal a.
arciform density
arcitome
  Hanna a.
Arc-T blade
arcuate
  a. Bjerrum scotoma
  a. commissure
  a. course
  a. field defect
  a. incision
  a. nerve fiber bundle
  a. retinal fold
  a. staining
  a. transverse keratotomy
arcus, pl. **arcus**
  a. adiposus
  corneal a.
  a. cornealis
  juvenile a.
  a. juvenilis
  a. lipoides
  a. lipoides corneae
  a. palpebralis inferior
  a. palpebralis superior
  a. parietooccipitalis
  a. senilis
  a. superciliaris
  unilateral a.
Arden grating
ARE
  acute red eye
area, pl. **areae, areas**
  aspheric lenticular a.
  Bjerrum a.
  Brodmann a.
  a. centralis
  a. choroidea
  a. of conscious regard
  cortical oculomotor a.
  corticooculocephalogyric a.
  a. cribrosa
  a. of critical definition

  fusion a.
  macular a.
  a. Martegiani
  medial superior temporal visual a.
  middle temporal visual a.
  mirror a.
  MST visual a.
  MT visual a.
  Panum fusion a.
  papillary a.
  parastriate a.
  pretectal a.
  spindle-shaped a.
  visual association a.
AREDS
  Age-Related Eye Disease Study
areflexia
  pupillary a.
areflexical mydriasis
areolar
  a. central choroiditis
  a. choroidopathy
ArF
  argon fluoride
  A. excimer laser
  A. excimer laser system
argamblyopia
argema
argon
  a. blue laser
  a. fluoride (ArF)
  a. green laser
  a. laser coagulator
  a. laser endophotocoagulation
  a. laser iridectomy
  a. laser peripheral iridoplasty (ALPI)
  a. laser photocoagulation
  a. laser retinal treatment
  a. laser trabeculopexy (ALT)
  a. laser trabeculoplasty (ALTP)
argon-fluoride excimer laser
argon-pumped tunable dye laser
Argyll
  A. Robertson instrument
  A. Robertson operation
  A. Robertson pupil (ARP)
  A. Robertson pupil sign
argyria
argyriasis
argyrism
Argyrol S.S.

NOTES

argyrosis
arida
  conjunctivitis a.
Arion
  A. operation
  A. sling
Aristocort
Aristospan
ARK
  Analysis of Radial Keratotomy
Arlt
  A. disease
  A. epicanthus repair
  A. eyelid repair
  A. lens
  A. lens loupe
  A. line
  A. operation
  A. pterygium
  A. recess
  A. scoop
  A. sinus
  A. trachoma
  A. triangle
Arlt-Jaesche
  A.-J. excision
  A.-J. operation
  A.-J. recess
  A.-J. sinus
  A.-J. trachoma
ARM
  age-related maculopathy
arm
  q a.
  Wiltmoser optical a.
Armaly cup/disk ratio
Armaly-Drance technique
ARMD
  age-related macular degeneration
    dry ARMD
    risk factors in ARMD
    wet ARMD
ARN
  acute retinal necrosis
  ARN syndrome
Arnold
  zygomatic foramen of A.
Arnold-Chiari malformation
AROA
  autosomal-recessive ocular albinism
ARP
  Argyll Robertson pupil
arrachement
array
  ordered a.
  radial vessel a.
Array multifocal intraocular lens

ARRON
  autoimmune-related retinopathy and optic
  neuropathy
  ARRON syndrome
Arrowhead operation
arrow-shaft silicone punctal plug
Arrowsmith corneal marker
Arroyo
  A. cataract extraction
  A. dacryostomy
  A. encircling suture
  A. expressor
  A. forceps
  A. implant
  A. keratoplasty
  A. operation
  A. protector
  A. sign
  A. tenotomy
  A. trephine
Arruga
  A. capsule forceps
  A. cataract extraction
  A. dacryostomy
  A. elevator retractor
  A. encircling suture
  A. expressor
  A. implant
  A. keratoplasty
  A. lacrimal trephine
  A. lens
  A. needle holder
  A. operation
  A. orbital retractor
  A. protector
  A. tenotomy
Arruga-Berens operation
Arruga-McCool capsule forceps
Arruga-Moura-Brazil implant
Arruga-Nicetic capsule forceps
arsenic amblyopia
arterial
  a. circle
  a. circle of greater iris
  a. circle of lesser iris
  a. dissection
  a. hypertension
  a. macroaneurysm
  a. occlusive change
  a. occlusive disease
arteriogram
  carotid a.
arteriography
  cerebral a.
arteriola
  a. macularis inferior
  a. macularis superior
  a. medialis retinae
  a. nasalis retinae inferior

a. nasalis retinae superior
a. temporalis retinae inferior
a. temporalis retinae superior
arteriolar
a. attenuation
a. narrowing
a. nicking
a. sclerosis
a. sheathing
arteriole
aneurysm of retinal a.
attenuated retinal a.
a. communication
copper-wire a.
inferior macular a.
macular a.
narrowed a.
narrowing of retinal a.
perifoveal a.
precapillary a.
retinal a.
silver-wire a.
superior macular a.
arteriolovenous (A-V)
a. crossing
arteriosclerosis (AS)
cerebral a.
a. of retina
arteriosclerotic
a. ischemic optic neuropathy
a. retinopathy
arteriosus
arteriovenous (AV)
a. aneurysm
a. communication
a. crossing defect
a. malformation
a. nicking
a. pattern
a. ratio
a. strabismus syndrome
arteritic anterior ischemic optic neuropathy
arteritis
cranial a.
giant cell a. (GCA)
occlusive retinal a.
pseudotemporal a.
temporal a. (TA)
artery
anterior cerebral a.
anterior ciliary a.

anterior conjunctival a.
anterior inferior cerebellar a. (AICA)
basilar a.
branch retinal a. (BRA)
calcarine a.
carotid a.
central retinal a. (CRA)
cerebellar a.
cerebral a.
ciliary a.
cilioretinal a.
conjunctival a.
copper-wire a.
corkscrew a.
dolichoectatic anterior cerebral a.
episcleral a.
ethmoidal a.
hyaline a.
hyaloid a.
hypophyseal a.
inferior nasal a.
inferior temporal a.
inferonasal a.
inferotemporal a.
infraorbital a.
internal carotid a.
intracavernous carotid a.
lacrimal a.
long posterior ciliary a.
middle cerebral a.
ophthalmic a.
optic a.
parietooccipital a.
posterior cerebral a.
posterior ciliary a.
posterior conjunctival a.
retinal a.
retrobulbar a.
short posterior ciliary a.
superior nasal a.
superior temporal a.
supraorbital a.
tarsal a.
temporal a.
temporooccipital a.
thrombosed a.
vertebrobasilar a.
zygomaticoorbital a.
artery-to-vein ratio (A/V)
arthrokinetic nystagmus

NOTES

arthroophthalmopathy
　　hereditary progressive a.
Arthus reaction
articularis
　　lentis a.
artifact
　　high-gain a.
artifactiously
artifactual
artificial
　　a. cornea
　　a. diabetes
　　a. divergence procedure
　　a. divergency surgery
　　a. eye
　　a. eye amplitude
　　a. eye motility
　　a. lens
　　a. pupil
　　a. silicone retina
　　a. silk keratitis
　　a. tears (AT)
　　a. UV radiation
　　a. vision
Artisan
　　A. iris-fixated phakic IOL
　　A. myopia lens
ARVO
　　Association for Research in Vision and
　　Ophthalmology
AS
　　arteriosclerosis
As
　　astigmatism
ASC
　　anterior subcapsular cataract
A-scan
　　contact A-s.
　　DGH 5000 A-s.
　　Jedmed A-s.
　　Jedmed/DGH A-s.
　　Ultra-Image A-s.
　　Ultrascan Digital 2000 contact
　　　ultrasound A-s.
　　A-s. ultrasonogram
　　A-s. ultrasonography
Ascaris lumbricoides
ascent phase
Ascher
　　A. aqueous-influx phenomenon
　　A. glass-rod phenomenon
　　A. syndrome
　　A. vein
Asch septal forceps
ASCO
　　American Society of Contemporary
　　Ophthalmology
Ascon instrument

ASCR
　　autologous stem cell rescue
ASCRS
　　American Society of Cataract and
　　Refractive Surgery
aseptic endophthalmitis
Aseptron II
ASFA
　　anterior segment fluorescein angiography
AsH
　　hyperopic astigmatism
ash leaf spot
ASICO
　　American Surgical Instrument Company
　　　ASICO capsulorrhexis forceps
　　　ASICO multiangled diamond knife
　　　ASICO multi incision system 10
　　　　facet blade
AsM
　　myopic astigmatism
aspartoacylase
aspartylglycosaminuria
aspergillosis uveitis
Aspergillus
　　A. *flavus*
　　A. *fumigatus*
　　A. *terreus*
aspheric
　　a. cataract lens
　　a. contact lens
　　a. cornea
　　a. lenticular area
　　a. spectacle lens
aspherical ophthalmoscopic lens
aspheric-viewing lens
aspirate
　　vitreoretinal a.
aspirating/irrigating vectis
aspirating lid speculum
aspiration
　　Alcon a.
　　cataract a.
　　a. of cortex
　　fine-needle a.
　　a. flow rate
　　irrigation and a. (I&A)
　　a. of lens
　　trabecular a.
　　vitreous a.
aspirator
　　Alcon a.
　　Castroviejo orbital a.
　　Cavitron a.
　　Cooper a.
　　Fibra Sonics phaco a.
　　Fink cataract a.
　　Kelman a.

Legacy Series 2000
Cavitron/Kelman
phacoemulsifier a.
Nugent soft cataract a.
Stat a.

aspirator/hydrodissector
Alpern cortex a.

assay
antiacetylcholine receptor
antibody a.
chemiluminescence a.
enzyme-linked immunosorbent a.
(ELISA)
immunofluorescent a.
Leber hereditary optic atrophy
reverse dot-blot a.
Lowry a.
mucous a.
Raji cell a.
Southern blot hybridization a.
TUNEL a.
urinary GAG a.
urinary glycosaminoglycan
measurement a.

assessment
Hirschberg reflex a.
Jacko Low Vision Interaction A.
(JLVIA)
ocular hemodynamic a.
quantitative haze a.

ASSI
Accurate Surgical and Scientific
Instruments
A. Accu-line surgical marking pen
A. air injection cannula
A. capsulorrhexis forceps
A. fixation hook
A. IOL inserter forceps
A. Phaco Chopper 90-degree angle
A. Polar-Mate coagulator
A. serrefine
A. triple marker
A. tubing introducer forceps
A. universal lens folding forceps

assistant
Certified Paraoptometric A. (CPOA)

associate
Prosthetic Orthotic A.'s

association
American Medical A. (AMA)
American Optometric A. (AOA)
CHARGE a.

A. for Research in Vision and
Ophthalmology (ARVO)
A. of Technical Personnel in
Ophthalmology (ATPO)
teratogenic a.

associative prosopagnosia

Ast
astigmatism

astemizole

asteroid
a. body
a. hyalitis
hyaloid a.
a. hyalosis

asteroides
Nocardia a.

asthenocoria

asthenometer

asthenope

asthenopia
accommodative a.
muscular a.
nervous a.
neurasthenic a.
retinal a.
tarsal a.

asthenopic

astigmagraph

astigmagraphic error

astigmatic
a. amblyopia
a. axis
a. clock
a. dial
a. dial chart
a. image
a. keratotomy (AK)
a. keratotomy enhancement
a. lens
a. marker
a. refractive error
a. vector analysis

astigmatism (As, Ast)
acquired a.
against-the-rule a.
asymmetric a.
ATR a.
central a.
complex a.
compound hyperopic a.
compound myopic a.
congenital a.

NOTES

astigmatism *(continued)*
    corneal a.
    a. correction
    cross-cylinder technique for
      correction of mixed a.
    direct a.
    hypermetropic a.
    hyperopic a. (AsH)
    inverse a.
    irregular a.
    keratometric a.
    lenticular a.
    mixed a.
    myopic a. (AM, AsM)
    oblique a.
    a. of oblique pencils
    pathological a.
    penetrating keratoplasty a.
    physiologic a.
    postoperative irregular a.
    pterygium-induced a.
    radial a.
    radical a.
    refractive a.
    regular a.
    residual a.
    reversed a.
    simple hyperopic a.
    simple myopic a.
    surgically induced a.
    "suture-out" a.
    symmetrical a.
    topographic a.
    total a.
    a. with the rule
    with-the-rule a.
    WTR a.
astigmatome
    Terry a.
astigmatometer, astigmometer
astigmatometry, astigmometry
astigmatoscope, astigmoscope
astigmatoscopy, astigmoscopy
astigmia
astigmic
astigmometer *(var. of* astigmatometer)
astigmometry *(var. of* astigmatometry)
astigmoscope *(var. of* astigmatoscope)
astigmoscopy *(var. of* astigmatoscopy)
ASTRA
    Advanced Shape Technology Refractive
    Algorithm
A-strabismus
ASTRAmax stereo topographer
astringent
astrocytic
    a. glioma
    a. hamartoma

astrocytoma
    juvenile pilocytic a.
    pilocytic a.
    retinal a.
asymmetric
    a. astigmatism
    a. papilledema
    a. refractive error
    a. surgery
asymmetry
    chromatic a.
asymptomatic optic neuritis
AT
    applanation tension
    applanation tonometry
    artificial tears
    Fluor-I-Strip AT
Atabrine
Atarax
ataxia
    cerebellar a.
    cone dystrophy-cerebellar a.
    familial episodic a.
    familial paroxysmal a.
    Friedreich a.
    hereditary cerebellar a.
    Marie a.
    ocular a.
    optic a.
    Pierre-Marie a.
    spinocerebellar a.
    vestibulocerebellar a.
ataxia-telangiectasia
    a.-t. syndrome
ataxic nystagmus
ATD
    aqueous tear deficiency
at distance and at near (D/N)
atenolol
Athens suture spreader
atheroembolism
atheroma
atherosclerosis
    diffuse a.
    ischemic a.
atherosclerotic ischemic neuritis
athetosis
    pupillary a.
Atkin lid block
Atkinson
    A. block
    A. corneal scissors
    A. 25-G short curved cystitome
    A. retrobulbar needle
    A. sclerotome
    A. single-bevel blunt-tip needle
    A. technique
    A. tip peribulbar needle

Atlas
    A. corneal topographer
    A. ophthalmic laser
Atlas-Elite laser
atonic
    a. ectropion
    a. entropion
    a. epiphora
atopic
    a. cataract
    a. conjunctivitis
    a. eczema keratoconjunctivitis
    a. line
atopy
atovaquone
ATPase
    actomyosin A.
ATPO
    Association of Technical Personnel in
    Ophthalmology
ATR
    against-the-rule
    ATR astigmatism
Atraloc suture
atresia
    a. iridis
    retinal a.
    tilting lens a.
atretoblepharia
atretopsia
Atropa belladonna
Atropair
atrophia
    a. bulbi
    a. bulborum hereditaria
    a. choroideae et retinae
    a. dolorosa
    a. gyrata
    a. striata et maculosa
atrophic
    a. age-related macular degeneration
    (AAMD)
    a. degenerative maculopathy
    a. excavation
    a. heterochromia
    a. hole
    a. macular degeneration
    a. polychondritis
    a. rhinitis
atrophy
    autosomal-dominant optic a.
    autosomal-recessive optic a.

band optic a.
Behr optic a.
bow-tie optic a.
bulbous a.
cavernous optic a.
central areolar choroidal a.
central gyrate a.
cerebral a.
choriocapillaris a.
chorioretinal a.
choroidal epithelial a.
choroidal gyrate a.
choroidal myopic a.
choroidal secondary a.
choroidal vascular a.
congenital optic a.
consecutive optic a.
diabetic optic a.
diffuse inflammatory eyelid a.
dominant optic a.
essential iris a.
essential progressive atrophy of a.
flat chorioretinal a.
Fuchs a.
geographic a.
glaucomatous a.
gray a.
growth retardation, alopecia,
    pseudoanodontia, and optic a.
    (GAPO)
gyrate a.
helicoid peripapillary a.
hemifacial a.
hereditary optic a.
heredodegenerative a.
heredofamilial optic a.
infantile optic a.
iris a.
ischemic choroidal a.
ischemic optic a.
juvenile optic a.
Kjer dominant optic a.
Leber hereditary optic a.
linear subcutaneous a.
morning glory optic a.
myopic choroidal a.
neuritic a.
neurogenic iris a.
nummular a.
olivopontocerebellar a. (OPCA)
optic disk a.
optic nerve a.

NOTES

atrophy *(continued)*
a. of optic nerve
opticoacoustic nerve a.
patchy a.
periorbital fat a.
peripapillary choroidal a.
peripheral chorioretinal a.
pigment a.
pigmented paravenous
chorioretinal a.
pigmented paravenous
retinochoroidal a.
postinflammatory a.
postpapilledema a.
primary optic a.
progressive choroidal a.
progressive encephalopathy with
edema, hypsarrhythmia and
optic a. (PEHO)
progressive hemifacial a.
progressive optic a.
retinal pigment epithelial a.
retinochoroidal a.
Schnabel optic a.
Schweninger-Buzzi macular a.
secondary optic a.
segmental iris a.
senile a.
sex-linked recessive optic a.
simple optic a.
subcutaneous fat a.
tabetic optic a.
traumatic a.
uveal a.

atropine
A Randomized Trial Comparing
Daily Atropine Versus
Weekend A.
A. Care
a. conjunctivitis
Isopto A.
prednisolone and a.
a. sulfate

atropinism
atropinization
Atropisol
attachment
Accuvac smoke evacuation a.
desmosomal cellular a.
MP video endoscopic lens a.
pathometer a.
photo-kerato a.
Planar Haag Streit a.
specular a.
vitreoretinal a.
zonular a.

attack
transient ischemic a. (TIA)

attention
a. reflex
a. reflex of the pupil
attentional dyslexia
attentiveness
visual a.
attenuated retinal arteriole
attenuation
arteriolar a.
focal a.
A-tuck
Atwood loupe
atypical
a. achromatopsia
a. coloboma
a. facial pain
a. monochromat
a. mycobacteria
Aubert phenomenon
audio
Eye Net A.
audiokinetic nystagmus
audito oculogyric reflex
auditory
a. oculogyric reflex
a. perceptual disability
a. stimulus
augmentation
periorbital volume a.
Augmentin
aural
a. nystagmus
a. scotoma
Aura Nd:YAG photodisruptor
Auranofin
Aureomycin
aureus
methicillin-resistant
Staphylococcus a. (MRSA)
Staphylococcus a.
auriasis
auricular glaucoma
Aurolate
Australia
A. antigen
Fellow of the Royal College of
Surgeons of A. (FRCSA)
Glaucoma Foundation of A.
Australian Corneal Graft Registry
auto
A. Ref-keratometer ARK-900
autorefractor and retinoscopy
autoantibody
antipericyte a.
circulating antipericyte a.
Autoclave Testing Service, Inc.
autoenucleation
autofluorescence
fundus a.

autofunduscope
autofunduscopy
autogenous
  a. dermis fat graft
  a. donor material
  a. hard palate eyelid spacer
  a. keratoplasty
autograft
  free conjunctival a.
  free skin a.
  full-thickness a.
  limbal-conjunctivitis a.
  skin a.
  split-thickness a.
autografting
  conjunctival rotation a.
  limbal a.
autoimmune
  a. corneal endotheliopathy
  a. demyelination
autoimmune-related retinopathy and optic neuropathy (ARRON)
autokeratometer
autokeratometry
autokeratoplasty
autokeratorefractometer
  KR-8000PA SUPRA a.
autokinesis visible light
autokinetic
  a. effect
  a. visible light phenomenon
AutoLensmeter
  Tomey Trooper A.
autologous
  a. chondrocyte transplantation
  a. ipsilateral rotating penetrating keratoplasty
  a. plasmin enzyme
  a. serum application
  a. stem cell rescue (ASCR)
autolysis
automated
  A. Corneal Shaper (ACS)
  A. Corneal Shaper microkeratome
  a. hemisphere perimeter
  a. lamellar keratoplasty-Excimer (ALK-E)
  a. lamellar therapeutic keratoplasty (ALTK)
  a. laser keratomileusis (ALK)
  A. Quantification of After-Cataract automated analysis system

  a. refractor
  a. static threshold perimetry
  a. tissue delamination technique
  a. trephine
  a. visual field
  a. vitrectomy
automatic
  a. infrared optometer
  a. refractor
  a. tonometry
  a. trephine
  a. twin syringe injector
autonomic
  a. nervous system
  a. nervous system disorder
Autonomous Technologies laser
autoophthalmoscope
autoophthalmoscopy
autopatch
  intralamellar a.
autoperimetry
  short wavelength a.
autophagic vacuole
Autophoro-Optimeter
  Clark A.-O.
Auto-Plot
Autoref
  Canon A. R-1
autorefraction (AR)
autorefractometer refraction
autorefractor
  6600 A.
  Canon Autoref R-1 a.
  Canon R-50+ a.
  HARK 599 a.
  Hoya AR-570 a.
  Nikon Retinomax K-Plus a.
  Retinomax 2 a.
  Retinomax cordless hand-held a.
  Subjective A.-7
  SureSight a.
  Tomey a.
  Welch Allyn SureSight a.
autorefractor/keratometer
  Retinomax K-Plus a.
autoregulation
autoshaped lamellar keratomileusis
autosomal-dominant
  a.-d. congenital cataract
  a.-d. hereditary optic neuropathy
  a.-d. oculocutaneous albinism
  a.-d. ophthalmoplegia

NOTES

autosomal-dominant *(continued)*
    a.-d. optic atrophy
    a.-d. retinitis pigmentosa
autosomal-recessive
    a.-r. hereditary optic neuropathy
    a.-r. ocular albinism (AROA)
    a.-r. ophthalmoplegia
    a.-r. optic atrophy
Autoswitch System
autotopographer
    Tomey a.
auxiliary
    a. fiber
    a. lens
auxometer
AV
    arteriovenous
    AV crossing defect
    AV nicking
    AV pattern
    AV strabismus syndrome
A-V
    arteriolovenous
    A-V crossing
    A-V nicking
A/V
    artery-to-vein ratio
avascular
    a. corneal stroma
    a. keratitis
    a. peripheral retina
    a. plaque
avascularity
Avellino dystrophy
average
    a. lens density (ALD)
    a. retinal image quality
Avit handpiece
avium
    Mycobacterium a.
Avonex
avulsion
    a. of caruncula lacrimalis
    a. of eyelid
    facial nerve a.
a-wave test
AWE
    advancing wave-like epitheliopathy
awl
    lacrimal a.
    Mustarde a.
axanthopsia
Axenfeld
    A. anomaly
    A. follicular conjunctivitis
    A. nerve loop
    A. suture
    A. syndrome
Axenfeld-Fieger syndrome

Axenfeld-Krukenberg spindle
Axenfeld-Reiger
    A.-R. anomaly (ARA)
    A.-R. syndrome
axial
    a. amblyopia
    a. ametropia
    a. anisometropia
    a. chamber
    a. cornea
    a. CT scan
    a. curvature map
    a. curvature mapping
    a. embryonal cataract
    a. fusiform developmental cataract
    a. hyperopia
    a. illumination
    a. length (AL)
    a. length/corneal radius (AL:CR)
    a. length/corneal radius ratio
    a. length of eye
    a. myopia
    a. partial childhood cataract
    a. point
    a. proptosis
    a. ray of light
    a. tomography
    a. view
axis, pl. **axes**
    achromatic a.
    anteroposterior a.
    astigmatic a.
    axis external a.
    a. bulbi externus
    a. bulbi internus
    corneal polarization a. (CPA)
    cylinder a.
    a. of cylindric lens (x)
    Fick a.
    a. fixation
    flat a.
    frontal a.
    geometric a.
    hypothalamic-pituitary-thyroid a.
    lens a.
    a. lentis
    longitudinal a.
    ocular a.
    a. oculi externa
    a. oculi interna
    optic a.
    optical a.
    a. opticus
    orbital a.
    principal optic a.
    pupillary a.
    red-green a.
    sagittal a.
    secondary a.

steep a.
tritan a.
vertical a.
visual a.
x a.
y a.
Axisonic II ultrasound
AXM
acetoxycyclohexamide
axometer
axon
fiber layer of a.
nerve fiber a.
preganglionic parasympathetic a.
retinal a.
axonal loss
axonometer
axoplasm
axoplasmic
a. flow
a. stasis

Azar
A. curved cystitome
A. lens
A. lens-holding forceps
A. lens-manipulating hook
A. lid speculum
azatadine
Azathioprine
azelastine hydrochloride ophthalmic solution
azidamfenicol
azidothymidine (AZT)
azithromycin
azlocillin
AZOOR
acute zonal occult outer retinopathy
Azopt
azotemic retinitis
AZT
azidothymidine

NOTES

β (*var. of* beta)
B
    amphotericin B
    bacitracin, neomycin, and
      polymyxin B
    B cell
    Fumidil B
    B measurement
    ultraviolet B (UVB)
2b
    interferon alfa-2b
BAB
    blood-aqueous barrier
baby
    b. Barraquer needle holder
Baciguent
bacillary layer
Bacillus
    B. anthracis
    B. cereus
    B. fragilis
    B. pyocyaneus
    B. subtilis
bacillus, pl. bacilli
    acid-fast b.
    gonococcal b.
    Koch-Weeks b.
    pneumococcal b.
    streptococcal b.
    tubercle b.
    Weeks b.
bacitracin
    b., neomycin, and polymyxin B
    b., neomycin, polymyxin B, and
      hydrocortisone
    zinc b.
    b. zinc
back
    b. optic zone radius (BOZR)
    b. surface debris (BSD)
    b. surface toric
    b. surface toric contact lens
    b. vertex power (BVP)
backcrack
backcracking
background
    b. diabetic retinopathy (BDR)
    b. illumination
    b. luminance
    tigroid b.
background-presented test target
Backhaus
    B. clamp
    B. syndrome
    B. towel clip

backscattering
bacteria
    gram-negative b.
    gram-positive b.
    saprophytic b.
bacterial
    b. blepharitis
    b. blepharoconjunctivitis
    b. collagenase
    b. conjunctivitis
    b. contamination
    b. corneal binding
    b. culture
    b. dacryoadenitis
    b. endophthalmitis
    b. infection
    b. infectious corneal infiltrate
    b. infectious corneal ulcer
    b. keratitis
    b. superinfection
    b. uveitis
bactericidal permeability-increasing
  protein (BPI)
bacteriocidal antibiotic
bacteriostatic antibiotic
Bacteroides
    B. fragilis
    B. melaninogenicus
Bacticort
Bactrim
Badal
    B. Lensmeter
    B. operation
    B. stimulus system
Baer nystagmus
Baerveldt
    B. filtering procedure
    B. glaucoma implant
    B. glaucoma implant tube
    B. seton implant
    B. shunt
    B. shunt tube
bag
    capsular b.
    mercury b.
    palpebral adipose b.
baggy eyelid
Bagley-Wilmer expressor
Bagolini
    B. lens
    B. striated glasses test
Bahn spud
Baikoff lens
Bailey
    B. chalazion forceps

Bailey *(continued)*
  B. foreign body remover
  B. lacrimal cannula
Bailey-Lovie
  B.-L. distance visual acuity
  B.-L. logMar chart
  B.-L. Near Test
  B.-L. visual acuity chart
Baillarger sign
Bailliart
  B. goniometer
  B. ophthalmodynamometer
  B. ophthalmoscope
Baird chalazion forceps
BAK
  benzalkonium chloride
Baker equation
balance
  Humphriss binocular b.
  meridional b.
  muscular b.
balanced
  b. saline solution
  b. salt solution (BSS)
Baldex
balding the limbus
Balint syndrome
ball
  ice b.
  Pinky b.
  retinal ice b.
  Super Pinky b.
ballast
  prism b.
  b. prism
ballasted contact lens
Ballen-Alexander
  B.-A. forceps
  B.-A. orbital retractor
Baller-Gerold syndrome
Ballet
  B. disease
  B. sign
balloon
  b. buckle
  b. degeneration
  endocapsular b.
  Honan b.
  Lincoff b.
ballottement
  ocular b.
Balo
  concentric sclerosis of B.
balsam
  Canada b.
Baltimore Eye Survey
Bamatter syndrome
Banaji irrigation cannula

band
  #40 b.
  A b.
  cellophane-like b.
  ciliary body b.
  circling b.
  encircling b.
  fascia b.
  H b.
  keratitis b.
  b. keratitis
  b. keratopathy
  M b.
  Mach b.
  b. optic atrophy
  retinal demarcation b.
  scleral expansion b.
  silicone b.
  Storz b.
  traction b.
  Watzke b.
  Z b.
  zonular b.
bandage
  binocle b.
  binocular b.
  Borsch b.
  Elastoplast b.
  monocular b.
  pressure b.
  b. scissors
  b. soft contact lens
bandelette
  keratitis b.
bandpass function
band-shaped
  b.-s. keratitis
  b.-s. keratopathy
Bangerter
  B. iris spatula
  B. method of pleoptics
  B. muscle forceps
  B. pterygium operation
Bangla Joy conjunctivitis
bank
  eye b.
  Lions Doheny Eye and Tissue
    Transplant B.
  New England Eye B.
banking
  venule b.
Bannayan syndrome
Banner
  B. enucleation snare
  B. forceps
  B. snare enucleator
Banophen Oral

Bansal
  B. irrigation cannula
  B. LASIK forceps
Baquacil
bar
  Berens prism b.
  horizontal prism b.
  prism b.
  b. prism
  b. reader
  skiascopy b.
  vertical prism b.
Bárány
  B. caloric test
  B. sign
Barbie retractor
barbital
Bardelli lid ptosis operation
Bardet-Biedl syndrome
Bard-Parker
  B.-P. blade
  B.-P. forceps
  B.-P. keratome
  B.-P. knife
  B.-P. razor
  B.-P. trephine
Bard sign
bare
  b. lymphocyte syndrome
  b. scleral technique
bared sclera
bare-sclera excision
baring
  b. of blind spot
  b. of sclera
Barkan
  B. double cyclodialysis operation
  B. goniolens
  B. gonioscopic lens
  B. goniotomy knife
  B. goniotomy lens
  B. goniotomy operation
  B. infant implant
  B. iris forceps
  B. light
  B. membrane
  B. theory
Barkan-Cordes linear cataract operation
Barlow syndrome
Barnes-Hind
  B.-H. contact lens cleaning and
    soaking solution

  B.-H. Gas Permeable Daily Cleaner
  B.-H. wetting solution
Baron-Bietti syndrome
Baron lens
barrage
  double-row diathermy b.
Barraquer
  B. applanation tonometer
  B. cannula
  B. cilia forceps
  B. conjunctival forceps
  B. corneal dissector
  B. corneal utility forceps
  B. corneoscleral scissors
  B. cryolathe
  B. curved holder
  B. enzymatic zonulolysis operation
  B. erysiphake
  B. eye shield
  B. eye speculum
  B. hemostatic mosquito forceps
  B. implant
  B. irrigator spatula
  B. keratomileusis
  B. keratomileusis operation
  B. keratoplasty knife
  B. lens
  B. method
  B. microkeratome
  B. needle
  B. needle carrier
  B. needle holder
  B. needle holder clamp
  B. operating room tonometer
  B. razor bladebreaker
  B. sable brush
  B. sweep
  B. trephine
  B. vitreous strand scissors
  B. wire speculum
  B. zonulolysis
Barraquer-Carriazo microkeratome
Barraquer-Colibri
  B.-C. forceps
  B.-C. speculum
Barraquer-de Wecker iris scissors
Barraquer-Krumeich-Swinger retractor
Barraquer-Krumeich test
Barraquer-Vogt needle
Barraquer-von Mandach capsule forceps
Barr body
barrel distortion

NOTES

B

Barré sign
Barrett hydrodelineation cannula
Barrie-Jones canaliculodacryorhinostomy
  operation
Barrier
  B. drape
  B. Phaco Extracapsular Pack
  B. sheet
barrier
  blood b.
  blood-aqueous b. (BAB)
  blood-eye b.
  blood-ocular b.
  blood-optic nerve b.
  blood-retinal b. (BRB)
  blood-vitreous b.
  epithelial b.
  ocular b.
  posterior capsular zonular b.
Barrio operation
Barron
  B. donor corneal punch
  B. epikeratophakia trephine
  B. marking corneal punch
  B. radial vacuum trephine
Barron-Hessburg corneal trephine
Barrow color shadow
Bartel spectacles
Bartholin syndrome
Bartonella henselae
bartonellosis
  ocular b.
Bartter syndrome
basal
  b. cell
  b. cell carcinoma (BCC)
  b. cell carcinoma of eyelid
  b. cell carcinoma of the medial
    canthus
  b. cell nevus
  b. cell nevus syndrome
  b. coil
  b. encephalocele
  b. epithelial nerve
  b. ganglia disease
  b. ganglia lesion
  b. ganglion
  b. iridectomy
  b. junction
  b. lamina
  b. lamina of choroid
  b. lamina of ciliary body
  b. laminar deposit (BLD)
  b. laminar drusen
  b. layer
  b. ophthalmoplegia
  b. phoria
  b. tear secretion

basalis
  b. choroideae lamina
  b. corporis ciliaris lamina
base
  cilia b.
  b. curve (BC)
  b. down
  b. in (BI)
  b. out (BO)
  b. plate
  prism b.
  sloughing b.
  b. up (BU)
  vitreous b.
baseball lens
Basedow disease
base-down (BD)
  b.-d. prism
base-in (BI)
  b.-i. prism
  b.-i. reserve
basement
  b. membrane (BM)
  b. membrane of choroid
  b. membrane of corneal epithelium
  b. membrane disorder
  b. membrane dystrophy
base-out (BO)
  b.-o. prism
  b.-o. reserve
basic
  b. esotropia
  b. exotropia
  b. secretion test
basilar
  b. artery
  b. artery aneurysm
  b. impression
  b. migraine
basin of inferior orbital fissure
basket
  Schultz fiber b.
basket-style scleral supporter speculum
Basol-S
basophilic
  b. adenoma
  b. intranuclear inclusion body
  b. reaction
Bassen-Kornzweig syndrome
Basterra operation
BAT
  Brightness Acuity Test
bathomorphic
Batimastat matrix metalloproteinase
  inhibitor
Batlle ICL manipulator
Batten
  B. disease
  B. syndrome

Batten-Mayou
B.-M. disease
B.-M. syndrome
battered-baby syndrome
battered-child syndrome
Battle sign
Baumgarten gland
Bausch
B. & Lomb LENSender
B. & Lomb manual keratometer
B. & Lomb Moisture Eyes Protect Lubricant Eye Drops
B. & Lomb Optima lens
B. & Lomb Surgical L161U lens
Bausch-Lomb-Thorpe slit lamp
bay
junctional b.
lacrimal b.
Bayadi lens
Baylisascaris procyonis
Baylor-Video Acuity Tester (BVAT)
bayonet forceps
BB shot forceps
BC
base curve
8.4 BC disposable lens
BCBC
bulbar conjunctival blood column
BCC
basal cell carcinoma
BCVA
best-corrected visual acuity
BD
base-down
Becton Dickinson and Company
BD K-3000 microkeratome
BD needle
BD prism
BDR
background diabetic retinopathy
bead
glass b.
beaded telangiectatic bulbar conjunctival vessel
beading
retinal venous b.
venous b.
beaked forceps
Béal
B. conjunctivitis
B. syndrome

beam
aiming b.
convergent b.
divergent b.
helium-neon b.
HeNe b.
proton b.
b. scatter
b. splitter
bear
b. tracks
b. track spots
Beard
B. knife
B. operation
Beard-Cutler operation
beaten-bronze appearance
beaten-copper appearance
beaten-metal appearance
Beaupre cilia forceps
Beaver
5435 B. blade
B. cataract cryoextractor
B. clear cornea incision system
B. Dam Eye Study
B. discission blade
B. eye blade
B. goniotomy needle knife
B. handle
B. keratome
B. Ocu-1 curved cystitome
B. Optimum blade
B. scleral Lundsgaard blade
B. Xstar knife
Beaver-Lundsgaard blade
Beaver-Okamura blade
Beaver-Ziegler needle blade
BEB
benign essential blepharospasm
Bechert
B. lens-holding forceps
B. 7-mm lens
B. nucleus rotator
Bechert-Kratz cannulated nucleus retractor
Bechert-McPherson angled tying forceps
Becker
B. corneal section spatulated scissors
B. goniogram
B. gonioscopic prism

NOTES

43

Becker *(continued)*
- B. phenomenon
- B. sign

Becker-Park speculum
Becton Dickinson and Company (BD)
bed
- capillary b.
- corneal stromal b.
- recipient b.
- retinal capillary b.
- stromal b.

bedewing
- corneal b.
- epithelial b.
- b. to wet

Beebe
- B. lens
- B. loupe

Beehler irrigating pupil expander
Beer
- B. blade
- B. canaliculus knife
- B. cataract knife
- B. Collyrium
- B. law
- B. operation

before meals (a.c.)
Behçet
- B. disease
- B. skin puncture test
- B. syndrome
- B. uveitis

Behler
- B. LASIK enhancement hook
- B. LASIK retreatment hook

Behr
- B. disease
- B. optic atrophy
- B. pupil
- B. syndrome

Behren rule
Bekhterev
- B. nystagmus
- B. reflex
- B. sign

Belin double-ended needle holder
Belix Oral
Bell
- B. erysiphake
- B. palsy
- B. phenomenon
- B. reflex
- B. sign

belladonna
- b. alkaloid
- *Atropa b.*

Bellows
- B. cryoextractor
- B. cryophake

bell-shaped curve
belly
- muscle b.
- b. of pterygium

belonoskiascopy *(var. of* velonoskiascopy)
Belz lacrimal sac rongeur
Benadryl Oral
Benazol
Bence Jones test
bench
- optical b.

bendazac
bender
- Watt stave b.

bending power
Benedict orbit operation
Benedikt syndrome
beneficial effect
bengal
- rose b.

benign
- b. anisocoria
- b. concentric anular macular dystrophy
- b. dyskeratosis
- b. essential blepharospasm (BEB)
- b. mucosal pemphigoid
- b. paroxysmal positional vertigo (BPPV)
- b. reactive lymphoid hyperplasia
- b. retinal vasculitis
- b. tumor

Bennett cilia forceps
benoxinate hydrochloride
Benson
- B. disease
- B. sign

bent
- b. blunt blade
- b. blunt needle
- b. 22-gauge needle

Benton Facial Recognition Test
benzalkonium chloride (BAK)
benzathine
- penicillin G b.

benzododecinium bromide
benzyl alcohol
Béraud valve
Bercovici wire lid speculum
Berens
- B. blade
- B. cataract knife
- B. conical implant
- B. corneal dissector
- B. corneal transplant forceps
- B. corneal transplant scissors
- B. corneoscleral punch
- B. dilator
- B. electrode

B. expressor
B. glaucoma knife
B. iridocapsulotomy scissors
B. keratoplasty knife
B. lens loupe
B. lid everter
B. lid retractor
B. marking calipers
B. muscle clamp
B. muscle forceps
B. orbital compressor
B. partial keratome
B. pinhole and dominance test
B. prism
B. prism bar
B. ptosis forceps
B. ptosis knife
B. pyramidal implant
B. refractor
B. scleral hook
B. sclerectomy operation
B. spatula
B. speculum
B. sterilizing case
B. suturing forceps
B. test object
B. three-character test
B. tonometer
Berens-Rosa scleral implant
Berens-Smith
B.-S. cul-de-sac restoration
B.-S. operation
Berens-Tolman ocular hypertension indicator
Berger
B. sign
B. space
B. symptom
Bergland-Warshawski phaco/cortex kit
Bergmeister papilla
Bergsma-Kaiser-Kupfer oculocutaneous albinism
Berke
B. approach
B. clamp
B. lid everter
B. operation
B. ptosis
B. ptosis forceps
Berke-Krönlein orbitotomy
Berkeley
B. Bioengineering bipolar cautery

B. Bioengineering brass scleral plug
B. Bioengineering infusion terminal port
B. Bioengineering mechanized scissors
B. Bioengineering ocutome
B. Bioengineering ptosis forceps
B. Bioengineering stiletto
B. optic zone marker
Berke-Motais operation
Berlin
B. disease
B. retinal edema
Berman
B. foreign body locator
B. localizer
Bernard-Horner syndrome
Bernard syndrome
Bernell
B. grid
B. tangent screen
Bernheimer fiber
Bernoulli law
berry
b. aneurysm
B. circle
Bertel position
besiclometer
best
B. degeneration
B. disease
b. ophthalmic correction
B. vitelliform macular dystrophy
best-corrected
b.-c. vision
b.-c. visual acuity (BCVA)
best-uncorrected
b.-u. visual acuity (BUVA)
beta, β
b. carotene
b. crystallin
b. radiation
b. therapy eye applicator
beta-1a
interferon b.
beta-blocker
Betadine
Betadine Sterile Ophthalmic Prep Solution

NOTES

45

Betagan
  B. Liquifilm
  B. R
Betalut
betamethasone phosphate eye drops
Beta-Ophtiole ophthalmic solution
Betaseron
BetaSite
betaxolol
  b. HCl
  b. hydrochloride
Betaxon
Bethke
  B. iridectomy
  B. operation
Betimol
  B. beta-blocker solution
  B. Ophthalmic
Betoptic
  B. S
  B. S Ophthalmic
better visual response
Bettman-Noyes fixation forceps
beveled-edge lens
Bezold-Brücke phenomenon
BFVW
  blood flow velocity waveform
BHP
  Bielschowsky head-tilt phenomenon
BI
  base in
  base-in
  BI prism
Bianchi
  B. sign
  B. valve
Biaxin
Biber-Haab-Dimmer
  B.-H.-D. corneal dystrophy
  B.-H.-D. degeneration
bibrocathol
bicanalicular tubing
bicarbonate
  sodium b.
bicentric
  b. grinding
  b. spectacle lens
Bick procedure
biconcave contact lens
biconvex
  b. lens
  b. optic
bicoronal scalp flap
bicurve contact lens
bicylindrical lens
b.i.d.
  twice daily
Bidwell ghost
Biedl disease

Bielschowsky
  B. disease
  B. head-tilt phenomenon (BHP)
  B. operation
  B. sign
  B. strabismus
  B. three-step head-tilt test
Bielschowsky-Jansky
  B.-J. disease
  B.-J. syndrome
Bielschowsky-Lutz-Cogan syndrome
Bielschowsky-Parks head-tilt three-step test
Biemond syndrome
Bietti
  B. corneal retinal dystrophy
  B. crystalline corneoretinal dystrophy
  B. crystalline retinopathy
  B. keratopathy
  B. lens
  B. syndrome
  B. tapetoretinal degeneration
bifermentans
  Clostridium b.
Bifidobacterium
bifixation
bifocal, pl. **bifocals**
  cement b.
  b. contact lens
  curved-top b.
  Emerson one-piece segment b.
  executive b.
  b. fixation
  flat top b.
  Franklin b.
  Ful-Vue b.
  b. glasses
  high-add b.
  b. intracorneal lens
  invisible b.
  Kryptok b.
  Morck cement b.
  Nokrome b.
  occupational b.
  one-piece b.
  Panoptic b.
  plastic b.
  progressive-add b.
  round top b.
  Schnaitmann b.
  b. segment
  b. spectacle lens
  b. spectacles
  straight-line b.
  Ultex b.
  Univis b.
bifoveal fixation
bifurcation

big blind spot syndrome
BIGH3 gene mutation
Bigliano tonometer
biguanide
 polyhexamethylene b.
 tropical polyhexamethylene b.
bilaminar membrane
bilateral
 b. altitudinal field defect
 b. homonymous altitudinal defect
 b. homonymous hemianopsia
 b. hypotony
 b. juxtafoveal telangiectasis (BJT)
 b. keratoconjunctivitis
 b. occipital lobe lesion
 b. ptosis
 b. simultaneous laser in situ
  keratomileusis
 b. simultaneous LASIK
 b. sporadic retinoblastoma
 b. strabismus
 b. uveal effusion syndrome
 b. uveitis
 b. visual field defect
biliaire
 masque b.
biloba
 ginkgo b.
bilobalide
Biltricide
bimatoprost ophthalmic solution
bimedial recession
binasal
 b. field defect
 b. hemianopsia
 b. quadrant field
bind
 vitronectin b.
binding
 bacterial corneal b.
Binkhorst
 B. collar stud lens implant
 B. four-loop iris-fixated implant
 B. four-loop iris-fixated lens
 B. intraocular lens
 B. iridocapsular lens
 B. irrigating cannula
 B. tip
 B. two-loop intraocular lens
  implant
 B. two-loop lens
Binkhorst-Fyodorov lens

BINO
 binocular internuclear ophthalmoplegia
binocle
 b. bandage
binocular
 b. accommodation
 b. amplitude
 b. aphakia
 b. bandage
 b. depth perception
 b. diplopia
 b. disparity
 b. eye patch
 b. field
 b. fixation
 b. fixation forceps
 b. function
 b. fusion
 b. hemianopsia
 b. heterochromia
 b. imbalance
 B. Indirect Ophthalmic Microscope
  (BIOM)
 b. indirect ophthalmoscope
 b. indirect ophthalmoscopy
 b. internuclear ophthalmoplegia
  (BINO)
 b. loupe
 b. luster
 b. microscope
 b. parallax
 b. perimetry
 b. polyopia
 b. rivalry
 b. single vision (BSV)
 b. strabismus
 b. visual acuity
 B. Visual Acuity Test
binocularity
binoculus
binophthalmoscope
binoscope
biochrome test
biocular VR-HMD
Bio-Eye ocular implant
biofilm
Biogel Sensor surgical glove
Biohist-LA
BioLon solution
BIOM
 Binocular Indirect Ophthalmic
 Microscope

B

NOTES

BIOM (*continued*)
    BIOM noncontact panoramic viewing system
    BIOM noncontact wide-angle viewing system
BioMask
Biomatrix ocular implant
Biomedics contact lens
Biometer
    Ophthasonic Ultrasonic B.
biometric ruler
biometry
    B-scan b.
    b. test
biomicroscope
    Haag-Streit slit-lamp b.
    high-frequency ultrasound b.
    Nikon FS-3 photo slit lamp b.
    slit lamp b.
    b. slit lamp
biomicroscopic indirect lens
biomicroscopy
    contact lens b.
    laser b.
    slit-lamp b.
    ultrasound b. (UBM)
Biom lens
Biomydrin
Bion
    B. Tears
    B. Tears eye drops
    B. Tears Solution
Bionic eye microdetector subretinal implant
Bio-Optics
    B.-O. Bambi Cell Analysis System
    B.-O. Bambi fixed-frame method
    B.-O. Bambi image analysis system
    B.-O. camera
    B.-O. specular microscope
    B.-O. telescope system
Bio-Pen biometric ruler
biophotometer
Biophysic
    B. Medical YAG laser
    B. Ophthascan S instrument
Biopore membrane
biopsy
    corneal b.
    greater superficial temporal artery b.
    temporal artery b.
    vitreous aspiration b.
biopter test
bioptic amorphic lens system
bioptics
biorbital angle
Biotic-O
biperiden

biphasic curve
biplate
    Ahmed glaucoma b.
bipolar
    b. cautery
    b. cone
    b. diathermy adapter clip
    b. electrode position
    b. forceps
    b. horizontal interaction
    b. retinal cell
    b. rod
biprism applanation tonometer
biprong muscle marker
Birbeck granule
Birch-Harman irrigator
Birch-Hirschfeld
    B.-H. entropion operation
    B.-H. lamp
Birch lamp
birdshot
    b. chorioretinitis
    b. chorioretinopathy
    b. choroiditis
    b. retinochoroiditis
    b. retinochoroidopathy
    b. retinopathy
    b. spot
birefractive
birefringence
    corneal b.
birefringent
Birkhauser test chart
Birks
    B. Mark II Colibri forceps
    B. Mark II grooved forceps
    B. Mark II hook
    B. Mark II instrument
    B. Mark II Instruments micro trabeculectomy scissors
    B. Mark II micro cross-action holder
    B. Mark II micro lock-type needle holder
    B. Mark II micro needle-holder forceps
    B. Mark II micro push/pull spatula
    B. Mark II microspatula
    B. Mark II straight forceps
    B. Mark II suture-tying forceps
    B. Mark II toothed forceps
Birks-Mathelone microforceps
Bishop-Harman
    B.-H. anterior chamber cannula
    B.-H. anterior chamber irrigator
    B.-H. bladebreaker
    B.-H. crisscross forceps
    B.-H. foreign body forceps
    B.-H. irrigating/aspirating unit

B.-H. knife
B.-H. Superblade
B.-H. tissue forceps
Bishop-Peter tendon tucker
Bishop tendon tucker
Bi-Soft lens
Bisolvon
bispherical lens
Bistouri blade
bitartrate
epinephrine b.
bite
16-b. nylon suture
bitemporal
b. disparity
b. field defect
b. fugax hemianopsia
b. hemianopic scotoma
biting rongeur
bitoric
b. contact lens
b. LASIK
Bitot
B. patch
B. spot
Bitumi monobjective microscope
bivariate analysis
bizygomatic
Bjerrum
B. area
B. scope
B. scotoma
B. scotometer
B. screen
B. sign
BJT
bilateral juxtafoveal telangiectasis
BK virus
black
b. braided nylon suture
b. braided silk suture
b. cataract
b. cornea
b. dot sign
b. eye
b. patch psychosis
b. reflex
b. silk bridle suture
b. silk sling suture
b. sunburst
b. sunburst sign
black-ball hyphema

blackout
visual b.
black/white occluder
blade
#15 b.
Accutome black diamond b.
Alfonso diamond corneal
transplant b.
Arc-T b.
ASICO multi incision system 10
facet b.
Bard-Parker b.
5435 Beaver b.
Beaver discission b.
Beaver eye b.
Beaver-Lundsgaard b.
Beaver-Okamura b.
Beaver Optimum b.
Beaver scleral Lundsgaard b.
Beaver-Ziegler needle b.
Beer b.
bent blunt b.
Berens b.
Bistouri b.
broken razor b.
Castroviejo razor b.
circular b.
ClearCut dual-bevel b.
crescent b.
Curdy b.
Curdy-Hebra b.
3D angled stainless phaco
trapezoid b.
Davidoff b.
Dean b.
diamond b.
diamond-dusted knife b.
Duotrak b.
Feather crescent tunnel b.
Feather round tunnel b.
b. gauge
Genesis diamond b.
Gill b.
Gill-Hess b.
Grieshaber b.
GS-9 b.
GSA-9 b.
Hansatome microkeratome b.
Hebra b.
Hoskins razor fragment b.
Katena double-edged sapphire b.
Keeler retractable b.

B

NOTES

blade *(continued)*
    Kellan sutureless incision b.
    Knapp b.
    b. knife
    Lange b.
    Lieberman-type speculum, reversible
      thin solid b.
    Lieberman-type speculum, thin
      solid b.
    Lieberman-type speculum with
      Kratz open wire b.
    Lieberman wire aspirating speculum
      with V-shape b.
    LRI diamond b.
    Martinez corneal trephine b.
    Mastel trifaceted diamond b.
    McPherson-Wheeler b.
    M4-400 freedom b.
    Micra double-edged diamond b.
    Micro-Sharp b.
    microvitreoretinal b.
    miniature b.
    multiincision 10-facet diamond b.
    MVB b.
    MVR b.
    Myocure b.
    myringotomy b.
    Optimum b.
    orbit b.
    Orca surgical b.
    Personna steel b.
    Planar b.
    razor b.
    rectangular b.
    replaceable b.
    Rhein 3-D trapezoid diamond b.
    ScalpelTec phaco keratome slit b.
    ScalpelTec wound-enlargement b.
    Scheie b.
    scleral b.
    Sharpoint spoon b.
    Sharpoint V-lance b.
    Sichel b.
    slimcut b.
    spoon b.
    Sputnik Russian razor b.
    stab incision angled b.
    Stealth DBO diamond b.
    Superblade No. 75 b.
    Surgistar ophthalmic b.
    Thornton arcuate b.
    Thornton tri-square b.
    trephine b.
    UltraThin surgical b.
    V-lance b.
    Wheeler b.
    Ziegler b.
bladebreaker
    Barraquer razor b.

    Bishop-Harman b.
    Castroviejo b.
    Castroviejo-style mini b.
    I-tech Castroviejo b.
    b. knife
    razor b.
    Swiss b.
    Troutman b.
    Vari b.
blade/knife
    V-lance b./k.
Blair
    B. epicanthus repair
    B. head drape
    B. operation
    B. retractor
    B. stiletto
Blairex
    B. Hard Contact Lens Cleaner
    B. Sterile Preserved Saline Solution
    B. sterile saline
    B. System
blanching of sclera
bland ophthalmic ointment
blank
    blocking of lens b.
    contact lens b.
    lens b.
    semifinished b.
    b. spot
Blasius lid flap operation
Blaskovics
    B. canthoplasty operation
    B. dacryostomy operation
    B. flap
    B. inversion of tarsus operation
    B. lid operation
    B. tarsectomy
Blaskovics-Berke ptosis
blastoma
    pineal b.
Blastomyces dermatitidis
blastomycosis
Blatt operation
Blaydes
    B. corneal forceps
    B. lens-holding forceps
BLD
    basal laminar deposit
bleb
    conjunctival b.
    b. cup
    b. disorder of the cornea
    encapsulated b.
    endothelial b.
    epithelial b.
    filtering b.
    flat filtration b.
    iron-leaking b.

B

ischemic b.
leaking filtering b.
b. migration
nonleaking b.
postcataract b.
bleb-associated endophthalmitis
blebitis
bleed
subarachnoid b.
vitreal b.
bleeding
intraoperative b.
intraretinal b.
limbal b.
Blefcon
Blenderm
B. tape
B. tape dressing
blennophthalmia
blennorrhagica
keratoderma b.
blennorrhea
b. adultorum
b. conjunctivalis
inclusion b.
neonatal inclusion b.
b. neonatorum
blennorrheal conjunctivitis
Bleph
Bleph-10
B.-10 Liquifilm
B.-10 Ophthalmic
B.-10 SOP
Blephamide
B. Ophthalmic
B. SOP
blepharadenitis
blepharal
blepharectomy
blepharedema
blepharelosis
blepharism
blepharitis
b. acarica
allergic b.
angular b.
b. angularis
bacterial b.
chlamydial b.
chronic b. (CB)
b. ciliaris
ciliary b.

clostridial b.
coliform b.
b. conjunctivitis
contact b.
demodectic b.
diplobacillary b.
eczematoid b.
b. follicularis
fungal b.
herpes simplex b.
marginal b.
b. marginalis
meibomian b.
nonulcerative b.
b. oleosa
parasitic b.
b. parasitica
pediculous b.
b. phthiriatica
pustular b.
rickettsial b.
b. rosacea
seborrheic b.
b. sicca
b. squamosa
squamous seborrheic b.
staphylococcal b.
streptococcal b.
b. ulcerosa
viral b.
blepharoadenitis
blepharoadenoma
blepharoatheroma
blepharochalasis
b. forceps
Kreiker b.
b. repair
blepharochromidrosis
blepharoclonus
blepharocoloboma
blepharoconjunctivitis
acne rosacea b.
allergic b.
angular b.
bacterial b.
chronic b.
herpes simplex b.
b. rosacea
staphylococcal b.
b. vaccinia
blepharodiastasis
blepharokeratoconjunctivitis

NOTES

51

blepharomelasma
blepharoncus
blepharopachynsis
blepharophimosis
    epicanthus b.
    b. inversus
    b. ptosis syndrome
blepharophyma
blepharoplast
blepharoplastic
blepharoplasty
    Ammon b.
    Davis-Geck b.
    transconjunctival lower eyelid b.
blepharoplegia
blepharoptosis, blepharoptosia
    b. adiposa
    false b.
    involutional b.
    b. repair
blepharopyorrhea
blepharorrhaphy
    Elschnig b.
blepharospasm, blepharospasmus
    benign essential b. (BEB)
    essential b.
    hemifacial b.
    nonorganic b.
    ocular b.
    primary infantile glaucoma b.
    reflex b.
    symptomatic b.
blepharospasm-oromandibular
    b.-o. dystonia
    b.-o. dystonia syndrome
blepharosphincterectomy
blepharostat
    Goldman scleral fixation ring
      and b.
    McNeill-Goldman b.
blepharostenosis
blepharosynechia
blepharotomy
blepharoxysis
Blessig
    B. cyst
    B. groove
    B. lacuna
    B. spaces
Blessig-Iwanoff
    B.-I. cyst
    B.-I. microcyst
blind
    color b.
    legally b.
    Royal National Institute for the B.
      (UK)
    b. spot
    b. spot enlargement

    b. spot of Mariotte
    b. spot reflex
    b. spot syndrome
blinding
    b. eye disease
    b. glare
blindness
    amnesic color b.
    blue b.
    bright b.
    cerebral b.
    color b.
    concussion b.
    congenital stationary night b.
    cortical psychic b.
    day b.
    deaf b.
    deuton color b.
    eclipse b.
    electric light b.
    epidemic b.
    factitious b.
    flash b.
    flight b.
    functional b.
    green b.
    hysterical b.
    Ishihara test for color b.
    legal b.
    letter b.
    mind b.
    miner's b.
    moon b.
    National Institute of Neurologic
      Diseases and B. (NINDB)
    night b.
    note b.
    nutritional b.
    object b.
    postoperative b.
    protan color b.
    psychic b.
    red b.
    red-green b.
    river b.
    Schubert-Bornschein congenital
      stationary night b.
    severe visual impairment and b.
      (SVI/BL)
    snow b.
    solar b.
    soul b.
    stationary night b.
    syllabic b.
    b. test
    text b.
    total b.
    transient b.
    twilight b.

word b.
X-linked congenital night b.
yellow b.
blindsight
blink
b. adequacy
b. inadequacy
b. out lagophthalmia
b. reflex
blinking
Blink-N-Clean
Blinx
BLL
brow, lids, lashes
Bloch-Stauffer syndrome
Bloch-Sulzberger syndrome
block
aphakic pupillary b.
Atkin lid b.
Atkinson b.
ciliary b.
ciliolenticular b.
ciliovitreal b.
ciliovitrectomy b.
cocaine b.
corneal b.
facial b.
Fine folding b.
b. glaucoma
lid b.
modified Van Lint b.
Nadbath facial b.
nerve b.
b. nerve
O'Brien lid b.
phakic pupillary b.
posterior peribulbar b.
punch b.
pupil b.
pupillary b.
regional b.
retrobulbar lid b.
reverse pupillary b.
Smith modification of Van Lint
lid b.
Spaeth b.
Stahl caliper b.
Tanne corneal cutting b.
Teflon b.
Van Lint b.
Van Lint-Atkinson lid akinetic b.
vitreous b.

blockade
nasolacrimal b.
pharmacological b.
blockage nystagmus
blocked fluorescence
blocker
H-1 b.
ultraviolet b.
blocking of lens blank
blond fundus
blood
b. barrier
b. cyst
extravasated b.
b. flow velocity waveform
(BFVW)
b. loss
b. oxygenation level-dependent
(BOLD)
b. oxygenation level-dependent
effect
retinal b.
b. staining
b. staining of cornea
subhyaloid b.
vitreous b.
blood-and-thunder retinopathy
blood-aqueous
b.-a. barrier (BAB)
b.-a. barrier breakdown
blood-eye barrier
blood-influx phenomenon
blood-ocular barrier
blood-optic nerve barrier
blood-retinal barrier (BRB)
Bloodshot WildEyes lens
blood-vitreous barrier
bloody tears
Bloomberg
B. SuperNumb anesthetic ring
B. trabeculotome set
blooming
b. of lens
b. spectacle lens
blot
b. hemorrhage
Western b.
blot-and-dot hemorrhage
blotchy positive staining
blow-in fracture
blown pupil

NOTES

blow-out
    b.-o. fracture
    b.-o. fracture of orbit
blue
    b. blindness
    b. cataract
    b. cone
    b. cone monochromasy
    b. cone monochromatism
    B. core PMMA
    Daimas B.
    b. field entoptic phenomenon
    b. field stimulation technique
    b. flash stimulus
    b. limbus
    b. line
    B. Mountain Eye Study
    b. nevus
    b. rubber bleb nevus syndrome
    b. sclera
    b. spike
    b. spot
    b. vision
    B. Vista
blue-dot cataract
blue-green argon laser
blue-yellow perimetry
Blumenthal
    B. anterior chamber maintainer
    B. push-pull irrigating cystitome
blunt
    b. needle
    b. trauma
blunted
    b. red reflex
    b. retinoscopic reflex
blur
    b. anatomy point source of light
    b. circle
    b. and clear exercise
    optical b.
    b. pattern
    b. point
    spectacle b.
    b. spot
    b. zone
blurred vision
blurring
    considerable b.
    mild b.
    b. of vision
BM
    basement membrane
B-mode handpiece
BO
    base-out
    base out
boat hook

bobbing
    converse b.
    inverse ocular b.
    ocular b.
    reverse b.
Boberg-Ans
    B.-A. lens
    B.-A. lens implant
Bochdalek valve
Bodian
    B. lacrimal pigtail probe
    B. mini lacrimal probe
Bodkin thread holder
body, pl. bodies
    adipose b.
    amyloid b.
    asteroid b.
    Barr b.
    basal lamina of ciliary b.
    basophilic intranuclear inclusion b.
    cellular inclusion b.
    ciliary b.
    colloid b.
    conjunctival foreign b.
    copper foreign b.
    cystoid b.
    cytoid b.
    cytoplasmic b.
    Dutcher b.
    electromagnetic removal of foreign b.
    Elschnig b.
    embryonal medulloepithelioma of ciliary b.
    embryonal tumor of ciliary b.
    eosinophilic intranuclear inclusion b.
    external geniculate b.
    foreign b. (FB)
    geniculate b.
    Goldmann-Larson foreign b.
    Guarnieri inclusion b.
    Halberstaedter-Prowazek inclusion b.
    Hassall b.
    Hassall-Henle b.
    Henderson-Patterson inclusion b.
    Henle b.
    Hensen b.
    Hollenhorst b.
    hyaline b.
    hyaloid b.
    inclusion b.
    intracytoplasmic inclusion b.
    intranuclear eosinophilic inclusion b.
    intraocular foreign b. (IOFB)
    intraorbital foreign b.
    ischemic necrosis of ciliary b.
    Landolt b.

lateral geniculate b. (LGB)
Leishman-Donovan b.
lenticular fossa of vitreous b.
Lewy b.
Lipschütz inclusion b.
multivesicular b.
nigroid b.
occult anular ciliary b.
pigmented layer of ciliary b.
pituitary b.
Prowazek-Greeff b.
Prowazek-Halberstaedter b.
Prowazek inclusion b.
psammoma b.
racquet b.
refractile b.
removal of foreign b.
retained foreign b. (RFB)
Rosenmüller b.
Rucker b.
Russell b.
Schaumann inclusion b.
sclerotomy removal of foreign b.
subconjunctival foreign b.
synaptic b.
trachoma b.
vitreous b.
vitreous foreign b.
wartlike b.
Weibel-Palade b.
body-referenced stimulus
Boeck sarcoid
boggy edema
Böhm operation
Bohr model
Boil-n-Soak
BOLD
blood oxygenation level-dependent
BOLD effect
bolus dressing
bombé
b. configuration
iris b.
Bonaccolto
B. fragment forceps
B. jeweler forceps
B. magnet tip forceps
B. monoplex orbital implant
B. scleral ring
B. trephine
B. utility and splinter forceps

Bonaccolto-Flieringa
B.-F. scleral ring
B.-F. scleral ring operation
B.-F. vitreous operation
Bondek suture
bone
b. cutter
ethmoid b.
foramen of sphenoid b.
frontal b.
glandular fossa of frontal b.
b. graft
lacrimal sulcus of lacrimal b.
maxillary b.
orbital arch of frontal b.
orbital border of sphenoid b.
orbital plane of frontal b.
orbital plate of ethmoid b.
orbital plate of frontal b.
orbital sulci of frontal b.
orbital wing of sphenoid b.
palatine b.
petrous b.
b. punch
b. removal decompression (BROD)
b. rongeur
sphenoid b.
supraorbital arch of frontal b.
supraorbital margin of frontal b.
temporal b.
b. trephine
uncinate process of lacrimal b.
zygomatic b.
bone-biting
b.-b. forceps
b.-b. punch
b.-b. trephine
Bonferroni test
Bonn
B. iris forceps
B. iris scissors
B. microiris hook
B. suturing forceps
Bonnet
B. capsule
B. enucleation operation
B. sign
Bonnet-DeChaume-Blanc syndrome
Bonnier syndrome
bony cataract

B

NOTES

Bonzel
B. blood staining of cornea
B. operation
boomerang-shaped lesion
borate
epinephrine b.
epinephryl b.
sodium b.
border
brushfire b.
corneoscleral b.
rolled-up epithelium with wavy b.
scalloped b.
b. tissue of Jacoby
Bordetella pertussis
Bordier-Fränkel sign
Bores
B. axis marker
B. optic zone marker
B. radial marker
B. twist fixation ring
boric
b. acid
b. acid solution
boring pain
Borrelia
B. burgdorferi
B. novyi
B. recurrentis
borreliosis
ocular lyme b.
Borsch
B. bandage
B. dressing
Borthen iridotasis operation
Boruchoff forceps
Bossalino blepharoplasty operation
Boston
B. Advance cleaner
B. Advance Comfort Formula
  Conditioning Solution
B. Advance reconditioning drops
B. 7 contact lens
B. Envision contact lens
B. EO, ES contact lens
B. II, IV contact lens
B. One Step Liquid Enzymatic
  Cleaner
B. Rewetting Drops
B. RXD contact lens
B. sign
B. Simplicity Multi-Action Solution
B. trephine
B. XO contact lens
both eyes (OU)
Botox
bottlemaker's cataract
botulin (BTX)

botulinum
b. A toxin
b. injection
b. toxin A (BTA)
botulism-induced
b.-i. blurred vision
b.-i. ptosis
botulismotoxin
Botvin-Bradford enucleator
Botvin iris forceps
bouche de tapir
bound-down muscle
bounding
b. mydriasis
b. pupil
bouquet of Rochon-Duvigneaud
Bourneville-Brissaud disease
Bourneville phakomatosis
boutons
b. en passant
b. terminaux
Bovie
B. electrocautery unit
B. electrosurgical unit
B. retinal detachment unit
B. wet-field cautery
bovied
bovina
facies b.
bovis
Moraxella b.
Mycobacterium b.
Bowen disease
Bower disease
bowl
Ganzfield b.
lenticular b.
Bowling lens
Bowman
B. capsule
B. cataract needle
B. lacrimal probe
B. lamina
B. layer
B. membrane
B. muscle
B. needle stop
B. operation
B. stop needle
B. tube
B. zone
bowstring
bow-tie
b.-t. hypoplasia
b.-t. knot
b.-t. optic atrophy
b.-t. stitch
boxcarring
boxing system

B

box measurement
Boyce needle holder
Boyd
  B. operation
  B. orbital implant
  B. zone
Boyden chamber technique
boydii
  Allescheria b.
  Petriellidum b.
  Pseudallescheria b.
Boynton needle holder
Boys-Smith laser lens
BOZR
  back optic zone radius
Bozzi foramen
BPI
  bactericidal permeability-increasing
    protein
BPPV
  benign paroxysmal positional vertigo
BQ
  Slit Lamp 900 B.
BRA
  branch retinal artery
brachial
  b. arch syndrome
  b. plexus palsy
brachium
  conjunctival b.
  b. conjunctivum
brachymetropia
brachymetropic
brachytherapy
  b. episcleral plaque
  orbital plaque b.
  palladium 103 ophthalmic
    plaque b.
  plaque b.
  radioactive plaque b.
  radon ring b.
Bracken
  B. anterior chamber cannula
  B. effect
  B. fixation forceps
  B. iris forceps
  B. irrigating/aspirating unit
Bradford snare enucleator
bradykinin
Braid
  B. effect
  B. strabismus

braided
  b. silk suture
  b. Vicryl suture
Brailey operation
braille
brailler
  Perkins b.
brain
  b. cortex
  b. damage
  b. dysfunction
  B. Heart infusion broth
  b. stem
  b. tumor
  b. tumor headache
brainstem, brain stem
  b. dysfunction
  b. lesion
  b. motor nucleus
branch
  b. retinal artery (BRA)
  b. retinal artery occlusion (BRAO)
  b. retinal vein (BRV)
  b. retinal vein occlusion (BRVO)
  B. Vein Occlusion Study
brancher enzyme deficiency
branching
  b. dendrite
  b. filament
  b. infiltration
  b. lesion
Branhamella catarrhalis
Brannon
  B. extracapsular cleaving forceps
  B. extracapsular removal forceps
BRAO
  branch retinal artery occlusion
brasiliensis
  Nocardia b.
brass scleral plug
Brawley
  B. refractor
  B. retractor
Brawner orbital implant
brawny
  b. edema
  b. scleritis
  b. tenonitis
  b. trachoma
Brayley
  polymorphic macular degeneration
    of B.

NOTES

Brazilian ophthalmia
BRB
    blood-retinal barrier
bread-crumb exudate
breadth of accommodation
break
    conjunctival b.
    giant retinal b.
    iatrogenic retinal b.
    b. phenomenon
    b. point
    retinal b.
    b. in retinal integrity
breakdown
    blood-aqueous barrier b.
    optical b.
    surface b.
breakpoint
    fusion b.
breakthrough
breakup
    b. phenomenon
    b. time (BUT)
    b. time of tear
    b. time test
Brems Astigmatism Marker with Level
breves
    nervi ciliares b.
Brevital
Brickner sign
bridge
    b. coloboma
    comfort b.
    keyhole b.
    B. operation
    b. pedicle flap
    b. pedicle flap operation
    saddle b.
    b. of spectacles
    b. suture
bridle suture
Brierley nucleus splitter
Briggs strabismus operation
bright
    b. blindness
    b. empty field
    B. eye
    b. staining
bright-field accommodation
brightness
    B. Acuity Test (BAT)
    b. comparison
    b. difference threshold
bright-sense
bright-white flash stimulus
brimonidine tartrate ophthalmic solution
brinzolamide ophthalmic suspension
British
    B. N system

    B. Standards Institution optotype
      set
Britt
    B. argon/krypton laser
    B. argon pulsed laser
    B. BL-12 laser
    B. krypton laser
brittle
    b. cornea syndrome
    b. diabetes
broad-beam ablation
broad-spectrum
    b.-s. antibiotic
    b.-s. heater (BSH)
Broca
    B. aphasia
    B. visual plane
brochure
    Kids, Computers & Vision b.
Brockhurst technique
BROD
    bone removal decompression
Broders grading
Brodmann area
broken razor blade
Brolene
Bromarest
Brombach perimeter
Brombay
bromhexine
bromide
    benzododecinium b.
    demecarium b.
    pancuronium b.
Bromley foreign body operation
bromocriptine
Bromphen
brompheniramine
bromvinyldeoxyuridine (BVDU)
Bronson foreign body removal
  operation
Bronson-Magnion
    B.-M. eye magnet
    B.-M. forceps
Bronson-Park speculum
Bronson-Turner foreign body locator
Bronson-Turtz
    B.-T. refractor
    B.-T. retractor
bronze diabetes
bronzing
    nuclear b.
Brooke tumor
broth
    Brain Heart infusion b.
    thioglycate b.
    trypticase soy b.
brow
    b. droop

b. fixation
b., lids, lashes (BLL)
b. tape

brown
b. cataract
B. insertion forceps
B. interchangeable lid speculum
B. limbal relaxing incision guide
B. pocket starter
B. sterile adhesive
B. technique of nuclear flipping
B. tendon
B. tendon sheath syndrome
B. vertical retraction syndrome

Brown-Beard technique
Brown-Dohlman Silastic corneal implant
Brown-Grabow capsulorrhexis cystitome forceps
Brown-Kelly sign
Brown-McLean syndrome
Brown-Pusey corneal trephine
broxyquinoline
Brucella suis
Bruch
B. gland
B. layer
B. membrane

Brücke
B. fiber
B. lens
B. line
B. muscle
B. reagent
B. tunica nervea

Brücke-Bartley phenomenon
Brückner reflex testing
Brueghel syndrome
Bruening forceps
Brunati sign
brunescens
cataracta b.

brunescent cataract
Bruns nystagmus
Brunsting-Perry cicatricial pemphigoid
brush
Alger b.
Barraquer sable b.
Cytobrush S b.
5139 flexible retinal b.
mechanical epithelial b.
rotating b.
Thomas b.

Brushfield spot
Brushfield-Wyatt syndrome
brushfire border
BRV
branch retinal vein
BRVO
branch retinal vein occlusion
BRVO knife
52.00 BRVO knife
B-Salt Forte
B-scan
B-s. biometry
contact B-s.
Humphrey B-s.
B-s. ultrasonogram
B-s. ultrasonography
BSD
back surface debris
BSH
broad-spectrum heater
BSS
balanced salt solution
BSS Plus
BSS Plus ophthalmic irrigating solution
BSS sterile irrigating solution
BSV
binocular single vision
BTA
botulinum toxin A
BTX
botulin
BU
base up
bubble
air b.
gas b.
intraocular gas b.
buckle
balloon b.
encircling band for scleral b.
encircling silicone b.
b. height
prominent b.
scleral b. (SB)
temporary balloon b.
Bücklers I, II, III dystrophy
buckling
Custodis scleral b.
b. procedure
b. sclera
scleral b.

NOTES

59

budding yeast cell
Budge
  ciliospinal center of B.
Budinger blepharoplasty operation
Buedding squeegee cortex extractor and polisher
Buettner-Parel vitreous cutter
buffer
  HEPES b.
  Tris-borate b.
buffy coat
bufilcon A
build-up implant
bulb
  b. of eye
  terminal b.
bulbar
  b. conjunctiva
  b. conjunctival blood column (BCBC)
  b. conjunctival scarring
  b. fascia
  b. paralysis
  b. sheath
bulbi (pl. of bulbus)
bulbocapnine
bulbous atrophy
bulbus, pl. bulbi
  atrophia bulbi
  camera vitrea bulbi
  capsula bulbi
  cholesterosis bulbi
  cyanosis bulbi
  endothelium camerae anterioris bulbi
  essential phthisis bulbi
  fascia lata musculares bulbi
  hemosiderosis bulbi
  lacertus musculi recti lateralis bulbi
  melanosis bulbi
  musculi bulbi
  musculus obliquus inferior bulbi
  musculus obliquus superior bulbi
  musculus rectus inferior bulbi
  musculus rectus lateralis bulbi
  musculus rectus medialis bulbi
  b. oculi
  phthisis bulbi
  siderosis bulbi
  Tenon fascia bulbi
  trochlea musculi obliqui superioris bulbi
  tunica fibrosa bulbi
  tunica interna bulbi
  tunica sensoria bulbi
  tunica vasculosa bulbi
  xanthelasmatosis bulbi
  xanthomatosis bulbi

bulge
  vitreous b.
bulla, pl. bullae
  epithelial b.
  ethmoid b.
  b. ethmoidalis ossis
  b. ossea
bulldog clamp
Buller eye shield
bullosa
  concha b.
  epidermolysis b.
  keratitis b.
  recessive dystrophic epidermolysis b.
bullosum
  erythema multiforme b.
bullous
  b. detachment
  b. disorder
  b. keratopathy
  b. pemphigoid
  b. retinoschisis
bull's
  b. eye
  b. eye macular lesion
  b. eye maculopathy
  b. eye retinopathy
Bumke pupil
bump
  jelly b.
bundle
  arcuate nerve fiber b.
  Drualt b.
  b. of Drualt
  inferior arcuate b.
  maculopapillary b.
  maculopapular b.
  nerve fiber b.
  papillomacular nerve fiber b.
  paracentral nerve fiber b.
  superior arcuate b.
Bunge evisceration spoon
Bunker implant
Bunsen grease spot photometer
Bunsen-Roscoe law
buphthalmia, buphthalmos, buphthalmus
bupivacaine
bupranolol
bur, burr
  aftercataract b.
  Alfonso guarded b.
  Allport cutting b.
  Burwell b.
  corneal foreign body b.
  cutting b.
  diamond b.
  foreign body b.
  lacrimal sac b.

Storz corneal b.
Wills spud and b.
Worst corneal b.
Yazujian b.
Buratto
B. contact lens spoon and spatula
B. flap forceps
B. flap protector
B. III acrylic implantation forceps
B. irrigating cannula
B. LASIK Forceps
B. ophthalmic forceps
Burch
B. calipers
B. eye evisceration operation
B. pick
Burch-Greenwood tendon tucker
Burch-Lester speculum
burgdorferi
Borrelia b.
Burian-Allen
B.-A. contact lens
B.-A. contact lens electrode
buried
b. disk drusen
b. suture
burn
acid b.
alkali b.
alkaline b.
ammonia alkali b.
ammonium hydroxide alkali b.
chemical b.
corneal alkali b.
foveal b.
laser b.
light argon laser b.
radiation b.
retinal b.
solar b.
b. spot size
thermal b.
ultraviolet b.
burnetii
Coxiella b.
Burns amaurosis
Burow flap operation
Burr
B. butterfly needle
B. cornea
B. corneal ring
B. silicone button

burr (*var. of* bur)
burst
b. hemiflip procedure
laser b.
Burton lamp
Burwell bur
Busacca nodule
BUT
breakup time
butacaine
Butazolidin
Butcher conjunctivitis
butterfly
b. macular dystrophy
b. needle
b. needle infusion port
b. pattern steepening of the cornea
b. test
butterfly-shaped pigment epithelial dystrophy
button
Burr silicone b.
collar b.
corneal b.
corneoscleral b.
Graether collar b.
penetrating keratoplasty b.
silicone b.
buttonhole
b. incision
b. iridectomy
button-tip manipulator
butyl
b. cyanoacrylate
b. cyanoacrylate glue
butyrate
cellulose acetate b. (CAB)
BUVA
best-uncorrected visual acuity
Buzard Diamond Barraqueratome Microkeratome System
Buzzi operation
b.v.
DORC International b.v.
BV100 needle
BVAT
Baylor-Video Acuity Tester
BVDU
bromvinyldeoxyuridine
BVI
BVI AXIS biometric ruler

NOTES

BVI *(continued)*
> BVI PAXIS biometric ruler and pachymeter

BVP
> back vertex power

b wave

b-wave amplitude
Byrne expulsive hemorrhage lens
Byron
> B. Smith ectropion operation
> B. Smith lazy T correction

C
contraction
cylinder
cylindrical lens
  adjunctive mitomycin C
  C loop
  C measurement
  mitomycin C (MMC)
  C value
CA
carbonic anhydrase
carcinoma
corneal abrasion
CAB
cellulose acetate butyrate
cable temple
cabufocon A
CAC
central anterior curve
CA/C
convergence accommodation
  CA/C ratio
CACT
computer-assisted corneal topography
caecum
punctum c.
caecutiens
  Onchocerca c.
Caenorhabditis elegans
caerulea
cataracta c.
caespitosus
  Streptomyces c.
CAG
closed-angle glaucoma
CAI
carbonic anhydrase inhibitor
Cairns
  C. operation
  C. procedure
  C. trabeculectomy
Cajal
interstitial nucleus of C.
calcareous
  c. cataract
  c. conjunctivitis
  c. degeneration
  c. degeneration of cornea
  c. deposit
calcarine
  c. artery
  c. cortex
  c. fissure
calcein-AM stain
calciferol

calcific
  c. band keratopathy
  c. phacolysis
calcification
  conjunctival c.
  lamellar c.
  optic disk drusen c.
  sclerochoroidal c.
  sellar c.
calcified retinoblastoma
calcinosis cutis, Raynaud phenomenon, esophageal motility disorder, sclerodactyly, and telangiectasia (CREST)
calcitriol
calcium
  c. alginate swab
  c. deposition
  c. hydroxide
calcium-containing opacity
calcoaceticus
  Acinetobacter c.
calcofluor
  c. white
  c. white stain
calculating equivalent defocus
calculation
  lens power c.
  power c.
calculus, pl. calculi
  lacrimal c.
Caldwell
  C. Suction Trephine
  C. view
Caldwell-Luc approach
Caldwell-Waters view
Calendar monthly disposable contact lens
Calhoun-Hagler
  C.-H. lens extraction operation
  C.-H. lens needle
Calhoun-Merz needle
Calhoun needle
Calibri forceps
caliculus ophthalmicus
caligation
caligo
  c. corneae
  c. lentis
  c. pupilla
calipers
  Berens marking c.
  Burch c.
  Castroviejo c.
  Green c.

C

calipers *(continued)*
Jameson c.
John Green c.
Machemer c.
Miyajima LASIK c.
Stahl c.
Storz c.
surgical c.
Thomas c.
Thorpe c.
Thorpe-Castroviejo c.
Callahan
C. fixation forceps
C. lens loupe
C. operation
Callender cell type classification
callipaeda
Thelazia c.
callosum
corpus c.
splenium of corpus c.
Calmette
C. conjunctival reaction
C. ophthalmic reaction
C. ophthalmoreaction
caloric
c. irrigation test
c. nystagmus
caloric-induced nystagmus
calotte
calvaria, pl. **calvariae**
Cambridge
C. acuity card
C. low-contrast grating
C. Research Systems (CRS)
camera, pl. **camerae, cameras**
Bio-Optics c.
c. bulbi anterior
c. bulbi posterior
Canon CF-60U fundus c.
Canon CF-60Z fundus c.
Carl Zeiss Jena Retinophot
fundus c.
CCD c.
Coburn c.
CooperVision c.
Cr6-45NMf retinal c.
Docustar fundus c.
Donaldson fundus c.
Eyecor c.
fiberoptic digital fundus c.
fundus c.
Garcia-Ibanez c.
hand-held fundus c.
Handy nonmydriatic video
fundus c.
Holofax Oxford retroillumination
cataract c.
House-Urban-Pentax c.

Kowa PRO II retinal c.
Kowa RC-XV fundus c.
c. lucida
Neitz CT-R cataract c.
Nidek 3Dx stereodisk c.
Nikon Retinopan fundus c.
NM-1000 digital non-mydriatic
fundus c.
c. obscura
c. oculi
c. oculi anterior
c. oculi posterior
Olympus fundus c.
PhotoScreener pediatric c.
RC-2 fundus c.
Reichert c.
RetCam 120 fiberoptic fundus c.
retinal c.
Retinopan 45 c.
telecentric fundus c.
Topcon 50IA c.
Topcon TRC-501A fundus c.
Topcon TRC-50VT retinal c.
Topcon TRC-50X retinal c.
Topcon TRV-50VT fundus c.
TRC-50IX ICG-capable fundus c.
TRC-SS2 stereoscopic fundus c.
c. vitrea bulbi
Zeiss FF450 fundus c.
Zeiss-Nordenson fundus c.
cAMP
cyclic adenosine monophosphate
cAMP final common pathway
cAMP mediated mechanism
Campbell
iris retraction syndrome of C.
C. refractor
C. retractor
C. slit lamp
campimeter
campimetry
Campodonico
C. canal
C. operation
CAM vision stimulator
Canada
C. balsam
Fellow of the Royal College of
Physicians of C. (FRCPC)
Canadian
C. Ophthalmology Society
C. Study of Health and Aging
canal
ampulla of lacrimal c.
Campodonico c.
central c.
ciliary c.
Cloquet c.
collateral pulp c.

Dorello c.
emissarial c.
ethmoid c.
fallopian c.
Ferrein c.
Fontana c.
Gartner c.
Hannover c.
Hovius c.
hyaloid c.
infraorbital c.
lacrimal c.
Lauth c.
nasal c.
nasolacrimal c.
c. of Nuck
optic c.
orbital c.
Petit c.
ruffed c.
Schlemm c.
scleral c.
scleroticochoroidal c.
semicircular c.
Sondermann c.
c. of Stilling
supraciliary c.
supraoptic c.
supraorbital c.
tarsal c.
zygomaticofacial c.
zygomaticotemporal c.
canalicular
c. disorder
c. duct
c. laceration
c. pathway
c. route
c. scissors
canaliculi (*pl. of* canaliculus)
canaliculitis
canaliculodacryocystostomy
canaliculodacryorhinostomy
canaliculorhinostomy
canaliculum
canaliculus, pl. canaliculi
common c.
inferior c.
c. infraorbitalis opticus
lacrimal c.
c. lacrimalis
lower c.

c. rod and suture
stenosis c.
superior c.
upper c.
canalis
c. hyaloideus
c. opticus
Canavan disease
cancer-associated retinopathy (CAR)
cancrum nasi
candela (cd)
c. laser
c. laser lithotriptor
C. videoimaging system
candela/m²
candela-sec/m²
Candida
C. *albicans*
C. *endophthalmitis*
C. *glabrata*
C. *krusei*
C. *parapsilosis*
C. *tropicalis*
candidal
c. conjunctivitis
c. endophthalmitis
c. granuloma
c. keratitis
c. retinitis
c. uveitis
candidiasis conjunctivitis
candle
foot c. (fc)
German Hefner c.
candle-guttering
candle-meter
candle-power
candlewax drippings
caniculotomy
surgical c.
canis
Toxocara c.
canities circumscripta
cannula
AE-7277 Rubenstein LASIK C.
air injection c.
Akahoshi hydrodissection c.
alpha-chymotrypsin c.
angled left/right c.
anterior chamber washout c.
ASSI air injection c.
Bailey lacrimal c.

C

NOTES

cannula *(continued)*
  Banaji irrigation c.
  Bansal irrigation c.
  Barraquer c.
  Barrett hydrodelineation c.
  Binkhorst irrigating c.
  Bishop-Harman anterior chamber c.
  Bracken anterior chamber c.
  Buratto irrigating c.
  Castroviejo cyclodialysis c.
  Chang hydrodissection c.
  coaxial irrigation/aspiration c.
  Cobra LASIK irrigating c.
  cortical cleaving hydrodissector c.
  Corydon expression c.
  Corydon hydroexpression c.
  cyclodialysis c.
  DeCamp viscoelastic c.
  De LaVega vitreous-aspirating c.
  Dischler irrigation c.
  Dishler type LASIK irrigating c.
  double irrigating/aspirating c.
  Drews irrigating c.
  Fasanella lacrimal c.
  Feaster K7-5460 hydrodissecting c.
  Galt aspirating c.
  Gans cyclodialysis c.
  Gass cataract-aspirating c.
  Gass vitreous-aspirating c.
  Ghormley double c.
  Gills double irrigating/aspirating c.
  Gills double Luer-Lok c.
  Gills-Welsh aspirating c.
  Gills-Welsh double-barreled
    irrigating/aspirating c.
  Gills-Welsh irrigating/aspirating c.
  Gills-Welsh olive-tip c.
  Gimbel fountain c.
  Girard irrigating c.
  Glaser microvitreoretinal c.
  Goldstein c.
  goniotomy knife c.
  Grizzard subretinal fluid c.
  Guell irrigation c.
  Guell LASIK c.
  Gulani triple function LASIK c.
  Healon aspirating c.
  Heyner double c.
  Hilton self-retaining infusion c.
  Hilton sutureless infusion c.
  Hoffer forward-cutting knife c.
  Hoffman irrigation c.
  Huang LASIK c.
  hydrodissection c.
  I/A c.
  infusion c.
  iris hook c.
  irrigating/aspirating c.
  irrigating J-hook c.

  irrigation/aspiration c.
  I-tech c.
  Jensen capsule polisher c.
  Jensen-Thomas
    irrigating/aspirating c.
  Johnson double c.
  Johnson hydrodelineation c.
  Johnson hydrodissection c.
  J-shaped irrigating/aspirating c.
  Kara cataract-aspirating c.
  Karickhoff double c.
  Keeler-Keislar lacrimal c.
  Kelman cyclodialysis c.
  Khouri Hydrodissection C.
  Klein curved c.
  Knolle anterior chamber
    irrigating c.
  Kraff cortex c.
  lacrimal irrigating c.
  Landers subretinal aspiration c.
  LASIK Banaji irrigating c.
  LASIK Burrato irrigating c.
  LASIK Guell irrigating c.
  LASIK Pettigrove irrigating c.
  Lewicky threaded infusion c.
  liquid vitreous-aspirating c.
  Look I/A coaxial c.
  Manche irrigation c.
  Manche-type LASIK irrigating c.
  Maumenee goniotomy knife c.
  Maumenee knife goniotomy c.
  McIntyre anterior chamber c.
  McIntyre-Binkhorst irrigating c.
  McIntyre coaxial c.
  Mendez-Freeman silicone oil c.
  Mendez-Goldbaum Tri-Port subtenon
    anesthesia c.
  model 177-33 viscocanalostomy c.
  Moehle c.
  Moncrieff c.
  Morris flexible c.
  Nichamin hydrodissection c.
  Nichamin LASIK irrigating c.
  Oaks double straight c.
  O'Gawa cataract-aspirating c.
  O'Gawa two-way aspirating c.
  olive-tip c.
  O'Malley-Heintz infusion c.
  Packo pars plana c.
  Pautler infusion c.
  Peacekeeper c.
  Pearce coaxial
    irrigating/aspirating c.
  Peczon I/A c.
  perfluorocarbon coaxial I/A c.
  Pettigrove irrigation c.
  Peyman silicone oil c.
  Pierce coaxial irrigating/aspirating c.
  Pierce I/A c.

quad-ported LASIK irrigating c.
Rainin air injection c.
Randolph cyclodialysis c.
reel aspiration c.
Rhein aspiration c.
Rhein irrigation c.
Roper alpha-chymotrypsin c.
Rowsey fixation c.
Rubenstein type LASIK
  irrigating c.
Rubinstein irrigation c.
Rycroft c.
Scheie anterior chamber c.
Scheie cataract-aspirating c.
Seibel LASIK flap irrigator and
  squeegee c.
self-retaining infusion c.
self-retaining irrigating c.
Shepard incision irrigating c.
Shepard radial keratotomy
  irrigating c.
side-port c.
sidewall infusion c.
Simcoe cortex extractor
  aspiration c.
Simcoe II PC double c.
Simcoe reverse aperture c.
Simcoe reverse
  irrigating/aspirating c.
Slade formed irrigation c.
smooth c.
soft-tipped c.
Steriseal disposable c.
subretinal aspiration c.
sub-Tenon anesthesia c.
Swets goniotomy knife c.
Tenner lacrimal c.
Thomas irrigating-aspirating c.
Thurmond nucleus-irrigating c.
Tri-Port sub-Tenon anesthesia c.
Troutman c.
TruPro lacrimal c.
Tulevech c.
two-way cataract-aspirating c.
Ulanday double c.
Vander vitreoretinal injection c.
Veirs c.
Vidaurri double irrigation c.
Visco expression c.
Viscoflow c.
Visitec irrigating/aspirating c.
vitreous-aspirating c.

Wagner silicone oil c.
Weil lacrimal c.
Weiss self-retaining c.
Welsh cortex stripper c.
Welsh flat olive-tip double c.
Wergeland double c.
West lacrimal c.
Yamagishi viscocanalostomy c.
Canon
  C. Auto Keratometer K-1
  C. Autoref R-1
  C. auto refraction keratometer
  C. auto refractometer
  C. Autoref R-1 autorefractor
  C. CF-60U fundus camera
  C. CF-60Z fundus camera
  C. perimeter
  C. R-5+ Auto Ref-Keratometer
  C. R-50+ autorefractor
  C. refractor
  C. RO-4000 slit lamp
  C. RO-5000 slit lamp
  C. SLO scanning laser
    ophthalmoscope
can-opener capsulotomy
Cantelli sign
Cantera-Olivieri
  C.-O. CB speculum
  C.-O. Hansa speculum
canthal
  c. hypertelorism
  c. keratinization
  c. ligament
  c. raphe
  c. recess
  c. tendon
canthaxanthin crystalline retinopathy
canthectomy
canthi (*pl. of* canthus)
canthitis
cantholysis
canthomeatal
canthopexy
canthoplasty
  Agnew c.
  Ammon c.
  Imre lateral c.
canthorrhaphy
  Elschnig c.
canthorum
  dystopia c.

NOTES

canthotomy
    external c.
    lateral c.
canthus, pl. **canthi**
    basal cell carcinoma of the
        medial c.
    inner c.
    c. inversus
    lateral c.
    medial c.
    nasal c.
    outer c.
    temporal c.
CAP
  Contoured Ablation Pattern
    VISX CAP
cap
    compliance c.
    corneal c.
    Gelfilm c.
    SupraCAPS quarter-globe c.
capillaritis
    retinal c.
capillary
    c. bed
    c. closure
    c. hemangioma
    c. hemangioma of eyelid
    c. lumen
    c. microaneurysm
    nonfenestrated c.
    c. nonperfusion
    c. perfusion
    c. plexus
    c. scaffolding
    c. tube plasma viscosimeter
capillary-free zone
capitis
    dolor c.
caplet
    TripTone C.'s
Caprogel
capsitis
capsomere
capsula, pl. **capsulae**
    c. bulbi
    c. lentis
capsular
    c. advancement
    c. bag
    c. bag distention syndrome
    c. cataract
    c. debris
    c. delamination
    c. exfoliation syndrome
    c. fixation
    c. glaucoma
    c. opacification
    c. support

capsular-zonular
capsulatum
    Histoplasma c.
capsule
    anterior lens c.
    Bonnet c.
    Bowman c.
    c. contraction syndrome
    crystalline c.
    curling of c.
    exfoliation of lens c.
    c. forceps technique
    c. fragment forceps
    c. fragment spatula
    leaves of c.
    lens c.
    ocular c.
    c. polisher
    pseudoexfoliation of lens c.
    Tenon c.
capsulectomy
    anterior c.
capsulitis
capsulolenticular cataract
capsulorrhexis
    c. capsulotomy
    continuous circular c.
    continuous curvilinear c. (CCC)
    c. forceps
    Kraff-Utrata c.
    minicircular c.
capsulotome
    Darling c.
capsulotomy
    anterior c.
    can-opener c.
    capsulorrhexis c.
    Castroviejo c.
    circular tear c.
    Darling c.
    Fugo blade c.
    posterior c.
    c. scissors
    triangular c.
    Vannas c.
    Verhoeff-Chandler c.
CAPT
    Complications of Age-Related Macular
        Degeneration Prevention Trial
capture
    iris c.
    pupillary c.
CAR
    cancer-associated retinopathy
    CAR syndrome
Carbacel
carbachol
    Isopto C.
carbacholine

Carbastat Ophthalmic
carbenicillin
carbinoxamine and pseudoephedrine
Carbiset Tablet
Carbiset-TR Tablet
Carbocaine
Carbodec
    C. Syrup
    C. TR Tablet
carbogen
carbomycin
carbon
    c. arc lamp
    c. dioxide laser
    c. monoxide retinopathy
carbonic
    c. anhydrase (CA)
    c. anhydrase inhibitor (CAI)
    c. anhydrase tomography
Carbopol
Carboptic Ophthalmic
carboxymethylcellulose sodium
carboxy termini
Carcholin
carcinoid tumor
carcinoma (CA)
    adenoid cystic c.
    basal cell c. (BCC)
    embryonal c.
    epidermoid c.
    c. of eyelid
    meibomian gland c.
    metastatic c.
    mucoepidermoid c.
    radiation-induced c.
    sebaceous cell c.
    sebaceous gland c.
    signet-ring c.
    squamous cell c.
carcinomatosis
    meningeal c.
carcinomatous meningitis
card
    Allen preschool c.
    Cambridge acuity c.
    digital acuity c.
    flash picture c.
    Howell phoria c.
    illuminated near c. (INC)
    Jaeger acuity c.
    microendoscopic test c.

    MIM c.
    reading c.
    reduced Snellen c.
    Rosenbaum c.
    Sherman c.
    Sloan reading c.
    Snellen near-vision c.
    Snellen reading c.
    standard near c.
    stigmatometric test c.
    Teller acuity c.
    test c.
    VSG 2/3F graphic c.
Cardec-S Syrup
cardinal
    c. diagnostic position of gaze
    c. direction of gaze
    c. field test
    c. ocular movement
    c. point
    c. position
    c. suture
Cardiobacterium
    Haemophilus sp., *Actinobacillus*
      actinomycetemcomitans, C.
    C. hominis
    C. hominis, *Eikenella corrodens*
      and *Kingella kingae*
Cardio-Green (CG)
    C.-G. dye
Cardona
    C. corneal prosthesis forceps
    C. corneal prosthesis trephine
    C. fiberoptic diagnostic lens
    C. focalizing fundus lens implant
    C. goniofocalizing implant
    C. laser
    C. threading forceps
Cardrase
care
    AoSept Clear C.
    Atropine C.
    monitored anesthesia c. (MAC)
carinii
    Pneumocystis c.
Carl
    C. Zeiss instrument
    C. Zeiss Jena Retinophot fundus
    camera
    C. Zeiss lens
    C. Zeiss lensometer

NOTES

Carl (*continued*)
    C. Zeiss tonometer
    C. Zeiss YAG laser
Carlo Traverso maneuver (CTM)
carnitine deficiency
carnosus
    pannus c.
Carones
    C. LASEK pump
    C. LASEK spatula
    C. 10.0 mm OZ chamber
carotene
    beta c.
carotid
    c. aneurysm
    c. angiography
    c. arteriogram
    c. artery
    c. artery occlusion
    c. artery stenosis
    c. artery thrombosis
    c. cavernous sinus fistula
    c. ischemia
    c. obstruction
    c. occlusive disease retinopathy
Carpel
    C. one-step trabeculectomy punch
    C. speculum
Carpenter syndrome
Carpine
    E C.
    Isopto C.
    P.V. C.
Carriazo-Barraquer
    C.-B. instrument set
    C.-B. microkeratome
    C.-B. principle
Carriazo-Pendular microkeratome
carrier
    Barraquer needle c.
    minus c.
    obligate c.
Cartella eye shield
carteolol
    c. HCl
    c. hydrochloride
Carter
    C. operation
    C. sphere
    C. sphere introducer
cartilage
    central c.
    ciliary c.
    palpebral c.
    tarsal c.
Cartman lens insertion forceps
Cartrol Oral

caruncle
    epicanthus c.
    lacrimal c.
caruncula, pl. **carunculae**
    lacrimal c.
    c. lacrimalis
    trichosis carunculae
caruncular papilloma
CAS
    congenital anterior staphyloma
Casanellas lacrimal operation
cascade
    phototransduction c.
Cascadeflo AC 1760 filtrator
case
    Berens sterilizing c.
    Contique contact lens c.
    Essilor storage c.
    Fine corneal carrying c.
    index c.
    Per-Protocol-Observed C.
    Titmus Washer storage c.
    trial c.
caseating
    c. orbital granuloma
    c. tubercle
Casebeer keratorefractive planning program
Casebeer-Lindstrom nomogram
case-control study
caseosa
    rhinitis c.
caseous necrosis
Casey operation
Caspar
    C. ring
    C. ring opacity
cast
    c. molding
    c. resin lens
Castallo
    C. refractor
    C. retractor
    C. speculum
castellanii
    Acanthamoeba c.
Castillejos LASIK retreatment spatula
Castroviejo
    C. acrylic implant
    C. angled keratome
    C. anterior synechia
    C. anterior synechia scissors
    C. bladebreaker
    C. blade holder
    C. calipers
    C. capsule forceps
    C. capsulotomy
    C. clip-applying forceps
    C. compressor

C. corneal dissector
C. corneal-holding forceps
C. corneal scissors with inside stop
C. corneal section scissors
C. corneal transplant marker
C. corneal transplant scissors
C. corneal transplant trephine
C. corneoscleral forceps
C. corneoscleral punch
C. cyclodialysis cannula
C. cyclodialysis spatula
C. discission knife
C. double-ended spatula
C. electro keratome
C. electrokeratotome
C. enucleation snare
C. erysiphake
C. fixation forceps
C. improved trephine
C. iridectomy
C. iridocapsulotomy scissors
C. keratectomy
C. keratoplasty scissors
C. lacrimal dilator
C. lacrimal sac probe
C. lens loupe
C. lens spoon
C. lid clamp
C. lid forceps
C. lid retractor
C. mini-keratoplasty
C. mucotome
C. needle holder
C. needle holder clamp
C. operation
C. orbital aspirator
C. radial iridotomy
C. razor blade
C. refractor
C. scleral fold forceps
C. scleral marker
C. scleral shortening clip
C. sclerotome
C. snare enucleator
C. speculum
C. suture forceps
C. suturing forceps
C. synechia scissors
C. synechia spatula
C. twin knife
C. tying forceps

C. vitreous aspirating needle
C. wide grip handle forceps
Castroviejo-Arruga forceps
Castroviejo-Barraquer needle holder
Castroviejo-Colibri forceps
Castroviejo-Galezowski dilator
Castroviejo-Kalt needle holder
Castroviejo-Scheie
C.-S. cyclodiathermy
C.-S. cyclodiathermy operation
Castroviejo-style mini bladebreaker
Castroviejo-Vannas capsulotomy scissors
catadioptric
Catalano
C. corneoscleral forceps
C. intubation set
C. muscle hook
C. tying forceps
catalase
Catalin
Catalyst machine
catamenialis
iritis c.
cataphoria
mature c.
cataplexy
Catapres
cataract
aculeiform c.
adherent c.
adolescent c.
adult-onset c.
age-related c.
aminoaciduria c.
anterior axial developmental c.
anterior axial embryonal c.
anterior axonal embryonal c.
anterior polar c.
anterior pyramidal c.
anterior subcapsular c. (ASC)
anular c.
arborescent c.
c. aspiration
atopic c.
autosomal-dominant congenital c.
axial embryonal c.
axial fusiform developmental c.
axial partial childhood c.
black c.
blue c.
blue-dot c.
bony c.

NOTES

71

cataract *(continued)*
    bottlemaker's c.
    brown c.
    brunescent c.
    calcareous c.
    capsular c.
    capsulolenticular c.
    central c.
    cerulean c.
    cheesy c.
    choroidal c.
    Christmas tree c.
    complete congenital c.
    complicated c.
    concussion c.
    congenital c.
    contusion c.
    copper c.
    Coppock c.
    coralliform c.
    coronary c.
    cortical spokes c.
    corticosteroid-induced c.
    crystalline c.
    cuneiform c.
    cupuliform c.
    cystic c.
    degenerative c.
    delayed onset c.
    dendritic c.
    dermatogenic c.
    developmental c.
    diabetic c.
    diabetic-osmotic c.
    diffuse c.
    dilacerated c.
    disk-shaped c.
    drug-induced c.
    dry-shelled c.
    early mature c.
    electric shock c.
    embryonal nuclear c.
    embryonic c.
    embryopathic c.
    evolutional c.
    extracapsular c. (ECC)
    extracapsular extraction of c.
    c. extraction (CE)
    extraction of intracapsular c.
    c. extraction operation
    c. extraction with intraocular lens
      (CE/IOL)
    fibrinous c.
    fibroid c.
    flap operation c.
    Fleischer c.
    floriform c.
    fluid c.
    furnacemen's c.

    fusiform c.
    galactose c.
    galactosemia c.
    general c.
    glassblower's c.
    c. glasses
    glassworker's c.
    glaucomatous c.
    global c.
    gray c.
    green c.
    hard c.
    heat-generated c.
    heat-ray c.
    hedger c.
    heterochromic c.
    hook-shaped c.
    hypermature c.
    hypocalcemic c.
    hypoglycemic c.
    immature c.
    incipient c.
    infantile c.
    infrared c.
    intracapsular extraction of c.
    intumescent c.
    irradiation c.
    juvenile developmental c.
    c. knife
    c. knife guard
    Koby c.
    lacteal c.
    lamellar developmental c.
    lamellar zonular perinuclear c.
    lenticular c.
    life-belt c.
    lightning c.
    Marner c.
    c. mask ring
    c. mask shield
    mature c.
    membranous c.
    metabolic syndrome c.
    milky c.
    mixed c.
    Morgagni c.
    morgagnian c.
    myotonic dystrophy c.
    c. needle
    NS c.
    nuclear developmental c.
    nuclear sclerotic c.
    nutritional deficiency c.
    O'Brien c.
    osmotic c.
    overripe c.
    partial c.
    pear c.
    c. pencil

perinuclear c.
peripheral c.
pisciform c.
poikiloderma atrophicans and c.
poisoning degenerative c.
polar c.
polymorphic c.
posterior polar c.
posterior subcapsular c. (PSC)
postinflammatory c.
postvitrectomy c.
C. PPO project
c. of prematurity
presenile c.
primary c.
probe c.
progressive c.
puddler's c.
punctate c.
pyramidal c.
radiation c.
reduplicated c.
ring-form congenital c.
ring-shaped c.
ripe c.
rubella c.
sanguineous c.
saucer-shaped c.
sclerotic c.
secondary c.
sector cortical c.
sedimentary c.
senescent cortical degenerative c.
senescent nuclear degenerative c.
senile nuclear sclerotic c.
c. senilis
shaped c.
siderosis c.
siderotic c.
siliculose c.
snowflake c.
snowstorm c.
Soemmering ring c.
soft c.
spear developmental c.
c. spectacles
c. spindle
spindle c.
spoke-like sutural c.
c. spoon
spurious c.

stationary c.
stellate c.
steroid-induced c.
subcapsular c.
sugar c.
sugar-induced c.
sunflower c.
supranuclear c.
c. surgery
sutural developmental c.
syndermatotic c.
syphilitic c.
tetany c.
thermal c.
total c.
toxic c.
traumatic degenerative c.
tremulous c.
umbilicated c.
vascular c.
Vogt c.
Volkmann c.
c. with Down syndrome
x-ray-induced c.
zonular nuclear c.
zonular pulverulent c.
zonular sutural c.
cataracta
    c. adiposa
    c. brunescens
    c. caerulea
    c. centralis pulverulenta
    c. cerulea
    c. complicata
    c. congenita membranacea
    c. coronaria
    c. dermatogenes
    c. electrica
    c. fibrosa
    c. membranacea accreta
    c. neurodermatica
    c. nigra
    c. nodiformis
    c. ossea
    c. syndermotica
    c. zonularis pulverulenta
cataract-aspirating needle
cataractogenesis
cataractogenic drug
cataractous
Catarase

C

NOTES

Catarex
>C. cataract removal system
>C. technology

catarrh
>sinus c.
>spring c.
>vernal c.

catarrhal
>c. conjunctivitis
>c. corneal ulcer
>c. marginal ulceration
>c. ophthalmia
>c. ulcerative keratitis

catarrhalis
>*Branhamella* c.
>*Moraxella* c.

catastrophic complication
catatonic pupil
catatropic image
caterpillar-hair ophthalmia
caterpillar ophthalmia
Catford visual acuity test
catgut suture
catheter
>C-flex c.
>French c.
>LacriCATH lacrimal duct c.
>lacrimal balloon c.
>Lincoff balloon c.
>red rubber c.
>Teflon injection c.

catheterization
>c. of lacrimal duct
>c. of lacrimonasal duct

catoptric
catoptroscope
cat's
>c. eye
>c. eye amaurosis
>c. eye effect
>c. eye pupil
>c. eye reflex
>c. eye syndrome

cat scratch disease neuroretinitis
CAU
>chronic anterior uveitis

caudate hemorrhage
Cauer chalazion forceps
cautery
>Alcon hand c.
>Berkeley Bioengineering bipolar c.
>bipolar c.
>Bovie wet-field c.
>Codman wet-field c.
>Colorado c.
>Concept disposable c.
>Concept hand-held c.
>disposable c.
>Eraser c.

>Fine micropoint c.
>Geiger c.
>Gonin c.
>Hildreth c.
>Ishihara I-Temp c.
>I-Temp c.
>Khosia c.
>Mentor wet-field c.
>Mira c.
>Mueller c.
>NeoKnife c.
>c. operation
>ophthalmic c.
>Op-Temp disposable c.
>Parker-Heath c.
>pencil c.
>phacoemulsification c.
>Prince c.
>punctal c.
>Rommel c.
>Rommel-Hildreth c.
>Scheie ophthalmic c.
>scleral c. (SC)
>thermal c.
>Todd c.
>ValleyLab c.
>von Graefe c.
>Wadsworth-Todd c.
>wet-field c.
>Wills c.
>Ziegler c.

cave
>myopic c.

cavern
>Schnabel c.

cavernous
>c. angioma
>c. optic atrophy
>c. orbital hemangioma
>c. portion of the oculomotor nerve
>c. sinus
>c. sinus aneurysm
>c. sinus fistula
>c. sinus/superior orbital fissure syndrome
>c. sinus syndrome
>c. sinus thrombosis

caviae
>*Nocardia* c.

cavinasi
cavitary uveal melanoma
cavitation
Cavitron
>C. aspirator
>C. I/A handpiece
>C. irrigation/aspiration system

Cavitron-Kelman irrigation/aspiration system

cavity
    laser c.
    opening of orbital c.
    optic papilla c.
    orbital c.
    schisis c.
    vitreous c.
CB
    chronic blepharitis
CBS
    Charles Bonnet syndrome
cc
    with correction
CCA
    central choroidal apposition
CCC
    continuous curvilinear capsulorrhexis
CCD
    choriocapillaris degeneration
        CCD camera
CCF
    critical corresponding frequency
c̄cl
    with contact lenses
CCT
    central corneal thickness
CCTS
    Collaborative Corneal Transplantation
    Studies
CCTV
    closed-circuit television vision
        enhancement system
C/D
    cup-to-disk ratio
cd
    candela
CD-5 needle
CD8 cell
CDCR
    conjunctivodacryocystorhinostomy
CDR
    cup-to-disk ratio
CDS
    Cornea Donor Study
CE
    cataract extraction
Ceclor
cecocentral
    c. depression
    c. scotoma
cecum
    punctum c.

CeeNU
CeeOn
    C. Edge
    C. Edge foldable IOL
    C. foldable lens
    C. heparin surface-modified lens
    C. intraocular lens
cefaclor
cefadroxil
cefamandole sodium
cefazaflur
cefazolin
cefmenoxime
cefoperazone
ceforanide
cefotaxime
cefsulodin
ceftazidime
Ceftin
ceftizoxime
ceftriaxone
cefuroxime
CE/IOL
    cataract extraction with intraocular lens
    CE/IOL implant
Celestone
Celita
    C. elite knife
    C. sapphire knife
cell
    c. adhesion
    air c.
    amacrine c.
    anticalbindin c.
    antigen-presenting c.
    B c.
    basal c.
    bipolar retinal c.
    budding yeast c.
    CD8 c.
    chick lens c.
    clump c.
    cluster of retinoblastoma c.'s
    collagen c.
    cone c.
    conjunctival epithelial c.
    conjunctival goblet c.
    corneal c.
    cytoxic T c.
    c. density
    endoneural c.
    endothelial c.

NOTES

cell *(continued)*
    eosin-Y c.
    epithelial c.
    epithelioid c.
    fat c.
    fiber c.
    c. and flare
    foam c.
    foreign body c.
    ganglion c.
    ghost c.
    giant epithelial c.
    goblet c.
    granulomatous inflammatory c.
    helper/inducer T c.
    heterogeneous c.
    horizontal c.
    inflammatory c.
    interplexiform c.
    killer c.
    Leber c.
    lens epithelial c. (LEC)
    leukemic c.
    limbal stem c.
    lipid c.
    c. lysis
    M c.
    magnocellular c.
    mast c.
    membrane lipid c.
    meningeal c.
    mesangial c.
    metaplastic epithelial c.
    Mueller c.
    Müller c.
    multinucleated giant epithelial c.
    mural c.
    myoepithelial c.
    myoid visual c.
    nests and strands of c.'s
    neural crest c.
    neural ganglionic c.
    nonneural ganglionic c.
    OFF-center bipolar c.
    ON-center bipolar c.
    Onodi c.
    paracentral c.
    parvocellular c.
    perineural c.
    perivascular stromal c.
    photoreceptor c.
    phytohemagglutinin c.
    pigment c.
    plasma c.
    polygonal pigmented c.
    polyhedral c.'s
    Reed-Sternberg c.
    reticulum c.
    retinal visual c.

    retinoblastoma c.
    rod c.
    satellite ganglionic c.
    Schwann c.
    sebaceous c.
    secretory epithelial c.
    somatic c.
    spillover c.
    spindle c.
    spindle-shaped c.
    squamous c.
    stem c. (SC)
    suppressor T c.
    Touton giant c.
    vascular endothelial c.
    visual c.
    vitreal c.
    vitreous c.
    water c.
    Wedl c.
    wet c.
    white c.
    wing c.
    X c.
    Y c.
cell-mediated immunity
cellophane
    crinkled c.
    c. macular reflex
    c. maculopathy
    c. retinopathy
cellophane-like band
Cell-Tak autologous fibrin
Cellufluor
Cellufresh Formula
cellula, pl. **cellulae**
    cellulae lentis
cellular
    c. aggregate
    c. debris
    c. inclusion body
cellularity
cellulite
    orbital c.
cellulitis
    amyloid c.
    herpes simplex c.
    orbital c.
    periorbital c.
    preseptal c.
celluloid frame
cellulosa
    tela c.
cellulose
    c. acetate
    c. acetate butyrate (CAB)
    c. acetate butyrate contact lens
    c. acetate frame
    hydroxyethyl c.

hydroxypropyl c.
c. nitrate
c. nitrate frame
c. surgical sponge
Celluvisc
Celsus
C. lid
C. spasmodic entropion operation
Celsus-Hotz
C.-H. entropion
C.-H. operation
cement
c. bifocal
Morck c.
center
distance between c.'s (DBC)
Dutch Ophthalmic Research C.
(DORC)
foveal c.
gaze c.
geometric c.
horizontal gaze c.
Lions Low Vision C.
optic c.
optical c.
pontine gaze c. (PGC)
pupillary c.
c. of rotation
c. of rotation distance
supranuclear gaze c.
vertical gaze c.
W.K. Kellogg Eye C.
centering ring
Centra-Flex lens
centrage
central
c. abrasion
c. achromatopsia
c. amaurosis
c. angiospastic retinitis
c. angiospastic retinopathy
c. anisocoria
c. anterior curve (CAC)
c. areolar choroidal atrophy
c. areolar choroidal dystrophy
c. areolar choroidal sclerosis
c. areolar pigment epithelial
dystrophy
c. astigmatism
c. canal
c. cartilage
c. cataract

c. chorioretinitis
c. choroidal apposition (CCA)
c. choroiditis
c. cloudy corneal dystrophy
c. cloudy dystrophy of François
c. cloudy parenchymatous dystrophy
c. corneal thickness (CCT)
c. corneal ulcer
c. crystalline dystrophy
c. crystalline dystrophy of
Schnyder
c. defect
c. discoid corneal dystrophy
c. disk-shaped retinopathy
c. dyslexia
c. edema
c. edema of cornea
c. endothelial photography
c. field loss (CFL)
c. fovea
c. fovea of retina
c. fusion
c. gyrate atrophy
c. illumination
c. iridectomy
c. island
c. island of vision
c. keyhole of vision
c. light
c. nervous system (CNS)
c. pigmentary retinal dystrophy
c. posterior curve (CPC)
c. posterior curve of contact lens
c. reflex stripe
c. retinal artery (CRA)
c. retinal artery occlusion (CRAO)
c. retinal degeneration
c. retinal lens
c. retinal vein (CRV)
c. retinal vein occlusion (CRVO)
c. retinal vein occlusion knife
c. scotoma
c. scotoma syndrome
c. serous chorioretinopathy (CSC, CSCR)
c. serous choroidopathy
c. serous retinitis
c. serous retinochoroidopathy
c. serous retinopathy (CSR)
c. speckled corneal dystrophy
c., steady and maintained (CSM)
c., steady and maintained fixation

NOTES

central *(continued)*
    c. steep zone
    c. stellate laceration
    c. striate keratopathy
    c. stromal infiltrate
    c. suppression
    c. thickness of contact lens
    C. Vein Occlusion Study (CVOS)
    c. vestibular imbalance
    c. vestibular nystagmus
    c. visual acuity
    c. visual field (CVF)
    c. yellow point
centralis
    amaurosis c.
    area c.
    fovea c.
centrally fixing eye
centration
    optical zone c.
centraxonial
centrifugal
    c. incision
    c. separation
centripetal
    c. incision
    c. movement
    c. nystagmus
centrocecal
    c. defect
    c. scotoma
centronuclear myopathy
centrophose
Centurion syndrome
CEOS
    Congenital Esotropia Observational Study
cepacia
    Pseudomonas c.
cephalexin
cephalgia
cephalic
cephaloorbital
cephalosporin
Cephalosporium
cephalothin
ceratectomy
cerclage operation
cerebellar
    c. artery
    c. astrocytoma tumor
    c. ataxia
    c. ataxia-cone dystrophy
    c. cortex
    c. dysfunction
    c. eye sign
    c. flocculus
    c. hemisphere
    c. hemorrhage
    c. lesion

    c. notch
    c. tonsil
    c. vermis
cerebellomedullary
cerebellopontine
    c. angle (CPA)
    c. angle lesion
    c. angle tumor
cerebelloretinal
cerebellospinal
cerebellotegmental
cerebellothalamic
cerebellum
cerebra (*pl. of* cerebrum)
cerebral
    c. abscess
    c. achromatopsia
    c. akinetopsia
    c. amaurosis
    c. amyloid angiopathy
    c. arteriography
    c. arteriosclerosis
    c. artery
    c. artery aneurysm
    c. atrophy
    c. blindness
    c. cortex
    c. cortex reflex
    c. diplopia
    c. dyschromatopsia
    c. edema
    c. giantism
    c. hemisphere lesion
    c. heterotopia
    c. infarction
    c. layer of retina
    c. metamorphopsia
    c. micropsia
    c. palsy
    c. phycomycosis
    c. polyopia
    c. ptosis
    c. radionuclide angiography
    c. stratum of retina
    c. tunnel vision
    c. venous drainage
    c. ventricle
cerebri
    idiopathic pseudotumor c.
    pseudotumor c. (PTC)
cerebritis
cerebrohepatorenal syndrome
cerebroocular
cerebroopthalmic
cerebropupillary reflex
cerebroretinal angiomatosis
cerebrospinal fluid (CSF)
cerebrotendinous xanthomatosis
cerebrum, pl. **cerebra, cerebrums**

cereus
> *Bacillus c.*

ceroid lipofuscinosis
certified
> C. Ophthalmic Medical
> Technologist (COMT)
> C. Ophthalmic Technologist (COT)
> C. Orthoptist (CO)
> C. Paraoptometric Assistant (CPOA)
> C. Paraoptometric Technician
> (CPOT)
> C. Registered Nurse in
> Ophthalmology (CRNO)

cerulea
> cataracta c.

ceruleae
> maculae c.

cerulean cataract
cervical
> c. ganglion
> c. lesion
> c. nystagmus

cervicoocular reflex (COR)
cervicooculoacoustic syndrome
Cestan
> C. sign
> C. syndrome

Cestan-Chenais syndrome
Cestan-Raymond syndrome
Cetamide
> Isopto C.
> C. Ophthalmic

Cetapred
> Isopto C.
> C. ophthalmic

Cetazol
Cetirizine
cetylpyridinium chloride
CF
> counting fingers

C3F8
> perfluoropropane gas
> C3F8 gas

C₃F₃ C_3F_3
> perfluoropropane

CFEOM
> congenital fibrosis of the extraocular
> muscles

CFF
> critical flicker frequency
> critical flicker fusion

CFL
> central field loss

C-flex catheter
CFTD
> congenital fiber-type disproportion

CG
> Cardio-Green

cGMP
> cyclic guanosine monophosphate

chafing
> iris c.

chagrin
> peau de c.

chain
> collagen alpha c.
> fenestrated c.
> sialylated c.

chalazion, pl. chalazia
> acute c.
> c. clamp
> collar-stud c.
> c. curette
> Desmarres c.
> c. forceps
> Meyhoeffer c.
> c. trephine

chalcosis
> cornea c.
> c. lentis

chalkitis
Challenger digital applanation tonometer
chamber
> air c.
> c. angle
> angle of anterior c.
> anterior c. (AC)
> aqueous c.
> axial c.
> Carones 10.0 mm OZ c.
> choroidal c.
> closed c.
> c. collapse
> depth of c.
> eye c.
> flat anterior c.
> hydrometric c.
> Moistair Humidifying C.
> moisture c.
> multicorneal perfusion c.
> parallel-plate flow c.
> post c.
> posterior c. (PC)

NOTES

chamber *(continued)*
    postoperative flat anterior c.
    quiet c.
    reformation of c.
    shallow c.
    shallowing of c.
    vitreous c.
chamber-deepening glaucoma
CHAMPS
    Controlled High Risk Subjects Avonex
    Multiple Sclerosis Prevention Study
chancre of conjunctiva
chancroid
Chandler
    C. iridectomy
    C. iris forceps
    C. syndrome
    C. vitreous operation
Chandler-Verhoeff
    C.-V. lens extraction
    C.-V. operation
Chang
    C. combination phaco chopper
    C. hydrodissection cannula
    C. Quick Chop Combo
change
    arterial occlusive c.
    contralateral disc c.
    cortical c.
    crossing c.
    fatty c.
    Keith-Wagener c.
    KW c.
    nuclear c.
    optic disc c.
    pigment c.
    senile choroidal c.
    skin c.
    surgically induced refractive c.
    trophic c.
changer
    Galilean magnification c.
    Littmann Galilean magnification c.
channel
    c. dissector
    lamellar c.
    scleral c.
characteristic
    determinants of optic discharge c.
    electron microscopic c.
Charcot
    C. sign
    C. triad
CHARGE
    coloboma, heart defects, atresia choanae,
    retarded growth, genital hypoplasia, and
    ear anomalies
        CHARGE association
        CHARGE syndrome

Charleaux
    C. oil droplet reflex
    C. oil droplet sign
Charles
    C. anterior segment sleeve
    C. Bonnet syndrome (CBS)
    C. flute needle
    C. hand-held infusion lens
    C. infusion sleeve
    C. intraocular lens
    C. irrigating/aspirating unit
    C. irrigating contact lens
    C. lensectomy
    C. vacuuming needle
    C. vitrector with sleeve
Charlin syndrome
chart
    aberrated acuity c.
    Amsler c.
    astigmatic dial c.
    Bailey-Lovie logMar c.
    Bailey-Lovie visual acuity c.
    Birkhauser test c.
    color c.
    contemporary nearpoint c.
    cross-Polaroid projection c.
    Donders c.
    Duane accommodation c.
    E c.
    eye c.
    Ferris c.
    Guibor c.
    Illiterate E c.
    Illiterate eye c.
    kindergarten eye c.
    Konig bar c.
    Lancaster-Regan dial 1, 2 c.
    Landolt broken-ring c.
    Landolt-C acuity c.
    Lea Symbol c.
    Lebensohn reading c.
    Lebensohn visual acuity c.
    Lighthouse ET-DRS acuity c.
    logMAR c.
    Low-Contrast Sloan Letter C.
      (LCSLC)
    pedigree c.
    Pelli-Robson contrast sensitivity c.
    Pelli-Robson letter c.
    picture c.
    pseudoisochromatic c.
    Randot c.
    reading c.
    Regan low-contrast acuity c.
    Reuss color c.
    Snellen c.
    sunburst dial c.
    Turtle c.
    unaberrated c.

University of Waterloo c.
vectograph c.
Vistech wall c.
charting
EyeSys c.
chatter line
Chavasse glass
Chayet type corneal LASIK marker
ChBFlow
choroidal blood flow
ChBVol
choroidal blood volume
checkerboard
c. hemianopsia
c. visual field
check ligament
Chédiak-Higashi
C.-H. anomaly
C.-H. syndrome
Chédiak-Steinbrinck-Higashi anomaly
cheek
c. clamp
c. flap
cheese wire
cheesewiring of sutures
cheesy cataract
chelonae
Mycobacterium c.
chelonei
Mycobacterium c.
chemical
c. burn
c. conjunctivitis
c. diabetes
Fluka C.
c. injury
c. vapor deposition (CVD)
chemically treated spectacle lens
chemiluminescence assay
chemofluorescent dye
chemoreduction
chemosis
conjunctival c.
chemotherapy drops
chemotic
cherry-red
c.-r. spot
c.-r. spot in macula
c.-r. spot myoclonus syndrome
chevron incision
Cheyne nystagmus
chi, χ

Chiari malformation
chiasm
glioma of optic c.
c. lesion
optic c.
chiasma
c. arachnoiditis
c. opticum
c. syndrome
chiasmal
c. aplasia
c. arachnoiditis
c. compression
c. disease
c. dysplasia
c. glioma
c. hypoplasia
c. lesion
c. metastasis
post c.
c. sulcus
c. syndrome
c. tumor
c. visual field loss
chiasmapexy
chiasmatic
c. cisterna
c. field defect
c. syndrome
chiasmatis
lupus c.
chiasmometer
Chiba eye needle
Chibroxin
chick lens cell
chief fiber
Chievitz
fiber layer of C.
transient layer of C.
child-friendly VDS test
childhood episcleritis
children
An Evaluation of Treatment of Amblyopia in C. 7-18
Refractive Error Study in C.
chip-and-flip phacoemulsification technique
Chiroflex C11UB lens
Chiron
C. ACS microkeratome
C. automated corneal shaper

NOTES

81

Chiron *(continued)*
    C. Hansatome
    C. Hansatome microkeratome
chiroscope
chisel
    cornea c.
    Freer c.
    lacrimal sac c.
    West lacrimal sac c.
chi-squared test
Chlamydia
    C. *psittaci*
    C. *trachomatis*
chlamydial
    c. blepharitis
    c. inclusion conjunctivitis
    c. infection
Chlo-Amine
Chloracol
chlorambucil
chloramphenicol
    c., polymyxin B, and
      hydrocortisone
    c. and prednisolone
Chlorate
chlordecone
chlordiazepoxide
chlorhexidine
chloride
    acetylcholine c.
    aluminum c.
    benzalkonium c. (BAK)
    cetylpyridinium c.
    edrophonium c.
    hexamethonium c.
    methacholine c.
    quaternary ammonium c.
    sodium c. (NaCl)
    tetraethylammonium c.
chlorisondamine
chloroacetophenone
chlorobutanol
Chlorofair
chloroform
chlorolabe
chloroma
Chloromycetin Hydrocortisone
Chloromyxin
chlorophane
chloropia
chloroprocaine
chloropsia
Chloroptic
    C. Ophthalmic
    C. SOP
Chloroptic-P Ophthalmic
chloroquine
    c. keratopathy

    c. retinopathy
    c. toxicity
chloroquine/hydroxychloroquine
    retinopathy
Chlorphed
chlorpheniramine maleate
chlorphentermine
Chlor-Pro
chlorpromazine
chlorpropamide
chlorprothixene
chlortetracycline
chlorthalidone
Chlor-Trimeton
chocolate agar
choked
    c. optic disk
    c. reflex
cholesterinosis
cholesterol
    c. emboli of retina
    c. granuloma
    c. plaque
cholesterolosis
cholesterosis bulbi
cholinergic
    c. drug
    c. mechanism
    c. neuron
    c. pupil
cholinesterase
chondrodystrophia calcificans congenita
    punctata
chondrodystrophic myotonia
chondroitin
    hyaluronate sodium with c.
    c. sulfate
    c. sulfate medium
chondroitinase
choo-choo chop and flip
    phacoemulsification
chop
    phaco quick c.
chopper
    AE-7618 Tsuneoka irrigating c.
    Agarwal irrigating phaco c.
    Chang combination phaco c.
    combination phaco c.
    Davidoff ambidextrous nucleus c.
    Dodick-Kammann bimanual c.
    Dodick nucleus irrigating c.
    Fine irrigating reverse actuating
      splitting c.
    Fine-Nagahara phaco c.
    Fine sideport actuating quick c.
    Fukasaku snap & split tip
      irrigating c.
    He Hook C.
    Inamura race c.

Katena MicroFinger tip irrigating c.
Koch c.
Koch-Minami c.
Langerman bi-directional phaco c.
Minardi phaco c.
Miyoshi c.
Nagahara karate c.
Nagahara phaco c.
Nagahara quick c.
Nichamin I and II nucleus
 quick c.
Nichamin triple c.
Nichamin vertical c.
Olson phaco c.
Olson quick c.
Seibel nucleus c.
Seibel vertical safety quick c.
Shepherd tomahawk c.
Steinert double-ended claw c.
Steinert II claw c.
Sung reverse nucleus c.
Vergés phaco c.
chopper/manipulator
Universal phaco c.
chord
c. diameter
c. incision
c. length
chordoma
clivus c.
choriocapillaris
c. atrophy
c. degeneration (CCD)
lamina c.
membrana c.
c. vascular network
choriocapillary layer
choriocele
chorioid
ischemic necrosis of c.
lymphatic sinusoid c.
chorioidea
chorionic vesicle
choriopathy
chorioretinal (C/R)
c. adhesion
c. atrophic spot
c. atrophy
c. coloboma
c. degeneration
c. fold
c. granuloma

c. lesion
c. scar
c. venous anastomosis
chorioretinitis
birdshot c.
central c.
luetic c.
miliary tuberculosis c.
peripheral multifocal c. (PMC)
salt-and-pepper c.
sclerosing panencephalitis c.
c. sclopetaria
senile c.
septic c.
syphilitic c.
Toxoplasma c.
toxoplasmosis c.
vitiliginous c.
chorioretinopathy
birdshot c.
central serous c. (CSC, CSCR)
disciform c.
idiopathic central serous c. (ICSC)
c. and pituitary dysfunction (CPD)
serous c.
choristoma
epibulbar limbal dermoid c.
epibulbar osseous c.
episcleral osteocartilaginous c.
limbal c.
osseous c.
phakomatous c.
c. tumor
choroid
basal lamina of c.
basement membrane of c.
c. coloboma
contusion of c.
crescent c.
c. fissure
knuckle of c.
malignant melanoma of the c.
peripapillary c.
reattachment of c.
vascular lamina of c.
c. vein
choroidal
c. amelanotic melanoma
c. blood flow (ChBFlow)
c. blood volume (ChBVol)
c. cataract
c. chamber

C

NOTES

choroidal *(continued)*
  c. coloboma
  c. detachment
  c. dystrophy
  c. edema
  c. effusion
  c. epithelial atrophy
  c. filling
  c. flush
  c. fold
  c. granuloma
  c. gyrate atrophy
  c. hemangioma
  c. hemorrhage
  c. hyperfluorescence
  c. infarct
  c. infiltration
  c. ischemia
  c. lesion
  c. mass
  c. melanocytic tumor
  c. metastasis
  c. myopic atrophy
  c. neoplasm
  c. neovascularization (CNV)
  c. neovascular membrane (CNVM)
  c. nevus
  c. osteoma
  c. primary sclerosis
  c. pulse
  c. ring
  c. rupture
  c. scan
  c. secondary atrophy
  c. tap
  c. thinning
  c. vascular atrophy
  c. vascular occlusion
  c. vasculature
  c. vessel
  c. watershed zone
choroidea
  area c.
choroideae
  complexus basalis c.
  lamina vasculosa c.
  tapetum c.
choroidectomy
choroideremia
choroiditis
  acute diffuse serous c.
  anterior c.
  areolar central c.
  birdshot c.
  central c.
  diffuse c.
  disseminated c.
  Douvas honeycombed c.
  Doyne familial honeycombed c.

  exudative c.
  focal c.
  Förster c.
  geographic peripapillary c.
  c. guttata senilis
  histoplasmic c.
  Holthouse-Batten superficial c.
  Hutchinson-Tays central guttate c.
  Jensen juxtapapillary c.
  juxtapupillary c.
  macular c.
  metastatic c.
  multifocal c. (MFC)
  c. myopia
  nongranulomatous c.
  posterior c.
  proliferative c.
  punctate inner c.
  recurrent c.
  senescent macular exudative c.
  senile macular exudative c.
  c. serosa
  serosa c.
  serpiginous c.
  suppurative c.
  syphilitic c.
  Tay c.
  toxoplasmic c.
  traumatic c.
  unifocal helioid c.
choroidocapillaris
  lamina c.
choroidocyclitis
choroidoiritis
choroidopathy
  areolar c.
  central serous c.
  Doyne honeycombed c.
  geographic helicoid peripapillary c.
  guttate c.
  helicoid c.
  inner punctate c.
  myopic c.
  peripapillary central serous c.
  punctate inner c. (PIC)
  senile guttate c.
  serpiginous c.
  systemic lupus erythematosus c.
choroidoretinal dystrophy
choroidoretinitis
choroidosis
choroidovitreal neovascularization
Choyce
  C. intraocular lens
  C. lens-inserting forceps
  C. Mark VIII implant
  C. Mark VIII lens
Christensen punch
Christmas tree cataract

chromatic
- c. asymmetry
- c. contrast threshold
- c. dispersion
- c. induction effect
- c. lens aberration
- c. perimetry
- c. spectrum
- c. vision

chromaticity
- complementary c.

chromatism
chromatometer
chromatopsia
chromatoptometer
chromatoptometry
chromatoskiameter
chromic
- c. catgut suture
- c. collagen suture
- c. gut suture

chromodacryorrhea
chromogranin antibody
chromometer
chromophane
chromophobe adenoma
chromophore
chromoscope
chromoscopy
Chromos imager system
chromostereopsis
chronic
- c. actinic keratopathy
- c. anterior uveitis (CAU)
- c. blepharitis (CB)
- c. blepharoconjunctivitis
- c. catarrhal conjunctivitis
- c. catarrhal rhinitis
- c. cicatricial conjunctivitis
- c. cicatrizing conjunctivitis
- c. cyclitis
- c. dacryocystitis
- c. demyelinating optic neuritis
- c. endophthalmitis
- c. follicular conjunctivitis
- c. immunogenic conjunctivitis
- c. myopia
- c. narrow-angle glaucoma
- c. open-angle glaucoma (COAG)
- c. optic disk swelling
- c. optic nerve compression
- c. papilledema
- c. primary angle-closure glaucoma (C-PACG)
- c. progressive external ophthalmoplegia (CPEO)
- c. serpiginous ulcer
- c. simple glaucoma
- c. superficial keratitis

CHRPE
- congenital hypertrophy of the retinal pigment epithelium

chrysiasis
chrysoderma
Chrysosporium parvum
Chu Foldable Lens Cutter
Churg-Strauss syndrome
Chvostek sign
Chymar
- Alpha C.

chymotrypsin
CI
- complete iridectomy
- convergence insufficiency

Ciaccio gland
CIBA
- C. TearSaver punctual gauging system
- C. Vision Cleaner
- C. Vision Daily Cleanser
- C. Vision lens drops
- C. Vision Saline

CibaSoft Visitint contact lens
Cibathin lens
Cibis
- C. conjunctivitis
- C. ectropion
- C. electrode
- C. entropion
- C. liquid silicone procedure
- C. operation
- C. pemphigoid
- C. ski needle

cibisotome
cicatrices (*pl. of* cicatrix)
cicatriceum
- ectropion c.
- entropion c.

cicatricial
- c. adhesion
- c. conjunctivitis
- c. ectropion
- c. entropion
- c. mass

NOTES

cicatricial *(continued)*
   c. pemphigoid
   c. pterygium
   c. retinopathy of prematurity
   c. retrolental fibroplasia
   c. shortening
   c. strabismus
cicatrix, pl. cicatrices
   cystoid c.
   filtering c.
cicatrization
cicatrizing
   c. conjunctivitis
   c. trachoma
CICE
   combined intracapsular cataract
   extraction
CID
   cytomegalic inclusion disease
cidofovir
   c. eye drops
   c. therapy
CIF4 needle
CIGTS
   Collaborative Initial Glaucoma Treatment
   Study
Cilco
   C. argon laser
   C. Frigitronics
   C. Frigitronics laser
   C. Hoffer Laseridge
   C. Hoffer Laseridge laser
   C. krypton laser
   C. lens forceps
   C. MonoFlex multi-piece PMMA
   intraocular lens
   C. perimeter
   C. Ultrasound unit
   C. vitrector
   C. YAG laser
Cilco/Lasertek
   C. A/K laser
   C. argon laser
   C. krypton laser
Cilco-Simcoe II lens
cilia (*pl. of* cilium)
ciliare
   corpus c.
ciliares
   plicae c.
   processus c.
ciliaris
   acne c.
   anulus c.
   blepharitis c.
   corona c.
   corpus c.
   fibrae circulares musculi c.
   fibrae longitudinales musculi c.

   fibrae meridionales musculi c.
   fibrae radiales musculi c.
   gangliosus c.
   musculus c.
   orbicularis c.
   pars plana corporis c.
   pars plicata corporis c.
   plica c.
   radix oculomotoria ganglii c.
   radix sympathica ganglii c.
   striae c.
   tylosis c.
   zona c.
   zonula c.
ciliariscope
ciliarotomy
ciliary
   c. apparatus
   c. artery
   c. blepharitis
   c. block
   c. block glaucoma
   c. body
   c. body band
   c. body coloboma
   c. body inflammation
   c. body melanoma
   c. body melanoma with extrascleral
   extension
   c. canal
   c. cartilage
   c. crown
   c. disk
   c. epithelium
   c. flush
   c. fold
   c. ganglion
   c. ganglionic plexus
   c. gland
   c. hyperemia
   c. injection
   c. ligament
   c. margin
   c. margin of iris
   c. muscle
   c. nerve
   c. procedure
   c. process
   c. reflex
   c. region
   c. ring
   c. spasm
   c. staphyloma
   c. sulcus
   c. vein
   c. vessel
   c. zone
   c. zonule
ciliate

C

ciliectomy
ciliochoroidal
   c. detachment
   c. effusion
   c. melanoma
ciliodestructive surgery
cilioequatorial fiber
ciliogenesis
ciliolenticular block
cilioposterocapsular fiber
cilioretinal
   c. artery
   c. artery occlusion
   c. collateral
   c. vein
cilioscleral
ciliosis
ciliospinal
   c. center of Budge
   c. reflex
ciliotomy
ciliovitreal block
ciliovitrectomy block
cilium, pl. **cilia**
   cilia base
   cilia ectopia
   cilia follicle
   cilia forceps
   intraocular cilia
cillo
cillosis
Ciloxan Ophthalmic
CIMA*flex* 411 foldable silicone lens
CIN
   conjunctival intraepithelial neoplasia
cinching operation
cinema eye
cine-magnetic resonance imaging
Cine-Microscope
Cipro
ciprofloxacin hydrochloride
circadian heterotropia
circinata
   retinitis c.
circinate
   c. exudate
   retinal c.
   c. retinitis
   c. retinopathy
circle
   arterial c.

   Berry c.
   blur c.
   c. diffusion
   c. of dispersion
   c. dissipation
   episcleral arterial c.
   c. of greater iris
   c. of Haller
   Hovius c.
   c. of least confusion
   least diffusion c.
   c. of lesser iris
   Minsky c.
   Randot c.
   Vieth-Mueller c.
   c. of Willis
   Wort c.
   c. of Zinn
   Zinn-Haller arterial c.
circlet
   Zinn c.
Circline magnifier
circling band
circular
   c. blade
   c. ciliary muscle
   c. ciliary muscle fiber
   c. dichroism
   c. nystagmus
   c. synechia
   c. tear capsulotomy
circularvection
circulating
   c. antipericyte autoantibody
   c. immune complex
circulation
   conjunctival c.
   episcleral c.
   foveolar choroidal c.
   perilimbic c.
   retinal c.
   sludging of c.
circulus, pl. **circuli**
   c. arteriosus halleri
   c. arteriosus iridis major
   c. arteriosus iridis minor
   c. vasculosus nervi optici
   c. zinnii
circumbulbar
circumciliary flush
circumcorneal injection

NOTES

circumduction
    c. of the eye
    c. hyperphoria
circumferential vascular plexus of the limbus
circumlental space
circumocular
circumorbital
circumpapillary
    c. light reflex
    c. telangiectatic microangiopathy
circumscribed episcleritis
circumscripta
    canities c.
circus senilis
cirsoid aneurysm
cirsophthalmia
cisterna
    chiasmatic c.
cisternography
CIT
    corneal impression test
Citelli rongeur
citrate
    Reynold lead c.
CK
    conductive keratoplasty
CL
    contact lens
Cladosporium
cladribine
Claforan
CLAMP
    Contact Lens and Myopia Progression
    CLAMP Study
clamp
    Alabama-Green c.
    Backhaus c.
    Barraquer needle holder c.
    Berens muscle c.
    Berke c.
    bulldog c.
    Castroviejo lid c.
    Castroviejo needle holder c.
    chalazion c.
    cheek c.
    cross-action towel c.
    curved mosquito c.
    Desmarres lid c.
    Erhardt c.
    Gladstone-Putterman transmarginal
      rotation entropion c.
    Halsted curved mosquito c.
    Halsted straight mosquito c.
    Hartmann c.
    Jones towel c.
    Kalt needle holder c.
    King c.

    Moria-France
      dacryocystorhinostomy c.
    mosquito c.
    muscle c.
    needle holder c.
    Prince muscle c.
    Putterman levator resection c.
    Putterman-Mueller blepharoptosis c.
    Putterman ptosis c.
    recession c.
    Robin chalazion c.
    Schaedel cross-action towel c.
    Schnidt c.
    serrefine c.
    straight mosquito c.
CLARE
    contact lens-induced acute red eye
ClariFlex
    C. foldable IOL
    C. OptiEdge foldable intraocular
      lens
Clarine
Claris
    C. Cleaning and Soaking Solution
    C. Rewetting Drops
clarithromycin
Claritin
clarity
    corneal c.
    optical c.
clariVit
    c. central mag lens
    c. wide angle lens
Clark
    C. Autophoro-Optimeter
    C. capsule fragment forceps
    C. probe
    C. speculum
Clark-Verhoeff capsule forceps
classic
    c. choroidal neovascularization
    c. dendritic keratitis
    c. flower petal pattern
classical congenital esophoria
classification
    Callender cell type c.
    Duane c.
    Gass macular hole c.
    Keith-Wagener-Barker c.
    KWB c.
    Leishman c.
    MacCallan c.
    Nelson c.
    Reese-Ellsworth c.
    Retina Society c.
    Roper-Hall c.
    Scheie c.
    Shaffer anterior angle c.
    Shaffer-Weiss c.

Spaeth c.
tear secretion c.
Tessier c.
Wagener-Clay-Gipner c.

Claude
C. Bernard-Horner syndrome
C. Bernard syndrome

Claude-Lhermitte syndrome
claudin
clavulanate
Clayman
C. guide
C. intraocular lens
C. lens-holding forceps
C. lens implant forceps
C. lens-inserting forceps
C. posterior chamber lens

Clayman-Knolle irrigating lens loop
CLBF-100 blood flowmeter
CLE
clear lens extraction

clean
Non-Allergenic Clear C.

cleaner
Allergan Enzymatic C.
Barnes-Hind Gas Permeable
Daily C.
Blairex Hard Contact Lens C.
Boston Advance c.
Boston One Step Liquid
Enzymatic C.
CIBA Vision C.
ComfortCare GP Dual Action
Daily C.
Complete Weekly Enzymatic C.
enzymatic c.
enzyme c.
gas-permeable daily c.
LC-6 Daily Contact Lens C.
LC-65 Daily Contact Lens C.
Lens Plus daily c.
MiraFlow Daily C.
Opti-Free Daily C.
Opti-Free Enzymatic C.
Optimum by Lobob Daily C.
Opti-Soak Daily C.
Opti-Zyme enzymatic c.
ProConcept Contact Lens C.
ProFree/GP weekly enzymatic c.
ReNu Effervescent enzymatic c.
ReNu 1 Step Enzymatic C.
ReNu Thermal enzymatic c.

Sensitive Eyes daily c.
Sensitive Eyes Enzymatic C.
Sereine C.
Soflens enzymatic contact lens c.
Soft Mate Enzyme Plus c.
Soft Mate Hands Off daily c.
Sterile Preserved Daily C.
Ultrazyme enzymatic c.
Vision Care enzymatic c.

Cleaner/Rinse
Pure Eyes C./R.

Cleaning/Disinfecting/Storage
Optimum by Lobob Gas
Permeable C./D./S.

Clean-N-Soak
Clean-N-Stow
cleanser
CIBA Vision Daily C.
Hibiclens antiseptic/antimicrobial
skin c.
OCuSoft eyelid c.

cleanup
cortical c.

clear
All C.
c. cornea angled CVD diamond
knife
c. corneal phacoemulsification
c. corneal step incision
c. corneal tunnel incision
c. crystalline lens
deep and c. (D&C)
C. Eyes
C. Eyes ACR
C. Image III
c. keratin sleeve
Lens c.
c. lensectomy
c. lens extraction (CLE)
c. lid vesicle
Swim'n C.
C. View hydrophilic shield
c. window

clearance
apical c.

ClearCut
C. dual-bevel blade
C. dual-bevel line knife
C. SatinSlit knife

clearing
media c.

Clearpath corneal diamond knife

NOTES

C

ClearView contact lens
Cleasby
    C. iridectomy operation
    C. spatula
    C. spatulated needle
cleavage syndrome
cleaver
    Haefliger c.
CLEERE
    Collaborative Longitudinal Evaluation in
    Ethnicity and Refractive Error
    CLEERE Study
cleft
    corneal c.
    cortical c.
    cyclodialysis c.
    excessive cyclodialysis c.
    facial c.
    sonolucent c.
    c. syndrome
clefting
    cortical c.
    Tessier c.
CLEK
    Collaborative Longitudinal Evaluation of
    Keratoconus
    CLEK Study
clemastine
Clens
Clerf needle holder
clerical spectacles
Clerz
    C. 2
    C. 2 Lubricating and Rewetting
    Drops
    C. Plus lens drops
click phenomenon
climatic
    c. droplet keratopathy
    c. proteoglycan stromal keratopathy
clindamycin
clinic
    Mayo C.
clinical
    c. applications of aberrometry
    c. conference
    C. Trial of Eye Prophylaxis in the
    Newborn
clinically viable methods maximum
  optimization of visual performance
clinicopathologic finding
Clinitex
    C. Charles endophotocoagulator
    probe
    C. photocoagulator
    C. photomydriasis
clinometer
clinoscope
clioquinol

clip
    AGV pars plana c.
    Backhaus towel c.
    bipolar diathermy adapter c.
    Castroviejo scleral shortening c.
    double tantalum c.
    Duraclose scleral c.
    Federov four-loop iris c.
    Friedman tantalum c.
    Halberg trial c.
    holding c.
    Janelli c.
    lens c.
    Platina c.
    scleral shortening c.
    tantalum c.
    trial c.
    two-way towel c.
clip-applying forceps
clip-on/tie-on occluder
clivus, pl. clivi
    c. chordoma
clobetasol propionate
clock
    astigmatic c.
    c. dial
clock-mechanism esotropia
clofazimine
C-loop
    C-l. intraocular lens
    C-l. IOL
    C-l. posterior chamber lens
Cloquet canal
closed
    c. chamber
    eyelids sutured c.
    c. loop
    c. surgery on eye
closed-angle glaucoma (CAG)
closed-circuit television vision
  enhancement system (CCTV)
closed-dissection technique
closed-eye surgery
closed-funnel vitreoretinopathy
closed-loop system
closed-system pars plana vitrectomy
clostridial
    c. blepharitis
    c. panophthalmitis
Clostridium
    C. bifermentans
    C. difficile
    C. histolyticum
    C. perfringens
    C. subterminale
    C. tetani
    C. welchii
closure
    capillary c.

crow-foot c.
endovascular c.
forced-eye c.
hallucination with eye c.
insufficiency of eyelid c.
synechial c.
wound c.
clotrimazole
clouding
corneal c.
feathery c.
hyaloid c.
retinal c.
vitreous c.
cloudy cornea
clove-hitch suture
cloxacillin
CLPU
contact lens-induced peripheral ulcer
cLSO
confocal laser scanning ophthalmoscopy
clump
c. cell
vortex-like c.
clumped
c. pigmentation
c. retinal pigment
clumping
pigment c.
pigmentary rarefaction and c.
cluster
c. headache
macular c.
c. of pigmented spots
c. of retinoblastoma cells
CMAP
compound muscle action potential
CMD
cystoid macular degeneration
CME
cystoid macular edema
CMID
cytomegalic inclusion disease
CMS AccuProbe 450 system
CMV
cytomegalovirus
macular CMV
CMV retinitis
CMV retinopathy
CN
cranial nerve
CN III

third cranial nerve
CN IV
fourth cranial nerve
CN V
fifth cranial nerve
CN VI
abducens nerve
abducent nerve
sixth cranial nerve
CN VII
seventh cranial nerve
CNS
central nervous system
CNTGS
Collaborative Normal Tension Glaucoma
Study
CNV
choroidal neovascularization
CNVM
choroidal neovascular membrane
CO
Certified Orthoptist
corneal opacity
CO₂
CO_2 Sharplan laser
COAG
chronic open-angle glaucoma
coagulating electrode
coagulation
disseminated intravascular c.
endodiathermy c.
endolaser c.
light c.
Meyer-Schwickerath light c.
coagulator
argon laser c.
ASSI Polar-Mate c.
Evergreen Lasertek c.
Grieshaber micro-bipolar c.
Laserflex c.
Meyer-Schwickerath c.
Walker c.
coagulopathy
coalescent mass
coal-mining lensectomy
coaptation bipolar forceps
coarse
c. punctate staining
c. stereopsis
c. vascular pattern
COAS
Complete Ophthalmic Analysis System

NOTES

C

coastal erysipelas
coast erosion
coat
  buffy c.
  sclerotic c.
  uveal c.
coated Vicryl suture
coater
  Polaron sputter c.
coating
  antireflection c.
  color c.
  edge c.
  c. material
  mirror c.
  nondeposited tear c.
  proteinaceous c.
  RLX c.
  Single-Vision Thin & Lite 1.67
    Semi-Finished Lens with hard c.
  c. for spectacle lens
Coats
  C. disease
  C. retinitis
  C. syndrome
  C. white ring
coaxial
  c. illumination
  c. irrigation/aspiration cannula
coaxially sighted corneal reflex
cobalt
  c. blue filter
  c. blue light
  c. therapy
cobalt-60 eye plaque
cobblestone
  c. appearance
  c. conjunctivitis
  c. papilla
  c. retinal degeneration
Cobra LASIK irrigating cannula
Coburn
  C. camera
  C. intraocular lens
  C. irrigation/aspiration system
  C. irrigation/aspiration unit
  C. lensometer
  C. refractor
  C. tonometer
Coburn-Rodenstock slit lamp
cocaine
  c. block
  crack c.
  c. hydrochloride
  c. methylphenidate
  c. test
cocci (pl. of coccus)
Coccidioides immitis

coccidioidomycosis
  c. immitis
  intraocular c.
coccus, pl. cocci
  gram-positive cocci
Cochet-Bonnet esthesiometer
cochleopupillary reflex
Cochran-Mantel-Haenszel analysis
Cockayne syndrome
cocoamidopropylamine oxide
cocoamidopropyl hydroxysultaine
co-contraction syndrome
codeine
  acetaminophen with c.
Codman wet-field cautery
CoEase viscoelastic
coefficient
  c. of facility of outflow
  c. of variation
  Zernike c.
Coerens tumor
Coffin-Lowry syndrome
Cogan
  C. congenital oculomotor apraxia
  C. disease
  C. interstitial keratitis
  C. lid twitch
  C. lid-twitch sign
  C. microcystic dystrophy
  C. microcystic dystrophy of the
    corneal epithelium
  C. patch
  C. syndrome
Cogan-Boberg-Ans lens implant
Cogan-Reese syndrome
cogwheel
  c. ocular movement
  c. pupil
  c. pursuit
  c. pursuit movement
Cohan-Barraquer microscope
Cohan-Vannas iris scissors
Cohan-Westcott scissors
Cohen
  C. corneal forceps
  C. needle holder
  C. syndrome
Coherent
  C. 920 argon/dye laser
  C. 900, 920 argon laser
  C. dye laser
  C. EPIC laser
  C. krypton laser
  C. 7910 laser
  C. LaserLink slit lamp
  C. Medical YAG laser
  C. Novus Omni multiwavelength
    laser
  C. photocoagulator

C. radiation argon/krypton laser
C. radiation argon model 800 laser
C. radiation Fluorotron
C. Schwind Keraton 2 laser
C. Selecta 7000 laser

coherent light
cohort study
coil
basal c.
electromagnetic scleral search c.
scleral search c.

coin gauge
colchicine
cold-opposite, warm-same (COWS)
Coleman retractor
Coleman-Taylor IOL forceps
colforsin
coli
Escherichia c.
Colibri
C. forceps
C. microforceps
coliform
c. blepharitis
c. organism
colistin
Collaborative
C. Corneal Transplantation Studies
(CCTS)
C. Initial Glaucoma Treatment
Study (CIGTS)
C. Longitudinal Evaluation in
Ethnicity and Refractive Error
(CLEERE)
C. Longitudinal Evaluation of
Keratoconus (CLEK)
C. Longitudinal Evaluation of
Keratoconus Study
C. Normal Tension Glaucoma
Study (CNTGS)
C. Ocular Melanoma Study
(COMS)
collagen
c. alpha chain
c. bandage lens
c. cell
c. fiber
c. fibril
c. fibril interweaving
c. lamella
c. plug
c. and rheumatoid-related disease

c. shield
c. vascular disease
c. wick procedure
collagenase
bacterial c.
collagenolysis
collagenolytic trabecular ring
collagenous trabecular ring
Collamer
C. 3-piece intraocular lens
C. 3-piece IOL
collapse
chamber c.
collar button
collarette
iris c.
collar-stud chalazion
collateral
cilioretinal c.
c. pulp canal
c. vessel
colliculus
superior c.
Collier
tucked lid of C.
C. tucked lid sign
Collin-Beard operation
Collin 140 color adaptometer
Collins syndrome
colliquation
colliquative
collision tumor
collodion dressing
colloid
c. body
c. cyst
c. deposit
collyr.
eye wash
collyrium
Beer C.
C. eye drops
C. Fresh Ophthalmic
Colmascope
coloboma, pl. colobomata
c. anomaly
atypical c.
bridge c.
chorioretinal c.
choroid c.
choroidal c.
ciliary body c.

NOTES

coloboma *(continued)*
  complete c.
  congenital optic nerve c.
  dysplastic c.
  eyelid c.
  fissure c.
  Fuchs inferior c.
  Fuchs spot c.
  c. of fundus
  c., heart defects, atresia choanae,
    retarded growth, genital
    hypoplasia, and ear anomalies
    (CHARGE)
  c. iridis
  iris c.
  c. of iris
  c. of lens
  c. lentis
  c. lobuli
  macular c.
  ocular c.
  c. of optic nerve
  optic nerve c.
  c. palpebrale
  peripapillary c.
  c. of retina
  c. retinae
  retinochoroidal c.
  typical c.
  c. of vitreous
  vitreous c.
colobomatous
  c. cyst
  c. microphthalmia
  c. optic disk
color
  c. aberration
  c. adaptation
  c. adaptometer
  c. agnosia
  c. amblyopia
  c. anomia
  C. Bar Schirmer strip
  C. Bar Schirmer Tear Test
  c. blind
  c. blindness
  c. chart
  c. coating
  c. comparison
  c. comparison test
  complementary c.
  confusion c.
  c. confusion
  c. constancy
  c. contrast
  c. defect
  deviant c.
  c. discrimination
  c. disk

  c. Doppler imaging
  end-point c.
  eye c.
  c. fusion
  incidental c.
  metameric c.
  c. mixing
  Munsell c.
  c. naming
  opponent c.
  c. perception
  c. perimetry
  primary c.
  pure c.
  reflected c.
  saturated c.
  c. saturation
  c. scotoma
  C. Screening Inventory
  c. sense
  simple c.
  solid c.
  c. spectrum
  c. theory
  c. triangle
  UltraCare Disinfecting
    Solution/Neutralizer with C.
  c. vision (CV)
  c. vision test
  C. Vision Testing Made Easy test
    (CVTMET)
  c. washout
Colorado
  C. cautery
  C. needle
ColorChecker
  Macbeth C.
color-contrast
  c.-c. sensitivity measurement
  c.-c. threshold
colorimeter
colossal agenesis
column
  bulbar conjunctival blood c.
    (BCBC)
  ocular dominance c.
columnar layer
Colvard handheld infrared pupillometer
Coly-Mycin S
COMA
  congenital ocular motor apraxia
coma
  c. aberration
  eyes-open c.
  metabolic c.
Comberg
  C. contact lens
  C. foreign body operation
  C. localization

Combiline System
combination phaco chopper
combined
c. cilioretinal artery and central retinal vein occlusions
c. dystrophy of Fuchs
c. exfoliation
c. fracture
c. intracapsular cataract extraction (CICE)
c. trabeculotomy-trabeculectomy
combined-mechanism glaucoma
Combo
Chang Quick Chop C.
comedo pattern
COMET
Correction of Myopia Evaluation Trial
comet scotoma
comfort
c. bridge
C. eye drops
C. Ophthalmic
C. Tears
C. Tears Solution
ComfortCare
C. GP Dual Action Daily Cleaner
C. GP One Step
C. GP Wetting and Soaking Solution
ComfortKone lens
comitance
comitant
c. esotropia
c. exodeviation
c. exophoria
c. exotropia
c. heterotropia
c. squint
c. strabismus
c. vertical deviation
comminuted orbital fracture
commissura, pl. **commissurae**
commissurae opticae
c. palpebrarum lateralis
c. palpebrarum medialis
c. palpebrarum nasalis
c. palpebrarum temporalis
commissure
arcuate c.
c. of Gudden
interthalamic c.
Meynert c.

nucleus of posterior c.
optic c.
palpebral c.
posterior chiasmatic c.
supraoptic c.
common
c. canaliculus
c. tendinous ring
commotio retinae
communicating
c. artery aneurysm
internal carotid-posterior c. (IC-PC)
communication
arteriole c.
arteriovenous c.
communis
anulus tendineus c.
community
professional c.
community-acquired corneal ulcer
Compak-200 mini-excimer
company
American Surgical Instrument C. (ASICO)
Neitz Instruments C.
comparison
brightness c.
color c.
c. eyepiece
compass
Mastel diamond c.
compensated
c. glaucoma
c. segment
compensating eyepiece
compensation
cornea-lens c.
competition swimmer's eyelid syndrome
complement
c. component
c. fixation test
c. system
complementary
c. afterimage
c. chromaticity
c. color
complement-fixing antibody
complete
c. achromatopsia
C. Blink-N-Clean Lens Drops
c. blood count

C

NOTES

95

complete *(continued)*
    c. but pupil-sparing oculomotor
        nerve paresis
    c. coloboma
    C. Comfort Plus Multi-Purpose
        Solution
    c. congenital cataract
    c. hemianopsia
    c. iridectomy (CI)
    c. iridoplegia
    C. Lubricating and Rewetting
        Drops
    C. Ophthalmic Analysis System
        (COAS)
    c. palsy
    c. vitrectomy
    C. Weekly Enzymatic Cleaner
complex
    AIDS-related c. (ARC)
    c. astigmatism
    circulating immune c.
    c. ectropion
    Golgi c.
    immune c.
    c. laceration
    major histocompatibility c. (MHC)
    c. motion tomography
    c. retinal detachment
    triple symptom c.
    tuberous sclerosis c. (TSC)
complexus basalis choroideae
compliance cap
complicata
    cataracta c.
complicated cataract
complication
    C.'s of Age-Related Macular
        Degeneration Prevention Trial
        (CAPT)
    catastrophic   c.
    serious corneal c.
component
    amyloid P c.
    complement c.
    quick left/right c.
composite
    Multiple Sclerosis Functional C.
        (MSFC)
composition of spectacle lens
compound
    c. eye
    Hurler-Scheie c.
    c. hyperopic astigmatism
    c. lens
    c. muscle action potential (CMAP)
    c. myopic astigmatism
    c. nevus
    quaternary ammonium c.
    silver c.

    skin cancer c.
    c. spectacles
    c. vesicle
compression
    chiasmal c.
    chronic optic nerve c.
    c. cyanosis
    c. dressing
    c. gonioscopy
    limbal c.
    c. molding
    optic tract c.
    prechiasmal c.
    c. retinopathy
    c. suture
compressive
    c. nystagmus
    c. optic nerve defect
    c. optic neuropathy
compressor
    Anthony orbital c.
    Berens orbital c.
    Castroviejo c.
    orbital enucleation c.
compulsive eye opening
Compuscan-P pachymeter
computed
    C. Anatomy Corneal Modeling
        System
    c. perimetry
    c. tomographic angiography
    c. tomography (CT)
    c. tomography scan
computer
    C. Eye Drops
    c. vision syndrome (CVS)
computer-assisted
    c.-a. corneal topography (CACT)
    c.-a. videokeratography
    c.-a. videokeratoscope
computerized
    c. corneal topography
    c. corneal videokeratography
    c. photokeratoscope
    c. tomography scan
Computon Microtonometer
COMS
    Collaborative Ocular Melanoma Study
    Cooperative Ocular Melanoma Study
COMT
    Certified Ophthalmic Medical
        Technologist
Con
    Eye C. 5
concave
    c. cylinder
    double c. (DCC)
    c. mirror

c. reflecting surface
c. spectacle lens
concavity
iris c.
concavoconcave lens
concavoconvex lens
concentration
c. deficit
immunoreactive adrenomedullin c.
steroid c.
concentric
c. constriction
c. fold
c. lesion
c. sclerosis of Balo
c. stria
concentrica
encephalitis periaxialis c.
concentrically
Concentrix Fluidics
concept
C. disposable cautery
C. hand-held cautery
concha bullosa
conclination
concomitance
concomitant
c. exophoria
c. heterotropia
c. strabismus
concretion
conjunctival c.
concussion
c. blindness
c. cataract
c. injury
c. of the retina
condensation
de-misting c.
vitreoretinal c.
condensing lens
condition
conjunctival cell c.
normal viewing c.
null c.
predisposing c.
test c.
conditioning film
conductive keratoplasty (CK)
cone
c. achromatopsia
apical c.

bipolar c.
blue c.
c. b-wave amplitude
c. b-wave implicit time
electroretinogram
c. cell
c. degeneration
distraction c.
c. dysfunction
c. dystrophy
c. dystrophy-cerebellar ataxia
c. fiber
c. function
c. granule
layer of rods and c.'s
McIntyre truncated c.
c. monochromat
monochromatic c.
c. monochromatism
muscle c.
ocular c.
c. opsin
pedicle c.
c. photopigment
c. response
retinal c.
28-ring Placido c.
Rochon-Duvigneaud bouquet of c.'s
rods and c.'s
triad of retinal c.
twin c.
c. vision
visual c.
X-linked c.
cone-rod
c.-r. degeneration
c.-r. dystrophy (CRD)
conference
clinical c.
configuration
bombé c.
Kratz-Sinskey loop c.
plateau iris c.
vacuolar c.
whorl-like c.
confluent
c. defect
c. drusen
confocal
c. laser scanning microscope
c. laser scanning ophthalmoscope

C

NOTES

confocal *(continued)*
- c. laser scanning ophthalmoscopy (cLSO)
- c. laser scanning topography
- c. microscopy
- c. microscopy identification of *Acanthamoeba* keratitis
- c. optics
- c. scanning laser (CSL)
- c. scanning laser Doppler flowmetry
- c. scanning laser polarimeter
- c. scanning laser tomography

conformer
- eye implant c.
- Fox c.
- McGuire c.
- Moore-Wilson hyperopic c.
- silicone c.
- Trokel hyperopia c.
- Universal c.

ConfoScan 2.0 slit corneal confocal microscope

confrontation
- c. field defect
- full to c. (FTC)
- c. method
- c. visual field
- c. visual field test
- c. visual field testing

confusion
- circle of least c.
- color c.
- c. color
- congenital c.
- visual c.

congenita
- dyskeratosis c.
- ectopia pupillae c.
- myotonia c.
- paramyotonia c.

congenital
- c. abducens facial paralysis
- c. abducens nerve lesion
- c. abducens nerve palsy
- c. abduction paralysis
- c. abnormality
- c. absence of abduction
- c. adduction palsy with synergistic divergence
- c. adherence syndrome
- c. amaurosis
- c. anomaly
- c. anophthalmos
- c. anterior staphyloma (CAS)
- c. anterior synechia
- c. astigmatism
- c. brain malformation
- c. bulbar paralysis
- c. cataract
- c. cleft of iris
- c. confusion
- c. conus
- c. crescent
- c. dacryocele
- c. dacryocystitis
- c. dermoid of limbus
- c. dichromatism
- c. dyschromatopsia
- c. dyskeratosis
- c. dystrophic ptosis
- c. dysversion
- c. ectropion
- c. entropion
- c. esophoria
- c. esotropia
- C. Esotropia Observational Study (CEOS)
- c. facial diplegia
- c. fiber-type disproportion (CFTD)
- c. fibrosis
- c. fibrosis of the extraocular muscles (CFEOM)
- c. fibrosis syndrome
- c. glaucoma
- c. grouped pigmentation of retina
- c. hemianopsia
- c. hereditary endothelial corneal dystrophy
- c. Horner syndrome
- c. hypertrophy of the retinal pigment epithelium (CHRPE)
- c. ichthyosis
- c. III nerve lesion
- c. impatency
- c. iris heterochromia
- c. juxtafoveolar syndrome
- c. lens dislocation
- c. lens opacity
- c. leukopathia
- c. limbal corneal dermoid
- c. limbal corneal dermoid tumor
- c. macrodisc
- c. macular degeneration
- c. medullated optic nerve fiber
- c. melanosis oculi
- c. miosis
- c. muscular dystrophy
- c. mydriasis
- c. myopathic eyelid retraction
- c. myopathic ptosis
- c. myopathy
- c. myotonic dystrophy
- c. nasolacrimal duct obstruction
- c. nystagmus
- c. ocular melanocytosis
- c. ocular motor apraxia (COMA)
- c. oculodermal melanocytosis

c. oculofacial paralysis
c. oculomotor nerve palsy
c. oculopalpebral synkinesia
c. optic atrophy
c. optic disk elevation
c. optic disk pigmentation
c. optic nerve coloboma
c. optic nerve pit
c. paradoxic gustolacrimal reflex
c. prepapillary vascular loop
c. pterygium
c. retinal fold
c. retinoschisis
c. rubella syndrome
c. stationary night blindness
c. superior oblique underaction
c. syphilis
c. syphilitic conjunctivitis
c. tilted disk syndrome
c. toxoplasmosis
congenitale
poikiloderma c.
congenitum
corestenoma c.
congested vessel
congestion
c. of conjunctiva
deep c.
superficial c.
transient c.
vascular c.
venous c.
congestive
c. glaucoma
c. orbitopathy
congruent point
congruity
congruous
c. field defect
c. hemianopsia
c. homonymous hemianopic scotoma
c. homonymous horizontal sectoranopia
c. homonymous quadruple sectoranopia
coni (*pl. of* conus)
conical
c. cornea
c. implant
c. protrusion

conjugacy
object/image c.
conjugate
c. disparity
c. focus
c. gaze
c. gaze palsy
c. horizontal deviation
c. horizontal eye movement
c. movement of eyes
c. nystagmus
c. ocular movement
c. paralysis
c. point
conjugately
conjunctiva, pl. **conjunctivae**
anulus of c.
bulbar c.
chancre of c.
congestion of c.
emphysema of c.
epitheliosis desquamativa conjunctivae
c. forceps
fornical c.
fornix c.
Förster c.
glandulae mucosae conjunctivae
leptotrichosis conjunctivae
limbal c.
lithiasis conjunctivae
marginal c.
ocular c.
orbital c.
pale c.
pallor of c.
palpebral c.
plica semilunaris conjunctivae
c. retractor
saccus conjunctivae
scleral c.
sebaceous gland of c.
semilunar folds of c.
siderosis conjunctivae
c. spreader
supertemporal bulbar c.
tarsal c.
tela c.
temporal bulbar c.
tunica c.
tyloma conjunctivae
upper palpebral c.

C

NOTES

conjunctiva *(continued)*
 upper tarsal c.
 xerosis conjunctivae
conjunctiva-associated lymphoid tissue
conjunctival
 c. abrasion
 c. advancement technique
 c. amyloidosis
 c. angioma
 c. artery
 c. bleb
 c. brachium
 c. break
 c. calcification
 c. cell condition
 c. chemosis
 c. ciliary injection
 c. circulation
 c. concretion
 c. contusion
 c. crystal
 c. cul-de-sac
 c. cyst
 c. deposit
 c. dermoid
 c. discharge
 c. dysplasia
 c. edema
 c. epithelial cell
 c. exudate
 c. flap
 c. follicle
 c. foreign body
 c. gland
 c. goblet cell
 c. goblet cell density
 c. granuloma
 c. hemangioma
 c. hemorrhage
 c. hyperemia
 c. impression cytology
 c. incision
 c. intraepithelial neoplasia (CIN)
 c. laceration
 c. limbus
 c. lipodermoid
 c. lithiasis
 c. lymphangioma
 c. lymphoid proliferation
 c. lymphoid tumor
 c. melanoma
 c. melanotic lesion
 c. membrane
 c. metaplasia
 c. necrosis
 c. NITFBUT
 c. nodule
 c. papilla
 c. papilloma
 c. patch graft
 c. phlyctenule
 c. phlyctenulosis
 c. pigmented nevus
 c. pseudomembrane
 c. pterygium
 c. reaction
 c. recession
 c. reflex
 c. rhinosporidiosis
 c. ring
 c. rotation autografting
 c. sac
 c. scarring
 c. scissors
 c. scraping
 c. semilunar fold
 c. slough
 c. smear
 c. sporotrichosis
 c. squamous cell neoplasia
 c. staining
 c. tear
 c. ulcer
 c. varix
 c. vascular engorgement
 c. vascularization
 c. vein
 c. vessel
 c. xerosis
conjunctivales
 glandulae ciliares c.
 glandulae sebaceae c.
 venae anteriores c.
 venae posteriores c.
conjunctivalis
 blennorrhea conjunctivalis
 nodulus c.
 saccus c.
conjunctiva-Mueller muscle excision
conjunctiva-Tenon flap
conjunctiviplasty *(var. of* conjunctivoplasty)
conjunctivitis
 acne rosacea c.
 actinic c.
 acute atopic c.
 acute catarrhal c.
 acute congestive c.
 acute contagious c.
 acute epidemic c.
 acute follicular c.
 acute hemorrhagic c.
 adenoviral c.
 adenovirus c.
 adult inclusion c.
 allergic c.
 anaphylactic c.
 angular c.

Apollo c.
arc-flash c.
c. arida
atopic c.
atropine c.
Axenfeld follicular c.
bacterial c.
Bangla Joy c.
Béal c.
blennorrheal c.
blepharitis c.
Butcher c.
calcareous c.
candidal c.
candidiasis c.
catarrhal c.
chemical c.
chlamydial inclusion c.
chronic catarrhal c.
chronic cicatricial c.
chronic cicatrizing c.
chronic follicular c.
chronic immunogenic c.
Cibis c.
cicatricial c.
cicatrizing c.
cobblestone c.
congenital syphilitic c.
contact c.
contagious granular c.
croupous c.
diphtheritic c.
diplobacillary c.
drug-induced cicatrizing c.
eczematous c.
Egyptian c.
Elschnig c.
epidemic c.
erythema multiforme major c.
exanthematous c.
factitious c.
follicular c.
giant papillary c. (GPC)
gonococcal c.
gonorrheal c.
gout c.
granular c.
hay fever c.
hemorrhagic c.
herpes simplex c.
herpes zoster c.
herpetic c.

hyperacute c.
immunological c.
inclusion c.
infantile purulent c.
infectious c.
Koch-Weeks c.
lacrimal c.
lagophthalmia c.
larval c.
ligneous c.
limbal c.
lithiasis c.
Lymphogranuloma venereum c.
c. medicamentosa
meibomian c.
membranous c.
meningococcus c.
microbiallergic c.
molluscum c.
Morax-Axenfeld c.
mucopurulent c.
c. necroticans infectiosus
necrotic infectious c.
neisserial c.
neonatal inclusion c.
newborn c.
c. nodosa
nodular c.
nonatopic allergic c.
ocular vaccinial c.
oculoglandular c.
papillary c.
Parinaud oculoglandular c.
Pascheff c.
c. petrificans
phlegmatous c.
phlyctenular c.
pinkeye c.
pneumococcal c.
prairie c.
pseudomembranous c.
pseudovernal c.
purulent c.
Reiter c.
rubeola c.
Samoan c.
Sanyal c.
scrofulous c.
seasonal allergic c.
shipyard c.
simple acute c.
Singapore epidemic c.

NOTES

C

conjunctivitis *(continued)*
 snow c.
 spring c.
 springtime c.
 squirrel plague c.
 staphylococcal c.
 superior tarsal papillary c.
 swimming pool c.
 Thygeson chronic follicular c.
 toxic follicular c.
 toxicogenic c.
 trachoma-inclusion c. (TRIC)
 trachomatous c.
 tuberculosis c.
 tularemic c.
 c. tularensis
 unilateral c.
 uratic c.
 vernal c.
 viral c.
 Wegener granulomatosus c.
 welder's c.
 Widmark c.
 Wucherer c.
 c. xeroderma pigmentosum
conjunctivochalasis
conjunctivodacryocystorhinostomy (CDCR)
conjunctivodacryocystostomy
conjunctivoma
conjunctivoplasty, conjunctiviplasty
conjunctivorhinostomy
conjunctivotarsal
conjunctivum
 brachium c.
Con-Lish polishing method
connection
 Luer c.
 synaptic c.
connective
 c. tissue
 c. tissue membrane
connector
 McIntyre nylon cannula c.
Connor
 C. angled wand
 C. capsulorrhexis peeler forceps
 C. curved wand
 C. straight irrigating wand
 C. straight nonirrigating wand
Conn syndrome
conoid
 c. lens
 c. of Sturm
conomyoidin
conophthalmus
conotruncal anomalies face syndrome
Conradi syndrome

Conrad orbital blowout fracture operation
consecutive
 c. anophthalmia
 c. esotropia
 c. exotropia
 c. optic atrophy
consensual
 c. light reflex
 c. light response
 c. pupillary reflex
 c. pupillary response
 c. reaction
Consept
 Soft Mate C.
considerable blurring
constancy
 color c.
constant
 c. esotropia
 c. exophoria
 c. exotropia
 c. hypertropia
 c. hypotropia
 c. monocular tropia
 c. nystagmus
 c. strabismus
constricted pupil
constriction
 concentric c.
 focal c.
constructional
 c. ability contact lens
 c. apraxia
consummatum
 glaucoma c.
ContaClair multi-purpose contact lens solution
contact
 c. angle
 arc of c.
 c. A-scan
 c. bandage lens
 c. blepharitis
 c. B-scan
 c. B-scan ultrasonography
 c. burns of globe
 c. conjunctivitis
 c. dermatoconjunctivitis
 eye c.
 c. glasses
 haptic c.
 c. illumination
 iridociliary process c.
 iridolenticular c.
 iridozonular c.
 c. lens (CL)
 c. lens biomicroscopy
 c. lens blank

c. lens chord diameter
c. lens curve
c. lens height
c. lens-induced acute red eye (CLARE)
c. lens-induced keratopathy
c. lens-induced peripheral ulcer (CLPU)
c. lens-induced warpage
C. Lens and Myopia Progression (CLAMP)
C. Lens and Myopia Progression Study
c. lens overwearing syndrome
c. lens overwear syndrome
c. lens-related microbial keratitis
c. lens thickness
c. lens training mirror
c. lens vertex power
c. low-vacuum lens
c. method
contact lens (CL) (*See also* lens)
AIRLens c. l.
anular bifocal c. l.
aphakic c. l.
aspheric c. l.
cellulose acetate butyrate c. l.
contour c. l.
decentration of c. l.
disposable c. l.
double slab-off c. l.
Dyer nomogram system of ordering c. l.
extended wear c. l. (EWCL)
finished c. l.
flexible-wear c. l.
fluorocarbon in c. l.
gas-permeable c. l. (GPCL)
Korb c. l.
lenticular c. l.
lenticular-cut c. l.
loose c. l.
microthin c. l.
minus carrier c. l.
polymethylmethacrylate c. l.
prism ballast c. l.
prolonged-wear c. l.
rigid gas-permeable c. l.
scratched c. l.
semifinished c. l.
silicone acrylate c. l.
single-cut c. l.

Soper cone c. l.
steep c. l.
thickness of c. l.
tight c. l.
toric c. l.
toroidal c. l.
wetting angle of c. l.
X chrom c. l.
zone of c. l.
contactologist
contactology
contactoscope
contagiosa
impetigo c.
contagiosum
ecthyma c.
keratitis molluscum c.
molluscum c.
contagious granular conjunctivitis
contaminant
wind-blown c.
contamination
bacterial c.
contemporary nearpoint chart
content
orbital c.
water c.
contiguous
c. fibers
c. pattern
Contino
C. epithelioma
C. glaucoma
continuous
c. circular capsulorrhexis
c. curvilinear capsulorrhexis (CCC)
c. fiber
c. laser
continuous-wave
c.-w. argon laser
c.-w. diode laser
Contique contact lens case
contour
c. contact lens
corneal c.
edge c.
eyelid c.
c. interaction
scalloped c.
c. stereo test
Contoured Ablation Pattern (CAP)

C

NOTES

contracted socket
contraction (C)
    anisocoria c.
    c. of cyclitic membrane
    c. and liquefaction
    c. of pupil
    pupillary sphincter c.
    vermiform c.
    vitreous c.
contracture
    socket c.
    spastic paretic facial c.
contraindication
contralateral
    c. antagonist
    c. disc change
    c. eye
contrapulsion
    saccadic c.
contrast
    color c.
    c. discrimination
    gallium citrate c.
    long-scale c.
    low c.
    c. material
    c. medium
    c. sensitivity
    c. sensitivity reduction
    c. sensitivity test (CST)
    short-scale c.
    simultaneous color c.
    successive c.
    c. threshold for motion perception
    (CTMP)
    c. visualization
contrecoup injury
control
    Integrated Light C. (ILC)
    supranuclear c.
Controlled High Risk Subjects Avonex Multiple Sclerosis Prevention Study (CHAMPS)
controller
    Siepser endocapsular c.
    viscous fluid c. (VFC)
contusion
    c. angle glaucoma
    c. cataract
    c. of choroid
    conjunctival c.
    corneal c.
    c. of eye
    c. of globe
    c. of orbit
    vitreoretinal c.
conular
conus, pl. **coni**
    congenital c.

distraction c.
inferior c.
lateral oblique c.
myopic c.
c. of optic disk
c. shell-type eye implant
supertraction c.
c. supertraction
underlying c.
conventional
    c. outflow
    c. shell implant
converge
convergence
    c. accommodation (CA/C)
    c. accommodation ratio
    accommodative c. (AC)
    c. amplitude
    c. angle
    c. excess
    c. excess esotropia
    far point of c.
    fusional c.
    c. insufficiency (CI)
    c. insufficiency exotropia
    near point of c. (NPC)
    negative c.
    c. paralysis
    c. point
    point of basal c. (PBC, PcB)
    c. position
    positive c.
    proximal c.
    punctum proximum of c. (PP)
    range of c.
    relative c.
    c. retraction
    c. retraction nystagmus
    c. spasm
    tonic c.
    unit of ocular c.
    voluntary c.
convergence-accommodative micropsia
convergence-evoked nystagmus
convergence-retractory nystagmus
convergency
    c. reflex
    voluntary c.
convergent
    c. beam
    c. deviation
    c. exercise
    c. lens
    c. light
    c. misalignment
    c. ray
    c. squint
    c. strabismus
    c. wavefront

convergent-divergent pendular oscillation
converging
    c. meniscus
    c. meniscus lens
    c. ray
convergiometer
converse
    c. bobbing
    C. double-ended alar retractor
convex
    double c. (DCx)
    high c.
    low c.
    c. mirror
    c. plano lens
    c. reflecting surface
    c. spectacle lens
convexity
convexoconcave lens
convexoconvex lens
convolution product
Conway lid retractor
Cook speculum
Cool Touch laser
Cooper
    C. aspirator
    C. blade fragment
    C. Clear DW contact lens
    C. I&A unit
    C. implant
    C. irrigating/aspirating unit
    C. 2000, 2500 laser
    C. Laser Sonics laser
    C. operation
    C. Toric contact lens
Cooperative Ocular Melanoma Study (COMS)
CooperVision
    C. argon laser
    C. balanced salt solution
    C. camera
    C. Diagnostic Imaging refractor
    C. Fragmatome
    C. I/A machine
    C. imaging perimeter
    C. irrigating/aspirating unit
    C. irrigating needle
    C. irrigation/aspiration unit
    C. microscope
    C. ocutome
    C. PMMA-ACL Flex lens

    C. refractive surgery
      photokeratoscope
    C. spatulated needle
    C. ultrasonography
    C. ultrasound
    C. vitrector
    C. YAG laser
Copaxone
Copeland
    C. implant
    C. radial panchamber intraocular lens
    C. radial panchamber UV lens
    C. retinoscopy
    C. streak retinoscope
Cophene-B
copiopia
copper
    c. cataract
    c. deposition
    c. foreign body
    c. wiring
copper-wire
    c.-w. arteriole
    c.-w. artery
    c.-w. effect
    c.-w. reflex
Coppock cataract
coquille plano lens
COR
    cervicoocular reflex
Coracin
coralliform cataract
Corbett spud
Corboy
    C. hemostat
    C. needle holder
Cordarone
cordless monocular indirect ophthalmoscope
cords of Schwann
core
    nerve c.
    c. vitrectomy
    c. vitreous
corecleisis, coreclisis
corectasia, corectasis
corectome
corectomedialysis
corectomy
corectopia
    midbrain c.

C

NOTES

coredialysis
corediastasis
corelysis
coremorphosis
corenclisis
coreometer
coreometry
coreoplasty
corepexy
corepraxy
corestenoma congenitum
coretomedialysis
coretomy
corkscrew
    c. artery
    c. visual field defect
cornea, gen. **corneae**
    c. abrader
    abrasio corneae
    abrasion of c.
    abscessus siccus corneae
    alkali burn of c.
    AlphaCor hydrogel synthetic c.
    c. anesthesia
    anterior epithelium corneae
    apical zone of c.
    arcus lipoides corneae
    artificial c.
    aspheric c.
    axial c.
    black c.
    bleb disorder of the c.
    blood staining of c.
    Bonzel blood staining of c.
    Burr c.
    butterfly pattern steepening of
      the c.
    calcareous degeneration of c.
    caligo corneae
    central edema of c.
    c. chalcosis
    c. chisel
    cloudy c.
    conical c.
    degeneration of c.
    deturgescence of c.
    diameter of c.
    donor c.
    C. Donor Study (CDS)
    dystrophia adiposa corneae
    dystrophia endothelialis corneae
    dystrophia epithelialis corneae
    dystrophy of c.
    ectatic c.
    edema of c.
    endothelial cell surface of c.
    epithelium anterius corneae
    epithelium posterius corneae
    facies anterior corneae

facies posterior corneae
c. farinata
fistula of c.
flat c.
floury c.
c. globosa
c. guttata
c. guttate lesion
herpes corneae
ichthyosis c.
indolent ulceration of the c.
inferior c.
infiltrate in c.
keratoconus c.
keratoglobus c.
lamina limitans anterior corneae
lamina limitans posterior corneae
lash abrasion of c.
lattice dystrophy of c.
lead incrustation of c.
leukoma corneae
ligamentum circulare corneae
limbus of c.
lipoidosis corneae
liquor corneae
macula corneae
marginal degeneration of c.
marginal ring ulcer of c.
meridian of c.
metaherpetic ulceration of the c.
natural c.
c. opaca
opalescent c.
oval c.
c. pachymetry
phthisis c.
pigmented line of c.
c. plana
c. plana congenita familiares
posterior conical c.
posterior epithelium of c.
recurrent erosion of c.
ring ulcer of c.
rust ring of c.
c. sensitivity
serpent ulcer of c.
spherical c.
substantia propria corneae
sugar-loaf c.
superficial line of c.
superior c.
transparent ulcer of the c.
transplantation of c.
trepanation of c.
trophic ulceration of the c.
ulceration of c.
ulcus serpens corneae
underlying c.
c. urica

c. verticillata
c. vesicle
Vogt c.
white ring of c.
xerosis of c.
cornea-holding forceps
corneal
  c. ablation plumes
  c. abrasion (CA)
  c. abscess
  c. abscission
  c. alkali burn
  c. apex
  c. arcus
  c. astigmatism
  c. bedewing
  c. biopsy
  c. birefringence
  c. block
  c. button
  c. cap
  c. cell
  c. clarity
  c. cleft
  c. clouding
  c. conjunctival intraepithelial neoplasia
  c. contact lens
  c. contact lens electrode
  c. contour
  c. contusion
  c. corpuscle
  c. crystal
  c. curette
  c. curvature (K)
  c. cylinder
  c. cyst
  c. débrider
  c. decompensation
  c. deep opacity
  c. dehydration
  c. dellen
  c. dendrite
  c. denervation
  c. deposit
  c. desiccation
  c. deturgescence
  c. diameter
  c. distortion
  c. dysgenesis
  c. dysplasia

  c. dystrophy of Waardenburg-Jonkers
  c. ectasia
  c. edema
  c. endothelial guttate dystrophy
  c. endothelial pigmentary dispersion
  c. endothelial touch
  c. endothelium
  c. enlargement
  c. epithelial barrier function
  c. epithelial scrape
  c. epithelial scraping
  c. epithelium
  c. erosion
  c. erysiphake
  c. facet
  c. fascia lata spatula
  c. filament
  c. fissure
  c. fistula
  c. fixation forceps
  c. fleck dystrophy
  c. foreign body bur
  c. furrow degeneration
  c. graft
  c. graft operation
  c. graft spatula
  c. graft step
  c. guttata
  c. guttate dystrophy
  c. guttering
  c. haze
  c. hook
  c. hydrops
  c. hypoesthesia
  c. implant
  c. impression test (CIT)
  c. incision
  c. inferior limbus
  c. inlay
  c. intercept
  c. iron line
  c. iron ring
  c. irregularity
  c. keratitis
  c. knife
  c. knife dissector
  c. laceration
  c. lamella
  c. lamellar groove
  c. lathing
  c. leakage

NOTES

corneal *(continued)*
    c. lens aberration
    c. leukoma
    c. light reflex
    c. light shield
    c. luster
    c. map
    c. marginal furrow
    c. melt
    c. melting
    c. meridian
    c. microscope
    C. Modeling System
    c. mushroom
    c. nebula
    c. needle
    c. neovascularization
    c. nerve
    c. nerve inflammation
    c. opacification
    c. opacity (CO)
    c. optical density
    c. pachometer
    c. pachymeter
    c. pachymetry
    c. pannus
    c. paracentesis track
    c. pellucid
    c. perforation
    c. phlyctenule
    c. phlyctenulosis
    c. pocket
    c. polarization axis (CPA)
    c. prosthesis forceps
    c. prosthesis trephine
    c. protrusion
    c. punch
    c. punctate infiltrate
    c. punctate lesion
    c. reflection
    c. reflection pupillometer (CRP)
    c. scar
    c. scarring
    c. section spatulated scissors
    c. sensation
    c. sensitivity
    C. Shaper microkeratome
    c. splinter forceps
    c. spot
    c. staining test
    c. staphyloma
    c. steepening
    c. storage medium
    c. stria
    c. stroma
    c. stromal bed
    c. stromal blood staining
    c. stromal disease
    c. stromal dystrophy

    c. stromal remodeling
    c. substance
    c. superinfection
    c. surgery
    c. swelling
    c. tattooing
    c. thinning
    c. topographic analysis
    c. topography
    c. topography system (CTS)
    c. transparency
    c. transplant
    c. transplantation
    c. transplant centering ring
    c. transplant marker
    c. trauma
    c. trepanation
    c. tube
    c. ulcer
    c. vascularization
    c. velum
    c. verticillata
    c. vesicle
    c. vortex dystrophy
    c. warpage
    c. xerosis
cornea-lens
    c.-l. compensation
    preexisting well-balanced c.-l.
cornealis
    arcus c.
    rima c.
Corneascope nine-ring photokeratoscope
CorneaSparing LTK system
corneitis
Cornelia de Lange syndrome
corneoblepharon
corneodysgenesis
Corneo-Gage PachKnife
corneoiritis
corneolenticular
corneolimbal ring graft
corneomandibular reflex
corneomental reflex
corneopterygoid reflex
corneosclera
corneoscleral
    c. border
    c. button
    c. forceps
    c. groove
    c. incision
    c. junction
    c. laceration
    c. lamella
    c. limbus
    c. melt
    c. punch
    c. right/left hand scissors

c. rim
c. spur
c. sulcus
c. trabeculum
corneoscleralis
pars c.
corners method
corneum
Nosema c.
cornpicker's pupil
corona
c. ciliaris
c. radiata
Zinn c.
coronal
c. CT scan
c. view
coronaria
cataracta c.
coronary cataract
coroparelcysis
coroplasty
coroscopy
Cor-Oticin
corotomy
corpus
c. adiposum orbitae
c. callosum
c. callosum lesion
c. ciliare
c. ciliaris
c. vitreum
corpuscle
corneal c.
hyaloid c.
Leber c.
Toynbee c.
Virchow c.
corrected
c. pattern standard deviation
(CPSD)
c. spectacle lens
c. visual acuity (Va$_{cc}$)
correction
aphakic c.
astigmatism c.
best ophthalmic c.
Byron Smith lazy T c.
dioptric c.
distance c.
epicanthal c.
c. of hyperopia

multistage c.
C. of Myopia Evaluation Trial
(COMET)
optical c.
spectacle c.
with c. (cc)
without c. (s̄c)
Yates c.
corrective movement
correspondence
abnormal harmonious retinal c.
abnormal unharmonious retinal c.
anomalous retinal c. (ARC)
dysharmonious c.
harmonious abnormal retinal c.
Hering law of motor c.
normal retinal c. (NRC)
c. point
retinal c.
sensory c.
corresponding retinal point
corridor incision
corrodens
Eikenella c.
corrugans
fibrosis choroideae c.
corrugated retinal detachment
corrugator muscle
Cort-Dome
Cortef
Delta C.
cortex, pl. cortices
aspiration of c.
brain c.
calcarine c.
cerebellar c.
cerebral c.
c. lentis
occipital c.
peristriate visual c.
primary visual c.
residual c.
striate visual c.
vestibular c.
visual c.
cortical
c. change
c. cleanup
c. cleaving hydrodissection
c. cleaving hydrodissector
c. cleaving hydrodissector cannula
c. cleft

C

NOTES

cortical *(continued)*
    c. clefting
    c. oculomotor area
    c. opacification
    c. opacity
    c. psychic blindness
    c. ptosis
    c. spokes cataract
    c. stripping
    c. substance of lens
    c. vacuole
    c. visual impairment
    c. visual insufficiency
    c. vitreous
corticolysis
corticonuclear fiber
corticooculocephalogyric area
corticopupillary reflex
corticosteroid
    c. drops
    ophthalmic c.
    c. therapy
    c. treatment
corticosteroid-induced
    c.-i. cataract
    c.-i. glaucoma
corticotropin
Cortimycin
cortisol
cortisone acetate
Cortisporin
    C. Ophthalmic Ointment
    C. Ophthalmic Suspension
Cortone Acetate
coruscation
Corydon
    C. expression cannula
    C. hydroexpression cannula
corymbifera
    Absidia c.
Corynebacterium
    C. diphtheriae
    C. keratitis
    C. pseudodiphtheriticum
    C. xerosis
cosegregation
Cosmegen
cosmesis
cosmetic
    c. contact shell implant
    c. defect
    c. iris
    c. shell contact lens
Cosmetica hand-painted contact lens
Cosopt ophthalmic solution
Costa Del Mar MP2 sunglasses
Costenbader incision spreader
cost-ineffective current screening
    technique

Coston-Trent iris retractor
COT
    Certified Ophthalmic Technologist
cotransmission of disease
cotton
    C. effect
    c. thread tear test
cottonoid
cotton-tipped applicator
cotton-wool
    c.-w. exudate
    c.-w. patch
    c.-w. spot (CWS)
couching needle
cough headache
count
    complete blood c.
    endothelial cell c.
    finger c.
    Kestenbaum capillary c.
counterpressor
    Amenabar c.
    angled c.
    Gill c.
counter rolling
countertorsion
    static c.
counting
    c. fingers (CF)
    c. fingers vision
coup injury
coupling
    c. of aberration
    c. agent
    c. of progressive power lens
course
    arcuate c.
    extramedullary c.
cover
    Expo Bubble eye c.
    Eye-Pak II c.
    prism and c. (P&C)
    c. test
cover-uncover test
Cowdry type A intranuclear inclusion
Cowen sign
cowhitch knot
cow horn-related ocular injury
COWS
    cold-opposite, warm-same
Cox
    C. II ocular laser shield
    C. rapid dry heat transfer sterilizer
Coxiella burnetii
Cozean-McPherson tying forceps
CPA
    cerebellopontine angle
    corneal polarization axis
    CPA lesion

C-PACG
  chronic primary angle-closure glaucoma
CPC
  central posterior curve
CPD
  chorioretinopathy and pituitary
  dysfunction
    CPD syndrome
CPEO
  chronic progressive external
  ophthalmoplegia
CPOA
  Certified Paraoptometric Assistant
CPOT
  Certified Paraoptometric Technician
CPSD
  corrected pattern standard deviation
CR
  cycloplegic refraction
    CR IV
C/R
  chorioretinal
CR-39 lens
Cr6-45NMf retinal camera
CRA
  central retinal artery
crack
    c. cocaine
    lacquer c.
crack-and-flip phacoemulsification
  technique
cracked windshield stromal lesion
cracker
    Dodick nucleus c.
    Ernest nucleus c.
    Newsom side port nucleus c.
    nucleus c.
cranial
    c. arteritis
    c. foramen
    c. nerve (CN)
    c. nerve palsy
    c. nerve testing
    c. stenosis syndrome
craniectomy
    suboccipital c.
craniocervical junction
craniofacial
    c. anomaly
    c. fibro-osseous tumor
    c. syndrome
cranioorbital surgery

craniopharyngioma
craniostenosis, pl. **craniostenoses**
craniosynostosis
craniotabes
craniotomy
    frontal c.
CRAO
  central retinal artery occlusion
crapulosa
  amblyopia c.
crassus
  pannus c.
crater depression
Crawford
    C. fascia
    C. fascial stripper
    C. forceps
    C. hook
    C. lacrimal intubation set
    C. method
    C. needle
    C. sling operation
    C. technique
    C. tube
crazing
CRD
  cone-rod dystrophy
cream
    Drysol c.
crease
    eyelid c.
    lid c.
    superior eyelid c.
Credé
    C. method
    C. prophylaxis
crepe bandage dressing
crescent
    c. blade
    c. choroid
    congenital c.
    c. corneal graft
    c. CVD diamond knife
    homonymous c.
    monocular temporal c.
    c. myopia
    myopic c.
    c. operation
    scleral c.
    c. scleral tunneler
    temporal c.
    c. tonofilm

C

NOTES

crescentic circumpapillary light reflex
CREST
    calcinosis cutis, Raynaud phenomenon,
    esophageal motility disorder,
    sclerodactyly, and telangiectasia
    CREST syndrome
crest
    lacrimal anterior c.
    lacrimal posterior c.
    neural c.
    orbital c.
cretinism
Creutzfeldt-Jakob disease
cribra
    c. orbitalia
    c. orbitalis of Welcker
cribriform
    c. field
    c. ligament
    c. spot
cribrosa
    area c.
    lamina c.
    scleral lamina c.
cri du chat syndrome
Crigler massage
Crile needle holder
crinkled cellophane
crisis, pl. **crises**
    glaucomatocyclitic c.
    myasthenic c.
    ocular c.
    oculogyric c.
    Pel c.
    Pel-Ebstein c.
cristallinus
    humor c.
Critchett operation
criterion, pl. **criteria**
    Dandy criteria
    Modified Dandy Criteria
    c. shift
criterion-free measurement
critical
    c. angle
    c. corresponding frequency (CCF)
    c. flicker frequency (CFF)
    c. flicker fusion (CFF)
    c. flicker fusion frequency
    c. flicker fusion test
    c. illumination
CRNO
    Certified Registered Nurse in
    Ophthalmology
Crock encircling operation
crocodile
    c. lens
    c. shagreen
    c. tears

crofilcon A
Crolom Ophthalmic Solution
cromoglycate
    sodium c.
cromolyn
    c. sodium
    c. sodium ophthalmic solution
Cronassial
Crookes
    C. glass
    C. lens
cross
    c. cover test
    c. cylinder
    c. fixation
    Lancaster C.
    optical c.
    C. retinoscopy
cross-action
    c.-a. capsule forceps
    c.-a. towel clamp
**cross-cylinder technique for correction
    of mixed astigmatism**
crossed
    c. amblyopia
    c. binasal quadrantanopia
    c. bitemporal quadrantanopia
    c. cylinder
    c. diplopia
    c. eyes
    c. fixation
    c. hemianopsia
    c. lens
    c. parallax
    c. reflex
cross-eyed
cross-fixation
crossing
    arteriolovenous c.
    A-V c.
    c. change
**crosslinked poly (HEMA) glaucoma
    filtration device**
cross-polarization photography
cross-Polaroid projection chart
cross-vector A-scan
croupous
    c. conjunctivitis
    c. rhinitis
Crouzon
    C. disease
    C. syndrome
crowding phenomenon
crow-foot closure
crown
    ciliary c.
    c. glass
    c. glass lens
    spectacle c.

CRP
  corneal reflection pupillometer
CRRT
  Cytomegalovirus Retinitis Retreatment
    Trial
CRS
  Cambridge Research Systems
  CRS Color Vision Test
cruciata
  amblyopia c.
crusher
  Lieberman phaco c.
crusting
  eyelid c.
  lid c.
crutch glasses
CRV
  central retinal vein
CRVO
  central retinal vein occlusion
  CRVO knife
  52.20 CRVO knife
  nonischemic CRVO
CRVRS
  Cytomegalovirus Retinitis and Viral
    Resistance Study
cryoablation
cryoapplication
Cryo-Barrages vitreous implant
cryocoagulation
cryoenucleator
  Gallie c.
cryoextraction
  open-sky c.
  c. operation
cryoextractor
  Alcon c.
  Amoils c.
  Beaver cataract c.
  Bellows c.
  Keeler c.
  Kelman c.
  Rubinstein c.
  Thomas c.
cryolathe
  Barraquer c.
cryopencil
  Amoils c.
  Mira endovitreal c.
cryopexy
  double freeze-thaw c.
  c. probe

retinal c.
transconjunctival c.
transscleral c.
cryophake
  Alcon c.
  Amoils c.
  Bellows c.
  Keeler c.
  Kelman c.
  Rubinstein c.
cryopreservation
cryoprobe
  Amoils c.
  cryoptor c.
  Rubinstein c.
  Thomas c.
cryoptor
  c. cryoprobe
  Thomas c.
cryoretinopexy
cryoretractor
  Thomas c.
CRYO-ROP
  Cryotherapy for Retinopathy of
    Prematurity
  CRYO-ROP Cooperative Group
CryoSeal FS System
cryostat
cryostylet, cryostylette
  C. 2000
cryosurgery
cryosurgical unit
Cryosystem
  Keeler-Amoils Ophthalmic C.
cryotherapy
  double freeze-thaw c.
  freeze-thaw c.
  c. operation
  c. probe
  retinal c.
  C. for Retinopathy of Prematurity
    (CRYO-ROP)
  C. for Retinopathy of Prematurity
    Cooperative Group
  transscleral c.
crypt
  Fuchs c.
  iris c.
cryptochrome
cryptococcal meningitis
cryptococcosis

C

NOTES

113

Cryptococcus
- *C. laurentii*
- *C. laurentii* keratitis
- *C. neoformans*

cryptoglioma

cryptophthalmus, cryptophthalmia, cryptophthalmos

crystal
- c. clear vision
- conjunctival c.
- corneal c.
- cystine c.
- refractile c.
- retinal c.

CrystaLens model AT-45 implant

crystallin
- alpha c.
- beta c.
- gamma c.

crystallina
- lens c.

crystalline
- c. capsule
- c. cataract
- c. corneal dystrophy
- c. deposit
- c. humor
- c. infiltrate
- c. keratopathy
- c. lens
- c. lens aberration
- c. lens equator
- c. opacity
- c. retinopathy

crystallitis

crystallizable
- fragment c. (Fc)

Csapody orbital repair operation

CSC
- central serous chorioretinopathy

C-Scan
- C-S. color-ellipsoid topometer
- C-S. corneal topography system
- TechnoMed C-S.

CSCR
- central serous chorioretinopathy

CSF
- cerebrospinal fluid

CSI Toric contact lens

CSL
- confocal scanning laser
  - CSL tomography

CSM
- central, steady and maintained
  - CSM fixation

CSR
- central serous retinopathy

CST
- contrast sensitivity test

CT
- computed tomography
  - CT 200 corneal topographer
  - CT scan of orbit

CTM
- Carlo Traverso maneuver

CTMP
- contrast threshold for motion perception

CTS
- corneal topography system

Cuban epidemic optic neuropathy

cube
- tumbling E c.

cuboidal

cuff
- fibrous tissue c.
- Honan c.
- opacified c.
- subretinal fluid c.
- Watzke c.

Cuignet
- C. method
- C. test

cul-de-sac
- conjunctival c.-d.-s.
- glaucomatous c.-d.-s.
- c.-d.-s. irrigating vectis
- c.-d.-s. irrigation T-tube
- c.-d.-s. irrigator
- ocular c.-d.-s.
- ophthalmic c.-d.-s.
- optic c.-d.-s.

Culler
- C. fixation forceps
- C. iris spatula
- C. lens spoon
- C. muscle hook
- C. speculum

culture
- bacterial c.
- c. medium
- organ c.
- vitreous c.

culturette
- Mini-tip c.

Cummings folding forceps

cuneate-shaped scotoma

cuneiform cataract

cup
- AoSept Lens Holder and C.
- bleb c.
- flat c.
- c. forceps
- Galin bleb c.
- glaucomatous c.
- large physiologic c.
- ocular c.
- ophthalmic c.
- optic c.

perilimbal suction c.
physiologic c.
slit-lamp c.
cup-disk ratio
cupped disk
Cupper-Faden operation
Cüppers
    C. method of pleoptics
    C. Visuscope
cupping
    glaucomatous c.
    optic disk c.
    c. of optic disk
    c. of optic nerve
    optic nerve c.
    pathologic c.
cup-to-disk ratio (C/D, CDR)
cupuliform cataract
cupulolithiasis
curb tenotomy
Curdy
    C. blade
    C. sclerotome
Curdy-Hebra blade
curette, curet
    Alvis c.
    chalazion c.
    corneal c.
    Fink c.
    Gifford corneal c.
    Gills-Welsh c.
    Green c.
    Heath chalazion c.
    Hebra c.
    Heyner c.
    Kraff capsule polisher c.
    Meyhoeffer chalazion c.
    Skeele c.
    Spratt mastoid c.
    Visitec capsule polisher c.
curlback shell implant
curling of capsule
curl temple
Curran knife needle
curvature
    c. aberration
    c. ametropia
    anterior corneal c.
    corneal c. (K)
    c. hyperopia
    c. of lens
    c. myopia

posterior corneal c.
radius of c.
curve
    anterior central c. (ACC)
    anterior peripheral c.
    base c. (BC)
    bell-shaped c.
    biphasic c.
    central anterior c. (CAC)
    central posterior c. (CPC)
    contact lens c.
    intermediate posterior c. (IPC)
    luminosity c.
    posterior central c.
    posterior intermediate c.
    posterior peripheral c. (PPC)
    c. response
    c. of spectacle lens
    Steiger c.
    Stromberg c.
    visibility c.
    c. width
curved
    c. iris forceps
    c. iris scissors
    c. mosquito clamp
    c. needle eye spud
    c. reflecting surface
    c. retinal probe
    c. scleral-limbal incision of Flieringa
    c. tenotomy scissors
    c. tying forceps
curved-top bifocal
Curvularia lunata
cushingoid appearance
Cushing syndrome
Cusick
    C. goniotomy knife
    C. operation
Cusick-Sarrail ptosis operation
Custodis
    C. nondraining procedure
    C. operation
    C. scleral buckling
    C. sponge
    C. suture
cut
    field c.
    sector c.
cutaneomucouveal syndrome

NOTES

cutaneous
  c. horn
  c. melanoma
  c. myiasis
  c. pupillary reflex
  c. tissue
cutdown incision
Cuterebra ophthalmomyiasis
cuticular
  c. layer
  c. stitch
Cutler
  C. implant
  C. lens spoon
  C. operation
Cutler-Beard
  C.-B. bridge flap
  C.-B. operation
cutter
  Alcon Accurus vitrectomy c.
  bone c.
  Buettner-Parel vitreous c.
  Chu Foldable Lens C.
  Douvas vitreous c.
  guillotine-type c.
  infusion suction cutter vitreous c.
  Katena soft IOL c.
  Kloti vitreous c.
  Koo foldable IOL c.
  Lightning high speed c.
  Machemer vitreous c.
  Maguire-Harvey vitreous c.
  Millennium vitreous c.
  O'Malley-Heintz vitreous c.
  Parel-Crock vitreous c.
  Premiere vitreous c.
  rotating-type c.
  soft IOL c.
  Tolentino vitreous c.
  Utrata foldable lens c.
  vitreoretinal infusion c.
  vitreous infusion suction c. (VISC)
cutting bur
CV
  color vision
CV232 square-round-edge IOL
CVD
  chemical vapor deposition
    CVD black diamond keratome line
    CVD diamond knife
CVF
  central visual field
CVOS
  Central Vein Occlusion Study
CVS
  computer vision syndrome
CVTMET
  Color Vision Testing Made Easy test

CWS
  cotton-wool spot
cyanoacrylate
  butyl c.
  ethyl c.
  c. retinopexy
  c. tissue adhesive
  c. tissue adhesive augmented tenoplasty
  c. tissue glue
cyanographic contrast material
cyanolabe
cyan opacification
cyanopsia, cyanopia
  c. retinae
cyanopsin
cyanosis
  c. bulbi
  compression c.
  c. retinae
cycle
  visual c.
cyclectomy
cyclic
  c. adenosine monophosphate (cAMP)
  c. esotropia
  c. guanidine monophosphate
  c. guanosine monophosphate (cGMP)
  c. ocular motor spasm
  c. oculomotor paresis
  c. strabismus
cyclicotomy
cyclitic membrane
cyclitis
  chronic c.
  Fuchs heterochromic c. (FHC)
  heterochromic Fuchs c.
  c. in pars planitis
  plastic c.
  pure c.
  purulent c.
  serous c.
cycloceratitis
cyclochoroiditis
cyclocoagulation
cyclocongestive glaucoma
cyclocryopexy
cyclocryotherapy
  YAG c.
cyclodamia
cyclodestruction
cyclodestructive procedure
cyclodeviation
cyclodextrin
cyclodialysis
  Allen c.
  c. cannula

c. cleft
Heine c.
c. spatula
cyclodiathermy
Castroviejo-Scheie c.
c. electrode
c. operation
cyclodiplopia
cycloduction
cycloelectrolysis
cyclofilcon A
cyclofusion
cyclogram
Cyclogyl
cyclohexylpiperidine
cyclokeratitis
Cyclomydril Ophthalmic
cyclopea
cyclopean eye
cyclopentolate hydrochloride
cyclophoria
accommodative c.
minus c.
plus c.
position c.
c. positive
cyclophorometer
cyclophosphamide
cyclophotocoagulation
endoscopic c. (ECP)
laser transscleral c.
Nd:YAG laser c.
transpupillary c.
transscleral laser c.
c. vitreoretinal surgery
YAG laser c.
cyclopia
cycloplegia
cycloplegic
c. refraction (CR)
topical c.
cyclorotary muscle
cycloscope
cycloscopy
cycloserine
cyclospasm
cyclosporin A
cyclosporine
efficacy of c.
safety of c.
cyclotherapy
laser c.

cyclotome
cyclotomy
cyclotorsion
cyclotropia
cyclovergence
cycloversion
cyclovertical muscle
cyl, cyl.
cylinder
Cylate
cylinder (C, cyl, cyl.)
anterior c.
c. axis
concave c.
corneal c.
cross c.
crossed c.
diopter c.
Jackson cross c.
minus c.
3-month postoperative refractive c.
c. retinoscopy
c. spectacle lens
cylindrical lens (C, cyl.)
cylindric refraction
Cylindrocarpon
cylindroma
CYP1B1 **gene**
cyproheptadine
cyst
Acanthamoeba c.
aneurysmal bone c.
arachnoidal c.
Blessig c.
Blessig-Iwanoff c.
blood c.
colloid c.
colobomatous c.
conjunctival c.
corneal c.
c. degeneration
dermoid c.
Echinococcus c.
epibulbar dermoid c.
epidermal inclusion c.
epidermoid c.
epithelial implantation c.
epithelial inclusion c.
foveal c.
Gartner c.
hematic c.
inclusion c.

NOTES

cyst *(continued)*
    infundibular c.
    intracorneal c.
    intraepithelial c.
    iris c.
    Iwanoff c.
    lacrimal ductal c.
    lacrimal gland c.
    meibomian c.
    Naegleria c.
    orbital c.
    pearl c.
    proteinaceous c.
    pupillary iris c.
    Rathke cleft c.
    retinal c.
    scleral c.
    sebaceous inclusion c.
    serous c.
    spontaneous congenital iris c.
    subconjunctival c.
    sudoriferous c.
    tarsal c.
    traumatic corneal c.
    traumatic scleral c.
    Vahlkampfia c.
cystadenoma
    Moll gland c.
cysteamine HCl
cystic
    c. amelanotic nevus
    c. cataract
    c. eye
    c. fibrosis
    c. hydrocystoma tumor
    c. microphthalmia
    c. retinal tuft
cysticerci (*pl. of* cysticercus)
cysticercoid
cysticercosis
cysticercus, pl. cysticerci
    intraocular c.
cysticum
    epithelioma adenoides c.
cystine crystal
cystinosis
    nephropathic c.
cystitome
    air c.
    Atkinson 25-G short curved c.
    Azar curved c.
    Beaver Ocu-1 curved c.
    Blumenthal push-pull irrigating c.
    double-cutting sharp c.
    Drews angled c.
    Graefe c.
    irrigating c.
    Kelman air c.
    kibisitome c.

    Knolle-Kelman cannulated c.
    Kratz angled c.
    Lewicky formed c.
    Lieppman c.
    Look c.
    McIntyre reverse c.
    Mendez c.
    Neuhann c.
    Nevyas double sharp c.
    Visitec double-cutting c.
    von Graefe c.
    Wheeler c.
    Wilder c.
cystitomy
cystoid
    c. body
    c. cicatrix
    c. cicatrix of limbus
    c. macular degeneration (CMD)
    c. macular dystrophy
    c. macular edema (CME)
    c. macular hole
    c. maculopathy
    c. retinal degeneration
Cytobrush S brush
CytoFluor II fluorometer
cytoid body
cytokeratin 7, 20 antibody
cytokine therapy
cytologic examination
cytology
    conjunctival impression c.
    impression c.
cytomegalic
    c. inclusion disease (CID, CMID)
    c. inclusion virus
cytomegalovirus (CMV)
    c. disease
    macular c.
    c. retinitis
    C. Retinitis Retreatment Trial (CRRT)
    C. Retinitis and Viral Resistance Study (CRVRS)
    c. retinopathy
cytophotocoagulation
cytoplasmic body
cytotoxic antibody
Cytovene
Cytoxan
    C. Injection
    C. Oral
cytoxic T cell
Czapski microscope
Czermak
    accommodation phosphene of C.
    C. keratome
    C. pterygium operation

D
dexter
diopter
D chromosome ring syndrome
hypervitaminosis D
D trisomy syndrome
3D
3D angled stainless phaco
trapezoid blade
3D i-Scan ophthalmic ultrasound
3D i-Scan ultrasound tomography
3D stainless steel knife
D-15
D-15 Hue Desaturated Panel test
D-15 test
d
day
Daclizumab
Dacriose
Dacron suture
dacryadenalgia
dacryadenitis
dacryadenoscirrhus
dacryagogatresia
dacryagogic
dacryagogue
dacrycystalgia
dacrycystitis
dacryelcosis
dacryoadenalgia
dacryoadenectomy operation
dacryoadenitis
bacterial d.
infectious d.
inflammatory d.
dacryoblennorrhea
dacryocanaliculitis
dacryocele
congenital d.
dacryocyst
dacryocystalgia
dacryocystectasia
dacryocystectomy operation
dacryocystitis
acute d.
chronic d.
congenital d.
phlegmonous d.
silent d.
syphilitic d.
trachomatous d.
tuberculous d.
dacryocystoblennorrhea
dacryocystocele
dacryocystoethmoidostomy

dacryocystogram
dacryocystography (DCG)
dacryocystoptosis, dacryocystoptosia
dacryocystorhinostenosis
dacryocystorhinostomy (DCR)
endonasal laser d. (ENL-DCR)
endoscopic laser d.
endoscopic laser-assisted d.
external d. (EXT-DCR)
intranasal endoscopic d.
d. operation
therapeutic d.
dacryocystostenosis
dacryocystostomy operation
dacryocystotome
dacryocystotomy
Ammon d.
d. operation
dacryogenic
dacryogram
dacryohelcosis
dacryohemorrhea
dacryolin
dacryolith
Desmarres d.
dacryolithiasis
dacryoma
dacryon
dacryops
dacryopyorrhea
dacryopyosis
dacryorhinocystotomy
dacryorrhea
dacryoscintigraphy
dacryosinusitis
dacryosolenitis
dacryostenosis
dacryostomy
Arroyo d.
Arruga d.
Dupuy-Dutemps d.
Kuhnt d.
dacryosyrinx
dactinomycin
DAF syndrome
Dailey operation
Dailies contact lens
daily
D. cataract needle
twice d. (b.i.d.)
daily-wear contact lens (DWCL)
Daimas Blue
Daisy irrigation/aspiration instrument
Dakrina Ophthalmic Solution
Dalalone

D

Dalcaine
Dalen-Fuchs nodule
Dalgleish operation
Dallas lens-inserting forceps
Dalrymple
    D. disease
    D. sign
daltonian
daltonism
damage
    brain d.
    dorsal rostral d.
    glaucomatous optic nerve d.
    (GOND)
    optic tract d.
    solar d.
    visual field d.
dammini
    Ixodes d.
Danberg iris forceps
Dan chalazion forceps
dancing eye
Dandy criteria
Dan-Gradle cilia forceps
Dannheim eye implant
dantrolene sodium
dapiprazole
    d. HCl
    d. hydrochloride
DAPS
    dark-adapted pupil size
dapsone
Daranide
Daraprim
Dardenne nucleus forceps
Darin lens
dark
    d. adaptation
    d. adaptometry
    d. disk
    d. empty field
    d. event
    d. retinoscopy
dark-adapted
    d.-a. eye
    d.-a. pupil size (DAPS)
dark-field
    d.-f. accommodation
    d.-f. examination
    d.-f. illumination
dark-ground illumination
dark-room
    d.-r. test
    d.-r. testing
Darling
    D. capsulotome
    D. capsulotomy
    D. Aron-Rosa lens-holding forceps
Dartmouth Eye Institute

DaSilva dermatome
data
    d. handling
    d. selection
datum line
Daubenton plane
daunorubicin
Davidoff
    D. ambidextrous nucleus chopper
    D. blade
Daviel
    D. lens spoon
    D. operation
    D. scoop
Davis
    D. forceps
    D. knife needle
    D. spud
    D. trephine
Davis-Geck
    D.-G. blepharoplasty
    D.-G. suture
day (d)
    1 d. Acuvue contact lens
    d. blindness
    90-d. glaucoma
    d. sight
    d. vision
Dazamide
dazzle
    monocular d.
    d. reflex
dazzling glare
dB
    decibel
DBC
    distance between centers
DBL
    distance between lenses
    distance between nasal lines
DC
    dermatochalasis
    discharge
    discontinue
D&C
    deep and clear
DCC
    double concave
DCG
    dacryocystography
DCR
    dacryocystorhinostomy
DCx
    double convex
DD
    disk diameter
    disk diffusion
dd
    disk diameter

DDHT
dissociated double hypertropia
DDLS
disk damage likelihood scale
DDMS
diamond dusted membrane scraper
Synergetics DDMS
DDT
dye disappearance test
de
de Grandmont operation
De Klair operation
de Lange syndrome
de Lapersonne operation
De LaVega lens pusher
De LaVega vitreous-aspirating
cannula
de Morsier-Gauthier syndrome
de Morsier syndrome
de Vincentiis operation
de Wecker anterior sclerotomy
de Wecker iris scissors
de Wecker operation
deaf blindness
deafness
diabetes insipidus, diabetes mellitus,
optic atrophy, d. (DIDMOAD)
lentigines, electrocardiogram
abnormalities, ocular hypertelorism,
pulmonary stenosis, abnormal
genitalia, retardation of growth,
and d. (LEOPARD)
Dean
D. blade
D. iris knife
D. knife holder
D. knife needle
death-to-preservation time
Deblasio LASIK marker
debrancher enzyme deficiency
débridement
epithelial d.
impression d.
wipe d.
débrider
corneal d.
Sauer corneal d.
debris
back surface d. (BSD)
capsular d.
cellular d.
desquamated epithelial d.

epithelial d.
phagocytosed cellular d.
seborrheic d.
tear film d.
debris-laden tear film
Decadron Phosphate
decalvans
keratosis follicularis spinulosa d.
DeCamp viscoelastic cannula
decenter
decentered
d. lens
d. spectacles
decentration
d. of contact lens
lens d.
decibel (dB)
Declaration of Helsinki
declination
decolorize
decompensated
d. accommodative esotropia
d. phoria
decompensation
corneal d.
endothelial d.
decomposition
Zernike d.
decompression
bone removal d. (BROD)
Dickson-Wright orbit d.
extracranial optic nerve d.
fat removal orbital d. (FROD)
intracranial optic nerve d.
lateral orbital d.
microvascular d.
Naffziger orbital d.
optic nerve sheath d. (ONSD)
orbital d.
d. of orbit operation
posterior fossa nerve d.
d. surgery
three-wall d.
transantral d.
decompressive surgery
decongestant
ocular d.
decrease
visual acuity d.
decreased corneal sensation
decreasing vision

NOTES

121

decussation
    oculomotor d.
    optic d.
deep
    d. blunt rake retractor
    d. and clear (D&C)
    d. congestion
    d. corneal stromal opacity
    d. dyslexia
    d. filiform dystrophy
    d. lamellar endothelial keratoplasty
      (DLEK)
    d. lamellar keratectomy
    d. parenchymatous dystrophy
    d. punctate keratitis
    d. pustular keratitis
    d. and quiet (D&Q)
    d. retina
    d. scleritis
    d. sclerotomy
defect
    acquired color d.
    afferent pupillary d. (APD)
    altitudinal visual field d.
    arcuate field d.
    arteriovenous crossing d.
    AV crossing d.
    bilateral altitudinal field d.
    bilateral homonymous altitudinal d.
    bilateral visual field d.
    binasal field d.
    bitemporal field d.
    central d.
    centrocecal d.
    chiasmatic field d.
    color d.
    compressive optic nerve d.
    confluent d.
    confrontation field d.
    congruous field d.
    corkscrew visual field d.
    cosmetic d.
    directional d.
    enzyme d.
    epithelial d. (ED)
    field d.
    functional d.
    glaucoma field d.
    gun-barrel field d.
    homonymous field d.
    hyperfluorescent window d.
    hysterical visual field d.
    incongruous field d.
    inferior altitudinal d.
    IOFB-caused d.
    iris transillumination d. (ITD)
    levator aponeurosis d.
    Marcus Gunn relative afferent d.
    monocular field d.

    nasal step d.
    nerve fiber bundle d.
    paracentral d.
    parietal lobe field d.
    patchy window d.
    persistent epithelial d.
    pie-in-the-sky d.
    pie-on-the-floor d.
    punctate corneal epithelial d.
    quadrantic d.
    radial transillumination d.
    relative afferent pupillary d.
      (RAPD)
    retinal pigment epithelial d.
    retrochiasmal visual field d.
    sector d.
    sector-shaped d.
    superior homonymous quadrantic d.
    temporal lobe field d.
    trophic d.
    vascular filling d.
    visual corkscrew d.
    visual field d.
    window d.
defective accommodation
deficiency
    acetylcholine receptor d.
    acetylcholinesterase d.
    acid maltase d.
    aqueous tear d. (ATD)
    brancher enzyme d.
    carnitine d.
    debrancher enzyme d.
    familial lecithin-cholesterol
      acyltransferase d.
    familial lipoprotein d.
    folic acid d.
    galactokinase d.
    iatrogenic limbal stem cell d.
    lecithin-cholesterol acyltransferase d.
    limbal stem-cell d.
    primary acetylcholine receptor d.
    supranuclear d.
    vitamin A d.
deficit
    abduction d.
    concentration d.
    hemisensory d.
    neurologic d.
definition
    area of critical d.
deflection
defocus
    calculating equivalent d.
defocus-induced ametropia
deformans
    osteitis d.
deformity
    d. angle

scleral d.
S-shaped d.
Defy
degeneratio
   d. hyaloidea granuliformis
   d. hyaloideoretinae hereditaria
   d. spherularis elaioides
degeneration
   aberrant d.
   advanced pellucid marginal d.
   age-related disciform macular d.
   age-related macular d. (AMD, ARMD)
   amyloid corneal d.
   anterograde d.
   atrophic age-related macular d. (AAMD)
   atrophic macular d.
   balloon d.
   Best d.
   Biber-Haab-Dimmer d.
   Bietti tapetoretinal d.
   calcareous d.
   central retinal d.
   choriocapillaris d. (CCD)
   chorioretinal d.
   cobblestone retinal d.
   cone d.
   cone-rod d.
   congenital macular d.
   d. of cornea
   corneal furrow d.
   cyst d.
   cystoid macular d. (CMD)
   cystoid retinal d.
   diabetic macular d.
   disciform macular d.
   Doyne familial colloid d.
   Doyne honeycombed d.
   dry senile macular d.
   ectatic marginal d.
   elastoid d.
   equatorial d.
   familial colloid d.
   familial pseudoinflammatory macular d.
   fine fibrillar vitreal d.
   furrow d.
   hepatolenticular d.
   hereditary d.
   heredomacular d.
   hyaline d.

hyaloideoretinal d.
hydropic d.
juvenile macular d.
keratinoid d.
Kozlowski d.
Kuhnt-Junius macular d.
lattice retinal d.
lenticular d.
lipid d.
macular disciform d.
marginal corneal d.
marginal furrow d.
myopic retinal d.
nodular corneal d.
nonneovascular age-related macular d.
opticocochleodentate d.
paraneoplastic cerebellar d.
paving-stone d.
pellucid corneal marginal d. (PCMD)
pellucid marginal corneal d.
pellucid marginal retinal d.
peripheral cystoid d.
peripheral disciform d.
peripheral tapetochoroidal d.
pigmentary perivenous chorioretinal d.
primary pigmentary d.
progressive cone d.
progressive myopic d.
Randomized Trial of Beta-Carotene and Macular D.
red cone d.
reticular cystoid d.
retinal lattice d.
retrograde transsynaptic d.
rod-cone d.
Salzmann nodular corneal d.
scleral d.
senescent disciform macular d.
senile disciform macular d.
senile exudative macular d.
senile furrow d.
Sorsby pseudoinflammatory macular d.
spheroid d.
spinocerebellar d.
striatal nigral d.
tapetochoroidal d.
tapetoretinal d.
Terrien marginal d.

D

NOTES

degeneration (*continued*)
    tractional retinal d.
    transneuronal d.
    transsynaptic d.
    trophic retinal d.
    vitelliform macular d.
    vitelline macular d.
    vitelliruptive d.
    vitreoretinal d.
    Vogt d.
    Wagner hereditary vitreoretinal d.
    Wagner hyaloid retinal d.
    wallerian d.
    wet macular d.
    Wilson d.
    xerotic d.
degenerative
    d. cataract
    d. cerebellar disease
    d. myopia
    d. ocular disease
    d. pannus
    d. retinal disease
    d. retinoschisis
degenerativus
    pannus d.
Degest 2 Ophthalmic
Degos syndrome
degradation
    image d.
degree
    prism d.
45-degree
    45-degree bent reform implant
    45-degree scissor with membrane
    pick
DeGrouchy syndrome
dehisced
dehiscence
    iris d.
    retinal d.
    traumatic wound d.
    wound d.
    Zuckerkandl d.
dehiscent
dehiscing
dehydration
    corneal d.
    d. injury
Dehydrex
dehydrogenase
    glucose 6-phosphate d.
    lactate d.
dehydroretinol
deinsertion
Deiter operation
Deitz incision depth gauge
Dejean syndrome
Deknatel silk suture

delacrimation
delamination
    capsular d.
delayed
    d. massive suprachoroidal
    hemorrhage
    d. mucous plaque
    d. onset cataract
    d. rectifier
    d. visual maturation
deletion mapping
delicate
    d. grasping forceps
    d. serrated straight dressing forceps
delimiting keratotomy
delivery system
Dell
    D. astigmatism marker
    D. fixation ring
dellen
    corneal d.
    d. of Fuchs
Deller modification
Delta Cortef
Deltasone
Del Toro operation
DEM
    Developmental Eye Movement
    DEM test
demarcated detachment
demarcation line of retina
demecarium bromide
demeclocycline
Demerol
de-misting condensation
demodectic blepharitis
Demodex folliculorum
demodicosis
demonstration
    d. eyepiece
    d. ophthalmoscope
demonstrator
    halo d.
Demours membrane
demyelinating
    d. disease
    d. optic neuropathy
    d. plaque
demyelination
    autoimmune d.
    nystagmus with d.
demyelinative disease
demyelinization
demyelinizing
Dendrid
dendriform
    d. corneal lesion
    d. epithelial lesion

d. keratitis
d. ulcer
dendrite
branching d.
corneal d.
epithelial d.
fragmented d.
herpetic d.
d. keratitis
VZV d.
dendritic
d. cataract
d. epithelial lesion
d. epitheliopathy
d. ghost
d. herpes simplex corneal ulcer
d. herpes zoster keratitis
d. keratopathy
dendritiform appearance
denervate
denervation
corneal d.
d. supersensitivity test
trigeminal d.
Dennie-Morgan fold
densa
lamina d.
dense
d. brunescent nucleus
d. core granule
d. opacity
d. vitreitis
densitometer
density
arciform d.
average lens d. (ALD)
cell d.
conjunctival goblet cell d.
corneal optical d.
endothelial cell d. (ECD)
Fas receptor d.
denudation
denuded corneal epithelium
deorsumduction
deorsumvergence
left d.
right d.
deorsumversion
depigmentation
periocular d.
depigmented spot
Depo-Medrol

deposit
adrenochrome d.
amorphous corneal d.
amyloid d.
basal laminar d. (BLD)
calcareous d.
colloid d.
conjunctival d.
corneal d.
crystalline d.
discrete micro gel d.
fibrillogranular d.
intraretinal lipid d.
iron d.
lipid d.
mutton-fat d.
posterior corneal d. (PCD)
protein d.
refractile d.
superficial retinal refractile d.
tear protein d.
deposition
calcium d.
chemical vapor d. (CVD)
copper d.
epithelial adrenochrome d.
iron d.
pigment d.
depot
sub-Tenon d.
depressed fracture
depression
cecocentral d.
crater d.
foveal d.
d. of orbital floor
posterior corneal d.
scleral d.
depressor
muscle d.
O'Connor d.
orbital d.
Schepens scleral d.
Schepens thimble d.
Schocket scleral d.
scleral d.
Simcoe scleral d.
Wilder scleral d.
deprimens oculi
deprivation
d. amblyopia
stimulus d.

D

NOTES

125

depth
    d. of chamber
    d. of field
    focal d.
    d. of focus
    d. gauge
    d. perception
    d. plate
    sagittal d.
Deq
    spherical equivalent
derangement
    pigment d.
Derby operation
Derf needle holder
derma
    epithelial d.
    stromal d.
Derma-K laser
dermal
    d. amyloid infiltration
    d. nevus
Dermalon suture
dermatan sulfate
dermatitidis
    Blastomyces d.
dermatitis, pl. dermatitides
    herpes simplex d.
    hyperkeratotic d.
    trigeminal herpes zoster d.
dermatoblepharitis
dermatochalasis (DC)
    eyelid d.
dermatoconjunctivitis
    contact d.
dermatogenes
    cataracta d.
dermatogenic cataract
dermatolysis palpebrarum
dermatome
    DaSilva d.
    Hall d.
dermatomyositis
dermatoophthalmitis
dermatosis
    papillopruritic d.
dermis
    acellular d.
    d. fat graft
    d. patch graft
dermochondral corneal dystrophy of François
dermoid
    congenital limbal corneal d.
    conjunctival d.
    d. cyst
    limbal d.
    d. of orbit
    orbital d.

    pedunculated congenital corneal d.
    d. tumor
dermolipoma
Dermostat implant
DES
    dry eye syndrome
desaturation
    red d.
Descartes law
Descemet
    D. fold
    D. membrane
    D. membrane detachment
    D. membrane punch
descemetitis
descemetocele ulcer
descemetopexy
    gas-exchange d.
desiccant
desiccate
desiccation
    corneal d.
    d. keratitis
design
    gripflex d.
Desmarres
    D. chalazion
    D. chalazion forceps
    D. corneal dissector
    D. dacryolith
    D. eyelid retractor
    D. fixation pick
    D. knife
    D. lamellar dissector
    D. law
    D. lid clamp
    D. lid elevator
    D. lid retractor
    D. marker
    D. operation
    D. refractor
    D. scarifier
desmopressin
desmosomal cellular attachment
desmosome
desquamated epithelial debris
DET
    dry eye test
    DET fluorescein strip
detached
    d. iris
    d. retina
    d. vitreous
detachment
    aphakic d.
    bullous d.
    choroidal d.
    ciliochoroidal d.
    complex retinal d.

corrugated retinal d.
demarcated d.
Descemet membrane d.
disciform retinal d.
extrafoveal retinal d.
exudative retinal d. (ERD)
exudative serous retinal d.
foveal retinal d.
foveolar retinal d.
funnel-shaped retinal d.
hemorrhagic choroidal d.
hyaloid membrane d.
d. infusion
late phase d.
macula-off rhegmatogenous
   retinal d.
macula-on rhegmatogenous
   retinal d.
macular d.
morning glory retinal d.
neurosensory retinal d.
nonrhegmatogenous retinal d.
open-funnel d.
perifoveal posterior vitreous d.
   (PPVD)
pigment epithelial d. (PED)
d. pocket
posterior vitreous d. (PVD)
pseudophakic d.
d. of retina
retinal d. (RD)
retinal pigment epithelium
   serous d.
rhegmatogenous retinal d. (RRD)
schisis-related d.
sensory d.
serous choroidal d.
serous macular d.
serous pigment epithelial d.
serous retinal pigment
   epithelium d.
shallow d.
tear-induced retinal d.
tractional retinal d. (TRD)
traction macular d.
Trbinger d.
vitreal d.
vitreous d.
Detamide
detectability
   ophthalmoscopic d.
detectable focus

detection
   d. acuity
   glaucoma d.
detector
   thermoluminescence d. (TLD)
deterenol HCl
**determinants of optic discharge
   characteristic**
deturgescence
   d. of cornea
   corneal d.
deturgescent state
deutan
deuteranoma
deuteranomalopia
deuteranomalous
deuteranomaly
deuteranope
deuteranopia, deuteranopsia
deuteranopic
deuton color blindness
Deutschman cataract knife
devascularization
development
   visual d.
developmental
   d. anomaly
   d. cataract
   D. Eye Movement (DEM)
   D. Eye Movement test
   d. prosopagnosia
   d. ptosis
deviant color
deviating eye
deviation
   angle of d.
   comitant vertical d.
   conjugate horizontal d.
   convergent d.
   corrected pattern standard d.
     (CPSD)
   dissociated vertical d.
   divergent d.
   downward d.
   esotropic d.
   forced downward d.
   frequency doubling technology
     mean d. (FDT-MD)
   frequency doubling technology
     pattern standard d. (FDT-PSD)
   global d. (GD)
   Hering-Hellebrand d.

D

NOTES

deviation *(continued)*
    heterotropic d.
    high-pass resolution perimetry global d. (HRP-GD)
    high-pass resolution perimetry local d. (HRP-LD)
    horizontal d.
    incomitant vertical d.
    intermittent d.
    latent d.
    local d. (LD)
    manifest d.
    mean d. (MD)
    minimum d.
    pattern standard d. (PSD)
    periodic alternating gaze d.
    primary d.
    right d.
    Roth-Bielschowsky d.
    secondary d.
    skew d.
    squint d.
    standard d. (SD)
    strabismal d.
    supranuclear d.
    tonic downward d.
    tonic upward d.
    torsional d.
    tropia d.
    tropic d.
    vertical comitant d.
deviational nystagmus
Devic disease
device
    Ahmed d.
    crosslinked poly (HEMA) glaucoma filtration d.
    doubling d.
    Envision TD ophthalmic drug delivery d.
    glaucoma drainage d. (GDD)
    Joseph d.
    Keratolux fixation d.
    Krupin d.
    laser-argon d.
    laser-ruby d.
    Look micropuncture d.
    M.A.T. postoperative comfort d.
    Microjet-based cutting and debriding d.
    oblique prism d.
    Ocusert d.
    OptiMed d.
    Panoramic200 Ultra-Widefield Ophthalmic Imaging D.
    Putterman-Chaflin ocular asymmetry d.
    retrieval d.
    Seton drainage d.

    spectacle-borne d.
    subjective d.
    Tano d.
    Venturi aspiration vitrectomy d.
    Welch four-drop d.
DeVilbiss
    D. irrigating/aspirating unit
    D. irrigator
deviometer
devitalized epithelium
Dexacidin
Dexacine ointment
Dexair
dexamethasone
    d. acetate
    neomycin, polymyxin B, and d.
    d. sodium phosphate
    d. solution
    tobramycin and d.
Dexasol
Dexasone L.A.
Dexasporin
Dexcaine
Dexchlor
dexchlorpheniramine
Dexedrine
Dexone LA
Dexon suture
Dexsol
Dexsone
dexter (D)
    oculus d. (right eye)
dextra
    tension oculus d. (tension of right eye) (TOD)
    visio oculus d. (vision of right eye) (VOD)
dextran medium
dextroclination
dextrocular
dextrocularity
dextrocycloduction
dextrocycloversion
dextrodepression
dextroduction
dextrogyration
dextrotorsion
dextroversion
Dey-Drop Ophthalmic Solution
Dey-Lube
DFP
    diisopropyl fluorophosphate
DGH
    DGH 2000 AP ultrasonic pachymeter
    DGH 5000 A-scan
DGH-500 Pachette
DHPG
    dihydrophenylethylene glycol

D&I
  dilation and irrigation
diabetes
  alloxan d.
  artificial d.
  brittle d.
  bronze d.
  chemical d.
  D. Control and Complications Trial
  experimental d.
  gestational d.
  gouty d.
  growth-onset d.
  d. innocens
  d. inositus
  d. insipidus
  d. insipidus, diabetes mellitus, optic
    atrophy, deafness (DIDMOAD)
  insulin-deficient d.
  juvenile d.
  ketosis-prone d.
  ketosis-resistant d.
  Lancereaux d.
  latent d.
  lipoatrophic d.
  lipoplethoric d.
  lipuric d.
  masked d.
  maturity-onset d.
  d. mellitus (DM)
  Mosler d.
  overflow d.
  overt d.
  pancreatic d.
  phlorhizin d.
  phosphate d.
  piqûre d.
  puncture d.
  renal d.
  skin d.
  steroid d.
  steroidogenic d.
  subclinical d.
  temporary d.
  toxic d.
  type 1, 2 d.
diabetic
  d. amaurosis
  d. Argyll Robertson pupil
  d. cataract
  d. iritis
  d. keratoepitheliopathy

  d. macular degeneration
  d. macular edema (DME)
  d. macular heterotopia
  d. maculopathy
  d. melanosis
  d. membrane
  d. optic atrophy
  d. papillopathy
  d. retinitis
  d. retinopathy (DR)
  D. Retinopathy Vitrectomy Study
    (DRVS)
  d. traction
diabetica
  rubeosis iridis d.
diabetic-osmotic cataract
diabeticus
  fundus d.
diagnosis
  neuroophthalmologic d.
  nonorganic disorder d.
diagnostic
  d. contact lens
  d. fiberoptic lens
  d. fitting set
  d. position of gaze
  d. program
dial
  astigmatic d.
  clock d.
  Mendez astigmatism d.
  Regan-Lancaster d.
  sunburst d.
dialer
  angled iris hook and IOL d.
  intraocular lens d.
  Lester lens d.
  Spadafora MemoryLens d.
  Visitec intraocular lens d.
dialysis
  d. retinae
  retinal d.
Diamatrix trapezoidal diamond knife
diameter
  anterior optic zone d.
  chord d.
  contact lens chord d.
  d. of cornea
  corneal d.
  disk d. (DD, dd)
  effective d. (ED)
  iris d.

D

NOTES

129

diameter *(continued)*
    large pupil d.
    minimal effective d. (MED)
    optical zone d.
    visible iris d. (VID)
Diamine T.D.
3,4-diaminopyridine
diamond
    d. blade
    d. blade knife
    d. bur
    d. dusted membrane scraper
    (DDMS)
    D. Dye
    d. laser knife
    d. micrometer
    d. phaco knife
    d. wound separator
diamond-bur polishing
diamond-dusted
    d.-d. knife
    d.-d. knife blade
Diamontek knife
Diamox Sequels
Dianoux operation
diaphanoscopy
DiaPhine trephine
diaphragm
    iris-lens d.
    lens-iris d.
    Potter-Bucky d.
diaphragma sellae
diapositive
    stereooptic disk d.
diaschisis
diastasis
    iris d.
diathermocoagulator
diathermy
    d. application
    d. electrode
    Mira d.
    d. operation
    d. point
    d. puncture
    d. tip
    transscleral d.
    d. unit
    wet-field d.
Diatracin
dibromopropamidine isethionate
dichlorphenamide
dichroic
dichroism
    circular d.
dichromasy
dichromat

dichromatic
    d. light
    d. vision
dichromatism
    congenital d.
dichromatopsia
dichromic
Dickey-Fox operation
Dickey operation
Dickson-Wright
    D.-W. operation
    D.-W. orbit decompression
diclofenac sodium
dicloxacillin
Dicon
    D. CT 200 corneal topographer
    D. ocular blood flow analyzer
dicoria
dictyoma *(var. of* diktyoma)
DIDMOAD
    diabetes insipidus, diabetes mellitus,
    optic atrophy, deafness
    DIDMOAD syndrome
Dieffenbach
    D. operation
    D. serrefine
diencephalic
    d. lesion
    d. syndrome
diencephalon
Difei glasses
difference
    frame d.
    light d.
difficile
    Clostridium d.
Diff-Quick stain
diffraction
    Fraunhofer d.
diffraction-limited pupil
diffusa
    encephalitis periaxialis d.
diffuse
    d. angiokeratoma
    d. anterior scleritis
    d. atherosclerosis
    d. cataract
    d. choroidal sclerosis
    d. choroiditis
    d. deep keratitis
    d. drusen
    d. endotheliitis
    d. granuloma
    d. illumination
    d. inflammatory eyelid atrophy
    d. lamellar keratitis
    d. Lewy body disease
    d. unilateral subacute neuroretinitis
    (DUSN)

diffusion
circle d.
disk d. (DD)
diffusion-weighted imaging/magnetic resonance imaging (DWI/MRI)
diffusum
angiokeratoma corporis d.
Diflucan
difumarate
emedastine d.
DiGeorge syndrome
digestion
enzymatic d.
Digilab
D. perimeter
D. tonometer
digital
d. acuity card
D. B System
D. B System ultrascan
d. fitting measurement
D. fundus imager
d. nonmydriatic fundus imaging
d. pressure
D. slit-lamp imager
d. subtraction indocyanine green angiography (DS-ICGA)
d. subtraction photokeratoscopy
d. tonometry
digital-imaging analysis
Digitalis purpurea
digitized video fundus image
digitoocular sign
dihydrophenylethylene glycol (DHPG)
diisopropyl fluorophosphate (DFP)
diktyoma, dictyoma
dilacerated cataract
dilaceration
Dilatair
dilatans
pseudo sinus d.
dilate
dilated
d. pupil
d. retinal examination
d. stereoscopic fundus examination
dilation
ectatic d.
d. and irrigation (D&I)
d. lag
pharmacological d.
d. of punctum

d. of punctum operation
pupil d.
transient unilateral d.
dilator
Berens d.
Castroviejo-Galezowski d.
Castroviejo lacrimal d.
French lacrimal d.
Galezowski lacrimal d.
Heath d.
Heyner d.
Hosford lacrimal d.
House lacrimal d.
iris d.
Jones punctum d.
Keuch Pupil D.
lacrimal d.
Muldoon lacrimal d.
d. muscle
d. muscle of pupil
Nettleship-Wilder d.
Peters pupil d.
punctal d.
punctum d.
pupil d.
Rolf d.
Ruedemann lacrimal d.
Weiss gold d.
Wilder lacrimal d.
Ziegler lacrimal d.
dilution
pigmentary d.
dimefilcon A
dimenhydrinate
dimensional
three d.
Dimetabs Oral
Dimetane Extentabs
dimethylaminoethanol
dimethylpolysiloxane
dimethyl sulfate
diminazene aceturate
Dimitry
D. chalazion trephine
D. erysiphake
Dimitry-Bell erysiphake
Dimitry-Thomas erysiphake
Dimmer nummular keratitis
dimness of vision
dimple
Fuchs d.
d. veil

D

NOTES

131

dimpling of eyeball
Dine digital scanner
diode
    d. endolaser
    d. endophotocoagulation
    d. laser
    d. laser trabeculoplasty (DLT)
    light-emitting d. (LED)
    D. microlaser
diolamine
    sulfisoxazole d.
diolipin antibody
diopsimeter
diopter, dioptre (D)
    d. cylinder
    66-d. iridectomy laser lens
    prism d. (PD)
    d. prism
    d. sphere (DS)
dioptometer, dioptrometer
dioptometry, dioptrometry
dioptoscope, dioptroscope
dioptoscopy, dioptroscopy
dioptre (var. of diopter)
dioptric
    d. aberration
    d. apparatus
    d. correction
    d. medium
    d. power
    d. system
dioptrometer (var. of dioptometer)
dioptrometry (var. of dioptometry)
Dioptron
    D. Nova
    D. Ultima
dioptroscope (var. of dioptoscope)
dioptroscopy (var. of dioptoscopy)
dioptry
Diphenhist
diphenhydramine hydrochloride
diphtheriae
    Corynebacterium d.
diphtheritic conjunctivitis
diphtheroid
dipivalyl epinephrine
dipivefrin HCl
diplegia
    congenital facial d.
diplexia
diplobacillary
    d. blepharitis
    d. conjunctivitis
diplocoria
diplopia
    binocular d.
    cerebral d.
    crossed d.
    direct d.

    heteronymous d.
    homonymous d.
    horizontal d.
    monocular d.
    paradoxical d.
    simple d.
    stereoscopic d.
    torsional d.
    uncrossed d.
    vertical d.
diplopiometer
diploscope
dipping
    ocular d.
    reverse d.
Diprivan
direct
    d. astigmatism
    d. carotid cavernous fistula
    d. chlamydial immunofluorescence
    test
    d. diplopia
    d. fluorescent antibody stain
    d. glare
    d. gonioscopic lens
    d. illumination
    d. image
    d. measurement
    d. method
    d. ophthalmoscope
    d. ophthalmoscopy
    d. parallax
    d. pupillary light reaction
    d. pupillary reflex
    d. pupillary response
    d. vision
direction
    angle of d.
    line of d.
    principal line of d.
    principal visual d.
    visual d.
directional
    d. defect
    d. preponderance
direct-light
    d.-l. reflex
    d.-l. refraction
    d.-l. response
director
    grooved d.
Dirofilaria repens
disability
    auditory perceptual d.
    glare d. (GD)
    motor-output d.
    visual d.
disc (var. of disk)
discharge (DC)

conjunctival d.
mucoid d.
mucous d.
socket d.
watery d.
Dischler irrigation cannula
disci (*pl. of* discus)
DisCide disinfecting towelettes
disciform
    d. chorioretinopathy
    d. degeneration of retina
    d. endotheliitis
    d. herpes simplex keratitis
    d. macular degeneration
    d. macular scar
    d. opacity
    d. process
    d. retinal detachment
disciformans
    retinitis d.
disciformis
    keratitis d.
discission
    d. hook
    d. knife
    d. of lens operation
    Moncrieff d.
    d. needle
    posterior d.
discitis
disclination
discoloration of pigment
disconjugate
    d. gaze
    d. nystagmus
    d. roving eye movement
discontinue (DC)
discontinuity
    zone of d.
discoria
discrete
    d. colliquative keratopathy
    d. granuloma
    d. micro gel deposit
discrimination
    color d.
    contrast d.
    light d.
    light-dark d. (LDD)
    spatial d.

two-light d.
visual d.
discus, pl. **disci**
    excavatio disci
    d. nervi optici
    d. opticus
discussion pallor
disease
    Aland eye d.
    Albers-Schönberg d.
    Albright d.
    allergic eye d.
    Alström d.
    angio-Behçet d.
    Apollo d.
    Arlt d.
    arterial occlusive d.
    Ballet d.
    basal ganglia d.
    Basedow d.
    Batten d.
    Batten-Mayou d.
    Behçet d.
    Behr d.
    Benson d.
    Berlin d.
    Best d.
    Biedl d.
    Bielschowsky d.
    Bielschowsky-Jansky d.
    blinding eye d.
    Bourneville-Brissaud d.
    Bowen d.
    Bower d.
    Canavan d.
    chiasmal d.
    Coats d.
    Cogan d.
    collagen and rheumatoid-related d.
    collagen vascular d.
    corneal stromal d.
    cotransmission of d.
    Creutzfeldt-Jakob d.
    Crouzon d.
    cytomegalic inclusion d. (CID, CMID)
    cytomegalovirus d.
    Dalrymple d.
    degenerative cerebellar d.
    degenerative ocular d.
    degenerative retinal d.
    demyelinating d.

NOTES

disease *(continued)*

demyelinative d.
Devic d.
diffuse Lewy body d.
Dyggve d.
Eales d.
entero-Behçet d.
epithelial basement membrane d.
epithelial herpetic d.
Erdheim-Chester d.
exogenous d.
extraorbital d.
Faber d.
Farber d.
Flajani d.
Flatau-Schilder d.
flecked retina d.
Förster d.
Franceschetti d.
Gaucher d.
Gerstmann-Straussler-Scheinker d.
Gierke d.
Goldflam d.
Goldflam-Erb d.
Goldmann-Favre d.
Gorham d.
Graefe d.
graft-versus-host d.
Graves d.
Hand-Schüller-Christian d.
Harada d.
Heerfordt d.
helminthic d.
herpetic ocular d.
Hippel d.
HSV ocular d.
HSV stromal d.
Hünermann d.
Hurler d.
infantile Refsum d.
infectious d.
inflammatory meibomian gland d.
International Study Group for
 Behçet D.
interpalpebral stromal d.
Jansky-Bielschowsky d.
Jensen d.
Kawasaki d.
Kikuchi-Fujimoto d.
Kimmelstiel-Wilson d.
Kjer d.
Koeppe d.
Krabbe d.
Krill d.
Kuhnt-Junius d.
Kyrle d.
Lauber d.
Leber d.
Leigh d.

Lindau d.
Lindau-von Hippel d.
lysosomal storage d.
Machado-Joseph d.
macular d.
Marsh d.
Masuda-Kitahara d.
medullary cystic d.
medullary optic d.
meibomian d.
midbrain d.
Mikulicz d.
miner's d.
mitochondrial d.
Möbius d.
multicore d.
multifactorial d.
multifocal chorioretinal d.
muscle-eye-brain d.
mycobacterial d.
neonatal onset multisystem
 inflammatory d. (NOMID)
neuro-Behçet d.
neuropathic d.
Niemann-Pick d.
Niemann-Pick d. type A, B
Norrie d.
Nunery classification of Graves d.,
 type I, II
occlusive vascular d.
ocular surface d. (OSD)
ocular syphilitic d.
oculoglandular d.
Oguchi d.
ophthalmic Graves d.
optic nerve d.
pancreatic d.
Parry d.
plus d.
prethreshold d.
primary demyelinating d.
primary ocular d.
pulseless d.
Purtscher d.
Randomized Trials of Vitamin
 Supplements and Eye D.
Recklinghausen d.
Reese-Ellsworth group Va, Vb d.
Refsum d.
Reis-Bücklers d.
Reiter d.
retinal d.
Rosai-Dorfman d.
Sanders d.
Schilder d.
shipyard d.
Sichel d.
Sjögren d.
Sneddon-Wilkinson d.

Spielmeyer-Sjögren d.
Spielmeyer-Stock d.
Spielmeyer-Vogt d.
Stargardt and Best d.
Steele-Richardson-Olszewski d.
Steinert d.
Strachan d.
stromal d.
Sturge-Weber d.
syphilitic ocular d.
Tangier d.
Tay d.
Tay-Sachs d.
threshold d.
Thygeson d.
thyroid eye d.
toxic-nutritional d.
van der Hoeve d.
vanishing bone d.
vascular cerebellar d.
vascular occlusive d.
venous occlusive d.
viral ocular d.
visual pathway d.
Vogt d.
Vogt-Koyanagi-Harada d.
Vogt-Spielmeyer d.
von Gierke d.
von Hippel d.
von Hippel-Lindau d.
von Recklinghausen d.
Wagner d.
Weil d.
Werdnig-Hoffmann d.
Westphal-Strümpell d.
Whipple d.
Wilson d.
zone 1 d.
disequilibrium
Dishler
　　D. Excimer Laser System for
　　　LASIK
　　D. type LASIK irrigating cannula
disinfectant
　　AoSept D.
disinfecting solution
disinserted
　　d. muscle
　　d. retina
disinsertion
　　levator aponeurosis d.
　　d. of retina

disjugate
　　d. movement
　　d. movement of eyes
disjunctive
　　d. movement
　　d. nystagmus
disk, disc
　　Airy d.
　　anangioid d.
　　anomalous d.
　　aperture d.
　　choked optic d.
　　ciliary d.
　　colobomatous optic d.
　　color d.
　　conus of optic d.
　　cupped d.
　　cupping of optic d.
　　d. damage likelihood scale (DDLS)
　　dark d.
　　d. diameter (DD, dd)
　　d. diffusion (DD)
　　doubling of the optic d.
　　dragged d.
　　d. drusen
　　d. drusen hemorrhage
　　d. edema
　　edema of optic d.
　　d. elevation
　　excavation of optic d.
　　d. forceps
　　gelatin d.
　　hypoplastic d.
　　d. intraocular lens
　　d. IOL
　　ischemic d.
　　Krill d.
　　Krupin eye d.
　　leukemic infiltration of the
　　　optic d.
　　micrometer d.
　　morning glory d.
　　nasal border of optic d.
　　neovascularization of d. (NVD)
　　d. neovascularization
　　d. neurovascular vessel
　　Newton d.
　　new vessel d.
　　d. new vessel
　　optic d.
　　pale optic d.
　　d. pallor

D

NOTES

disk *(continued)*
pinhole d.
pink eye d.
Placido d.
planoconvex-shaped d.
posterior lamellar d.
Rekoss d.
stenopeic d.
stroboscopic d.
swelling of d.
tilted d.
d. vasculature
Whipple d.
disk-fovea distance
disk-shaped cataract
dislocated
d. lens
ocular circulation d.
dislocation
congenital lens d.
intraocular lens d.
lens d.
posterior d.
dislocator
Kirby lens d.
dismutase
manganese superoxide d.
disodium hydrogen phosphate
disorder
accommodation d.
adrenal d.
autonomic nervous system d.
basement membrane d.
bullous d.
canalicular d.
epithelial bleb d.
extraocular muscle d.
d. of eye
eyelid d.
eye movement d.
hemorrhagic d.
histiocytic d.
hyperkeratotic d.
infranuclear d.
lacrimation d.
motion perception d.
myelin d.
myopathic d.
neurologic d.
neuromuscular d.
ocular motility d.
oculodermal d.
oculomotor d.
ophthalmic d.
optic nerve d.
outflow d.
parathyroid d.
peroxisomal d.

postsynaptic congenital
myasthenic d.
prechiasmal d.
presynaptic congenital
myasthenic d.
pupil d.
pupillary d.
retinal d.
Sanders d.
sensorimotor d.
spatial perception d.
supranuclear d.
tear film d.
thyroid gland d.
vascular d.
visuospatial d.
vitreoretinal d.
disorganized globe
disorientation
topographic d.
disparate retinal point
disparity, pl. **disparities**
d. angle
binocular d.
bitemporal d.
conjugate d.
fixation d.
horizontal retinal d.
retinal d.
Dispase
dispenser
Drop-Tainer d.
optical d.
4 x 4 gauze d.
dispersing lens
dispersion
chromatic d.
circle of d.
corneal endothelial pigmentary d.
peripheral retinal pigment d.
pigment d.
point of d.
d. prism
d. syndrome
displacement
image d.
macular d.
object d.
d. threshold
display
point-of-purchase d.
virtual reality head-mounted d.
(VR-HMD)
Virtual Retinal D. (VRD)
Yorktown-style designer series d.
disposable
d. cautery
d. contact lens

d. ocutome
d. trephine
disproportion
congenital fiber-type d. (CFTD)
disruption
posterior capsular zonular d.
YAG laser d.
dissecting scissors
dissection
arterial d.
open-sky d.
visco d.
dissector
Barraquer corneal d.
Berens corneal d.
Castroviejo corneal d.
channel d.
corneal knife d.
Desmarres corneal d.
Desmarres lamellar d.
Green corneal d.
d. knife
LASEK bow d.
Martinez d.
Troutman corneal d.
Troutman nonincisional lamellar d.
Wagner epiretinal membrane d.
disseminated
d. asymptomatic unilateral
neovascularization
d. choroiditis
d. intravascular coagulation
d. nonosteolytic myelomatosis
dissimilar
d. image test
d. segment
d. target test
dissipation
circle d.
dissociated
d. alkaloid
d. double hypertropia (DDHT)
d. hyperdeviation
d. position
d. vertical deviation
d. vertical divergence (DVD)
d. vertical nystagmus
dissociation
light-near d.
perception d.
d. of visual perception

distal
d. optic nerve syndrome
d. optic neuropathy
distance
angular d.
d. between centers (DBC)
d. between lenses (DBL)
d. between nasal lines (DBL)
center of rotation d.
d. correction
disk-fovea d.
egocentric fixation d.
equivalent d.
focal d. (FD)
frame papillary d.
geometric center d. (GCD)
infinite d.
intercanthal d. (ICD)
interpupillary d. (IPD)
intraocular d.
marginal reflex d. (MRD)
d. and near
object d.
pupillary d. (PD)
test d.
vertex of d.
d. vision
d. visual acuity (DVA)
d. visual performance
distant
d. direct ophthalmoscopy
d. gaze
distantial aberration
distichia, distichiasis
acquired d.
distometer
Haag-Streit d.
distortion
d. aberration
barrel d.
corneal d.
d. of lens
pin cushion d.
d. of vision
Xeroscope grid d.
distraction
d. cone
d. conus
distribution
gaussian d.
normal d.
districhiasis

NOTES

disturbance
    equilibrium d.
    sensation d.
    tear-film d.
    visual d.
diurnal
    d. fluctuation
    d. intraocular pressure measurement
    d. variation
divergence
    d. amplitude
    congenital adduction palsy with
      synergistic d.
    dissociated vertical d. (DVD)
    d. excess
    d. excess exotropia
    fusional d.
    d. insufficiency
    d. insufficiency exotropia
    negative vertical d.
    d. nystagmus
    d. paralysis
    d. paresis
    point of d.
    positive vertical d.
    relative d.
    d. reserve
    strabismus d.
    synergistic d.
    vertical d.
divergent
    d. beam
    d. cut angle
    d. deviation
    d. lens
    d. light
    d. ray
    d. squint
    d. strabismus
diverging
    d. meniscus
    d. meniscus lens
divers' spectacles
diverticulum
    lacrimal sac d.
divide-and-conquer
    d.-a.-c. method
    d.-a.-c. technique
divided spectacles
Dix foreign body spud
Dix-Hallpike test
Dixon Mann sign
Dixon-Thorpe vitreous foreign body
  forceps
Dk, DK
    oxygen permeability
      Dk IOL insertion forceps
      Dk value

Dk/L
    oxygen transmissibility
DLEK
    deep lamellar endothelial keratoplasty
DLT
    diode laser trabeculoplasty
DM
    diabetes mellitus
DME
    diabetic macular edema
DMV II contact lens remover
D/N
    at distance and at near
Doctor Ergo
Docustar fundus camera
Dodick
    D. lens-holding forceps
    D. nucleus cracker
    D. nucleus irrigating chopper
    D. photolysis
    D. photolysis probe
    D. photolysis system
Dodick-Kammann bimanual chopper
Doherty
    D. sphere
    D. sphere implant
Dohlman plug
dolichoectasia
dolichoectatic anterior cerebral artery
Döllinger tendinous ring
doll's
    d. eye
    d. eye maneuver
    d. eye reflex
    d. eye sign
    d. head maneuver
    d. head phenomenon
dolor capitis
dolorosa
    atrophia d.
D'ombrain operation
Domeboro solution
dome receptacle
dominance
    ocular d.
dominant
    d. cystoid macular dystrophy
    d. eye
    d. gene
    d. optic atrophy
    d. progressive foveal dystrophy
    d. slowly progressive macular
      dystrophy
Donaldson
    D. eye patch
    D. fundus camera
    D. stereoviewer
Donaldson-Fitzpatrick oculocutaneous
  albinism

Donders
  D. chart
  D. glaucoma
  D. law
  D. line
  D. procedure
  D. ring
Donnenfeld striae removal instrument
donor
  d. cornea
  d. eye
  d. graft
  d. material
  d. tissue
donut-cut flap
donut-shaped flap
Doppler
  D. flowmetry measure
  Hadeco intraoperative D.
  Siemens Quantum 2000 Color D.
  transcranial D. (TCD)
  D. ultrasonogram
  D. ultrasonography
  D. ultrasound
  D. velocimeter
Doran pattern stimulator
  ophthalmoscope
DORC
  Dutch Ophthalmic Research Center
  DORC backflush instrument
  DORC fast freeze cryosurgical
    system
  DORC handle
  DORC Hexon Illumination System
    1266 XII
  DORC illuminated diamond knife
  DORC International b.v.
  DORC microforceps and
    microscissors
  DORC subretinal instrument set
Dorello canal
Dorsacaine
dorsal
  d. midbrain syndrome
  d. rostral damage
  d. vermis
dorsalis
  tabes d.
Doryl
dorzolamide
  d. hydrochloride

  d. hydrochloride ophthalmic
    solution
  d. hydrochloride-timolol maleate
    ophthalmic solution
dose
  Lacrivisc unit d.
  mean episcleral heat d.
dot
  d. dystrophy
  Gunn d.
  d. hemorrhage
  Horner-Trantas d.
  lamina d.
  Marcus Gunn d.
  d. method
  Mittendorf d.
  Morgan d.
  Trantas d.
  white d.
4-dot
  Worth 4-d. (W4D)
dot-and-blot hemorrhage
dot-and-fleck retinopathy
dot-like lens
double
  d. arcuate scotoma
  d. concave (DCC)
  d. concave lens
  d. convex (DCx)
  d. convex lens
  d. dissociated hypertropia
  d. elevator palsy
  d. freeze-thaw cryopexy
  d. freeze-thaw cryotherapy
  d. graft
  d. homonymous hemianopsia
  d. irrigating/aspirating cannula
  d. lid eversion
  d. lower lid fold
  d. Maddox rod test
  d. refraction
  d. slab-off contact lens
  d. spatula
  d. tantalum clip
  d. vision (DV)
double-armed suture
double-barreled injector-aspirator
double-blind study
double-contrast visualization
double-cutting sharp cystitome
double-pronged forceps
double-quadrant testing

D

NOTES

double-row diathermy barrage
double-running penetrating keratoplasty
  suture
doublet
    achromatic d.
    Wollaston d.
doubling
    d. device
    d. of the optic disk
Doubra lens
Dougherty
    D. irrigating/aspirating unit
    D. irrigator
Douglas cilia forceps
douloureux
    tic d.
Douvas
    D. honeycombed choroiditis
    D. rotoextractor
    D. vitreous cutter
Douvas-Barraquer speculum
down
    base d.
    endothelial cell side d.
    d. to finger-counting
    D. syndrome
downbeat nystagmus
down-gaze saccade
downgrowth
    epithelial d.
    stromal d.
downward
    d. deviation
    d. gaze
    d. squint
doxycycline
Doyne
    D. familial colloid degeneration
    D. familial honeycombed choroiditis
    D. guttate iritis
    D. honeycombed choroidopathy
    D. honeycombed degeneration
    D. honeycombed dystrophy
    D. syndrome
D&Q
    deep and quiet
DR
    diabetic retinopathy
Draeger
    D. forceps
    D. high vacuum erysiphake
    D. modified keratome
    D. tonometer
dragged
    d. disk
    d. macula
    d. retina
dragging
    macular d.

    optic disk d.
    retinal d.
drain
    Mentor precut d.
drainage
    d. angle
    aqueous humor d.
    cerebral venous d.
    indirect argon laser d.
    lacrimal d.
    d. of lacrimal gland
    d. of lacrimal gland operation
    d. of lacrimal sac
    d. of lacrimal sac operation
    lymphatic d.
    quadrantic sclerectomy with
     internal d.
    sclerotomy with d.
    subretinal fluid d.
    tear d.
    uveovertex d.
Drance hemorrhage
drape
    1021 d.
    Alcon disposable d.
    Barrier d.
    Blair head d.
    Eye-Pak II d.
    Hough d.
    miniophthalmic d.
    3M Steri-Drape d.
    Opraflex d.
    Pro-Ophtha d.
    Steri-Drape d.
    Surgikos disposable d.
    Visi-Drape Elite ophthalmic d.
    Visi-Drape mini aperture d.
    Visi-Drape mini incise d.
    Visiflex d.
Drechslera
dressing
    Blenderm tape d.
    bolus d.
    Borsch d.
    collodion d.
    compression d.
    crepe bandage d.
    Elastoplast d.
    Expo Bubble d.
    eye pad d.
    fluff d.
    fluffed gauze d.
    d. forceps
    Harman eye d.
    lens d.
    moistened fine mesh gauze d.
    monocular d.
    pressure patch d.
    Pro-Ophtha d.

ribbon gauze d.
saline-saturated wool d.
sterile adhesive bubble d.
Telfa plastic film d.
tie-over Sellotape d.
tulle gras d.
wet d.
wool saturated in saline d.

Drews
    D. angled cystitome
    D. capsule polisher
    D. cataract needle
    D. cilia forceps
    D. inclined prism
    D. irrigating/aspirating unit
    D. irrigating cannula
    D. lens
    D. syndrome

Drews-Knolle reverse irrigating vectis
Drews-Rosenbaum
    D.-R. iris retractor
    D.-R. irrigating/aspirating unit

Drews-Sato
    D.-S. suture-pickup hook
    D.-S. suture-pickup spatula
    D.-S. tying forceps

drift
    d. movement
    post saccadic d.

drill
    ophthalmic d.

drippings
    candlewax d.

droop
    brow d.
    lid d.

drooping of eyelid
droopy lid
droperidol
dropout
    acinar d.
    nerve fiber layer d.
    pigmentary d.
    retinal pigment epithelium d.

dropped-socket appearance
dropper
    eye d.
    undine d.

drops
    AC eye d.
    Acular d.
    Akwa Tears lubricant eye d.

Allerest eye d.
Allergy D.
Alomide d.
Bausch & Lomb Moisture Eyes
    Protect Lubricant Eye D.
betamethasone phosphate eye d.
Bion Tears eye d.
Boston Advance reconditioning d.
Boston Rewetting D.
chemotherapy d.
CIBA Vision lens d.
cidofovir eye d.
Claris Rewetting D.
Clerz 2 Lubricating and
    Rewetting D.
Clerz Plus lens d.
Collyrium eye d.
Comfort eye d.
Complete Blink-N-Clean Lens D.
Complete Lubricating and
    Rewetting D.
Computer Eye D.
corticosteroid d.
Dry Eyes lubricant eye d.
eye d.
Focus Lens D.
GenTeal Mild lubricant eye d.
hypertonic d.
HypoTears Select lubricant eye d.
Lens Drops lubricating and
    rewetting d.
Lens Plus rewetting d.
lubricating d.
Mallazine eye d.
Moisture ophthalmic d.
Neosporin d.
Opcon Maximum Strength
    Allergy D.
Opti-Free Rewetting D.
Optimum by Lobob Wetting and
    Rewetting D.
Opti-One Rewetting D.
Optique 1 Eye D.
placebo eye d.
Prefrin Liquifilm Vasoconstrictor
    and Lubricant Eye D.
proparacaine ophthalmic d.
Refresh Endura eye d.
Refresh Liquigel eye d.
Refresh Plus lubricant eye d.
Refresh Tears eye d.
ReNu Rewetting D.

D

NOTES

drops *(continued)*
    Rondec D.
    Sensitive Eyes d.
    Similasan eye d.
    sympathomimetic eye d.
    Tears Again eye d.
    Tears Naturale Forte eye d.
    Tears Naturale Free eye d.
    Tears Naturale II Polyquad eye d.
    TheraTears lubricant eye d.
    trifluridine eye d.
    Twenty/Twenty d.
    Viva-Drops eye d.
Drop-Tainers
    Alcaine D.-T.
    D.-T. dispenser
droxifilcon A
Drualt
    bundle of D.
    D. bundle
drug
    d. abuse retinopathy
    adrenergic d.
    amphiphilic d.
    antiadrenergic d.
    anticataract d.
    anticholinergic d.
    cataractogenic d.
    cholinergic d.
    immunosuppressive d.
    d. interaction
    light-activated d.
    neuroloptic d.
    neuromuscular blocking d.
    neuromuscular disorder-causing d.
    nonsteroidal antiinflammatory d.
    ophthalmic d.
    parasympatholytic d.
    parasympathomimetic d.
    sulfa d.
    sympatholytic d.
    systemic d.
    topical d.
drug-induced
    d.-i. cataract
    d.-i. cicatrizing conjunctivitis
    d.-i. glaucoma
    d.-i. nystagmus
    d.-i. ptosis
drum
    optokinetic d.
drusen
    basal laminar d.
    buried disk d.
    confluent d.
    diffuse d.
    disk d.
    equatorial d.
    familial d.

    giant d.
    hard d.
    intrapapillary d.
    macular d.
    nerve head d.
    optic disk d.
    optic nerve head d. (ONHD)
    d. of optic papilla
    retinal d.
    soft d.
    visible d.
DRVS
    Diabetic Retinopathy Vitrectomy Study
dry
    d. ARMD
    D. Eye questionnaire
    D. Eyes
    D. Eyes lubricant eye drops
    D. Eyes lubricant ointment
    D. Eyes solution
    d. eye syndrome (DES)
    d. eye test (DET)
    D. Eye Therapy Solution
    d. fold
    d. senile degenerative maculopathy
    d. senile macular degeneration
    d. spot
    D. Therapy
Drysdale nucleus manipulator
dry-shelled cataract
Drysol cream
DS
    diopter sphere
DS-9 needle
D-shaped keratometric reflection
DS-ICGA
    digital subtraction indocyanine green
    angiography
dual
    d. aspiration pump system
    d. lens
Dualoop
Dual-Wet
Duane
    D. accommodation chart
    D. classification
    D. classification of squint
    D. retraction syndrome
    D. retractor
duboisii
    Histoplasma d.
Duchenne
    D. dystrophy
    D. paralysis
Duchenne-Erb paralysis
Ducournau fine gripping forceps
duct
    ampulla of lacrimal d.
    canalicular d.

catheterization of lacrimal d.
catheterization of lacrimonasal d.
excretory d.
Gartner d.
lacrimal d.
lacrimonasal d.
meibomian d.
nasal d.
nasolacrimal d. (NLD)
probing lacrimonasal d.
stenon d.
tear d.
d. T-tube lacrimal
ductal orifice obliteration
duction
forced d.
full versions and d.'s
ocular d.
passive d.
d. test
d.'s and versions (D&V)
vertical d.
ductional
ductus
d. lacrimales
d. nasolacrimalis
Duddell membrane
Duke-Elder
D.-E. lamp
D.-E. operation
Dulaney
D. LASIK Marker
D. lens
Dunnington operation
duochrome test
Duo-Flow
Duolube
Duotrak blade
DuoVisc viscoelastic system
duplex scan
duplicity theory of vision
Dupuy-Dutemps
D.-D. dacryocystorhinostomy dye
test
D.-D. dacryostomy
D.-D. operation
dura
DURAcare II
Duraclose scleral clip
dural
d. arteriovenous malformation
d. carotid cavernous fistula

d. cavernous sinus fistula
d. sheath
d. shunt
d. shunt syndrome
Duralone
Duralube
Duramist Plus
Duranest
D. HCl
D. HCl with epinephrine
Durasoft
D. 2 ColorBlends lens
D. 3 Optifit Toric Colorblends
contact lens
D. 2 Optifit Toric for light eyes
contact lens
Duratears Naturale
Dura-T lens
Durazyme
Duredge knife
Durette external laser shield
Durham tonometer
Duricef
Durr operation
DUSN
diffuse unilateral subacute neuroretinitis
dusting
fibrin d.
iris pigment d.
dust-like opacity
Dutch
D. Ophthalmic Research Center
(DORC)
D. Ophthalmic USA
Dutcher body
Duverger-Velter operation
DV
double vision
D&V
ductions and versions
DVA
distance visual acuity
DVCPRO digital video recorder
DVD
dissociated vertical divergence
DWCL
daily-wear contact lens
Dwelle Ophthalmic Solution
DWI/MRI
diffusion-weighted imaging/magnetic
resonance imaging
dyclonine

D

NOTES

143

dye

Alizarin Red S d.
Cardio-Green d.
chemofluorescent d.
Diamond D.
d. disappearance test (DDT)
fluorescein d.
Haag-Streit fluorescein d.
indocyanine green d.
materials primary d.
pooling of d.
tricarbocyanine d.
vital d.
d. yellow laser

Dyer

D. nomogram system of lens ordering
D. nomogram system of ordering contact lens

Dyggve disease
Dymadon
Dynacin
dynamic

d. accommodation insufficiency
d. refraction
d. scanning laser ophthalmoscopy
d. stabilization
d. strabismus
d. visual acuity

Dynosol
Dyonics syringe injector
dysacusia
dysaptation, dysadaptation
dysautonomia

familial autonomic d.

dyscephalic

d. syndrome
d. syndrome of François

dyschromasia
dyschromatopsia

acquired d.
cerebral d.
congenital d.

dysconjugate gaze
dyscoria
dyscrasia

retinopathy of blood d.

dyscrinic rhinitis
dysesthesia

glaucoma filtering bleb d.

dysfunction

anterior visual pathway d.
brain d.
brainstem d.
cerebellar d.
chorioretinopathy and pituitary d. (CPD)
cone d.
familial autonomic d.

foveal outer retinal d.
intraorbital nerve d.
isolated oculomotor nerve d.
meibomian gland d. (MGD)
minimal brain d.
neurologic d.
oblique d.
oculosympathetic d.
optic nerve d.
photoreceptor d.
pontomesencephalic d.
primary cone d.
rod-cone d.

dysgenesis

corneal d.
iridocorneal mesodermal d.
mesenchymal d.
mesodermal d.
posterior amorphous corneal d.

dysharmonious correspondence
dyskeratosis

benign d.
d. congenita
congenital d.
hereditary benign intraepithelial d.
intraepithelial d.
malignant d.

dyslexia

attentional d.
central d.
deep d.
endogenous d.
hemianopic d.
neglect d.
surface d.

dysmegalopsia
dysmetria

flutter d.
ocular d.
saccadic d.

dysmetropsia
dysmorphopsia
dysopia, dysopsia

d. algera

dysoric retinopathy
dysplasia

chiasmal d.
conjunctival d.
corneal d.
encephaloophthalmic d.
fibromuscular d.
fibrous d.
forebrain d.
hereditary renal-retinal d.
macular d.
OAV d.
oculoauricular d.
oculoauriculovertebral d.
oculodentodigital d.

oculovertebral d.
ODD d.
ophthalmomandibulomelic d.
optic disk d.
optic nerve d.
orodigitofacial d.
retinal d.
septooptic d.
vitreoretinal d.

dysplastic
d. coloboma
d. retina

Dysport
dysproteinemic retinopathy
dysthyroid
d. ophthalmopathy
d. optic neuropathy
d. orbitopathy

dysthyroidism
dystonia
blepharospasm-oromandibular d.
focal d.

dystopia
d. canthorum
foveal d.
orbital d.

dystrophia
d. adiposa corneae
d. endothelialis corneae
d. epithelialis corneae

dystrophica
elastosis d.
myotonia d.

dystrophy
adult-onset foveomacular d. (AOFMD)
amorphous corneal d.
anterior basement membrane d. (ABMD)
anular macular d.
Avellino d.
basement membrane d.
benign concentric anular macular d.
Best vitelliform macular d.
Biber-Haab-Dimmer corneal d.
Bietti corneal retinal d.
Bietti crystalline corneoretinal d.
Bücklers I, II, III d.
butterfly macular d.
butterfly-shaped pigment epithelial d.
central areolar choroidal d.

central areolar pigment epithelial d.
central cloudy corneal d.
central cloudy parenchymatous d.
central crystalline d.
central discoid corneal d.
central pigmentary retinal d.
central speckled corneal d.
cerebellar ataxia-cone d.
choroidal d.
choroidoretinal d.
Cogan microcystic d.
cone d.
cone-rod d. (CRD)
congenital hereditary endothelial corneal d.
congenital muscular d.
congenital myotonic d.
d. of cornea
corneal endothelial guttate d.
corneal fleck d.
corneal guttate d.
corneal stromal d.
corneal vortex d.
crystalline corneal d.
cystoid macular d.
deep filiform d.
deep parenchymatous d.
dominant cystoid macular d.
dominant progressive foveal d.
dominant slowly progressive macular d.
dot d.
Doyne honeycombed d.
Duchenne d.
ectatic corneal d.
endothelial cell d.
endothelial corneal d. (ECD)
epithelial basement membrane d.
Favre d.
Fehr macular d.
fenestrated sheen macular d.
filiform d.
fingerprint corneal d.
flecked corneal d.
Fleischer d.
foveomacular vitelliform d.
Franceschetti d.
François d.
François-Neetens d.
Fuchs combined corneal d.
Fuchs endothelial corneal d.
Fuchs epithelial corneal d.

D

NOTES

dystrophy *(continued)*
    Fuchs epithelial-endothelial d.
    furrow d.
    gelatino-lattice corneal d.
    gelatinous d.
    Goldmann-Favre d.
    granular corneal d.
    Grayson-Wilbrandt anterior
     corneal d.
    Groenouw corneal d.
    Groenouw type I, II d.
    gutter d.
    hereditary anterior membrane d.
    hereditary epithelial corneal d.
    hereditary hemorrhagic macular d.
    hereditary vitelliform d.
    honeycomb d.
    infantile neuroaxonal d. (INAD)
    juvenile corneal epithelial d.
    keratoconus d.
    lattice corneal d.
    lattice corneal d. type IIIA
     (LCDIIIA)
    Lefler-Wadsworth-Sidbury foveal d.
    Lisch corneal d.
    macroreticular d.
    macular corneal d.
    Maeder-Danis d.
    map d.
    map-dot corneal d.
    map-dot-fingerprint corneal
     epithelial d.
    marginal crystalline d.
    MDF corneal d.
    Meesman epithelial corneal d.
    Meesman juvenile epithelial d.
    microcystic corneal d.
    microcystic epithelial d.
    muscular d.
    myotonic d.
    North Carolina macular d.
    oculocerebrorenal d.
    oculopharyngeal d.
    ophthalmoplegic muscular d.
    parenchymatous corneal d.
    pattern d.
    pericentral rod-cone d.

    pigment epithelial d.
    Pillat d.
    polymorphous d.
    posterior amorphous corneal d.
    posterior polymorphic d. (of
     cornea) (PPMD)
    posterior polymorphous corneal d.
    progressive cone d.
    progressive cone-rod d.
    progressive foveal d.
    progressive macular d.
    progressive tapetochoroidal d.
    pseudoendothelial d.
    pseudoinflammatory macular d.
    Reis-Bücklers ring-shaped d.
    Reis-Bücklers superficial corneal d.
    reticular d.
    retinal cone d.
    retinal pigmentary d.
    ring-like corneal d.
    ring-shaped d.
    rod-cone d.
    Salzmann nodular corneal d.
    Schlichting d.
    Schnyder crystalline corneal d.
    sheen d.
    Sjögren reticular d.
    Sorsby pseudoinflammatory
     macular d.
    speckled corneal d.
    Stargardt d.
    Stocker-Holt d.
    Stocker-Holt-Schneider d.
    stromal corneal d.
    tapetochoroidal d.
    Thiel-Behnke corneal d.
    unilateral corneal lattice d.
    vitelliform macular d.
    vitelliruptive macular d.
    vitreotapetoretinal d.
    vortex corneal d.
    d. of Waardenburg-Jonkers
    Wagner vitreoretinal d.
    X-linked cone d.
dysversion
    congenital d.

E

E Carpine
E chart
E Clips prescription computer lens
E game
E syndrome
E test

E′

esophoria
apolipoprotein E′
Illiterate E′

E¹

esophoria at near

500e

Model A-Scan DGH 500e

EA-290

Toctron EA-290

Eagle FlexPlug
EaglePlug tapered-shaft punctum plug
EagleVision Freeman punctum plug
Eales disease
early

e. antigen
e. lens opacity
E. Manifest Glaucoma Trial (EMGT)
e. mature cataract
e. postoperative suture adjustment (EPSA)
e. receptor potential
e. receptor potential mottling
E. Treatment Diabetic Retinopathy Study (ETDRS)
E. Treatment for Retinopathy of Prematurity Study (ETROP)

early-onset

e.-o. myope
e.-o. myopia

early-phase reaction
EAS-1000 anterior eye segment analysis system
easily everted upper eyelid
Easterman visual function
Easy Eyes
Easyloupes

Oculus E.

Eaton-Lambert syndrome
EBAA

Eye Bank Association of America

Eber needle-holder forceps
EBV

Epstein-Barr virus
EBV nuclear antigen

EBV-associated antigen
EC-5000 excimer laser

ECC

extracapsular cataract

ECCE

extracapsular cataract extraction

eccentric

e. ablation
e. fixation
e. gaze
e. gaze-holding
e. limitation
e. photorefraction
e. vision

eccentricity

angle of e.

ecchymosis of eyelid
ECD

endothelial cell density
endothelial corneal dystrophy

ECF

epicanthic fold

Echinococcus

E. cyst
E. granulosus

echinophthalmia
Echodide
echogram

intraoperative B-scan e.

echography

kinetic e.
ocular e.
orbital e.
quantitative e.
topographic e.

echoophthalmogram
echoophthalmography
EchoScan by Nidek
echothiophate

e. iodide
e. pholine

Eckardt

E. Heme-Stopper instrument
E. temporary keratoprosthesis

eclamptic hypertensive retinopathy
eclipse

e. amblyopia
e. blindness
e. retinopathy
e. scotoma

ECM

extracellular matrix

Econochlor
Econopred

E. Ophthalmic
E. Plus

E

ECP
> endoscopic cyclophotocoagulation
> eosinophil cationic protein

ectasia, ectasis
> corneal e.
> iris e.
> e. of sclera
> scleral e.
> stromal e.

ectatic
> e. cornea
> e. corneal dystrophy
> e. dilation
> e. marginal degeneration

ecthyma
> e. contagiosum
> e. gangrenosum

ectiris

ectochoroidea

ectocornea

ectopia
> cilia e.
> e. iridis
> e. lentis
> e. lentis et pupillae
> e. maculae
> macular e.
> posterior pituitary e.
> e. pupillae congenita

ectopic
> e. eyelash
> e. tissue

ectropion, ectropium
> Adams operation for e.
> atonic e.
> Cibis e.
> e. cicatriceum
> cicatricial e.
> complex e.
> congenital e.
> eyelid e.
> flaccid e.
> inflammatory e.
> involutional senile e.
> e. irides
> e. iridis
> lid e.
> e. luxurians
> mechanical e.
> medial e.
> paralytic e.
> e. paralyticum
> pigment layer e.
> punctal e.
> e. sarcomatosum
> senescent e.
> senile e.
> e. senilis
> spastic e.

> e. spasticum
> tarsal e.
> e. uveae

ectropionize

eczematoid blepharitis

eczematosa
> ophthalmia e.

eczematosus
> pannus e.

eczematous
> e. conjunctivitis
> e. pannus

ED
> effective diameter
> epithelial defect

edema
> aphakic cystoid macular e.
> Berlin retinal e.
> boggy e.
> brawny e.
> central e.
> cerebral e.
> choroidal e.
> conjunctival e.
> e. of cornea
> corneal e.
> cystoid macular e. (CME)
> diabetic macular e. (DME)
> disk e.
> endothelial cell e.
> epithelial e.
> eyelid e.
> focal vasogenic e.
> foveal e.
> graft e.
> hereditary corneal e.
> high altitude cerebral e. (HACE)
> ischemic e.
> Iwanoff retinal e.
> lid e.
> macular e.
> microcystic e.
> mucinous e.
> optic disk e.
> e. of optic disk
> periorbital e.
> periretinal e.
> phakic cystoid macular e.
> pseudocystoid macular e.
> Randomized Trial of Acetazolamide
>   for Uveitis-Associated Cystoid
>   Macular E.
> retinal e.
> Stellwag brawny e.
> stromal e.
> subconjunctival e.
> tractional diabetic macular e.
>   (TDME)

edge
    CeeOn E.
    e. coating
    e. contour
    epithelial rolled e.
    fimbriated e.
    e. glare
    E. III hydrogel contact lens
    e. stand-off
EdgeAhead
    E. crescent knife
    E. microsurgical knife
    E. phaco slit knife
edge-light pupil cycle time
edger
edging of spectacle lens
Edinger
    E. fiber
    E. nucleus
Edinger-Westphal nucleus
edipism
edrophonium
    e. chloride
    e. chloride test
EDSS
    Expanded Disability Status Scale
EDTA
    ethylenediaminetetraacetate
Edwards syndrome
EEG
    electroencephalography
effect
    Abney e.
    autokinetic e.
    beneficial e.
    blood oxygenation level-
      dependent e.
    BOLD e.
    Bracken e.
    Braid e.
    cat's eye e.
    chromatic induction e.
    copper-wire e.
    Cotton e.
    experimental secondary e.
    Faden e.
    histopathologic e.
    lens flexure e.
    E.'s of Light Reduction on
      Retinopathy of Prematurity
    Lythgoe e.
    McCollough e.

    Mizuo-Nakamura e.
    muscarinic cholinergic side e.
    myotonic dystrophy e.
    neuromuscular e.
    ocular motility e.
    optical side e.
    pantoscopic e.
    prismatic e.
    Pulfrich e.
    pupillary e.
    Purkinje e.
    radiation e.
    Raman e.
    silver wire e.
    Stiles-Crawford e.
    sunburst e.
    telephoto e.
    threshold e.
    Tyndall e.
    venturi e.
    Zeeman e.
effective diameter (ED)
effectiveness
efferent
    e. fiber
    e. nerve
efficacy of cyclosporine
efficiency
    visual e. (VE)
effusion
    choroidal e.
    ciliochoroidal e.
    e. light pipe
    serous choroidal e. (SCE)
    uveal e.
Eflone
Efricel
EGb 761
Egger line
egilops
Egna-Neumarkt Study
egocentric fixation distance
Egyptian
    E. conjunctivitis
    E. ophthalmia
Ehlers-Danlos
    E.-D. syndrome
    E.-D. syndrome VI, VII
Ehrhardt lid forceps
Ehrlich-Türck line
Ehrmann test
eiconometer (*var. of* eikonometer)

E

NOTES

eidoptometry
eight-ball
    e.-b. hemorrhage
    e.-b. hyphema
eighth cranial nerve
Eikenella corrodens
eikonometer, eiconometer
Eisenmenger syndrome
EKC
    epidemic keratoconjunctivitis
EKV
    erythrokeratodermia variabilis
elaioides
    degeneratio spherularis e.
E-LASIK
    epithelial laser-assisted intrastromal
    keratomileusis
elastic pseudoxanthoma
elasticum
    pseudoxanthoma e. (PXE)
    xanthoma e.
elastodysplasia
elastodystrophy
elastoid degeneration
Elastoplast
    E. bandage
    E. dressing
    E. eye occlusor
elastorrhexis
elastosis
    e. dystrophica
    senescent e.
    senile e.
elastotic band keratopathy
El Bayadi-Kajiura lens
elbow
    Hofmann e.
Eldridge-Green lamp
electric
    e. light blindness
    e. ophthalmia
    e. retinopathy
    e. shock cataract
electrica
    cataracta e.
    ophthalmia e.
electrocauterizer
electrocautery
    Fine micropoint e.
    Geiger e.
    Hildreth e.
    Mentor wet-field e.
    Mira e.
    Mueller e.
    ophthalmic e.
    Op-Temp disposable e.
    Parker-Heath e.
    Prince e.
    Rommel e.

    Rommel-Hildreth e.
    Scheie e.
    Todd e.
    Valilab e.
    von Graefe e.
    Wadsworth-Todd e.
    wet-field e.
    Ziegler e.
electrocoagulation
electrode
    Berens e.
    Burian-Allen contact lens e.
    Cibis e.
    coagulating e.
    corneal contact lens e.
    cyclodiathermy e.
    diathermy e.
    gold disk Grass e.
    Gradle e.
    Grass e.
    Guyton e.
    Kronfeld e.
    Pischel e.
    Schepens e.
    Walker e.
    Weve e.
electrodiaphake
electroencephalogram
electroencephalography (EEG)
electroepilation
electrokeratotome
    Castroviejo e.
electromagnetic
    e. energy
    e. radiation
    e. removal of foreign body
    e. scleral search coil
    e. spectrum
electromucotome
    Steinhauser e.
electron
    e. interferometer
    e. interferometry
    e. microscope
    e. microscopic characteristic
electronegative
electronic tonometer
electronystagmogram (ENG)
electronystagmograph
electronystagmography (ENG)
electrooculogram (EOG)
    monocular e.
electrooculograph
electrooculography (EOG)
electroparacentesis
electroperimeter
electroretinogram (ERG)
    cone b-wave implicit time e.
    flash e. (fERG)

flicker e.
focal e.
full-field e.
multifocal e.
pattern e.
pattern-evoked e. (PERG)
peak latencies of pattern e.
rod e.
topographical e.
electroretinograph
Ganzfeld e.
electroretinography (ERG)
foveal cone e.
multifocal e. (MFE)
topographic e.
electrostatic interaction
elegans
Caenorhabditis e.
element
encircling e.
Kollmorgen e.
Mira encircling e.
retinal e.
elephantiasis oculi
Eletrohome Marquee 8500 Ultra graphics projector
elevation
e. angle
congenital optic disk e.
disk e.
immediate e.
parafoveal serous retinal e.
sensory e.
e. topography
e. topography map
elevator
Desmarres lid e.
Freer periosteal e.
Joseph periosteal e.
e. muscle
e. palsy
Sayre e.
Tenzel e.
Eliasoph lid retractor
Elimite
Eliprodil
ELISA
enzyme-linked immunosorbent assay
ELISA antibody
ELK
endothelial lamellar keratoplasty
Ellingson syndrome

Elliot
E. corneal trephine
E. operation
E. sign
E. trephine handle
ellipse
superimposed e.
ellipsoidal back surface
ellipsometer
retinal e.
elliptic
e. nystagmus
e. pupil
elliptical
e. nystagmus
e. trephination
Ellis
E. astigmatism marker
E. foreign body needle
E. foreign body spud
E. foreign body spud needle probe
E. needle holder
El-Naggar
E.-N. recession muscle hook
E.-N. resection double hook
Elrex
Elschnig
E. blepharorrhaphy
E. body
E. canthorrhaphy
E. canthorrhaphy operation
E. capsule forceps
E. cataract knife
E. central iridectomy
E. conjunctivitis
E. corneal knife
E. cyclodialysis spatula
E. extrusion needle
E. fixation forceps
E. keratoplasty
E. pearl
E. pterygium knife
E. refractor
E. retractor
E. spoon
E. spot
E. syndrome
E. trephine
Elschnig-O'Brien forceps
Elschnig-O'Connor fixation forceps
Elschnig-Weber loupe
Ely operation

E

NOTES

EM-1000 specular microscope
EMA
   epithelial membrane antigen
Emadine
embolic retinopathy
embolism
   retinal e.
embryonal
   e. carcinoma
   e. epithelial cyst of iris
   e. medulloepithelioma
   e. medulloepithelioma of ciliary body
   e. nuclear cataract
   e. tumor of ciliary body
embryonic
   e. cataract
   e. fixation syndrome
   e. plate
embryopathic cataract
embryotoxon
   anterior e.
   posterior e.
Emcee lens
emedastine
   e. difumarate
   e. difurmarate ophthalmic solution
emergence
   angle of e.
emergency light reflex
emergent
   e. ray
   e. ray of light
Emerson one-piece segment bifocal
Emery lens
EMGT
   Early Manifest Glaucoma Trial
EMI digital imaging system
emissarial canal
emittance
   radiant e.
emmetrope
emmetropia
emmetropic
emmetropization process
EMP
   epiretinal membrane proliferation
emphysema
   e. of conjunctiva
   e. of orbit
   orbital e.
   subconjunctival e.
Empire needle
empty
   optically e.
   e. sella
   e. sella syndrome
Emsley reduced eye
E-Mycin

encanthis
encapsulated bleb
encephalitis
   e. periaxialis concentrica
   e. periaxialis diffusa
   Schilder e.
Encephalitozoon hellem
encephalocele
   basal e.
   orbital e.
   transsphenoidal e.
encephalofacial angiomatosis
encephalomyelitis
encephalomyelopathy
   subacute necrotizing e.
encephalomyopathy
encephaloophthalmic dysplasia
encephalopathy
   hypertensive e.
   lead e.
   Leigh e.
   Wernicke e.
encephalotrigeminal angiomatosis
encircling
   e. band
   e. band for scleral buckle
   e. element
   e. explant
   e. of globe operation
   e. implant
   e. polyethylene tube
   e. of scleral buckle operation
   e. silicone buckle
Encore monthly disposable contact lens
endarteritis obliterans
end-gaze nystagmus
end-gripping forceps with standard jaw
endocapsular
   e. balloon
   e. phacoemulsification
endocrine
   e. exophthalmos
   e. lid retraction
   e. myopathy
   e. ophthalmopathy
endocrine-inactive adenoma
endocryopexy
endocryoretinopexy
endodiathermy coagulation
endogenous
   e. bacterial endophthalmitis
   e. dyslexia
   e. uveitis
endoillumination
endoilluminator
   Grieshaber e.
endokeratoplasty
endolase
   neuron-specific e. (NSE)

endolaser
    e. coagulation
    diode e.
    e. probe tip
endolenticular phacoemulsification
endonasal laser dacryocystorhinostomy
  (ENL-DCR)
endoneural cell
endonucleus
Endo Optiks MicroProbe
endophlebitis of retinal vein
endophotocoagulation
    argon laser e.
    diode e.
endophthalmitis
    Acanthamoeba e.
    aseptic e.
    bacterial e.
    bleb-associated e.
    Candida e.
    candidal e.
    chronic e.
    endogenous bacterial e.
    exogenous e.
    fungal e.
    granulomatous e.
    infectious e.
    Klebsiella e.
    latent e.
    metastatic e.
    nocardial e.
    e. ophthalmia nodosa
    Ovadendron sulphureo-ochraceum e.
    e. phacoallergica
    phacoanaphylactic e.
    e. phacoanaphylactica
    phacoantigenic e.
    pneumococcal e.
    postoperative e.
    Propionibacterium acnes e.
    sterile e.
    systemic bacterial e.
    toxocariasis e.
    traumatic e.
    E. Vitrectomy Study (EVS)
endophthalmodonesis
endophytum
    glioma e.
endoplasmic reticulum
EndoProbe
endoresection
endoretinal

endoscope
    Insight 4000 e.
    MicroProbe integrated laser e.
    ophthalmic e.
endoscopic
    e. cyclophotocoagulation (ECP)
    e. laser-assisted
    dacryocystorhinostomy
    e. laser dacryocystorhinostomy
    e. raking
Endosol Extra
endothelial
    e. bleb
    e. cell
    e. cell analysis
    e. cell basement membrane
    e. cell count
    e. cell density (ECD)
    e. cell dystrophy
    e. cell edema
    e. cell side down
    e. cell surface of cornea
    e. corneal dystrophy (ECD)
    e. decompensation
    e. exudate
    iridocorneal e. (ICE)
    e. lamellar keratoplasty (ELK)
    e. plaque
    e. rejection line
    vesiculosus linear e.
endothelialitis
endotheliitis
    diffuse e.
    disciform e.
    HSV e.
    linear e.
    peripheral e.
endothelioma
    Sidler-Huguenin e.
endotheliopathy
    autoimmune corneal e.
    idiopathic corneal e.
    progressive herpetic corneal e.
endothelitis
endothelium
    e. camerae anterioris bulbi
    corneal e.
    monolayered e.
    e. oculi
endotracheal
    e. anesthesia
    e. tube

E

NOTES

endovascular closure
EndoView Sapphire Lens
end piece
end-point
    e.-p. color
    e.-p. nystagmus
end-position nystagmus
Endrate
endrysone
energy
    electromagnetic e.
    radiant e.
enflurane
enfolding
ENG
    electronystagmogram
    electronystagmography
engine
    Silicon Graphics Crimson
    Reality E.
engorgement
    conjunctival vascular e.
    episcleral vascular e.
    venous e.
enhancement
    astigmatic keratotomy e.
Enhydrina schistosa
enlargement
    blind spot e.
    corneal e.
    orbital e.
ENL-DCR
    endonasal laser dacryocystorhinostomy
enophthalmia
enophthalmos, enophthalmus
    senescent e.
    e. wedge implant
enoxacin
Enroth sign
Enterobacter aerogenes
entero-Behçet disease
Enterococcus faecalis
enteropathica
    acrodermatitis e.
entochoroidea
entocornea
entophthalmia
entopic foveal avascular zone
  measurement
entoptic phenomenon
entoptoscope
entoptoscopy
entoretina
entrance pupil
entrapment
    extraocular muscle e.
    pupillary e.
entropion, entropium
    acquired e.

    acute spastic e.
    atonic e.
    Celsus-Hotz e.
    Cibis e.
    e. cicatriceum
    cicatricial e.
    congenital e.
    eyelid e.
    e. forceps
    Hotz e.
    involutional lower eyelid e.
    involutional senile e.
    marginal e.
    noncicatricial e.
    Poulard e.
    senescent e.
    senile e.
    spastic e.
    e. spasticum
    e. uveae
    uveal e.
entropionize
entry
    implant e.
enucleate
enucleated
enucleation
    e. of eyeball operation
    Foix e.
    e. scissors
    e. scoop
    e. spoon
    whole-globe e.
    e. wire snare
enucleator
    Banner snare e.
    Botvin-Bradford e.
    Bradford snare e.
    Castroviejo snare e.
    Foster snare e.
    snare e.
Enuclene
env gene
environment
    telepresence e.
Envision TD ophthalmic drug delivery
  device
enzymatic
    e. cleaner
    e. cleaner for extended wear
    e. digestion
    e. galactosemia
    e. glaucoma
    e. sclerostomy
    e. zonulolysis
enzyme
    antioxidant e.
    autologous plasmin e.
    e. cleaner

e. defect
e. glaucoma
proteolytic e.
enzyme-linked immunosorbent assay (ELISA)
EOG
electrooculogram
electrooculography
EOM
extraocular movement
extraocular muscle
EOMI
extraocular movement intact
eosinophil cationic protein (ECP)
eosinophilic
e. globule
e. granuloma
e. intranuclear inclusion body
e. reaction
e. response
eosin-Y cell
ependymoma tumor
ephaptic transmission
epiblepharon
epibulbar
e. dermoid cyst
e. Fordyce nodule
e. lesion
e. limbal dermoid choristoma
e. osseous choristoma
e. tissue
epicanthal
e. correction
e. inversus
e. skin fold
epicanthic fold (ECF)
epicanthus
e. blepharophimosis
e. caruncle
e. inversus
e. palpebralis
e. supraciliaris
e. tarsalis
epicapsular lens star
Epicar
epicauma
epicenter
epiciliary proliferative tissue
Epic laser
epicorneascleritis
epidemic
e. blindness

e. conjunctivitis
e. keratoconjunctivitis (EKC)
e. typhus
epidermal inclusion cyst
epidermidis
Staphylococcus e.
epidermis
Staphylococcus e.
epidermoid
e. carcinoma
e. cyst
epidermolysis
e. bullosa
e. bullosa acquisita
e. bullosa simplex
epidiascope
Epifrin
epikeratophakia
epikeratophakic keratoplasty
epikeratoplasty
e. lenticule
tectonic e.
epikeratoprosthesis
epilation
epilator
epilens
epileptic nystagmus
E-Pilo
epimacular
e. membrane
e. proliferation
epimysium
Epinal
Epinastine
epinephrine
e. bitartrate
e. borate
dipivalyl e.
Duranest HCl with e.
e. HCl
lidocaine with e.
Lidoject-1 with e.
Marcaine HCl with e.
Nervocaine with e.
e. and pilocarpine
pilocarpine and e.
Sensorcaine with e.
Xylocaine with e.
epinephryl borate
epinucleus
epipapillaris
membrana e.

NOTES

epipapillary membrane
Epi-peeler
 Sloane E.-p.
epiphora
 atonic e.
epiretinal
 e. membrane (ERM)
 e. membrane formation
 e. membrane proliferation (EMP)
 e. membrane traction
episclera
episcleral
 e. angioma
 e. arterial circle
 e. artery
 e. blood vessel
 e. circulation
 e. explant
 e. eye plaque
 e. fibrosis
 e. hemangioma
 e. injection
 e. lamina
 e. nevus
 e. osteocartilaginous choristoma
 e. rheumatic nodule
 e. scarring
 e. space
 e. tissue
 e. vascular engorgement
 e. vein
 e. venous pressure (EVP)
episclerale
 spatium e.
 venae e.
episcleritis, episclerotitis
 childhood e.
 circumscribed e.
 gouty e.
 e. multinodularis
 nodular e.
 e. partialis fugax
 e. periodica fugax
 simple e.
 syphilitic e.
episode
 ischemic e.
 stroke-like e.
episodic unilateral mydriasis
episphaeria
 Fusarium e.
epitarsus pterygium
epithelia (*pl. of* epithelium)
epithelial
 e. adrenochrome deposition
 e. barrier
 e. basement layer
 e. basement membrane
 e. basement membrane disease

 e. basement membrane dystrophy
 e. bedewing
 e. bleb
 e. bleb disorder
 e. bulla
 e. cell
 e. débridement
 e. debris
 e. defect (ED)
 e. dendrite
 e. derma
 e. diffuse keratitis
 e. downgrowth
 e. dystrophy of Fuchs
 e. edema
 e. erosion
 e. herpetic disease
 e. hyperplasia
 e. hypertrophy
 e. implantation cyst
 e. inclusion
 e. inclusion cyst
 e. infectious crystalline keratopathy
 e. ingrowth
 e. invasion
 e. iron line
 e. laser-assisted intrastromal keratomileusis (E-LASIK)
 e. LASIK
 e. membrane antigen (EMA)
 e. microcyst
 e. migration
 e. mitosis
 e. nerve plexus
 e. nevus
 e. orientation
 e. plug
 e. punctate haze
 e. punctate keratitis
 e. rolled edge
 e. scrape
 e. scraper
 e. scraping
 e. slide
 e. transplantation
 e. trephine
 e. tumor
 e. turnover
epithelialization
epitheliitis
 e. focal retinal pigment
 pigment e.
 retinal pigment e.
epitheliocapsularis
 fibrillopathia e.
epithelioid
 e. cell
 e. hemangioma
epithelioma, pl. **epitheliomata**

e. adenoides cysticum
Contino e.
intraepithelial e.
Malherbe calcifying e.
malignant ciliary e.

epitheliopathy
acute multifocal placoid pigment e.
(AMPPE)
acute posterior multifocal placoid
pigment e. (APMPPE)
advancing wave-like e. (AWE)
dendritic e.
multifocal posterior pigment e.
pigment e.
placoid pigment e.
posterior pigment e.
retinal pigment e.

epithelioplasty
epitheliosis desquamativa conjunctivae
epithelium, pl. **epithelia**
e. anterius corneae
basement membrane of corneal e.
ciliary e.
Cogan microcystic dystrophy of the
corneal e.
congenital hypertrophy of the
retinal pigment e. (CHRPE)
corneal e.
denuded corneal e.
devitalized e.
graft e.
iris pigment e. (IPE)
lens e.
e. lentis
migrating e.
nonpigmented ciliary e.
pigment e. (PE)
e. pigmentosum iridis
placoid pigmentation of e.
e. posterius corneae
retinal pigment e. (RPE)
serous pigment e.
stratified squamous e.
subcapsular e.
syngeneic e.

epithelium-deprived orthotopic corneal
allograft
Epitrate
epizootic keratoconjunctivitis
Eppendorf tube
Eppy/N

EPS
exophthalmos-producing substance
EPSA
early postoperative suture adjustment
Epstein
E. collar stud acrylic implant
E. collar stud acrylic lens
E. symptom
Epstein-Barr virus (EBV)
equal
pupils round, regular, and e.
(PRRE)
equation
Baker e.
equator
anatomic e.
e. bulbi oculi
crystalline lens e.
e. of crystalline lens
eyeball e.
geometric e.
lens e.
e. lentis
equatorial
e. degeneration
e. drusen
e. lentis
e. meridian
e. ring scotoma
e. staphyloma
equilateral hemianopsia
equilibrating operation
equilibrium disturbance
equipment
laser e.
Volk Plus noncontact adapter cap
and e.
equivalence
therapeutic e.
equivalent
e. distance
mean spherical e. (MSE)
migraine e.
e. oxygen percentage value
e. power
e. refracting plane
spherical e. (Deq)
Er
erbium
eraser
E. cautery
Mentor curved e.

E

NOTES

eraser *(continued)*
    Mentor wet-field e.
    Tano e.
Erbakan inferior fornix operation
Erb-Duchenne paralysis
erbium (Er)
    e. laser
erbium:yttrium-aluminum-garnet (Er:YAG)
Erb paralysis
ERD
    exudative retinal detachment
Erdheim-Chester disease
erect illumination
ERG
    electroretinogram
    electroretinography
        photopic ERG
ERG-Jet disposable contact lens
Ergo
    Doctor E.
ergograph
ergonovine
ergot alkaloid
ErgoTec vitreoretinal instrument system
Erhardt
    E. clamp
    E. lid forceps
ERM
    epiretinal membrane
Ernest-McDonald soft intraocular lens-folding forceps
Ernest nucleus cracker
erosion
    coast e.
    corneal e.
    epithelial e.
    punctate epithelial e.
    recurrent corneal e.
    recurrent epithelial e.
    sphincter e.
erosive vitreoretinopathy
erroneous projection
error
    astigmagraphic e.
    astigmatic refractive e.
    asymmetric refractive e.
    Collaborative Longitudinal
      Evaluation in Ethnicity and
      Refractive E. (CLEERE)
    field of view e.
    inborn e.
    myopic e.
    position e.
    refractive e.
    retinal e.
    sampling e.
    spherical refractive e.

    velocity e.
    wavefront e.
eruptio
    zoster sine e.
eruptive keratoacanthoma
Er:YAG
    erbium:yttrium-aluminum-garnet
    Er:YAG laser
    Er:YAG laser phacoemulsification
    Er:YAG phacolase
erysipelas
    coastal e.
erysiphake
    Barraquer e.
    Bell e.
    Castroviejo e.
    corneal e.
    Dimitry e.
    Dimitry-Bell e.
    Dimitry-Thomas e.
    Draeger high vacuum e.
    Esposito e.
    Floyd-Grant e.
    Harrington e.
    Johnson e.
    Johnson-Bell e.
    Kara e.
    Maumenee e.
    New York e.
    Nugent-Green-Dimitry e.
    oval cup e.
    Post-Harrington e.
    Sakler e.
    Searcy oval cup e.
    Simcoe nucleus e.
    Storz-Bell e.
    e. technique
    Viers e.
    Welch rubber bulb e.
    Welsh silastic e.
erythema
    e. chronicum migrans
    e. multiforme
    e. multiforme bullosum
    e. multiforme exudativum
    e. multiforme major
    e. multiforme major conjunctivitis
erythematous pouting of the punctum
Erythrocin
erythroclastic glaucoma
erythrocyte
    ghost e.
erythrokeratodermia variabilis (EKV)
erythrolabe
erythrometer
erythrometry
erythromycin
erythrophagocytosis
erythropsia, erythropia

escape
    e. phenomenon
    pupillary e.
Escapini cataract operation
Eschenbach
    E. low vision rehabilitation guide
    E. monocular telescope
    E. Optik lens
Escherichia coli
Esenbach Highlighter
eserine
    Isopto E.
    e. sulfate
esocataphoria
esodeviation
    e. accommodation
    accommodative e.
    incomitant e.
    nonaccommodative e.
esophoria (E′)
    accommodative e.
    e. at near (E^1)
    A Trial of Bifocals in Myopic Children with E.
    classical congenital e.
    congenital e.
    near-point e.
    nonaccommodative e.
esophoric
esotropia (ET, ST)
    e. accommodation
    accommodative e.
    acquired e.
    alternate day e.
    alternating e.
    A-pattern e.
    basic e.
    clock-mechanism e.
    comitant e.
    congenital e.
    consecutive e.
    constant e.
    convergence excess e.
    cyclic e.
    decompensated accommodative e.
    essential infantile e.
    idiopathic congenital e.
    infantile e.
    intermittent e. (E(T))
    late-onset e.
    left e.
    mixed e.

    near e. (ET′)
    nonaccommodative e.
    nonrefractive accommodative e.
    periodic e.
    refractive accommodative e.
    right e.
    sensory deprivation e.
    V-pattern e.
esotropic
    e. amblyopia
    e. deviation
Espaillat-Deblasio nucleus rotator
Esposito erysiphake
essential
    e. anisocoria
    e. blepharospasm
    e. hypertension
    e. hypotony
    e. infantile esotropia
    e. iris atrophy
    e. phthisis
    e. phthisis bulbi
    e. progressive atrophy of iris
    e. telangiectasia
Esser inlay operation
Essilor storage case
ester
    unoprostone isopropyl e.
Esterman scale
esthesiometer, aesthesiometer
    Cochet-Bonnet e.
    noncontact corneal e. (NCCA)
    noncontact pneumatic e.
esthesioneuroblastoma
Estivin II Ophthalmic
estropia
ET
    esotropia
ET′
    near esotropia
E(T)
    intermittent esotropia
etabonate
    loteprednol e.
etafilcon A lens
ETDRS
    Early Treatment Diabetic Retinopathy Study
ethambutol
ether
    e. guard
    e. theory of light

E

NOTES

Ethicon
>   E. BV-75-3 needle
>   E. micropoint suture
>   E. Sabreloc suture

Ethicon-Atraloc suture
ethidium homodimer stain
ethmoid
>   e. bone
>   e. bulla
>   e. canal
>   e. exenteration
>   e. sinus

ethmoidal
>   e. artery
>   e. incisure
>   e. lacrimal fistula
>   e. region
>   e. sinus

ethmoidalis
>   lamina orbitalis ossis e.

ethmoiditis
ethmoidolacrimalis
>   sutura e.

ethmoidomaxillaris
>   sutura e.

ethoxyzolamide
ethyl
>   e. alcohol amblyopia
>   e. cyanoacrylate
>   e. cyanoacrylate glue

ethylenediamine
>   naphthyl e.

ethylenediaminetetraacetate (EDTA)
ethylene glycol
etidocaine
etiopurpurin
>   tin ethyl e. (SnET2)

ETROP
>   Early Treatment for Retinopathy of
>   Prematurity Study

EUA
>   exam under anesthesia

eucatropine
euchromatopsy
European Contact Lens Society of Ophthalmologists
Euro Precision Technology submicron lathe machine
euryopia
euthyphoria
evagination
>   optic e.

evaluation
>   An E. of Treatment of Amblyopia
>   in Children 7-18
>   Low Vision Functional Status E.
>   (LVFSE)
>   E. of Posterior Capsular
>   Opacification system

reproducibility of e.
>   Statpac-like Analysis for
>   Glaucoma E. (SAGE)
>   Structure And Function E. (SAFE)
>   telemedical e.
>   visual function e.

evanescent corneal epithelial opacity
evasion
>   macular e.

event
>   dark e.
>   independent e.

Evergreen
>   E. Lasertek coagulator
>   E. Lasertek laser

Eversbusch operation
eversion
>   double lid e.
>   e. of eyelid
>   lid e.
>   e. of punctum
>   single lid e.

everted
>   e. eyelid
>   e. punctum

everter
>   Berens lid e.
>   Berke lid e.
>   lid e.
>   Roveda lid e.
>   Schachne-Desmarres lid e.
>   Struble lid e.
>   Walker lid e.

evisceration
>   e. of eyeball
>   e. operation
>   e. spoon

evisceroneurotomy
E-Vista
evoked
>   e. nystagmus gaze
>   e. potential

evolutional cataract
EVP
>   episcleral venous pressure

EVS
>   Endophthalmitis Vitrectomy Study
>   endophthalmitis Vitrectomy Study

evulsion
evulsio nervi optici
Ewald law
EWCL
>   extended wear contact lens

Ewing
>   E. capsule forceps
>   E. operation
>   E. sarcoma

ex
> e. amblyopia
> e. anopsia

examination
> anterior segment e.
> cytologic e.
> dark-field e.
> dilated retinal e.
> dilated stereoscopic fundus e.
> e. of eye
> flashlight e.
> fundus e.
> funduscopic e.
> glaucoma e.
> neurologic e.
> neuroophthalmologic e.
> ophthalmic e.
> ophthalmoscopic e.
> slit-lamp e. (SLE)
> Woods light e.

exam under anesthesia (EUA)
exanthematous conjunctivitis
excavated optic disk anomaly
excavatio
> e. disci
> e. papillae nervi optici

excavation
> atrophic e.
> glaucomatous e.
> e. of optic disk
> physiologic e.
> retinal e.

excess
> convergence e.
> divergence e.
> e. esotropia convergence

excessive
> e. accommodation
> e. cyclodialysis cleft
> e. lacrimation
> e. rebound uveitis

exchange
> air-fluid e.
> fluid-air e.
> fluid-gas e.
> gas-fluid e. (GFE)
> intraocular lens e.
> lens e.
> presbyopic lens e. (PRELEX)

ExciMed
> E. UV200 excimer laser
> E. UV200LA laser

excimer
> e. laser
> e. laser ablation
> e. laser, 193193-nm
> e. laser photorefractive keratectomy
> e. laser phototherapeutic keratectomy
> e. laser transepithelial photoablation
> e. laser trephination

excision
> Arlt-Jaesche e.
> bare-sclera e.
> conjunctiva-Mueller muscle e.
> e. of lacrimal gland operation
> e. of lacrimal sac operation
> pentagonal block e.

excitation
> L-cone e.
> M cone e.
> paradoxic levator e.
> S cone e.

exciting eye
exclusion of pupil
excretory duct
excycloduction
excyclophoria
excyclotorsion
excyclotropia
excyclovergence
executive
> e. bifocal
> e. spectacle lens
> e. trifocal

exenteration
> ethmoid e.
> eyelid-splitting orbital e.
> Iliff e.
> orbital e.
> e. of orbital contents operation

exenteratio orbitae
exercise
> antisuppression e.
> blur and clear e.
> convergent e.
> pleoptic e.

exertional amblyopia
Exeter ophthalmoscope
exfoliation
> combined e.
> e. glaucoma
> e. of lens
> e. of lens capsule

E

NOTES

exfoliation *(continued)*
    e. syndrome (XFS)
    true e.
exfoliative
    e. glaucoma
    e. keratitis
exit pupil
exocataphoria
exodeviation
    comitant e.
exogenous
    e. disease
    e. endophthalmitis
    e. ochronosis
exophoria (X, XP)
    alternating e.
    comitant e.
    concomitant e.
    constant e.
    near-point e.
exophoric
exophthalmic
    e. goiter
    e. ophthalmoplegia
exophthalmogenic
exophthalmometer
    Hertel e.
    LICO Hertel e.
    Luedde e.
    Marco prism e.
exophthalmometric
exophthalmometry
    Hertel e.
    Krahn e.
exophthalmos, exophthalmus
    e. due to pressure
    e. due to tower skull
    endocrine e.
    malignant e.
    ophthalmoplegic e.
    postural e.
    pulsatile e.
    pulsating e.
    recurrent e.
    substance e.
    thyroid e.
    thyrotoxic e.
    thyrotropic e.
    transient early e.
exophthalmos-producing substance (EPS)
exophytic papillary capillary hemangioma
exoplant
    scleral e.
exorbitism
exotropia (XT)
    alternating e.
    A-pattern e.
    basic e.

    comitant e.
    consecutive e.
    constant e.
    convergence insufficiency e.
    divergence excess e.
    divergence insufficiency e.
    flick e.
    intermittent e. (X(T))
    left e.
    paralytic pontine e.
    periodic e.
    right e.
    secondary e.
    sensory deprivation e.
    V-pattern e.
exotropic
Expanded Disability Status Scale (EDSS)
expander
    Beehler irrigating pupil e.
    field e.
    Graether pupil e.
    irrigating pupil e.
    scleral e.
expansion
    normalized Zernike e.
expedition
    Surgical Eye E.'s (SEE)
experience
    microbiologic e.
experiment
    Mariotte e.
    Scheiner e.
experimental
    e. apparatus
    e. diabetes
    e. secondary effect
explant
    encircling e.
    episcleral e.
    Molteno episcleral e.
    posterior e.
    scleral e.
    segmental e.
    silicone sponge e.
    sponge e.
    trypsin-digested e.
exploration
    sclerotomy with e.
Expo
    E. Bubble dressing
    E. Bubble eye cover
    E. Bubble eye shield
exposure
    e. keratitis
    e. keratopathy
expression
    e. of chemokine receptor
    nuclear e.

expressor
    Arroyo e.
    Arruga e.
    Bagley-Wilmer e.
    Berens e.
    Heath e.
    Heyner e.
    hook e.
    e. hook
    Hosford e.
    Kirby hook e.
    Kirby intracapsular lens e.
    lens e.
    e. loop
    McDonald e.
    meibomian gland e.
    nucleus e.
    ring lens e.
    Rizzuti lens e.
    Smith e.
    Stahl nucleus e.
    Verhoeff lens e.
    Wilmer-Bagley e.
expulsive hemorrhage
EXT-DCR
    external dacryocystorhinostomy
extended
    e. round needle
    e. wear contact lens (EWCL)
    e. wear hydrogel
    e. wear infection
extended-range keratometry
extender
    Ahmed tube e.
extension
    ciliary body melanoma with
     extrascleral e.
    finger-like e.
    orbital e.
Extentabs
    Dimetane E.
Extenzyme
externa
    axis oculi e.
    folliculitis e.
    membrana granulosa e.
    membrana limitans e.
    ophthalmoplegia e.
external
    e. ankyloblepharon
    e. axis of eye
    e. beam radiation therapy

    e. beam radiation treatment
    e. canthotomy
    e. dacryocystorhinostomy (EXT-
    DCR)
    e. exudative retinopathy
    e. geniculate body
    e. hordeolum
    e. limiting membrane
    e. limiting membrane of retina
    e. ophthalmopathy
    e. ophthalmoplegia
    e. orbital fracture
    e. palsy
    e. pterygoid levator synkinesis
    e. rectus muscle
    e. route
    e. squint
    e. strabismus
externi
    insufficiency of e.
externo
    ab e.
externum
    hordeolum e.
externus
    axis bulbi e.
extinction
    e. phenomenon
    visual e.
extirpation
extorsion
extort
extra
    AMO Endosol E.
    Endosol E.
    Ocuvite E.
extracanthic
extracapsular
    e. aphakia
    e. cataract (ECC)
    e. cataract extraction (ECCE)
    e. cataract extraction operation
    e. extraction of cataract
    e. phacoemulsification
extracellular matrix (ECM)
extraciliary fiber
extraconal fat reticulum
extracranial optic nerve decompression
extractable nuclear antigen
extraction
    Arroyo cataract e.
    Arruga cataract e.

E

NOTES

extraction *(continued)*
cataract e. (CE)
Chandler-Verhoeff lens e.
clear lens e. (CLE)
combined intracapsular cataract e. (CICE)
extracapsular cataract e. (ECCE)
e. flap
foreign body e.
intracapsular cataract e. (ICCE)
e. of intracapsular cataract
intraocular cataract e.
magnetic e.
planned extracapsular cataract e.
extractor
irrigating C-hook e.
irrigating cortex e.
Krwawicz cataract e.
Look cortex e.
Smirmaul nucleus e.
Visitec cortex e.
Welsh cortex e.
extrafoveal retinal detachment
extramacular binocular vision
extramedullary
e. course
e. segment
extraocular
e. movement (EOM)
e. movement intact (EOMI)
e. muscle (EOM)
e. muscle disorder
e. muscle entrapment
e. muscle palsy
e. muscles of Tillaux
e. muscle testing
extraorbital disease
extrapyramidal
e. syndrome
e. system
extrarectus
extraretinal
e. fibrovascular proliferation
e. neovascularization
extrascleral outgrowth
Extra-Strength
MiraFlow E.-S.
extrastriate cortex lesion
extravasated blood
extravisual zone
extrinsic muscle
extrusion
implant e.
e. needle
pellet e.
exudate
bread-crumb e.
circinate e.
conjunctival e.

cotton-wool e.
endothelial e.
fatty e.
fibrin e.
fibrinous e.
foaming e.
hard lipid e.
lipid e.
retinal e.
snow-bank e.
soft e.
waxy e.
exudation
proteinaceous aqueous e.
exudativa
retinitis e.
exudative
e. AMD
e. choroiditis
e. eye
e. idiopathic polypoidal choroidal vasculopathy
e. retinal detachment (ERD)
e. retinitis
e. retinopathy
e. senile maculopathy
e. serous retinal detachment
e. vitreoretinopathy
exudativum
erythema multiforme e.
eye
aberrated e.
accessory organ of e.
acute red e. (ARE)
alkali burn to e.
amaurotic cat's e.
anterior pole of the e.
anterior segment of e.
aphakic e.
appendage of e.
aqueous humor e.
artificial e.
e. axial length
axial length of e.
e. bank
E. Bank Association of America (EBAA)
black e.
both e.'s (OU)
Bright e.
bulb of e.
bull's e.
E. Cap Ophthalmic Image Capture System
cat's e.
centrally fixing e.
e. chamber
e. chart
cinema e.

circumduction of the e.
Clear E.'s
closed surgery on e.
e. color
compound e.
E. Con 5
conjugate movement of e.'s
e. contact
contact lens-induced acute red e.
  (CLARE)
contralateral e.
contusion of e.
crossed e.'s
cyclopean e.
cystic e.
dancing e.
dark-adapted e.
deviating e.
disjugate movement of e.'s
disorder of e.
doll's e.
dominant e.
donor e.
e. dropper
e. drops
E. Drops AC
E. Drops Regular
Dry E.'s
Easy E.'s
Emsley reduced e.
examination of e.
exciting e.
external axis of e.
exudative e.
fellow e.
fibrous coat of e.
fixating e.
fixing e.
focus image quality of e.
following e.
fundus of e.
gas-filled e.
Gullstrand reduced e.
Gullstrand schematic e.
hare's e.
heavy e.
Helmholtz schematic e.
e. holder
hop e.
hot e.
e. implant conformer
e. infarction

e. infirmary
inflammatory target site of e.
e. injury
internal axis of e.
iris e.
e. irrigating solution
Klieg e.
e. knife guard
lazy e.
left e. (LE, OS)
e. lens
light-adapted e.
Listing reduced e.
Listing schematic e.
e. magnet
master e.
master-dominant e.
medial angle of e.
micromovement of e.
model e.
Moisture E.
monochromatic e.
e. movement
e. movement disorder
muscle of e.
e. muscle surgery
Nairobi e.
near-emmetropic e.
E. Net Audio
nondominant e.
normal e.
e. occluder
old e.
orbicular muscle of e.
oval e.
e. pad
e. pad dressing
parietal e.
patch e.
phakic e.
photopic e.
phthisical e.
pineal e.
pink e.
e. plaque
e. plaque surgery
e. point
Pontocaine E.
posterior pole of e.
posterior segment of the e.
Preflex for Sensitive E.'s
Preservative-Free Moisture E.'s

NOTES

E

eye (*continued*)
    e. pressing
    primary e.
    e. protector
    protruding e.'s
    pseudophakic e.
    E. Quip Keratron Scout topography system
    raccoon e.'s
    red e.
    reduced e.
    e. reflex
    e. removed in toto
    e. restored to normotensive pressure
    right e. (OD)
    rolling of e.'s
    e. rotated inferiorly
    e. rotation
    rudimentary e.
    saccadic movements of e.
    sagittal axis of e.
    E. Scan corneal analyzer
    schematic e.
    scotopic e.
    secondary e.
    Sensitive E.'s
    e. shield
    shipyard e.
    e. size
    Snellen reform e.
    Soft Mate Comfort Drops for Sensitive E.'s
    Soft Mate Saline for Sensitive E.'s
    Soothe e.
    e. speculum
    e. spot
    e. spud
    squinting e.
    stony-hard e.
    e. strain
    E. Stream
    E. Stream sterile eye irrigating solution
    suspensory ligament of e.
    e. suture scissors
    e. sweep
    sympathizing e.
    tension of e.
    test e.
    tumor of interior of e.
    vertical axis of e.
    e. wall
    E. Wash
    e. wash (collyr.)
    E. Wash solution
    e. was quiet
    watery e.
    web e.
    wet e.
    white of e.
    wobbly e.
    worse e.

eyeball
    e. compression reflex
    dimpling of e.
    e. equator
    evisceration of e.
    fibrous tunic of e.
    luxation of e.
    meridian of e.
    pigmented layer of e.
    posterior pole of e.
    e. sheath
    vascular coat of e.

eyeball-heart reflex

eyebrow
    e. fixation
    e. laceration

EyeClose
    E. Adhesive strip
    E. external eyelid weight

eye-closure reflex

Eye-Cool

Eyecor camera

Eye-Cort

eyecup

eye/ear plane

eyeFix speculum system

Eye-Gene

eyeglasses

eyegrounds

eye-head
    e.-h. movement
    e.-h. shift

eyeing

eyelash
    ectopic e.
    piebald e.

eyelash-induced leak

eyelid
    e. abnormality
    angular junction of e.
    e. apraxia
    avulsion of e.
    baggy e.
    basal cell carcinoma of e.
    capillary hemangioma of e.
    carcinoma of e.
    e. coloboma
    e. contour
    e. crease
    e. crusting
    e. dermatochalasis
    e. disorder
    drooping of e.
    easily everted upper e.
    ecchymosis of e.

e. ectropion
e. edema
e. entropion
eversion of e.
everted e.
e. fissure
floppy e.
e. flutter
e. fold
e. forceps
free margin of e.
e. fusion
gland of e.
incision into e.
inflammation of e.
insufficiency of e.
e. keratosis
lateral commissure of e.
levator muscle of upper e.
e. lichenification
lower e.
e. lymphangioma
e. margin
medial commissure of e.
melanoma of e.
e. milia
e. molluscum contagiosum infection
e. muscle
e. myokymia
e. neurilemoma
e. neurofibroma
e. nevus
e. nystagmus
one-stage reconstruction of eye
   socket and e.'s
orbital portion of e.
e. papilloma
paradoxical movement of e.
e. plaque
plastic repair of e.
pseudobaggy e.
e. ptosis
reconstruction of e.
e. retraction
e. retractor
e. rhytid
sign of edema of lower e.
sluggish movements of eyes and
   e.'s
e. spacer
e. speculum
squamous cell carcinoma of e.

e. strawberry hemangioma
e. surgery
e.'s sutured closed
suturing of e.
e. syringoma
e. taping
tarsal portion of e.
tumor of e.
e. tumor
unilateral ptosis of e.
upper e.
e. vesiculation
xanthelasma around e.
eyelid-closure reflex
eyelid-splitting orbital exenteration
EyeLite photocoagulator
Eye-Lube-A Solution
EyeMap EH-290 corneal topography
   system
Eye-Mo
Eye-Pak
   E.-P. II cover
   E.-P. II drape
   E.-P. II sheet
eyepiece
   comparison e.
   compensating e.
   demonstration e.
   Huygenian e.
   negative e.
   position e.
   positive e.
   Ramsden e.
   wide-field e.
eye-popping reflex
eye-referenced stimulus
eye-refractometer
Eyes-CIBA
   Pure E.-C.
Eye-Scrub
Eye-Sed solution
eyeshot
eyesight
Eyesine
   E. Ophthalmic
   E. solution
eyes-open coma
EyeSys
   E. charting
   E. corneal analysis system
   E. 2000 corneal topographic
      mapping system

E

NOTES

EyeSys *(continued)*
    E. corneal topography system
    E. surface topography system
    E. System 2000
    E. Technologies corneal topography
    E. videokeratograph
    E. videokeratoscope

eyewash *(var. of* eye wash)
eyewear
    Timex TMX optical e.
eyewire
EZ.1 multifocal contact lens
EZE-FIT IOL system
EZVUE violet haptic intraocular lens

F
- filial generation
- focus
- visual field

F2 Color Vision test

FA
- fluorescein angiography

FAAO
- Fellow of the American Academy of Ophthalmology
- Fellow of the American Academy of Optometry

Faber disease

Fab fragment

Fabry syndrome

face
- hyaloid f.
- intact anterior hyaloid f.
- f. line
- f. shield
- vitreous f.

face-down position

facet, facette
- corneal f.

facetted
- f. avascular disciform opacity
- f. corneal scar

facial
- f. anomaly
- f. block
- f. cleft
- f. fracture
- f. hemangioma
- f. movement
- f. movement abnormality
- f. myokymia
- f. nerve
- f. nerve avulsion
- f. nerve lesion
- f. nerve misdirection
- f. nerve palsy
- f. nerve trunk
- f. neuroma
- f. pain
- f. paralysis
- f. perception
- f. spasm
- f. synkinesis
- f. vein
- f. vision

facialis
- vena f.

facies, pl. **facies**
- f. anterior corneae
- f. anterior iridis
- f. anterior lentis
- f. anterior palpebrarum
- f. antonina
- f. bovina
- Hutchinson f.
- mask-like f.
- f. orbitalis alae magnae
- f. orbitalis alae majoris
- f. orbitalis ossis frontalis
- f. orbitalis ossis zygomatici
- f. posterior corneae
- f. posterior iridis
- f. posterior lentis
- f. posterior palpebrarum

facility
- f. of outflow
- vergence f.

facioauriculovertebral spectrum

FACS
- Fellow of the American College of Surgeons

FACT
- Functional Acuity Contrast Test

factitious
- f. blindness
- f. conjunctivitis
- f. mydriasis

factor
- macrophage migration inhibitory f. (MMIF)
- nerve growth f.
- pigment epithelium-derived f. (PEDF)
- risk f.
- vascular endothelial growth f. (VEGF)

facultative
- f. hyperopia
- f. suppression

faculty
- fusion f.

Faden
- F. effect
- F. operation
- F. procedure
- F. suture

fading time

faecalis
- *Enterococcus f.*
- *Streptococcus f.*

FA/ICGA
- fluorescein angiography/indocyanine green angiography
- Heidelberg retina angiograph FA/ICGA

F

failed
    f. graft
    f. ptosis surgery
failure
    lacrimal pump f.
    late endothelial f.
    primary graft f.
    sympathetic innervation f.
faint flare
falciform
    f. fold of retina
    f. retinal fold
Falcon lens
fallopian canal
Falls-Kertesz syndrome
false
    f. blepharoptosis
    f. image
    f. macula
    f. negative
    f. orientation
    f. positive
    f. projection
    f. ptosis
    f. scotoma
    f. vision
false-negative result
false-positive result
FAMA
    fluorescent-antibody-to-membrane
      antigen
famciclovir
familial
    f. arteriolar tortuosity
    f. autonomic dysautonomia
    f. autonomic dysfunction
    f. colloid degeneration
    f. drusen
    f. episodic ataxia
    f. exudative retinopathy (FER)
    f. exudative vitreoretinopathy
      (FEVR)
    f. fibrosis
    f. foveal retinoschisis (FFR)
    f. juvenile systemic granulomatosis
    f. lecithin-cholesterol acyltransferase
      deficiency
    f. lipoprotein deficiency
    f. paroxysmal ataxia
    f. periodic paralysis
    f. pseudoinflammatory macular
      degeneration
    f. pseudoinflammatory maculopathy
    f. retinoblastoma
familiares
    cornea plana congenita f.
Famvir
Fanconi syndrome

Fanta
    F. cataract operation
    F. speculum
fantascope
FAP
    fatter add plus
far
    f. phoria
    f. point
    f. point of accommodation (FPA)
    f. point of convergence
    f. sight
Farber disease
farinaceous epithelial keratitis
farinata
    cornea f.
Farkas-Bracken fixation forceps
Farnsworth
    F. D-15 panel
    F. Panel D-15 test
Farnsworth-Munsell
    F.-M. 100-hue color vision test
farsighted
farsightedness
Fary anterior chamber maintainer
Fas
    F. interaction
    F. liquid protein
    F. receptor density
Fasanella
    F. lacrimal cannula
    F. operation
    F. retractor
Fasanella-Servat
    F.-S. procedure
    F.-S. ptosis operation
fascia, pl. fasciae
    f. band
    bulbar f.
    Crawford f.
    f. lata frontalis
    f. lata frontalis sling
    f. lata musculares bulbi
    f. lata musculares oculi
    f. lata sling for ptosis operation
    f. lata stripper
    muscular f.
    orbital f.
    fasciae orbitales
    palpebral f.
fascicle
    abducens nerve f.
    oculomotor nerve f.
fascicular
    f. keratitis
    f. ophthalmoplegia
    f. ulcer
fasciculus
    inferior longitudinal f.

longitudinal f.
maculary f.
medial longitudinal f. (MLF)
rostral interstitial medial
   longitudinal f.
fasciitis
nodular f.
orbital f.
fashion
in-tumbling f.
McLean f.
stepwise f.
X-linked f.
FasL interaction
Fast Grind 2200
FastPac
F. algorithm
F. 24-2 test
fat
f. adherence syndrome
f. cell
f. embolism of retina
f. graft
herniating orbital f.
mutton f.
orbital f.
f. pad
f. removal orbital decompression
   (FROD)
f. reticulum
suborbicularis oculi f. (SOOF)
fatigable ptosis
fatigue
f. nystagmus
f. phenomenon
fatter add plus (FAP)
fatty
f. change
f. exudate
Faulkner
F. folder
F. lens holding forceps
Favre dystrophy
FAZ
foveal avascular zone
FB
foreign body
Fc
fragment crystallizable
Fc fragment
fc
foot candle

FCT
fluorescein clearance test
FD
focal distance
FDACL
first definite apical clearance lens
FDT
frequency doubling technology
FDT perimetry
FDT-MD
frequency doubling technology mean
deviation
FDT-PSD
frequency doubling technology pattern
standard deviation
Feaster
F. Accura diamond knife
F. Dualens lens
F. K7-5460 hydrodissecting cannula
F. radial keratotomy knife
Feather
F. clear cornea knife
F. crescent tunnel blade
F. incision scalpel
F. keratome
F. round tunnel blade
F. Touch CO_2 laser
feathery
f. appearance
f. clouding
feature
felt-like f.
Fechtner
F. conjunctiva forceps
F. intraocular lens
F. ring forceps
Federov
F. four-loop iris clip
F. four-loop iris clip lens implant
F. type I, II intraocular lens
F. type I, II lens implant
feeder-frond technique
feeder vessel
feet
f. motion at 3 f. (HM/3ft)
Müller end f.
Fehr macular dystrophy
Feldman
F. adaptometer
F. buffer solution
F. RK optical center marker

NOTES

171

fellow
>F. of the American Academy of Ophthalmology (FAAO)
>F. of the American Academy of Optometry (FAAO)
>F. of the American College of Surgeons (FACS)
>f. eye
>F. of the Royal College of Physicians (FRCP)
>F. of the Royal College of Physicians of Canada (FRCPC)
>F. of the Royal College of Surgeons (FRCS)
>F. of the Royal College of Surgeons of Australia (FRCSA)

felt
>f. disk polisher
>f. pad

felt-like feature

femtosend pulse intrastromal laser microkeratome

fenestra, pl. **fenestrae**

fenestrated
>f. chain
>f. sheen macular dystrophy

fenestration
>optic nerve sheath f. (ONSF)

Fenhoff external and anterior segment

fenretinide

fentanyl

Fenzel
>F. angled manipulating hook
>F. insertion hook
>F. lens-manipulating hook

FER
>familial exudative retinopathy

Féréol-Graux palsy

fERG
>flash electroretinogram

Ferguson implant

Fergus operation

ferning
>tear mucus f.

Ferree-Rand perimeter

Ferrein canal

ferric
>f. ferrocyanide
>f. hyaluronate gel

Ferris chart

Ferris-Smith
>F.-S. refractor
>F.-S. retractor

Ferris-Smith-Sewall
>F.-S.-S. refractor
>F.-S.-S. retractor

ferrocholinate

ferrocyanide
>ferric f.

ferrous sulfate

Ferry line

Ferry-Porter law

fetal
>f. fibrovascular sheath
>f. hydantoin syndrome
>f. trimethadione syndrome
>f. warfarin syndrome
>f. Y suture

fever
>pharyngoconjunctival f.

FEVR
>familial exudative vitreoretinopathy

fexofenadine

F&F
>fix and follow

FFF
>flicker fusion frequency test

FFR
>familial foveal retinoschisis

FFSS
>Fluorouracil Filtering Surgery Study

FGCRT
>Foscarnet-Ganciclovir CMV Retinitis Trial

FHC
>Fuchs heterochromic cyclitis

fiber
>accessory f.
>auxiliary f.
>Bernheimer f.
>Brücke f.
>f. cell
>chief f.
>cilioequatorial f.
>cilioposterocapsular f.
>circular ciliary muscle f.
>collagen f.
>cone f.
>congenital medullated optic nerve f.
>contiguous f.'s
>continuous f.
>corticonuclear f.
>Edinger f.
>efferent f.
>extraciliary f.
>fibrillenstruktur f.
>Gratiolet radiating f.
>Henle f.
>interciliary f.
>intraocular myelination of retinal nerve f.
>f. layer of axon
>f. layer of Chievitz
>lens f.
>longitudinal f.
>main f.
>medullated nerve f.

meridional ciliary muscle f.
Monakow f.
Müller f.
myelinated retinal nerve f.
myoclonic epilepsy with ragged-
    red f.
nerve f.
oblique f.
optic nerve f.
f. orbicularis oculi
orbiculoanterocapsular f.
orbiculociliary f.
orbiculoposterocapsular f.
parasympathetic f.
peripapillary retinal nerve f.
postganglionic f.
principal f.
pupilloconstrictor f.
pupillomotor f.
radial f.
ragged-red f.
Ritter f.
rod f.
Sappey f.
sensory f.
sphincter f.
sustentacular f.
trabecular f.
vitreous f.
zonular f.
Fiberlite microscope
fiberoptic
    f. diagnostic lens
    f. digital fundus camera
    f. light projector
    f. pick
    f. videoendoscope
fiberscope
fibra, pl. **fibrae**
    fibrae circulares musculi ciliaris
    fibrae lentis
    fibrae longitudinales musculi ciliaris
    fibrae meridionales musculi ciliaris
    fibrae radiales musculi ciliaris
    fibrae zonulares
Fibra Sonics phaco aspirator
fibril
    collagen f.
fibrillar material
fibrillenstruktur fiber
fibrillin-1
fibrillogranular deposit

fibrillogranuloma
fibrillopathia epitheliocapsularis
fibrin
    Cell-Tak autologous f.
    f. dusting
    f. exudate
    f. gel
    intravitreal f.
    f. layer
    postvitrectomy f.
    f. pupillary block glaucoma
    f. strand
    f. thrombus
fibrinogen glue
fibrinoid necrosis
fibrinolysis
    local intraarterial f. (LIF)
fibrinous
    f. aqueous
    f. cataract
    f. exudate
    f. iritis
    f. rhinitis
fibroblast
    Tenon f.
fibroblastic
    f. ingrowth
    f. meningioma
fibroglial membrane
fibroid cataract
fibroma
    orbital f.
fibromatosis
    orbital f.
fibromuscular dysplasia
fibroosseous tumor
fibroplasia
    cicatricial retrolental f.
    retrolental f. (RLF)
fibroproliferative membrane
fibrosa
    cataracta f.
    pseudophakia f.
fibrosarcoma
    orbital f.
fibrosclerosis
    multifocal f.
fibrosis
    f. choroideae corrugans
    congenital f.
    cystic f.
    episcleral f.

F

NOTES

fibrosis *(continued)*
    familial f.
    preretinal macular f.
    subepithelial f.
    f. syndrome
fibrous
    f. coat of eye
    f. dysplasia
    f. frond
    f. proliferans
    f. tissue cuff
    f. tunic
    f. tunic of eyeball
fibrovascular
    f. frond
    f. membrane
    f. pannus
    f. proliferation
    f. sheath
    f. tunic
Fick
    anteroposterior axis of F.
    F. axis
    F. halo
    longitudinal axis of F.
    F. phenomenon
    sagittal axis of F.
    transverse axis of F.
    vertical axis of F.
    Z axis of F.
field
    altitudinal f.
    automated visual f.
    binasal quadrant f.
    binocular f.
    bright empty f.
    central visual f. (CVF)
    checkerboard visual f.
    confrontation visual f.
    cribriform f.
    f. cut
    dark empty f.
    f. defect
    depth of f.
    f. diaphragm setting
    f. expander
    f. of fixation
    Forel f.
    frontal eye f.
    f. of gaze
    Humphrey visual f. (HVF)
    hysteric f.
    hysterical constricted f.
    keyhole f.
    f. lens
    f. loss
    paracentral visual f.
    peripheral visual f.
    receptive f.

    remaining visual f.
    spiral f.
    star-shaped f.
    superonasal paracentral visual f.
    surplus f.
    Swiss-cheese visual f.
    temporal island of visual f.
    tubular visual f.
    tunnel f.
    f. of view
    f. of view error
    f. of vision
    visual f. (F, VF)
    wide f. (WF)
Fiessinger-Leroy-Reiter syndrome
fifth cranial nerve (CN V)
figure
    Allen f.
    fortification f.
    Kanizsa f.
    Purkinje f.
    Rey-Osterreith Complex F.
    Stifel f.
    Zöllner f.
figure-of-eight suture
filament
    Ammon f.
    branching f.
    corneal f.
    f. keratitis
    myosin f.
filamentary
    f. keratitis (FK)
    f. keratome
    f. keratopathy
filamentosa
    keratitis f.
filamentous fungus
filariasis
Filatov
    F. keratoplasty
    F. operation
Filatov-Marzinkowsky operation
filial generation (F)
filiform dystrophy
filling
    choroidal f.
    retinal arterial f.
film
    absorbable gelatin f.
    aqueous layer of tear f.
    conditioning f.
    debris-laden tear f.
    gelatin f.
    precorneal tear f.
    preocular tear f. (POTF)
    proteinolipidic f.
    tear f.

filmtab
Rondec F.
filter
cobalt blue f.
f. glasses for color testing
Haag-Streit 900 cobalt blue f.
interference f.
Interferenzfilter 675FS20-12.5 f.
Millex f.
Millipore f.
neutral density f.
OP-05 hollow fiber f.
pocket red f.
Polaroid f.
red f.
red-free f.
ultraviolet f.
UV blocking f.
Whatman f.
Wrattan f.
filtering
f. bleb
f. cicatrix
f. implant
f. operation
f. procedure
f. valve
f. wick
filtration
f. angle
f. surgery
Van Herick f.
filtrator
Cascadeflo AC 1760 f.
Rheofilter AR 2000 f.
fimbriated
f. edge
f. margin
Finalite 1.6
final threshold
finding
clinicopathologic f.
fine
F. bimanual handpiece set
F. corneal carrying case
F. crescent fixation ring
F. dissecting forceps
f. fibrillar vitreal degeneration
F. Finesse Triamond
F. folding block
F. gripping forceps
F. III inserter

f. iris process
F. irrigating capsulorrhexis forceps
F. irrigating reverse actuating splitting chopper
F. magnetic implant
F. micropoint cautery
F. micropoint electrocautery
f. punctate keratopathy
f. retinal fold
F. sideport actuating quick chopper
F. sideport capsulorrhexis forceps
F. suture scissors
F. suture-tying forceps
F. Toric/LRI marker
Fine-Castroviejo suturing forceps
Fine-Nagahara phaco chopper
fine-needle aspiration
Fine-Thornton scleral fixation ring
fine-toothed forceps
fine-wire speculum
finger
f. count
counting f.'s (CF)
f. mimicking
f. tension
f. vision
finger-counting
down to f.-c.
f.-c. vision
finger-like extension
fingerprint
f. body myopathy
f. corneal dystrophy
f. line
finished
f. contact lens
f. glass
Fink
F. biprong marker
F. cataract aspirator
F. cul-de-sac irrigator
F. curette
F. irrigating/aspirating unit
F. lacrimal retractor
F. muscle marker
F. oblique muscle hook
F. operation
F. refractor
F. tendon tucker
Fink-Jameson muscle forceps
Fink-Weinstein two-way syringe

F

NOTES

Finnoff transilluminator
first definite apical clearance lens (FDACL)
first-degree relative
first-grade fusion
Fisher
   F. exact test
   F. eye needle
   F. lid retractor
   F. spoon
   F. spud
   F. syndrome
Fisher-Arlt iris forceps
Fisher-Smith spatula
fishmouthing
fishmouth tear
Fison indirect binocular ophthalmoscope
fissura, pl. fissurae
   f. orbitalis inferior
   f. orbitalis superior
fissuratum
   acanthoma f.
fissure
   Ammon f.
   basin of inferior orbital f.
   calcarine f.
   choroid f.
   f. coloboma
   corneal f.
   eyelid f.
   inferior orbital f.
   interpalpebral f.
   lid f.
   orbital superior f.
   palpebral f.
   pterygomaxillary f.
   sphenoccipital f.
   sphenoid f.
   sphenoidal f.
   sphenomaxillary f.
   superior orbital f. (SOF)
   water f.
   f. zone
fistula, pl. fistulae, fistulas
   carotid cavernous sinus f.
   cavernous sinus f.
   f. of cornea
   corneal f.
   direct carotid cavernous f.
   dural carotid cavernous f.
   dural cavernous sinus f.
   ethmoidal lacrimal f.
   internal lacrimal f.
   intraocular f.
   lacrimal f.
   f. lacrimalis
   scleral f.
   f. test
fistulizing surgery

fitting
   Model 201-20 high-flow 0.20-mm filter Luer lock f.
   f. triangle
Fitz-Hugh-Curtis syndrome
Fitzpatrick sun-sensitivity scale
fix and follow (F&F)
fixate
fixating eye
fixation
   anomalous f.
   axis f.
   bifocal f.
   bifoveal f.
   binocular f.
   f. binocular forceps
   brow f.
   capsular f.
   central, steady and maintained f.
   cross f.
   crossed f.
   CSM f.
   f. disparity
   eccentric f.
   eyebrow f.
   field of f.
   four-point f.
   graft f.
   Guyton-Noyes f.
   f. hook
   f. instrument
   f. light
   line of f.
   locus of f.
   f. mechanism
   microplate f.
   monocular f.
   near f.
   f. nystagmus
   f. object
   f. pick
   pigtail f.
   point of f.
   f. point
   f. reflex
   f. ring
   saccadic f.
   split f.
   sulcus f.
   f. suture
   f. target
   transscleral suture f.
fixational ocular movement
fixation/anchor
   f. forceps
   f. pick
   f. ring
fixed
   f. dilated pupil

f. fold
f. forceps
f. mydriasis
f. point
fixing eye
fixus
strabismus f.
vertical strabismus f.
Fizeau-Tolansky interferometer
FK
filamentary keratitis
flaccid
f. canaliculus syndrome
f. ectropion
FLAIR
fluid-attenuated inversion recovery
FLAIR MRI
Flajani
F. disease
F. operation
flame
f. photometer
f. spot
flame-shaped hemorrhage
flammeus
nevus f.
flap
advancement f.
bicoronal scalp f.
Blaskovics f.
bridge pedicle f.
cheek f.
conjunctival f.
conjunctiva-Tenon f.
Cutler-Beard bridge f.
donut-cut f.
donut-shaped f.
extraction f.
fornix-based conjunctival f.
galeal f.
Gunderson conjunctival f.
hinged corneal f.
Hughes tarsoconjunctival f.
Imre sliding f.
f. irregularity
limbal-based f.
limbus-based conjunctival f.
Mustarde rotational cheek f.
f. operation cataract
partial conjunctival f. (PCF)
pedicle f.
pediculated f.

retinal f.
f. retraction
scalp f.
scleral f.
skin f.
sliding f.
swinging lid f.
tarsoconjunctival f.
f. tear
Tenon f.
Tenzel rotational cheek f.
total conjunctival f. (TCF)
trabeculectomy f.
Truc f.
Van Lint f.
FlapMaker
F. disposable microkeratome
F. microkeratome system
flare
aqueous f.
cell and f.
faint f.
f. response
flared ABS tip
Flarex
flash
f. blindness
f. electroretinogram (fERG)
f. keratoconjunctivitis
f.'s of light
f. ophthalmia
f. picture card
f. stimulus
f. visual-evoked potential (fVEP)
flashlamp-pumped microsecond pulse-dye laser
flashlight
f. examination
f. test
flask
Primaria tissue culture f.
flat
f. anterior chamber
f. axis
f. chorioretinal atrophy
f. contact lens
f. cornea
f. cup
f. demarcation line
f. eye spud
f. filtration bleb
f. hook

F

NOTES

flat *(continued)*
  f. top bifocal
  f. top spectacles
Flatau-Schilder disease
flat-edge lens
flattening
  keratometric f.
flavimaculatus
  fundus f.
Flavobacterium
  F. *indoltheticum*
  F. *meningosepticum*
flavus
  Aspergillus f.
fleck
  intraretinal f.
flecked
  f. corneal dystrophy
  f. retina
  f. retina disease
  f. retina of Kandori
  f. retina syndrome
flecken glaucoma
Fleischer
  F. cataract
  F. dystrophy
  F. keratoconus ring
  F. vortex
Fleischer-Strumpell ring
Flex-Care
flexible
  f. loop
  5139 f. retinal brush
  f. translimbal iris retractor
flexible-wear contact lens
Flexlens lens
flexneri
  Shigella f.
Flexner-Wintersteiner rosette
Flexner-Worst iris claw lens
FlexPlug
  Eagle F.
Flexsol
flicher-fusion frequency technique
flick
  f. exotropia
  f. hypertropia
  f. movement
flicker
  f. amplitude
  f. electroretinogram
  f. fusion
  f. fusion frequency test (FFF)
  f. fusion stimulus
  f. fusion test
  f. perimetry
  f. perimetry test
  f. phenomenon
  f. photometer

Flieringa
  curved scleral-limbal incision of F.
  F. scleral fixation ring
Flieringa-Kayser
  F.-K. copper ring
  F.-K. fixation ring
Flieringa-LeGrand fixation ring
flight blindness
flint glass
flint-glass lens
flipping
  Brown technique of nuclear f.
flittering scotoma
floater
  F. eye model
  meniscus f.
  pigment f.
  pupillary f.
  vitreous f.
flocculus, pl. **flocculi**
  cerebellar f.
  f. syndrome
floor
  depression of orbital f.
  f. fracture
  orbital f.
floppy
  f. eyelid
  f. eyelid syndrome
flora
  ocular f.
Florentine iris
Floresoft
florid xanthelasma
floriform cataract
Floropryl Ophthalmic
Flouren law
floury cornea
flow
  aqueous humor f.
  axoplasmic f.
  choroidal blood f. (ChBFlow)
  laminar f.
  retinal capillary blood f.
  reversed ophthalmic artery f.
    (ROAF)
  tear f.
  total steady-state tear f.
flower petal pattern
flowgraphy
  laser speckle f.
flowmeter
  CLBF-100 blood f.
  Heidelberg retinal f.
  laser Doppler f.
flowmetry
  confocal scanning laser Doppler f.
Floxin
floxuridine

Floyd-Barraquer wire speculum
Floyd-Grant erysiphake
Flucaine
fluconazole
fluctuation
　　diurnal f.
flucytosine
fluff
　　f. dressing
　　vitreous f.
fluffed gauze dressing
fluffy appearance
Fluftex gauze roll
fluid
　　aqueous f.
　　f. cataract
　　cerebrospinal f. (CSF)
　　f. contact lens
　　heavy f.
　　Hylan biopolymer f.
　　intraocular f.
　　f. lamellar keratoplasty
　　f. mechanics
　　perioptic cerebrospinal f.
　　subarachnoid f.
　　submembrane f.
　　subretinal f. (SRF)
　　viscous ochre f.
　　viscous xanthochromic f.
　　Vitreon sterile intraocular f.
　　xanthochromic f.
fluid-air exchange
fluid-attenuated inversion recovery
　　(FLAIR)
fluid-gas exchange
fluidic ILM separation
Fluidics
　　Concentrix F.
fluidless contact lens
Fluka Chemical
Fluocinolone
Fluoracaine
fluorescein
　　f. angiogram
　　f. angiogram test
　　f. angiography (FA)
　　f. angiography/indocyanine green
　　　angiography (FA/ICGA)
　　f. clearance test (FCT)
　　f. dilution test
　　f. dye
　　f. dye disappearance test

f. dye and stain solution
f. fundus angioscopy
f. instillation test
intravenous f.
f. isothiocyanate
parafoveal f.
f. pooling
sodium f. (NaFl)
f. sodium
f. stain
f. staining
f. stick
f. strip test
fluorescein-potentiated argon laser
　　therapy (FPAL)
fluorescence
　　blocked f.
　　f. microscopy
　　f. retinal photography
fluorescent
　　f. antibody test
　　f. lamp
　　f. treponemal antibody absorption
fluorescent-antibody-to-membrane antigen
　　(FAMA)
Fluorescite
Fluoresoft
Fluorets fluorescein sodium strips
Fluorex 300, 500 contact lens
fluorexon
fluoride
　　argon fluoride (ArF)
Fluor-I-Strip AT
fluorite
fluorobiprofen
fluorocarbon in contact lens
fluorometer
　　CytoFluor II f.
fluorometholone (FML)
　　f. acetate
　　f. ophthalmic suspension
　　sulfacetamide sodium and f.
fluorometholone/sulfacetamide (FML-S)
fluorometry
　　noninvasive corneal redox f.
Fluor-Op
fluorophosphate
　　diisopropyl f. (DFP)
fluorophotometer
　　Fluorotron Master f.
　　slit-lamp f.

F

NOTES

fluorophotometry
    vitreous f.
Fluoroplex
fluoroquinolone antibiotic
Fluorotron
    Coherent radiation F.
    F. Master fluorophotometer
5-fluorouracil (5-FU)
    topical 5-f.
Fluorouracil Filtering Surgery Study (FFSS)
Fluorox
flurbiprofen sodium
Fluress
flush
    choroidal f.
    ciliary f.
    circumciliary f.
    hemifacial f.
flute
    f. needle
    f. pipe
flutter
    f. dysmetria
    eyelid f.
    ocular f.
flux
    f. incident
    luminous f.
    oxygen f.
    radiant and luminous f.
    unit of luminous f.
fly
    f. test
    Titmus stereo f.
Flynn lens loop
FM-500
    Kowa F.
F/M base curve contact lens
FM-100 hue test
FML
    fluorometholone
    FML Forte
    FML SOP
FML-S
    fluorometholone/sulfacetamide
    FML-S Ophthalmic Suspension
foam cell
foaming exudate
focal
    f. attenuation
    f. choroiditis
    f. constriction
    f. depth
    f. distance (FD)
    f. dystonia
    f. electroretinogram
    f. granuloma
    f. illumination

    f. image point
    f. interval
    f. laser photocoagulation
    f. laser treatment
    f. length
    f. myasthenia
    f. scotoma
    f. staining
    f. vasogenic edema
foci (*pl. of* focus)
focimeter
focofilcon A
focus, pl. **foci (F)**
    aplanatic f.
    conjugate f.
    F. DAILIES Toric contact lens
    depth of f.
    detectable f.
    f. image quality of eye
    image-space f.
    F. Lens Drops
    F. Night & Day contact lens
    object-space f.
    principal f.
    real f.
    virtual f.
fogged manifest refraction
fogging
    f. retinoscopy
    f. system of refraction
fog test
foil sheet
Foix
    F. enucleation
    F. syndrome
fold
    arcuate retinal f.
    chorioretinal f.
    choroidal f.
    ciliary f.
    concentric f.
    congenital retinal f.
    conjunctival semilunar f.
    Dennie-Morgan f.
    Descemet f.
    double lower lid f.
    dry f.
    epicanthal skin f.
    epicanthic f. (ECF)
    eyelid f.
    falciform retinal f.
    fine retinal f.
    fixed f.
    f. forceps
    glabellar f.
    Hasner f.
    iridial f.
    lacrimal f.
    Lange f.

meridional f.
mongolian f.
nasojugal f.
nasolabial f.
palpebral f.
palpebronasal f.
papillomacular retinal f.
primary retinal f.
retinal fixed f.
retrotarsal f.
semilunar f.
star f.
stiff retinal f.

foldable
f. disk intraocular lens
f. intraocular lens surgery
f. IOP
f. plate-haptic silicone intraocular lens

folder
Faulkner f.

folding spectacles

folic
f. acid antagonist
f. acid deficiency

folinic acid

follicle
cilia f.
conjunctival f.
limbal f.
lymphoid f.
necrotic f.

follicular
f. conjunctivitis
f. hypertrophy
f. iritis
f. plugging
f. trachoma

follicularis
blepharitis f.
keratosis f.

folliculitis
f. externa
f. interna

folliculorum
Demodex f.

folliculosis
follow
fix and f. (F&F)

following
f. eye
f. movement

followup
Foltz valve
fomepizole
fomivirsen sodium
Fontana
F. canal
F. space

foot
f. candle (fc)
f. candle meter
f. lambert

footplate
Müller cell f.

footprints of HSV
foramen, pl. **foramina**
Bozzi f.
cranial f.
inferior zygomatic f.
infraorbital f.
f. infraorbitale
lacerate anterior f.
lacerate middle f.
lacerate posterior f.
f. lacerum anterius
optic f.
f. opticum
orbitomalar f.
rotundum f.
f. of sclera
Soemmering f.
f. sphenoidalis
f. of sphenoid bone
supraorbital f.
f. supraorbitale
zygomatic f.
zygomaticofacial f.
zygomaticoorbital f.
f. zygomatico-orbitale
zygomaticotemporal f.

force
muscle f.
Neurofibromatosis Type 1 Optic Pathway Glioma Task F.
shear f.

forced
f. choice preferential looking
f. downward deviation
f. duction
f. generation
f. generation test

F

NOTES

181

forced-duction
  f.-d. test
  f.-d. testing
forced-eye closure
forceps
  Adson f.
  Akahoshi acrylic intraocular lens f.
  Akahoshi acrylic IOL loading f.
  Akahoshi implantation f.
  Alabama tying f.
  Alabama University utility f.
  Alfonso nucleus f.
  Allen-Braley f.
  Allis f.
  Alvis fixation f.
  Ambrose suture f.
  Amenabar capsule f.
  angled capsule f.
  Anis lens-holding f.
  Arroyo f.
  Arruga capsule f.
  Arruga-McCool capsule f.
  Arruga-Nicetic capsule f.
  Asch septal f.
  ASICO capsulorrhexis f.
  ASSI capsulorrhexis f.
  ASSI IOL inserter f.
  ASSI tubing introducer f.
  ASSI universal lens folding f.
  Azar lens-holding f.
  Bailey chalazion f.
  Baird chalazion f.
  Ballen-Alexander f.
  Bangerter muscle f.
  Banner f.
  Bansal LASIK f.
  Bard-Parker f.
  Barkan iris f.
  Barraquer cilia f.
  Barraquer-Colibri f.
  Barraquer conjunctival f.
  Barraquer corneal utility f.
  Barraquer hemostatic mosquito f.
  Barraquer-von Mandach capsule f.
  bayonet f.
  BB shot f.
  beaked f.
  Beaupre cilia f.
  Bechert lens-holding f.
  Bechert-McPherson angled tying f.
  Bennett cilia f.
  Berens corneal transplant f.
  Berens muscle f.
  Berens ptosis f.
  Berens suturing f.
  Berkeley Bioengineering ptosis f.
  Berke ptosis f.
  Bettman-Noyes fixation f.
  binocular fixation f.

  bipolar f.
  Birks Mark II Colibri f.
  Birks Mark II grooved f.
  Birks Mark II micro needle-
    holder f.
  Birks Mark II straight f.
  Birks Mark II suture-tying f.
  Birks Mark II toothed f.
  Bishop-Harman crisscross f.
  Bishop-Harman foreign body f.
  Bishop-Harman tissue f.
  Blaydes corneal f.
  Blaydes lens-holding f.
  blepharochalasis f.
  Bonaccolto fragment f.
  Bonaccolto jeweler f.
  Bonaccolto magnet tip f.
  Bonaccolto utility and splinter f.
  bone-biting f.
  Bonn iris f.
  Bonn suturing f.
  Boruchoff f.
  Botvin iris f.
  Bracken fixation f.
  Bracken iris f.
  Brannon extracapsular cleaving f.
  Brannon extracapsular removal f.
  Bronson-Magnion f.
  Brown-Grabow capsulorrhexis
    cystitome f.
  Brown insertion f.
  Bruening f.
  Buratto flap f.
  Buratto III acrylic implantation f.
  Buratto LASIK F.
  Buratto ophthalmic f.
  Calibri f.
  Callahan fixation f.
  capsule fragment f.
  capsulorrhexis f.
  Cardona corneal prosthesis f.
  Cardona threading f.
  Cartman lens insertion f.
  Castroviejo-Arruga f.
  Castroviejo capsule f.
  Castroviejo clip-applying f.
  Castroviejo-Colibri f.
  Castroviejo corneal-holding f.
  Castroviejo corneoscleral f.
  Castroviejo fixation f.
  Castroviejo lid f.
  Castroviejo scleral fold f.
  Castroviejo suture f.
  Castroviejo suturing f.
  Castroviejo tying f.
  Castroviejo wide grip handle f.
  Catalano corneoscleral f.
  Catalano tying f.
  Cauer chalazion f.

chalazion f.
Chandler iris f.
Choyce lens-inserting f.
Cilco lens f.
cilia f.
Clark capsule fragment f.
Clark-Verhoeff capsule f.
Clayman lens-holding f.
Clayman lens implant f.
Clayman lens-inserting f.
clip-applying f.
coaptation bipolar f.
Cohen corneal f.
Coleman-Taylor IOL f.
Colibri f.
conjunctiva f.
Connor capsulorrhexis peeler f.
cornea-holding f.
corneal fixation f.
corneal prosthesis f.
corneal splinter f.
corneoscleral f.
Cozean-McPherson tying f.
Crawford f.
cross-action capsule f.
Culler fixation f.
Cummings folding f.
cup f.
curved iris f.
curved tying f.
Dallas lens-inserting f.
Danberg iris f.
Dan chalazion f.
Dan-Gradle cilia f.
Dardenne nucleus f.
D. Aron-Rosa lens-holding f.
Davis f.
delicate grasping f.
delicate serrated straight dressing f.
Desmarres chalazion f.
disk f.
Dixon-Thorpe vitreous foreign body f.
Dk IOL insertion f.
Dodick lens-holding f.
double-pronged f.
Douglas cilia f.
Draeger f.
dressing f.
Drews cilia f.
Drews-Sato tying f.
Ducournau fine gripping f.

Eber needle-holder f.
Ehrhardt lid f.
Elschnig capsule f.
Elschnig fixation f.
Elschnig-O'Brien f.
Elschnig-O'Connor fixation f.
entropion f.
Erhardt lid f.
Ernest-McDonald soft intraocular lens-folding f.
Ewing capsule f.
eyelid f.
Farkas-Bracken fixation f.
Faulkner lens holding f.
Fechtner conjunctiva f.
Fechtner ring f.
Fine-Castroviejo suturing f.
Fine dissecting f.
Fine gripping f.
Fine irrigating capsulorrhexis f.
Fine sideport capsulorrhexis f.
Fine suture-tying f.
fine-toothed f.
Fink-Jameson muscle f.
Fisher-Arlt iris f.
fixation/anchor f.
fixation binocular f.
fixed f.
fold f.
foreign body f.
Förster iris f.
Francis spud chalazion f.
Fuchs capsule f.
Fuchs extracapsular f.
Fuchs iris f.
Furniss cornea-holding f.
Gaskin fragment f.
25-gauge intraocular f.
Gelfilm f.
Gifford fixation f.
Gifford iris f.
Gill-Arruga capsular f.
Gill-Colibri f.
Gill-Hess iris f.
Gill iris f.
Gills-Welsh capsule f.
Girard corneoscleral f.
Goldmann capsulorrhexis f.
Grabow f.
Gradle cilia f.
Graefe eye dressing f.
Graefe fixation f.

F

NOTES

forceps *(continued)*

Graefe iris f.
Graefe tissue f.
grasping f.
Grayson corneal f.
Grazer blepharoplasty f.
Green capsule f.
Green chalazion f.
Green fixation f.
Grieshaber diamond-coated f.
Grieshaber internal limiting
  membrane f.
Grieshaber iris f.
f. guard
Guist fixation f.
Gunderson muscle f.
Guyton-Clark fragment f.
Guyton-Noyes fixation f.
Halberg contact lens f.
Halsted curved mosquito
  hemostatic f.
Harman fixation f.
Harms-Colibri f.
Harms corneal f.
Harms-Tubingen tying f.
Harms tying f.
Hartmann mosquito hemostatic f.
Hasner lid f.
Heath chalazion f.
hemostatic f.
Henry cilia f.
Hersh LASIK retreatment f.
Hertel stone f.
Hess f.
Hess-Barraquer f.
Hessburg lens f.
Hessburg lens-inserting f.
Hess-Horwitz f.
Heyner f.
Hirschman lens f.
Hirschman lens-inserting f.
Holth f.
Hoskins beaked Colibri f.
Hoskins-Dallas intraocular lens-
  inserting f.
Hoskins fine straight f.
Hoskins fixation f.
Hoskins-Luntz f.
Hoskins miniaturized micro
  straight f.
Hoskins-Skeleton fine f.
Hoskins-Skeleton micro-grooved
  broad-tipped f.
Hoskins straight microiris f.
Hoskins suture f.
host tissue f.
House miniature f.
Hubbard corneoscleral f.
Hunt chalazion f.

Hyde corneal f.
Hyde double-curved f.
Ikeda microcapsulorrhexis f.
Ilg capsule f.
Ilg curved microtying f.
Ilg insertion f.
Inamura small incision
  capsulorrhexis f.
intraocular f.
Iowa State fixation f.
iris bipolar f.
I-tech intraocular foreign body f.
I-tech splinter f.
I-tech tying f.
Jacob capsule fragment f.
Jacobson hemostatic f.
Jaffe capsulorrhexis f.
Jaffe suturing f.
Jameson muscle f.
Jansen-Middleton septotomy f.
Jensen intraocular lens f.
Jensen lens-inserting f.
Jervey capsule fragment f.
Jervey iris f.
jeweler's bipolar f.
John Weiss f.
Jones f.
Judd f.
Kalt f.
Kansas fragment lens f.
Katena capsulorrhexis f.
Katzin-Barraquer f.
Kawai capsulorrhexis f.
Keeler extended round tip f.
Keeler intraocular foreign body
  grasping f.
Kelman-McPherson corneal f.
Kelman-McPherson lens-holding f.
Kelman-McPherson suturing f.
Kelman-McPherson tying f.
Kerrison f.
Kershner butterfly capsulorrhexis f.
Kershner LASIK flap f.
Kershner One-Step Micro
  capsulorrhexis f.
Kevorkian-Younge f.
King-Prince muscle f.
Kirby capsule f.
Kirby corneoscleral f.
Kirby iris f.
Kirby tissue f.
Knapp f.
Knolle-Shepard lens-holding f.
Knolle-Volker lens-holding f.
Koby cataract f.
Kraff fixation f.
Kraff intraocular utility f.
Kraff lens-holding f.
Kraff lens-inserting f.

Kraff suturing f.
Kraff tying f.
Kraff-Utrata capsulorrhexis f.
Kraff-Utrata intraocular utility f.
Kraft f.
Kratz lens-inserting f.
Kremer corneal fixation f.
Kremer two-point fixation f.
Kronfeld suturing f.
Krukenberg pigment spindle f.
Kuhnt fixation f.
Kulvin-Kalt f.
Lalonde hook f.
Lambert chalazion f.
Lambert hook f.
large-angled f.
Leahey chalazion f.
Leigh capsule f.
lens-holding f.
lens-threading f.
Lester fixation f.
lid f.
Lieberman lens-holding f.
Lieberman micro-ring lens f.
Lieberman-Pollock double corneal f.
Lindstrom lens-insertion f.
Linn-Graefe iris f.
Lister f.
Littauer cilia f.
Livernois lens-holding f.
Livernois pickup and folding f.
Llobera fixation f.
Lordan chalazion f.
Lucae dressing f.
Machemer diamond-dust-coated
  foreign body f.
Malis f.
Manche LASIK f.
Manhattan Eye & Ear suturing f.
marginal chalazion f.
Masket capsulorrhexis f.
matte black f.
Maumenee capsule f.
Maumenee-Colibri corneal f.
Maumenee corneal f.
Maumenee Suregrip f.
Max Fine f.
McCullough suturing f.
McDonald lens-folding f.
McDonald soft IOL folding f.
McGregor conjunctival f.
McGuire marginal chalazion f.

McLean capsule f.
McLean muscle recession f.
McPherson angled f.
McPherson bent f.
McPherson corneal f.
McPherson irrigating f.
McPherson microiris f.
McPherson microsuture f.
McPherson suturing f.
McPherson tying iris f.
McQueen vitreous f.
MedOne Ducournau fine
  gripping f.
MedOne ILM f.
Mendez multi-purpose LASIK f.
Mentor-Maumenee Suregrip f.
Mermoud nonpenetrating
  glaucoma f.
Metico f.
micro Colibri f.
microserrated Tano asymmetrical
  peeling f.
miniature f.
Moehle corneal f.
Moody fixation f.
Moore lens f.
Moore lens-inserting f.
mosquito hemostatic f.
muscle f.
Neubauer f.
Nevyas lens f.
Newman collagen plug inserter f.
New Orleans Eye & Ear
  fixation f.
New York Eye & Ear Hospital
  fixation f.
Noble f.
Noyes f.
Nugent fixation f.
Nugent superior rectus f.
O'Brien-Elschnig fixation f.
O'Brien fixation f.
Ochsner cartilage f.
Ochsner tissue f.
Ochsner tissue/cartilage f.
O'Connor-Elschnig fixation f.
O'Connor iris f.
O'Connor lid f.
O'Connor sponge f.
O'Gawa suture-fixation f.
Ogura cartilage f.
Ogura tissue f.

F

NOTES

forceps *(continued)*

Ogura tissue/cartilage f.
Osher foreign body f.
Packo conjunctiva f.
Passarelli one-pass capsulorrhexis f.
Paton anterior chamber lens implant f.
Paton capsule f.
Paton corneal transplant f.
Paton suturing f.
Paton tying/stitch removal f.
Paufique suturing f.
Pavlo-Colibri corneal f.
Penn-Anderson scleral fixation f.
Perone LASIK Flap F.
Perritt double-fixation f.
Peyman-Green vitreous f.
Phillips fixation f.
Pierse corneal Colibri-type f.
Pierse fixation f.
Pierse-Hoskins f.
Pierse-type Colibri f.
Pley extracapsular f.
Pollock f.
pre-chopping f.
Primbs suturing f.
Prince muscle f.
ptosis f.
Puntenney f.
pupil spreader/retractor f.
Quevedo fixation f.
Quevedo suturing f.
Quire mechanical finger f.
recession f.
Reese muscle f.
Reisinger lens-extracting f.
Rhein Artisan lens-holding f.
Rhein capsulorrhexis cystitome f.
Rhein fine foldable lens-insertion f.
Rhein LASIK flap f.
ring f.
ring-tip f.
Ritch-Krupin-Denver eye valve-insertion f.
Rizzuti-Furniss cornea-holding f.
Rizzuti rectus f.
Rizzuti scleral fixation f.
Rolf f.
roller f.
Russian f.
Rycroft tying f.
Sachs tissue f.
Sanders-Castroviejo suturing f.
Sandt f.
Sattler advancement f.
Sauer suture f.
Saupe cilia f.
Schaaf foreign body f.
Schaefer fixation f.
Scheie-Graefe fixation f.
Schepens f.
Schweigger capsule f.
Schweigger extracapsular f.
scleral twist-grip f.
Scott lens-insertion f.
series five f.
serrated conjunctival f.
Sewall f.
Shaaf cilia foreign body f.
Shea f.
Sheets lens-inserting f.
Sheets-McPherson tying f.
Shepard intraocular lens f.
Shepard intraocular lens-holding f.
Shepard intraocular utility f.
Shepard lens-inserting f.
Shepard-Reinstein f.
Shepard tying f.
Shields f.
Shoemaker intraocular lens f.
S5-1804-HUMER lens-folding f.
silicone rod and sleeve f.
silicone sponge f.
Simcoe lens implant f.
Simcoe lens-inserting f.
Simcoe nucleus f.
Simcoe posterior chamber lens f.
Sinskey lens-holding f.
Sinskey micro-tying f.
Sinskey-Wilson foreign body f.
Skeleton fine f.
sleeve spreading f.
Smart f.
Smith-Leiske cross-action intraocular lens f.
smooth grasping f.
Snellen entropion f.
Snyder corneal spring f.
Sourdille f.
Spaleck f.
Spencer chalazion f.
Spero f.
splaytooth f.
Starr fixation f.
Stephens soft IOL-inserting f.
Stern-Castroviejo locking f.
Stern-Castroviejo suturing f.
Stevens iris f.
stitch-removal f.
Stolte capsulorrhexis f.
Storz-Bonn suturing f.
Storz capsule f.
Storz cilia f.
Storz corneal f.
Storz-Utrata f.
strabismus f.
straight-tip bipolar f.
straight tying f.

Strow corneal f.
superior rectus f.
suturing f.
Takahashi iris retractor f.
Tennant-Colibri corneal f.
Tennant lens-inserting f.
Tennant titanium suturing f.
Tennant-Troutman superior rectus f.
Tennant tying f.
Tenner titanium suturing f.
Tenzel f.
Terson capsule f.
Terson extracapsular f.
Thomas fixation f.
Thornton fixation f.
Thorpe-Castroviejo corneal f.
Thorpe-Castroviejo fixation f.
Thorpe-Castroviejo vitreous foreign
  body f.
Thorpe conjunctival f.
Thorpe corneal f.
Thorpe foreign body f.
Thrasher lens implant f.
three-toothed f.
tissue f.
titanium suturing f.
toothed f.
Troutman-Barraquer corneal
  fixation f.
Troutman-Barraquer corneal
  utility f.
Troutman-Castroviejo corneal
  fixation f.
Troutman-Llobera fixation f.
Troutman rectus f.
Troutman tying f.
tubing introducer f.
tying f.
tying/stitch removal f.
Universal II f.
Utrata capsulorrhexis f.
Utrata-Kershner capsulorrhexis
  cystitome f.
Verhoeff capsule f.
vertical f.
Vickerall round ringed f.
Vickers f.
vitreous foreign body f.
von Graefe fixation f.
von Graefe iris f.
von Graefe tissue f.

von Mondak capsule fragment-
  clot f.
Wadsworth lid f.
Wainstock suturing f.
Waldeau fixation f.
Watzke f.
Weaver chalazion f.
Welsh pupil-spreader f.
Whitney superior rectus f.
Wies chalazion f.
Wilde f.
Wilkerson intraocular lens-
  insertion f.
Wills Hospital utility f.
Wills utility eye f.
Wolfe f.
Worst implantation f.
Worth strabismus f.
Wullstein-House cup f.
Zaldivar iridectomy f.
Zaldivar micro acrylic lens
  implantation f.
Zaldivar reverse capsulorrhexis f.
Ziegler cilia f.
Zurich suturing f.
Fordyce nodule
forebrain dysplasia
foreign
  f. body (FB)
  f. body bur
  f. body cell
  f. body extraction
  f. body forceps
  f. body locator
  f. body needle
  f. body sclerotomy
  f. body spud
foreign-body sensation
Forel field
foreshortening
  fornical f.
Forker retractor
form
  f. perception
  f. sense
  f. vision
format
  tagged image file f. (TIFF)
formation
  epiretinal membrane f.
  macular hole f.
form-deprivation myopia

NOTES

F

forme fruste
FormFlex
    F. lens
    F. lens loupe
formula, pl. formulas, formulae
    Cellufresh F.
    Hoffer-Colenbrander f.
    Holladay f.
    Icaps Lutein & Zeaxanthin F.
    lens-maker f.
    Lepper-Trier f.
    MaxiVision Ocular F.
    MaxiVision Whole Body F.
    Sanders-Retzlaff-Kraff f.
    SRK f.
fornical
    f. conjunctiva
    f. foreshortening
fornix, pl. fornices
    f. approach
    f. conjunctiva
    inferior conjunctival f.
    lacrimal f.
    f. reformation
    f. sacci lacrimalis
    superior conjunctival f.
fornix-based conjunctival flap
Forsius-Eriksson syndrome
forskolin
Forssman carotid syndrome
Förster
    F. choroiditis
    F. conjunctiva
    F. disease
    F. enucleation snare
    F. iris forceps
    F. lacrimal sac
    F. operation
    F. photometer
    F. photoptometer
    F. sacci lacrimalis
    F. uveitis
Förster-Fuchs black spot
Forte
    AK-Sulf F.
    B-Salt F.
    FML F.
    Inflamase F.
    Lipo-Tears F.
    Liquifilm F.
    Naphcon F.
    Ocu-Pred F.
    Pred F.
    Predair F.
    Prednefrin F.
    Sulfair F.
    Tears Naturale F.

fortification
    f. figure
    f. spectrum
fortified antibiotic
fortuitum
    Mycobacterium f.
forward
    f. light scatter
    f. traction test
Foscarnet-Ganciclovir CMV Retinitis Trial (FGCRT)
foscarnet sodium
Foscavir
fossa, pl. fossae
    f. glandulae lacrimalis
    hyaloid f.
    f. hyaloidea
    interpeduncular f.
    lacrimal gland f.
    lacrimal sac f.
    lenticular f.
    optical f.
    f. sacci lacrimalis
    trochlear f.
    f. trochlearis
    f. tumor
fossette
Foster
    F. enucleation snare
    F. Kennedy syndrome
    F. snare enucleator
    F. suture
Foucault
    F. knife
    F. knife edge test
Fould entropion operation
foundation
    Fred Hollow's F.
four base-out prism testing
four-dot test
Fourier harmonic analysis
four-loop
    f.-l. iris clip implant
    f.-l. iris fixated implant
    f.-l. lens
four-mirror
    f.-m. goniolens
    f.-m. goniolens lens
four-point fixation
four-sided cutting needle
fourth
    f. cranial nerve (CN IV)
    f. nerve palsy
fovea, pl. foveae
    central f.
    f. centralis
    obscured f.
    trochlear f.
    f. trochlearis

foveal
    f. avascular zone (FAZ)
    f. burn
    f. center
    f. cone electroretinography
    f. cyst
    f. depression
    f. dystopia
    f. edema
    f. flicker fusion frequency
    f. image
    f. ischemia
    f. outer retinal dysfunction
    f. outer retinal function
    f. pit
    f. pseudocyst
    f. reflex
    f. retina
    f. retinal detachment
    f. sparing
    f. splitting
    f. traction
    f. translocation
    f. vision
foveating saccades
foveola, pl. **foveolae**
    f. ocularis
    retinal f.
foveolar
    f. choroidal circulation
    f. reflex
    f. retinal detachment
foveomacular
    f. cone dysfunction syndrome
    f. retinitis
    f. retinopathy
    f. vitelliform dystrophy
Foville syndrome
Foville-Wilson syndrome
fowleri
    Naegleria f.
Fox
    F. aluminum shield
    F. conformer
    F. eye shield
    F. irrigating/aspirating unit
    F. irrigator
    F. LASIK spatula
    F. operation
    F. speculum
    F. sphere implant

FOZR
    front optic zone radius
FP
    fundus photo
FPA
    far point of accommodation
FPAL
    fluorescein-potentiated argon laser
     therapy
FR3
    third framework region
fraction
    Snellen f.
fracture
    apex f.
    blow-in f.
    blow-out f.
    combined f.
    comminuted orbital f.
    depressed f.
    external orbital f.
    facial f.
    floor f.
    midfacial f.
    nasoorbital f.
    f. of orbit
    orbital blow-out f.
    orbital floor f.
    orbital rim f.
    orbital wall f.
    pediatric orbital floor f.
    roof f.
    trap-door f.
    tripod f.
    zygomatic f.
fragilis
    Bacillus f.
    Bacteroides f.
fragilitas ossium
Fragmatome
    CooperVision F.
    F. flute syringe
    Gill-Hess F.
    Girard F.
fragment
    Cooper blade f.
    Fab f.
    Fc f.
    Hoskins razor blade f.
fragmentation
    proportional f.

F

NOTES

fragmentation/aspiration handpiece
fragment crystallizable (Fc)
fragmented dendrite
fragmentor
>Lieberman f.

frame
>celluloid f.
>cellulose acetate f.
>cellulose nitrate f.
>f. difference
>Lucite f.
>molded f.
>MTL trial f.
>nylon f.
>Oculus trial f.
>optical f.
>Optyl f.
>f. papillary distance
>f. PD
>Perspex f.
>plastic f.
>Plexiglas f.
>polymethylmethacrylate f.
>rimless f.
>f. scotoma
>spectacle f.
>Stryker f.
>trial f.

frame-mounted pump
framework
>scleral f.
>uveal f.

Franceschetti
>F. coreoplasty operation
>F. corepraxy operation
>F. deviation operation
>F. disease
>F. dystrophy
>F. keratoplasty operation
>F. pupil deviation operation
>F. syndrome

Franceschetti-Klein syndrome
Francis
>F. spud
>F. spud chalazion forceps

Francisella tularensis
François
>central cloudy dystrophy of F.
>dermochondral corneal dystrophy of F.
>dyscephalic syndrome of F.
>F. dystrophy
>F. syndrome

François-Neetens dystrophy
frank corneal ulceration
Frankfort horizontal plane
Franklin
>F. bifocal

>F. glasses
>F. spectacles

Franklin-style bifocal lenses
Fraser syndrome
Fraunfelder "no touch" technique
Fraunhofer
>F. diffraction
>F. line

Frazier
>F. dura hook
>F. suction tube

FRCP
>Fellow of the Royal College of Physicians

FRCPC
>Fellow of the Royal College of Physicians of Canada

FRCS
>Fellow of the Royal College of Surgeons

FRCSA
>Fellow of the Royal College of Surgeons of Australia

freckle
>iris f.

Frederick sleeve spreader
Fred Hollow's Foundation
free
>f. conjunctival autograft
>f. margin of eyelid
>f. operculum
>f. running mode
>f. skin autograft
>Tears Naturale F.
>f. tenotomy

Freeman
>F. punctum plug
>F. solution

Freeman-Sheldon syndrome
Freer
>F. chisel
>F. periosteal elevator

freeze
>Keeler-Amoils f.

freezer
>Wallach cryosurgery f.

freeze-thaw cryotherapy
Frelex lens
French
>F. catheter
>F. hook spatula
>F. lacrimal dilator
>F. lacrimal probe
>F. lacrimal spatula
>F. needle holder
>F. pattern spatula

Frenkel anterior ocular traumatic syndrome

Frenzel
F. goggles
F. lens
frequency
critical corresponding f. (CCF)
critical flicker f. (CFF)
critical flicker fusion f.
f. doubling illusion
F. Doubling Perimeter test
f. doubling perimetry
f. doubling technique
f. doubling technology (FDT)
f. doubling technology mean
deviation (FDT-MD)
f. doubling technology pattern
standard deviation (FDT-PSD)
foveal flicker fusion f.
fusion f.
F. 38 monthly disposable contact
lens
relevant spatial f.
fresh
Lens F.
FreshLook ColorBlends lens
Fresnel
F. lens
F. membrane
F. optics
F. press-on prism
F. principle
Frey
F. syndrome
F. tunneled implant
Fricke operation
Fridenberg stigmatometric card
Friedenwald
F. funduscope
F. law
F. operation
F. ophthalmoscope
F. syndrome
Friedenwald-Guyton operation
Friede operation
Friedlander incision marker
Friedman
F. hand-held Hruby lens
F. Phaco/IOL manipulator
F. tantalum clip
F. test
Friedman-Hruby lens
Friedmann visual field analyzer

Friedreich
F. ataxia
F. syndrome
Frigitronics
Cilco F.
F. cryosurgical unit
F. freeze-thaw cryopexy probe
F. nitrous oxide cryosurgery
apparatus
F. vitrector
frill
iris f.
plaited f.
Frin
Isopto F.
fringe
interference f.
Moiré f.
Frisby stereoacuity test
Fritz vitreous transplant needle
FROD
fat removal orbital decompression
frog cortex remover
frond
fibrous f.
fibrovascular f.
sea f.
vascular f.
f. of vessel
front
f. build-up implant
f. optic zone radius (FOZR)
f. surface toric contact lens
f. vertex
f. vertex power
frontal
f. axis
f. bone
f. craniotomy
f. diploic vein
f. eye field
f. incisure
f. lobe
f. lobe unilateral cerebral
hemisphere lesion
f. nerve
f. sinus
f. sinusitis
f. triangle
f. tuber
frontalis
facies orbitalis ossis f.

F

NOTES

frontalis (*continued*)
    fascia lata f.
    f. fascia lata suspension
    incisura ethmoidalis ossis f.
    margo supraorbitalis ossis f.
    f. muscle
    f. muscle sling
    pars orbitalis ossis f.
    f. sling technique
    sulcus orbitales lobi f.
    vena diploica f.
frontolacrimalis
    sutura f.
frontolacrimal suture
frontoparietal bilateral cerebral hemisphere lesion
frontosphenoid suture
frontozygomatic suture
Frost
    F. scissors
    F. suture
frosted branch angiitis
Frostig Development Test of Visual Perception
Frost-Lang operation
frozen
    f. globe
    f. tissue
fruste
    forme f.
    keratoconus f.
FTC
    full to confrontation
5-FU
    5-fluorouracil
Fuchs
    F. adenoma
    angle of F.
    F. aphakic keratopathy
    F. atrophy
    F. black spot
    F. canthorrhaphy operation
    F. capsule forceps
    F. combined corneal dystrophy
    combined dystrophy of F.
    F. crypt
    dellen of F.
    F. dimple
    F. endothelial corneal dystrophy
    F. epithelial corneal dystrophy
    epithelial dystrophy of F.
    F. epithelial-endothelial dystrophy
    F. extracapsular forceps
    F. heterochromia
    F. heterochromic cyclitis (FHC)
    F. heterochromic iridocyclitis
    F. inferior coloboma
    F. iris bombe transfixation operation

    F. iris forceps
    F. keratitis
    lamella of F.
    F. lancet-type keratome
    F. retinal detachment syringe
    F. spot coloboma
    F. spur
    F. syndrome
    F. two-way syringe
    F. uveitis
Fuchs-Kraupa syndrome
fucidic acid gel
Fucidin gel
fugax
    amaurosis partialis f.
    episcleritis partialis f.
    episcleritis periodica f.
    hemianopsia bitemporalis f.
    keratitis periodica f.
    saburral amaurosis f.
Fugo blade capsulotomy
Fukala operation
Fukasaku
    F. small pupil snapper hook
    F. snap & split tip irrigating chopper
    F. spatula
Fukuyama LRI marker
Ful-Glo fluorescein strip
fulguration
full
    f. to confrontation (FTC)
    f. thickness macular hole
    f. versions and ductions
full-arc depth-dependent astigmatic keratotomy
full-dimpled Lucite implant
Fuller silicone sponge
Fullerview iris retractor
full-field
    f.-f. electroretinogram
    f.-f. system
full-thickness
    f.-t. autograft
    f.-t. corneal graft
    f.-t. corneal laceration
    f.-t. keratoplasty
fulminans
    glaucoma f.
fulminant
    f. abscess
    f. glaucoma
    f. myasthenia gravis
    f. ocular toxoplasmosis
Ful-Vue
    F.-V. bifocal
    F.-V. ophthalmoscope
    F.-V. spot retinoscope
    F.-V. streak retinoscope

fumagillin
fumarate
    ketotifen f.
Fumidil B
fumigatus
    Aspergillus f.
function
    bandpass f.
    binocular f.
    cone f.
    corneal epithelial barrier f.
    Easterman visual f.
    foveal outer retinal f.
    medial rectus f.
    modulation transfer f.
    motor f.
    neural transfer f.
    optical transfer f.
    peripheral rod f.
    response f.
    rod f.
    spread f.
    transfer f.
    visual f.
    wavefront aberration f.
    f. of Zernike mode
functional
    F. Acuity Contrast Test (FACT)
    f. amblyopia
    f. blindness
    f. defect
    f. visual loss
fundal reflex
fundectomy
fundus, pl. **fundi**
    albinotic f.
    albipunctate f.
    f. albipunctatus
    f. autofluorescence
    blond f.
    f. camera
    coloboma of f.
    f. contact lens
    f. diabeticus
    f. examination
    f. of eye
    f. flavimaculatus
    f. focalizing lens
    Kowa f.
    f. laser lens
    leopard f.
    f. microscopy

    mottling of f.
    normal f.
    f. oculi
    optic f.
    pepper-and-salt f.
    f. photo (FP)
    f. photograph
    f. polycythemicus
    prismatic f.
    f. reflex
    salt-and-pepper f.
    sunset f.
    tessellated f.
    f. tigré
    tigroid f.
    tomato-ketchup f.
    f. xerophthalmicus
Funduscein
Funduscein-10, -25
funduscope
    Friedenwald f.
funduscopic examination
funduscopy
fundusectomy
fungal
    f. blepharitis
    f. corneal ulcer
    f. endophthalmitis
    f. infection
    f. keratitis
    f. uveitis
Fungizone
fungus, pl. **fungi**
    filamentous f.
    hyaline f.
    moniliaceous filamentous f.
    nonfilamentous f.
funnel
    muscular f.
    vascular f.
funnel-shaped retinal detachment
furnacemen's cataract
Furniss cornea-holding forceps
furrow
    corneal marginal f.
    f. degeneration
    f. dystrophy
    f. keratitis
    marginal f.
    palpebral f.
    scleral f.
    superior palpebral f.

F

NOTES

furrowing
Fusarium
 F. episphaeria
 F. moniliforme
 F. oxysporum
 F. solani
fusca
 lamina f.
 membrana f.
fuscin
fused
 f. bifocal lens
 f. multifocal lens
fusiform
 f. aneurysm
 f. cataract
fusion
 amplitude of f.
 f. area
 binocular f.
 f. breakpoint
 central f.
 color f.
 critical flicker f. (CFF)
 eyelid f.
 f. faculty
 first-grade f.
 flicker f.

 f. frequency
 f. grade
 motor f.
 peripheral f.
 f. reflex
 second-grade f.
 sensory f.
 tenacious distance f.
 tenacious proximal f.
 third-grade f.
 f. tube
 f. with accommodation
 f. with amplitude
 Worth concept of f.
fusional
 f. convergence
 f. convergence amplitude
 f. divergence
 f. divergence amplitude
 f. movement
 f. reserve
 f. vergence
fusion-free position
fusionis
 horror f.
Fusobacterium necrophorum
fVEP
 flash visual-evoked potential

G
    aqueous crystalline penicillin G
    penicillin G
Gaffee speculum
gag gene
Gaillard-Arlt suture
galactokinase deficiency
galactose cataract
galactosemia
    g. cataract
    enzymatic g.
Galardin
Galassi pupillary phenomenon
galeal flap
Galen vein
galeropia
galeropsia
Galezowski lacrimal dilator
Galilean
    G. magnification changer
    G. microscope
    G. telescope
Galin
    G. bleb cup
    G. intraocular implant lens
Gallie cryoenucleator
gallium
    g. citrate contrast
    g. citrate contrast material
    g. scan
    g. scanning
Galt aspirating cannula
galvanic nystagmus
Gamboscope
game
    E g.
    The Pointing G.
gamma
    g. angle
    g. crystallin
    g. irradiation
ganciclovir
    g. cyclic phosphate
    G. Implant Study for
        Cytomegalovirus Retinitis
    g. sodium
    g. therapy
**Ganciclovir-Cidofovir CMV Retinitis
    Trial (GCCRT)**
ganglia (*pl. of* ganglion)
ganglioglioma
ganglioma
ganglion, pl. **ganglia**
    basal g.
    g. cell

g. cell layer
cervical g.
ciliary g.
gasserian g.
geniculate g.
g. layer of optic nerve
g. layer of retina
lenticular g.
long root of ciliary g.
motor root of ciliary g.
oculomotor root of ciliary g.
ophthalmic g.
optic g.
orbital g.
pterygopalatine g.
retinal g.
Schacher g.
sensory root of ciliary g.
short root of ciliary g.
sphenopalatine g.
g. stratum of optic nerve
superior cervical g.
trigeminal sensory g.
ganglioneuroma
ganglionic
    g. layer of optic nerve
    g. layer of retina
    g. stratum of optic nerve
    g. stratum of retina
ganglionitis
ganglioside
gangliosidosis
gangliosus ciliaris
gangraenescens
    granuloma g.
gangrenosa
    vaccinia g.
gangrenosum
    ecthyma g.
gangrenous rhinitis
Gans cyclodialysis cannula
Gantrisin
Ganzfeld
    G. electroretinograph
    G. illumination
Ganzfield bowl
gape
    wound g.
GAPO
    growth retardation, alopecia,
        pseudoanodontia, and optic atrophy
    GAPO syndrome
Garamycin
Garcia-Ibanez camera
Garcia-Novito eye implant

G

Gardner syndrome
garter
    Goffman eye g.
Gartner
    G. canal
    G. cyst
    G. duct
    G. phenomenon
    G. tonometer
Garway-Heath reasoning
gas
    g. bubble
    C3F8 g.
    g. discharge lamp
    heavy g.
    hexafluoride g.
    inspired g.
    intraocular g.
    ISPAN intraocular g.
    laughing g.
    long-acting g.
    mustard g.
    octafluoropropane g.
    perfluorocarbon g.
    perfluoropropane g. (C3F8)
    SF6 g.
    sulfur g.
    sulfurhexafluoride g.
    g. tamponade
    tear g.
gas-exchange descemetopexy
gas-filled eye
gas-fluid exchange (GFE)
Gaskin fragment forceps
gas-permeable
    g.-p. contact lens (GPCL)
    g.-p. daily cleaner
    rigid g.-p. (RGP)
Gass
    G. cataract-aspirating cannula
    G. corneoscleral punch
    G. dye applicator
    G. irrigating/aspirating unit
    G. macular hole classification
    G. muscle hook
    G. retinal detachment hook
    G. scleral marker
    G. scleral punch
    G. sclerotomy punch
    G. syndrome
    G. vitreous-aspirating cannula
gasserian ganglion
GAT
    Goldmann applanation tonometer
gatifloxacin
Gaucher disease
gauge
    blade g.
    coin g.

    Deitz incision depth g.
    depth g.
    Grandon rotatable radial marker
      and degree g.
    25-g. intraocular forceps
    Katena depth g.
    Marco radius g.
    Mendez degree g.
    30-g. needle
    radius g.
    Reichert radius g.
    Shepard incision depth g.
    Stahl lens g.
    Steinert-Deacon incision g.
    20-g. straight bipolar pencil
    V-groove g.
    Zaldivar degree g.
Gaule
    G. pit
    G. spot
Gault reflex
gaussian
    g. distribution
    g. optical system
    g. optics
Gayet operation
gaze
    apraxia of g.
    cardinal diagnostic position of g.
    cardinal direction of g.
    g. center
    conjugate g.
    diagnostic position of g.
    disconjugate g.
    distant g.
    downward g.
    dysconjugate g.
    eccentric g.
    evoked nystagmus g.
    field of g.
    horizontal g.
    lateral g.
    left g.
    midline position of g.
    g. movement
    near fixation position of g.
    g. nystagmus
    g. palsy
    parallelism of g.
    paralysis of g.
    ping-pong g.
    primary position of g.
    right g.
    spasticity of conjugate g.
    superior g.
    supranuclear paresis of vertical g.
    upward g.
    vertical g.

gaze-evoked
- g.-e. amaurosis
- g.-e. nystagmus
- g.-e. tinnitus

gaze-holding
- eccentric g.-h.

gaze-paretic nystagmus

G-banding

GC
- goniocurettage

GCA
- giant cell arteritis

GCCRT
- Ganciclovir-Cidofovir CMV Retinitis Trial

GCD
- geometric center distance

GCM
- good, central, maintained

GCNM
- good, central, not maintained

GD
- glare disability
- global deviation

GDD
- glaucoma drainage device

GDx nerve fiber analyzer

Geggel corneal transplant marker

Geiger
- G. cautery
- G. electrocautery

gel
- Aquasonic 100 g.
- ferric hyaluronate g.
- fibrin g.
- fucidic acid g.
- Fucidin g.
- GenTeal lubricant eye g.
- Gonio G.
- H.P. Acthar G.
- Night & Day Tears Again sterile lubricant g.
- Pilopine HS g.
- silica g.
- vitreous g.

gelatin
- g. disk
- g. film

gelatino-lattice corneal dystrophy

gelatinous
- g. dystrophy
- g. mass
- g. material
- g. scleritis

gelatinous-appearing limbal hypertrophy

Gel-Clean

Gelfilm
- G. cap
- G. forceps
- G. plate
- G. retinal implant
- Schepens G.

Gel Flex lens

gel-fluid
- Hylan biopolymer g.-f.

Gelfoam

gellan
- timolol g.

Gemella
- *Gemella haemolysans*
- *Gemella morbillorum*

gene
- a-crystallin/small heat-shock g.
- *CYP1B1* g.
- dominant g.
- env g.
- gag g.
- *LMX1B* g.
- g. locus
- metallothionein g.
- MHC g.
- myoclin g.
- nonpenetrant g.
- OCLM g.
- OPTN g.
- PEDF g.
- penetrant g.
- peripherin/RDS g.
- pol g.
- retinal degeneration slow (RDS) g.
- retinitis pigmentosa GTPase regulator g. (RPGR)
- retinoblastoma g.
- syntenic g.
- *TIGR* g.

general
- g. anesthesia
- g. anesthetic
- g. cataract

generalized
- g. essential telangiectasia (GET)
- g. vaccinia

generating spectacle lens

NOTES

G

generation
  filial g. (F)
  forced g.
Genesis
  G. diamond blade
  G. lens
Geneva lens measure
Geneye Ophthalmic
geniculate
  g. body
  g. ganglion
  g. hemianopsia
  g. nucleus
geniculocalcarine
  g. radiation
  g. tract
genome synthesis
Genoptic S.O.P. ophthalmic
Gentacidin ophthalmic
Gentadexa
Gentafair
Gentak ophthalmic
gentamicin
  prednisolone and g.
  g. sulfate
gentamicin-induced vestibulotoxicity
Gentasol
GenTeal
  G. lubricant eye gel
  G. Mild
  G. Mild lubricant eye drops
  G. Moderate
Gentex PDQ polycarbonate lens
gentian violet marking pen
GentleLASE laser
Gentrasul
geographic
  g. atrophy
  g. helicoid peripapillary
    choroidopathy
  g. herpes simplex corneal ulcer
  g. keratitis
  g. lesion
  g. peripapillary choroiditis
  g. ulceration
geometric
  g. axis
  g. center
  g. center distance (GCD)
  g. equator
  g. optics
Geopen
geotropic nystagmus
Gerlach network
German Hefner candle
gerontopia
gerontoxon lentis
Gerstmann-Straussler-Scheinker disease
Gerstmann syndrome

gestational
  g. diabetes
  g. diabetes mellitus
  g. injury
GET
  generalized essential telangiectasia
**Getman-Henderson-Marcus visual
  manipulation test**
Geuder
  G. implanter
  G. keratoplasty needle
GFAP
  glial fibrillary acidic protein
GFE
  gas-fluid exchange
Ghormley double cannula
ghost
  Bidwell g.
  g. cell
  g. cell glaucoma
  dendritic g.
  g. erythrocyte
  g. image
  g. ophthalmoscope
  g. scarring
  g. vessel
GHT
  Glaucoma Hemifield Test
Gianelli sign
giant
  g. aneurysm
  g. axonal neuropathy
  g. cell arteritis (GCA)
  g. cyst of retina
  g. drusen
  g. epithelial cell
  g. melanosome
  g. papilla
  g. papillary conjunctivitis (GPC)
  g. papillary hypertrophy (GPH)
  g. retinal break
  g. retinal tear (GRT)
giantism
  cerebral g.
Giardet corneal transplant scissors
Gibralter headrest
Gibson
  G. irrigating/aspirating unit
  G. irrigator
Giemsa stain
Gierke disease
Gifford
  G. applicator
  G. corneal curette
  G. delimiting keratotomy operation
  G. fixation forceps
  G. iris forceps
  G. needle holder

G. reflex
G. sign
Gifford-Galassi reflex
Gilbert-Behçet syndrome
Gill
G. blade
G. corneal knife
G. counterpressor
G. incision spreader
G. intraocular implant lens
G. iris forceps
G. scissors
Gill-Arruga capsular forceps
Gill-Colibri forceps
Gill-Fine corneal knife
Gill-Hess
G.-H. blade
G.-H. Fragmatome
G.-H. iris forceps
G.-H. knife
G.-H. scissors
Gillies scar correction operation
Gills
G. double irrigating/aspirating cannula
G. double Luer-Lok cannula
G. pop-up arcuate diamond knife
Gills-Welsh
G.-W. aspirating cannula
G.-W. capsule forceps
G.-W. capsule polisher
G.-W. curette
G.-W. double-barreled irrigating/aspirating cannula
G.-W. guillotine port
G.-W. irrigating/aspirating cannula
G.-W. knife
G.-W. olive-tip cannula
G.-W. scissors
G.-W. spatula
Gills-Welsh-Vannas angled micro scissors
Gilmore intraocular implant lens
Gimbel
G. fountain cannula
G. stabilization ring
G. stabilizing ring
ginkgo biloba
Ginsberg eye speculum
Girard
G. anterior chamber needle
G. cataract-aspirating needle

G. corneoscleral forceps
G. corneoscleral scissors
G. Fragmatome
G. irrigating cannula
G. irrigating tip
G. keratoprosthesis operation
G. phacofragmatome needle
G. phakofragmatome
G. procedure
G. scleral-expander ring
G. ultrasonic unit
Girard-Swan knife needle
Giraud-Teulon law
girdle
limbal g.
limbus g.
Vogt white limbal g.
Gish micro YAG laser
Gitelman syndrome
Givner lid retractor
glabella
glabellar fold
glabellum
glabrata
Candida g.
Torulopsis g.
Gladstone-Putterman transmarginal rotation entropion clamp
gland
accessory lacrimal g.
acinar lacrimal g.
apocrine g.
Baumgarten g.
Bruch g.
Ciaccio g.
ciliary g.
conjunctival g.
drainage of lacrimal g.
g. of eyelid
Harder g.
harderian g.
Henle g.
inferior lacrimal g.
Krause lacrimal g.
lacrimal g.
Manz g.
meibomian sebaceous g.
Moll g.
Mueller g.
nasolacrimal g.
palpebral g.
pineal g.

NOTES

gland (*continued*)
pituitary g.
Rosenmüller g.
salivary g.
sebaceous glands of conjunctiva g.
superior lacrimal g.
tarsal g.
tarsoconjunctival g.
tear g.
trachoma g.
g. trachoma
Waldeyer g.
g. of Wolfring
Wolfring lacrimal g.
Zeis g.
g. of Zeis
zeisian g.
glandula, pl. **glandulae**
glandulae ciliares conjunctivales
glandulae lacrimales accessoriae
g. lacrimalis
g. lacrimalis inferior
g. lacrimalis superior
glandulae mucosae conjunctivae
glandulae sebaceae conjunctivales
glandulae tarsales
glandular fossa of frontal bone
glare
blinding g.
dazzling g.
direct g.
g. disability (GD)
g. disability measurement
edge g.
peripheral g.
specular g.
g. test
veiling g.
g. vision
glarometer
Glaser microvitreoretinal cannula
glass
g. bead
Chavasse g.
Crookes g.
crown g.
finished g.
flint g.
High-Lite g.
g. lens
optical g.
semifinished g.
g. sphere implant
glassblower's cataract
Glasscock scissors
glasses
bifocal g.
cataract g.
contact g.

crutch g.
Difei g.
Franklin g.
Grafco magnifying g.
Hallauer g.
hemianopic g.
hyperbolic g.
magnifying g.
Masselon g.
presbyopia g.
reading g.
red-green g.
safety g.
self-adjusted g.
snow g.
striated g.
trifocal g.
without g. (VS)
glassine strand
glass-rod
g.-r. negative phenomenon
g.-r. positive phenomenon
glassworker's cataract
glassy
g. membrane
g. sheet
glatiramer acetate
glaucoma
absolute g.
g. absolutum
acute angle-closure g. (AACG)
acute chronic g.
acute congestive g.
acute intermittent primary angle-closure g. (A/I-PACG)
acute primary angle-closure g. (APACG)
air-block g.
alpha-chymotrypsin-induced g.
angle-closure g. (ACG)
angle-recession g.
aphakic g.
apoplectic g.
aqueous misdirected g.
auricular g.
block g.
capsular g.
chamber-deepening g.
chronic narrow-angle g.
chronic open-angle g. (COAG)
chronic primary angle-closure g. (C-PACG)
chronic simple g.
ciliary block g.
closed-angle g. (CAG)
combined-mechanism g.
compensated g.
congenital g.
congestive g.

g. consummatum
Contino g.
contusion angle g.
corticosteroid-induced g.
cyclocongestive g.
90-day g.
g. detection
Donders g.
g. drainage device (GDD)
drug-induced g.
enzymatic g.
enzyme g.
erythroclastic g.
g. examination
exfoliation g.
exfoliative g.
fibrin pupillary block g.
g. field defect
g. filtering bleb dysesthesia
g. filtering surgery
g. filtration surgery
flecken g.
G. Foundation of Australia
g. fulminans
fulminant g.
ghost cell g.
G. Hemifield Test (GHT)
hemolytic g.
hemorrhagic g.
herpes zoster g.
high-tension g. (HTG)
hypersecretion g.
g. imminens
infantile g.
inflammatory g.
intermittent angle-closure g.
iris-block g.
juvenile g.
juvenile-onset high pressure g.
juvenile open-angle g. (JOAG)
laser-induced g.
G. Laser Trial (GLT)
G. Laser Trial Followup Study
  (GLTFS)
latent angle-closure g.
lens exfoliation g.
lens-induced secondary open-
  angle g.
lens particle g.
lens protein g.
lenticular g.
low-pressure g.

low-tension g.
malignant g.
melanomalytic g.
monocular g.
mydriatic test for angle-closure g.
narrow-angle g. (NAG)
neovascular angle-closure g.
noncongestive g.
normal-pressure g.
normal-tension g. (NTG)
obstructive g.
ocular hypertension g.
ocular hypertensive g.
open-angle g. (OAG)
g. pencil
penetrating keratoplasty and g.
  (PKPG)
phacogenic g.
phacolytic g.
phacomorphic g.
phakic g.
pigmentary dispersion g.
primary angle-closure g.
primary infantile g.
primary open-angle g. (POAG)
prodromal g.
pseudoexfoliative g. (PEXG)
pseudoexfoliative capsular g.
pupil block g.
pupillary block g.
recessed-angle g.
recession-angle g.
retrobulbar hemorrhage g.
rubeotic g.
scleral shell g.
secondary angle-closure g.
secondary neovascular g.
simple g.
simplex g.
g. simplex
steroid g.
steroid-induced g.
g. suspect
trabeculitis g.
transscleral neodymium:yttrium-
  aluminum-garnet
  cyclophotocoagulation for g.
traumatic g.
uveitic g.
vitreociliary g.
vitreous block g.
wide-angle g.

NOTES

G

Glaucoma-Scope
glaucomatocyclitic crisis
glaucomatologist
glaucomatosa
    iritis g.
glaucomatous
    g. atrophy
    g. cataract
    g. cul-de-sac
    g. cup
    g. cupping
    g. damage detection by retinal thickness mapping
    g. excavation
    g. habit
    g. halo
    g. nerve-fiber bundle scotoma
    g. optic nerve damage (GOND)
    g. optic neuropathy
    g. pannus
    g. ring
    g. visual field loss
Glaucon
glaucosis
Glaucotest
GlaucTabs
glaukomflecken of Vogt
GLCIA **locus**
glia
glial
    g. fibrillary acidic protein (GFAP)
    g. fibrillary acidic protein antibody
    g. proliferation
    g. ring
glial-neural hamartoma
glide
    Hessburg intraocular lens g.
    intraocular lens g.
    lens g.
    Sheets lens g.
glioblastoma multiforme
gliocyte
    retinal g.
glioma
    anterior visual pathway g.
    astrocytic g.
    chiasmal g.
    g. endophytum
    hypothalamic g.
    intracranial g.
    g. of optic chiasm
    optic nerve g.
    orbital g.
    peripheral g.
    g. of retina
    retinal g.
    g. sarcomatosum
    telangiectatic g.
gliomatosis

gliomatous
glioneuroma
gliosarcoma
    retinal g.
gliosis
    neonatal g.
    premacular g.
    preretinal g.
    retinal g.
    traumatic g.
gliotic
    g. membrane
    g. strip
glissade
glissadic
Gln368Stop mutation
global
    g. cataract
    g. deviation (GD)
globe
    contact burns of g.
    contusion of g.
    disorganized g.
    frozen g.
    luxation of g.
    g. perforation
    ruptured g.
globosa
    cornea g.
globule
    eosinophilic g.
    Morgagni g.
    morgagnian g.
    ora g.
globus pallidus (GP)
glomerulonephritis
    membranoproliferative g. type II
glove
    Biogel Sensor surgical g.
glower
    Nernst g.
GLP
    grid laser photocoagulation
GLT
    Glaucoma Laser Trial
GLTFS
    Glaucoma Laser Trial Followup Study
Glucantime
glucocorticoid
    ophthalmic g.
    systemic g.
    topical g.
glucose 6-phosphate dehydrogenase
glue
    butyl cyanoacrylate g.
    cyanoacrylate tissue g.
    ethyl cyanoacrylate g.
    fibrinogen g.
    Histoacryl g.

methyl cyanoacrylate g.
N-butyl-2-cyanoacrylate g.
g. patch
g. patch leak
glued-on hard contact lens
glutamyltransferase
glycerin
glycerin-preserved graft
glycerol
anhydrase g.
glyceryl monostearate
glycocalyx matrix
glycogen granule
glycol
dihydrophenylethylene g. (DHPG)
ethylene g.
polyethylene g.
propylene g.
glycoprotein
mucin-like g.
glycosaminoglycan
Glyrol
GMS
Gomori methenamine silver
goblet
g. cell
g. cell hyperplasia
Goethe color shadow
Goffman eye garter
goggles
Frenzel g.
night-vision g.
pinhole g.
plethysmographic g.
swimmer's g.
goiter
exophthalmic g.
gold
g. disk Grass electrode
g. dust retinopathy
G. eyelid load implant
g. eye plaque
g. salts
g. sodium thiomalate
g. sphere implant
g. tattoo pigment
g. weight
Goldberg
G. side-port splitter
G. syndrome
Goldenhar-Gorlin syndrome
Goldenhar syndrome

golden tapetal-like fundus reflex
Goldflam disease
Goldflam-Erb disease
Goldmann
G. applanation tonometer (GAT)
G. capsulorrhexis forceps
G. Coherent radiation
G. contact lens prism
G. diagnostic contact lens
G. fundus contact lens
G. goniolens
G. kinetic perimetry
G. kinetic technique
G. macular contact lens
G. manual projection perimeter
G. multi-mirror lens
G. serrated knife
G. static technique
G. three-mirror contact diagnostic lens
G. three-mirror implant
G. three-mirror prism
G. visual field test
Goldmann-Favre
G.-F. disease
G.-F. dystrophy
G.-F. retinoschisis
G.-F. syndrome
Goldmann-Larson
G.-L. foreign body
G.-L. foreign body operation
Goldmann-Weekers dark adaptometer
Goldman scleral fixation ring and blepharostat
Gold-Mules implant
Goldstein
G. anterior chamber syringe
G. cannula
G. golf-club spud
G. lacrimal sac retractor
G. lacrimal syringe
G. refractor
golf-club eye spud
Golgi
G. apparatus
G. complex
G. I, II neuron
Goltz-Gorlin syndrome
Goltz syndrome
Gomborg-Nielsen keratoderma
Gomez-Marquez lacrimal operation

G

NOTES

Gomori
  G. methenamine silver (GMS)
  G. methenamine silver stain
Gonak
GOND
  glaucomatous optic nerve damage
gondii
  Toxoplasma g.
Gonin
  G. cautery
  G. cautery operation
  G. marker
Gonin-Amsler marker
Gonio
  G. Gel
  G. soft
goniocurettage (GC)
goniodysgenesis
goniofocalizing lens
goniogram
  Becker g.
goniolaser
  Thorpe four-mirror g.
goniolens
  Allen-Thorpe g.
  Barkan g.
  four-mirror g.
  Goldmann g.
  Koeppe g.
  g. lens
  P.F. Lee pediatric g.
  single-mirror g.
  Thorpe-Castroviejo g.
  Thorpe four-mirror g.
  Zeiss g.
goniometer
  Bailliart g.
goniophotocoagulation
goniophotography
gonioplasty
gonioprism
  Posner diagnostic g.
  Posner surgical g.
  Swan-Jacob g.
goniopuncture knife
gonioscope
  Jacob-Swann g.
  Lovac g.
  Sussman four-mirror g.
  Thorpe surgical g.
  Troncoso g.
  Zeiss g.
gonioscopic
  g. implant
  g. lens
  g. prism
gonioscopy
  compression g.

  indentation g.
  Koeppe g.
Goniosol
goniosynechia
goniosynechialysis (GSL)
goniotomy
  g. knife
  g. knife cannula
  g. needle holder
  g. operation
  photoablative laser g. (PLG)
gonoblennorrhea
gonococcal
  g. bacillus
  g. conjunctivitis
  g. keratitis
  g. ophthalmia
gonorrheal
  g. conjunctivitis
  g. ophthalmia
gonorrhoeae
  Neisseria g.
good
  g., central, maintained (GCM)
  g., central, not maintained (GCNM)
  G. retractor
Goppert sign
Gorham
  G. disease
  massive osteolysis of G.
Gorham-Stout syndrome
gossamer scarring
gouge
  lacrimal sac g.
  spud and g.
  g. spud
  Todd g.
  West g.
Gould intraocular implant lens
gout conjunctivitis
gouty
  g. diabetes
  g. episcleritis
  g. iritis
Gower sign
GP
  globus pallidus
GPC
  giant papillary conjunctivitis
GPCL
  gas-permeable contact lens
GPH
  giant papillary hypertrophy
Grabow forceps
graceful swirling rod
grade
  fusion g.
Gradenigo syndrome

gradient
   hydrostatic g.
   g. method
grading
   Broders g.
   g. of retinal nerve fiber layer
Gradle
   G. cilia forceps
   G. corneal trephine
   G. electrode
   G. keratoplasty operation
   G. refractor
   G. retractor
graduated tenotomy
Graefe
   G. cataract knife
   G. cystitome
   G. cystitome knife
   G. disease
   G. eye dressing forceps
   G. fixation forceps
   G. iris forceps
   G. needle
   G. operation
   G. sign
   G. strabismus hook
   G. syndrome
   G. test
   G. tissue forceps
Graether
   G. button hook
   G. collar button
   G. collar-button micro-iris retractor
   G. mushroom hook
   G. pupil expander
   G. refractor
Grafco
   G. eye shield
   G. magnifying glasses
graft
   Amsler corneal g.
   anular corneal g.
   autogenous dermis fat g.
   bone g.
   g. carrier spoon
   conjunctival patch g.
   corneal g.
   corneolimbal ring g.
   crescent corneal g.
   dermis fat g.
   dermis patch g.
   donor g.

   double g.
   g. edema
   g. epithelium
   failed g.
   fat g.
   g. fixation
   full-thickness corneal g.
   glycerin-preserved g.
   g. infection
   lamellar corneal g.
   lamellar patch g.
   Marquez-Gomez conjunctival g.
   mucous membrane g.
   mushroom corneal g.
   Mustarde g.
   patch g.
   pattern-cut corneal g.
   penetrating full-thickness corneal g.
   piggyback g.
   g. preservation solution
   retroauricular complex g.
   scleral patch g.
   skin g.
   snowman g.
   split-calvarial bone g.
   tarsoconjunctival composite g.
   tectonic corneal g.
   Tenon patch g.
   Tudor-Thomas g.
   Wolfe g.
graft-host interface
grafting
   surgical patch g.
graft-versus-host disease
gramicidin
   neomycin, polymyxin B, and g.
gram-negative
   g.-n. bacteria
   g.-n. medium
gram-positive
   g.-p. bacteria
   g.-p. bacterial keratitis
   g.-p. cocci
Grandon
   G. eye speculum
   G. rotatable radial marker and
     degree gauge
   G. T-incision marker
granular
   g. appearance
   g. conjunctivitis
   g. corneal dystrophy

G

NOTES

205

granular *(continued)*
    g. lid
    g. ophthalmia
    g. trachoma
granularity
granule
    Birbeck g.
    cone g.
    dense core g.
    glycogen g.
    keratohyaline g.
    Langerhans g.
    neurosecretory g.
    pigment g.
    rod g.
    scintillating g.
granuliformis
    degeneratio hyaloidea g.
granulocytic sarcoma
granuloma
    candidal g.
    caseating orbital g.
    cholesterol g.
    chorioretinal g.
    choroidal g.
    conjunctival g.
    diffuse g.
    discrete g.
    eosinophilic g.
    focal g.
    g. gangraenescens
    intracranial g.
    g. iridis
    lethal midline g.
    midline g.
    noncaseating conjunctival g.
    orbital g.
    palisading orbital g.
    peripheral g.
    pyogenic g.
    reparative giant cell g.
    sclerosing orbital g.
    zonal g.
granulomatosis
    familial juvenile systemic g.
    juvenile systemic g.
granulomatous
    g. anterior uveitis
    g. endophthalmitis
    g. inflammatory cell
    g. iridocyclitis
    g. keratic precipitate
    g. keratoconjunctivitis
    g. panuveitis
    g. vasculitis
granulosus
    Echinococcus g.
graph
    shadow g.

grasping forceps
Grass electrode
grating
    g. acuity
    Arden g.
    Cambridge low-contrast g.
    sine-wave g.
    sinusoidal g.
Gratiolet radiating fiber
Graves
    G. disease
    G. hyperthyroidism
    G. ophthalmopathy
    G. orbitography
    G. orbitopathy
    G. strabismus
gravidarum
    retinitis g.
gravidic
    g. retinitis
    g. retinopathy
gravid retinitis
gravis
    fulminant myasthenia g.
    myasthenia g.
Grawitz tumor
gray
    g. atrophy
    g. cataract
    g. line
    G. photochromic lens
    g. plaque
    G. Standardized Oral Reading
      Paragraphs
graying
    g. of macula
    macular g.
gray-line incision
gray-scale ultrasonogram
Grayson corneal forceps
Grayson-Wilbrandt anterior corneal
  dystrophy
gray-white corneal scar
Grazer blepharoplasty forceps
Great Big Barbie retractor
greater
    g. ring of iris
    g. superficial petrosal nerve
    g. superficial temporal artery
      biopsy
    g. wing of sphenoid
Greaves operation
green
    g. blindness
    G. calipers
    G. capsule forceps
    g. cataract
    G. cataract knife
    G. chalazion forceps

G. corneal dissector
G. corneal knife
G. corneal marker
G. curette
G. double spatula
G. eye shield
G. fixation forceps
indocyanine g. (ICG)
G. iris replacer
g. laser
G. lens spatula
lissamine g.
G. muscle hook
G. muscle tucker
G. needle holder
G. refractor
G. replacer spatula
G. strabismus hook
G. strabismus tucker
G. trephine
g. vision
Green-Kenyon corneal marker
Gregg syndrome
Greig syndrome
Greither syndrome
Grey-Hess screen
grid
Amsler g. (AG)
Bernell g.
HIRCAL g.
Hirji-Callandar g.
g. laser photocoagulation (GLP)
g. method
Gridley intraocular lens
Grieshaber
G. blade
G. calibrated trephine
G. corneal trephine
G. diamond-coated forceps
G. endoilluminator
G. flexible iris retractor
G. internal limiting membrane
forceps
G. iris forceps
G. keratome
G. micro-bipolar coagulator
G. needle holder
G. ophthalmic needle
G. power injector system
G. ruby knife
G. three-function manipulator

G. two-function manipulator
G. ultrasharp knife
G. ultrasharp microsurgery
instrument
G. vertical cutting scissors
G. vitreous scissors
Griess reaction
Griffith
G. scale
G. sign
Grimsdale operation
grind
Fast G. 2200
grinding
bicentric g.
slab-off g.
grip
scleral g.
gripflex design
grittiness
Grizzard subretinal fluid cannula
Grocco sign
**Grocott-Gomori methenamine silver
nitrate**
Groenholm
G. refractor
G. retractor
Groenouw
G. corneal dystrophy
G. type I, II dystrophy
G. type II maculopathy
Grolman photographic system
Grönblad-Strandberg syndrome
groove
Blessig g.
corneal lamellar g.
corneoscleral g.
infraorbital g.
lacrimal g.
lamellar g.
limbal g.
nasolacrimal g.
optic g.
peptide-binding g.
g. suture
Verga lacrimal g.
grooved
g. director
g. incision
g. silicone implant
g. silicone sponge

G

NOTES

Gross
>G. retractor
>G. stereopsis

Grossmann operation
ground-glass sheet
group
>g. B *Streptococcus*
>CRYO-ROP Cooperative G.
>Cryotherapy for Retinopathy of Prematurity Cooperative G.
>nonocular muscle g.
>Pediatric Eye Disease Investigator G. (PEDIG)

growth-onset diabetes
growth retardation, alopecia, pseudoanodontia, and optic atrophy (GAPO)
GRT
>giant retinal tear

Gruber syndrome
Gruening magnet
Grunert spur
GS
GS-9
>G. blade
>G. needle

GSA-9 blade
GSL
>goniosynechialysis

gt
>gutta (drop)

GTS
>Guided Trephine System

gtt
>guttae (drops)

guard
>cataract knife g.
>ether g.
>eye knife g.
>forceps g.
>Hansen keratome g.
>keratome g.
>knife g.
>LASIK eye g.
>scalpel g.

guarded filtration procedure
Guardian scalpel with myoguard depth resistor
guarding ptosis
Guarnieri inclusion body
Gudden
>commissure of G.

Gueder keratoplasty needle
Guell
>G. irrigation cannula
>G. LASIK cannula
>G. type LASIK speculum

Guibor
>G. chart

>G. duct tube
>G. shield
>G. Silastic tube

guide
>Brown limbal relaxing incision g.
>Clayman g.
>Eschenbach low vision rehabilitation g.
>Lu-Mendez LRI g.
>vacuum-centering g.

Guided Trephine System (GTS)
Guillain-Barré syndrome
guillotine
>g. cutting tip
>g. vitrectomy instrument
>g. vitrector

guillotine-type cutter
Guimaraes
>G. flap spatula
>G. ICL manipulator
>G. implantable contact lens manipulator
>G. ophthalmic spatula

Guist
>G. enucleation hemostat
>G. enucleation scissors
>G. fixation forceps
>G. speculum
>G. sphere implant

Guist-Bloch speculum
Gulani
>G. globe stabilizer and flap restrainer
>G. triple function LASIK cannula

Gullstrand
>G. law
>G. lens
>G. loupe
>G. monograph
>G. ophthalmoscope
>G. reduced eye
>G. schematic eye
>G. six-surface eye model
>G. slit lamp

gummate
gummatous meningitis
gun-barrel field defect
Gunderson
>G. conjunctival flap
>G. muscle forceps

Gunn
>G. dot
>G. jaw-winking phenomenon
>Marcus G. (MG)
>no Marcus G. (NMG)
>G. pupil
>G. pupillary reflex
>G. sign
>G. syndrome

gustatolacrimal reflex
gustatory lacrimation
Guthrie fixation hook
gutta, pl. **guttae**
    g. amaurosis
    g. serena
gutta (drop) (gt)
guttae (drops) (gtt)
guttat.
    guttatim (drop by drop)
guttata
    absent g.
    cornea g.
    corneal g.
guttate choroidopathy
guttatim (drop by drop) (guttat.)
gutter dystrophy
guttering
    corneal g.
    limbal g.
    limbus g.
Gutzeit dacryostomy operation
guy suture
Guyton
    G. corneal transplant trephine
    G. electrode
    G. ptosis operation

Guyton-Clark fragment forceps
Guyton-Friedenwald suture
Guyton-Lundsgaard
    G.-L. cataract knife
    G.-L. keratome
    G.-L. scalpel
    G.-L. sclerotome
Guyton-Maumenee speculum
Guyton-Minkowski potential acuity meter
Guyton-Noyes
    G.-N. fixation
    G.-N. fixation forceps
Guyton-Park
    G.-P. eye speculum
    G.-P. lid speculum
GV
    Healon GV
gymnastics
    ocular g.
gyrata
    atrophia g.
gyrate
    g. atrophy
    g. atrophy of choroid and retina
gyrus
    angular g.

NOTES

G

H
    hyperopia
    hyperopic
    hyperphoria
      H band
h
    hour
H-1 blocker
HA
    headache
    hydroxyapatite
Haab
    H. knife needle
    H. magnet
    H. reflex
    H. scleral resection knife
    H. stria
Haag-Streit
    H.-S. Biomicroscope 900 slit lamp
    H.-S. 900 cobalt blue filter
    H.-S. distometer
    H.-S. fluorescein dye
    H.-S. keratometer
    H.-S. ophthalmometer
    H.-S. slit-lamp biomicroscope
HAART
    highly active antiretroviral therapy
habit
    glaucomatous h.
HACE
    high altitude cerebral edema
HACEK group organism
Hadeco intraoperative Doppler
Haefliger cleaver
haemolysans
    Gemella h.
haemolyticus
    Staphylococcus h.
Haemophilus
    H. aegypticus
    H. influenzae
    H. parainfluenzae
    H. par aphrophilus
Haemophilus **sp.,** *Actinobacillus*
    actinomycetemcomitans, Cardiobacterium
haemorrhagica
    retinitis h.
Haenel symptom
Haenig irrigating scissors
Hagberg-Santavuori syndrome
Hague cataract lamp
Haidinger brush test
Haik implant

hair
    h. bulb incubation test
    h. follicle tumor
halation
Halberg
    H. contact lens forceps
    H. indirect ophthalmoscope
    H. trial clip
    H. trial clip occluder
Halberstaedter-Prowazek inclusion body
Haldrone
half-eye spectacles
half-field
    visual h.-f. (VHF)
half-glasses
half-glass spectacles
half-moon syndrome
half vision
HALK
    hyperopic automated lamellar
      keratoplasty
Hallauer
    H. glasses
    H. spectacles
Hall dermatome
Haller
    circle of H.
    H. layer
    H. membrane
halleri
    circulus arteriosus h.
Hallermann-Streiff-Francois syndrome
Hallermann-Streiff syndrome
Hallervorden-Spatz syndrome
Hallgren syndrome
Hallpike maneuver
hallucination
    hypnagogic h.
    hypnopompic h.
    irritative h.
    migrainous h.
    peduncular h.
    release h.
    visual h.
    h. with eye closure
hallucinogenic
halo
    h. demonstrator
    Fick h.
    glaucomatous h.
    parafoveal h.
    h. phenomenon
    pigmentary h.
    h. saturninus
    senescent h.

H

halo *(continued)*
    senile h.
    h. sheathing
    h. symptom
    h. vision
    visual h.
halogen
    h. Finoff transilluminator
    h. ophthalmoscope
halogenated hydroxyquinoline
halogram
halometer
halometry
halophilic noncholera *Vibrio* **species**
haloscope
    phase difference h.
halothane
Halpin operation
HALS
    Health and Activity Limitations Survey
Halsey needle holder
Halsted
    H. curved mosquito clamp
    H. curved mosquito hemostatic
    forceps
    H. hemostat
    H. strabismus scissors
    H. straight mosquito clamp
Haltia-Santavuori type of Batten
syndrome
hamartoblastoma
hamartoma
    astrocytic h.
    glial-neural h.
    melanocytic h.
    orbit h.
    orbital h.
    retinal astrocytic h.
    smooth muscle h.
    uveal tract h.
    vascular h.
hamartomatosis
hamartomatous lesion
hammock pupil
hamular procedure
hamulus, pl. **hamuli**
    h. lacrimalis
    trochlear h.
hand
    h. motion (HM)
    h. movement
    Winter Helping H.
hand-held
    h.-h. eye magnet
    h.-h. fundus camera
    h.-h. Hruby lens
    h.-h. infusion lens
    h.-h. magnifier
    h.-h. magnifying reticle

    h.-h. rotary prism
    h.-h. trephine
handle
    Beaver h.
    DORC h.
    Elliot trephine h.
    Stolte prechopper, angled h.
    Stolte prechopper, straight h.
    Storz h.
handling
    data h.
hand-motion
    h.-m. vision (HMV)
    h.-m. visual acuity test
hand-movement visual acuity test
handpiece
    AMO Series 4 phaco h.
    Avit h.
    B-mode h.
    Cavitron I/A h.
    fragmentation/aspiration h.
    Kelman irrigating h.
    Lightning high-speed vitrectomy h.
    MicroSeal ophthalmic h.
    Packer Wick extrusion h.
    phacoemulsification h.
    ProFinesse II ultrasonic h.
    SITE Phaco II h.
    soft-tipped extrusion h.
    Storz h.
    Vit Commander h.
Hand-Schüller-Christian
    H.-S.-C. disease
    H.-S.-C. syndrome
Handy nonmydriatic video fundus
camera
Hanna
    H. arcitome
    H. trephine
Hannover canal
Hansa speculum
Hansatome
    Chiron H.
    H. microkeratome
    H. microkeratome blade
    H. 8.5 mm suction ring
Hansen
    H. keratome
    H. keratome guard
haplopia
haploscope
    mirror h.
haploscopic
    h. test
    h. vision
haptic
    h. angulation
    h. contact
    lamellar h.

h. loop
h. plate lens
Slant h.
violet h.
HAR
high altitude retinopathy
Harada
H. disease
H. syndrome
Harada-Ito procedure
hard
h. cataract
h. contact lens (HCL)
h. drusen
h. lipid exudate
hardened spectacle lens
hardening of lens
Harder gland
harderian gland
Hardesty
H. tendon hook
H. tenotomy hook
hard-finger tension
Hardten double-ended LASIK flap lifter and spatula
Hardy
H. lensometer
H. punch
Hardy-Rand-Ritter
H.-R.-R. pseudoisochromatic plate
H.-R.-R. screening plate
H.-R.-R. test
hare's eye
HARK 599 autorefractor
Harman
H. eye dressing
H. fixation forceps
H. operation
harmonious abnormal retinal correspondence
Harms
H. corneal forceps
H. trabeculotome
H. trabeculotomy probe
H. tying forceps
Harms-Colibri forceps
Harms-Dannheim trabeculotomy operation
Harms-Tubingen tying forceps
Harrington
H. erysiphake

H. retractor
H. tonometer
Harrington-Flocks
H.-F. multiple pattern
H.-F. test
Harrison
H. retractor
H. scissors
Harrison-Stein nomogram
Hartinger Coincidence refractionometer
Hartmann
H. clamp
H. mosquito hemostatic forceps
Hartmann-Shack (HS)
H.-S. wavefront aberrometer
H.-S. wavefront sensor system
Hart pediatric three-mirror lens
Hartstein
H. irrigating/aspirating unit
H. irrigating iris retractor
H. irrigator
H. refractor
Hashimoto thyroiditis
Hasner
H. fold
H. lid forceps
H. operation
valve of H.
H. valve
Hassall body
Hassall-Henle
H.-H. body
H.-H. wart
Hawes-Pallister-Landor syndrome
hay fever conjunctivitis
Hay-Wells syndrome
haze
aerial h.
corneal h.
epithelial punctate h.
interface h.
late-onset corneal h.
reticular h.
stromal h.
subepithelial corneal h.
vitreous h.
haziness
HBO
hyperbaric oxygen therapy
HC
Ocutricin HC
Tri-Thalmic HC

NOTES

213

HCDVA
>high-contrast distance visual acuity

HCL
>hard contact lens

HCl
>hydrochloride
>>antazoline phosphate and
>>>naphazoline HCl
>>apraclonidine HCl
>>betaxolol HCl
>>carteolol HCl
>>cysteamine HCl
>>dapiprazole HCl
>>deterenol HCl
>>dipivefrin HCl
>>Duranest HCl
>>epinephrine HCl
>>levobunolol HCl
>>levocabastine HCl
>>Marcaine HCl
>>mepivacaine HCl
>>naboctate HCl
>>naphazoline HCl
>>oxymetazoline HCl
>>pheniramine maleate and
>>>naphazoline HCl
>>pilocarpine HCl
>>proparacaine HCl
>>proxymetacaine HCl 0.5%

He
>He Hook chopper
>He hook chopper in titanium

head
>Mastel Finish for application to
>>microkeratome h.
>h. mirror
>h. nystagmus
>optic nerve h. (ONH)
>h. tremor

headache (HA)
>brain tumor h.
>cluster h.
>cough h.
>migraine h.
>muscle contraction h.
>postherpetic h.
>posttraumatic h.
>retroorbital h.
>sinus h.

head-mounted video magnifier LVES
head-nodding
headrest
>Gibralter h.

head-tilt test
head-turning reflex
healing
>stromal wound h.

Healon
>H. aspirating cannula

>H. GV
>H. solution

Healon5
Health and Activity Limitations Survey (HALS)
Health-Related Quality of Life (HRQOL)
healthy
>h. control participant
>h. subject

hearing loss
heater
>broad-spectrum h. (BSH)
>infrared h.

heat-generated cataract
Heath
>H. chalazion curette
>H. chalazion forceps
>H. dilator
>H. expressor

heat-ray cataract
heavy
>h. eye
>h. fluid
>h. gas
>h. ion irradiation
>h. ion radiation

Hebra
>H. blade
>H. curette
>H. hook

hedger cataract
Hedges Corneal Wetting Pak
HEDS1
>Herpetic Eye Disease Study I

HEDS2
>Herpetic Eye Disease Study II

Heerfordt
>H. disease
>H. syndrome

hefilcon A
Heidelberg
>H. laser tomographic scanner
>H. retina angiogram (HRA)
>H. retina angiograph digital
>>scanning laser ophthalmoscope
>H. retina angiograph FA/ICGA
>H. retinal angiography
>H. retinal flowmeter
>H. retinal tomography
>H. retina tomograph (HRT)
>H. retina tomograph II (HRT-II)

Heidenhain
>H. syndrome
>H. variant

height
>buckle h.
>contact lens h.
>orbital h.

peripapillary retinal h.
sagittal h.
segment h.
Heine
    H. cyclodialysis
    H. HSL 100 hand-held slit lamp
    H. Lambda 100 retinometer
    H. operation
    H. penlight
Heisrath operation
helcoma
helical computed tomography
helicoid
    h. choroidopathy
    h. peripapillary atrophy
helium-ion aiming laser
helium-neon (HeNe)
    h.-n. aiming laser
    h.-n. beam
hellem
    Encephalitozoon h.
Helmholtz
    H. keratometer
    H. line
    H. ophthalmoscope
    H. schematic eye
    H. theory of accommodation
    H. theory of color vision
helminthic disease
helper/inducer T cell
Helsinki
    Declaration of H.
Helveston
    H. Big Barbie tissue retractor
    H. Great Big Barbie retractor
    H. hook
    H. scleral marking ruler
HEMA
    hydroxyethylmethacrylate
hemagglutination
    immune adherence h. (IAH)
    Treponema pallidum h.
hemangioblastoma
    optic nerve h.
hemangioendothelioma
    orbital h.
hemangioma
    capillary h.
    cavernous orbital h.
    choroidal h.
    conjunctival h.
    episcleral h.

epithelioid h.
exophytic papillary capillary h.
eyelid strawberry h.
facial h.
juxtapapillary endophytic
    capillary h.
orbital h.
osseous metaplasia over the
    choroidal h.
papillary capillary h.
periorbital h.
racemose h.
strawberry h.
uveal tract h.
venous h.
hemangiomatosis
    racemose h.
hemangiopericytoma
    lacrimal sac h.
    meningeal h.
    orbital h.
hematic cyst
hematogenous
    h. metastasis
    h. pigmentation
    h. sepsis
hematoma
    orbital h.
    subdural h.
hematopoietic metastasis
hematopsia
hemeralopia
hemeranopia
hemiachromatopsia
hemiakinesia
    pupillary h.
hemiakinetopsia
hemialexia
hemiamblyopia
hemianopic
    h. dyslexia
    h. glasses
    h. scotoma
    h. spectacles
hemianopsia, hemianopia
    absolute h.
    altitudinal h.
    bilateral homonymous h.
    binasal h.
    binocular h.
    bitemporal fugax h.
    h. bitemporalis fugax

NOTES

H

hemianopsia *(continued)*
   checkerboard h.
   complete h.
   congenital h.
   congruous h.
   crossed h.
   double homonymous h.
   equilateral h.
   geniculate h.
   heteronymous h.
   homonymous h.
   horizontal h.
   incomplete h.
   incongruous h.
   lateral h.
   lower h.
   nasal h.
   postgeniculate congenital
    homonymous h.
   quadrant h.
   quadrantic h.
   relative h.
   temporal h.
   true h.
   unilateral h.
   uniocular h.
   upper h.
   vertical h.
hemianoptic
hemianosmia
hemiastigmatism
hemichiasma
hemichromatopsia
hemicrania
hemicraniosis
hemi-CRVO
hemifacial
   h. atrophy
   h. blepharospasm
   h. flush
   h. spasm
hemifield
   H. glaucoma test
   h. slide phenomenon
hemihydrate
   timolol h.
hemimicropsia
hemiopalgia
hemiopia
hemiopic
   h. hypoplasia
   h. pupillary reaction
hemiplegia
   alternating oculomotor h.
hemiplegic migraine
hemiscotosis
hemi-seesaw nystagmus

hemisensory
   h. deficit
   h. loss
hemisphere
   cerebellar h.
   h. eye implant
   h. projection perimetry
   silicone h.
hemispherical
hemocytic mesenchyme
hemodynamically significant carotid
  artery stenosis (HSCAS)
hemolytic glaucoma
hemophthalmia
hemophthalmos, hemophthalmus
hemorrhage
   arachnoid h.
   blot h.
   blot-and-dot h.
   caudate h.
   cerebellar h.
   choroidal h.
   conjunctival h.
   delayed massive suprachoroidal h.
   disk drusen h.
   dot h.
   dot-and-blot h.
   Drance h.
   eight-ball h.
   expulsive h.
   flame-shaped h.
   hyperfluorescent h.
   intralenticular h.
   intraocular h.
   intraorbital h.
   intraretinal h.
   intraventricular h. (IVH)
   intravitreal h.
   kissing suprachoroidal h.
   h. and microaneurysm (h/ma)
   mild periocular h.
   nerve fiber layer h.
   ochre h.
   orbital h.
   perihemangioma subretinal h.
   peripheral intraretinal h.
   premacular subhyaloid h.
   prepapillary h.
   preretinal h.
   punctate h.
   retinal h.
   retinopathy h.
   retrobulbar h.
   retrohyaloid premacular h.
   round h.
   salmon-patch h.
   splinter disk h.
   spontaneous retrobulbar h.
   subarachnoid h.

subchoroidal h.
subconjunctival h.
subhyaloid h.
subinternal limiting membrane h.
subretinal h.
suprachoroidal h. (SCH, SH)
vitreal h.
vitreous h. (VH)
vitreous breakthrough h.
white-centered h.
yellow-ochre h.

hemorrhagic
    h. choroidal detachment
    h. conjunctivitis
    h. disciform lesion
    h. disorder
    h. glaucoma
    h. iritis
    h. retinopathy
    h. RPE
    h. sarcoma

hemorrhagica
    Leber lymphangiectasia h.

hemosiderosis bulbi

hemostat
    Corboy h.
    Guist enucleation h.
    Halsted h.
    Kelly h.

hemostatic forceps

Henderson-Patterson inclusion body

HeNe
    helium-neon
    HeNe beam
    HeNe laser

Henle
    H. body
    H. fiber
    H. fiber layer
    H. gland
    H. layer of the macula
    H. membrane
    H. wart

Hennebert sign

Henry cilia forceps

henselae
    Bartonella h.

Hensen body

Henson CFS 2000 perimeter

heparin
    h. surface-modified intraocular lens
    (HSM-IOL)

    h. surface-modified polymethyl
    methacrylate

heparin-surface-modified

hepatica
    ophthalmia h.

hepatolenticular degeneration

HEPES buffer

herapathite

Herbert
    H. operation
    H. peripheral pit

Herbit pit

hereditaria
    atrophia bulborum h.
    degeneratio hyaloideoretinae h.

hereditary
    h. anterior membrane dystrophy
    h. benign intraepithelial dyskeratosis
    h. benign intraepithelial dyskeratosis
    syndrome
    h. cerebellar ataxia
    h. corneal edema
    h. degeneration
    h. epithelial corneal dystrophy
    h. hemorrhagic macular dystrophy
    h. hemorrhagic telangiectasia
    h. hyperferritinemia-cataract
    syndrome
    h. optic atrophy
    h. optic atrophy syndrome
    h. optic neuropathy
    h. progressive arthroophthalmopathy
    h. renal-retinal dysplasia
    h. vitelliform dystrophy

heredity maculopathy

heredodegeneration
    macular h.

heredodegenerative
    h. atrophy
    h. neurologic syndrome

heredofamilial optic atrophy

heredomacular degeneration

Hering
    H. after-image mechanism
    H. law
    H. law of equal innervation
    H. law of equivalent innervation
    H. law of motor correspondence
    H. law of simultaneous innervation
    H. test
    H. theory
    H. theory of color vision

NOTES

H

Hering-Bielschowsky after-image test
Hering-Hellebrand deviation
Hermann grid illusion
Hermansky-Pudlak syndrome
hernia
> h. of iris
> orbital h.
> vitreous h.

herniating orbital fat
herniation
> hippocampal gyrus h.
> vitreous h.

Herpchek
herpes
> h. corneae
> h. epithelial tropic ulceration
> h. follicular keratoconjunctivitis
> h. iridis
> ocular h.
> h. panuveitis
> h. simplex blepharitis
> h. simplex blepharoconjunctivitis
> h. simplex cellulitis
> h. simplex conjunctivitis
> h. simplex corneal ulcer
> h. simplex dermatitis
> h. simplex iridocyclitis
> h. simplex keratitis
> h. simplex keratoconjunctivitis
> h. simplex keratouveitis
> h. simplex retinitis
> h. simplex scar
> h. simplex scleritis
> h. simplex uveitis
> h. simplex virus (HSV)
> h. simplex virus type I
> h. zoster conjunctivitis
> h. zoster glaucoma
> h. zoster iridocyclitis
> h. zoster keratitis
> h. zoster keratoconjunctivitis
> h. zoster ophthalmicus
> h. zoster oticus
> h. zoster virus

herpesvirus
herpete
> zoster sine h.

herpetic
> h. conjunctivitis
> h. dendrite
> H. Eye Disease Study
> H. Eye Disease Study I (HEDS1)
> H. Eye Disease Study II (HEDS2)
> h. fungal keratitis
> h. keratoconjunctivitis
> h. necrotizing retinopathy
> h. ocular disease
> h. ocular infection

> h. stromal keratitis
> h. ulcer

herpetoid lesion
Herplex
> H. Liquifilm
> H. Ophthalmic

Herrick
> H. lacrimal plug
> H. silicone lacrimal implant

Hersh
> H. LASIK retreatment forceps
> H. LASIK retreatment spatula

Hertel
> H. exophthalmometer
> H. exophthalmometry
> H. stone forceps

Hertwig-Magendie
> H.-M. phenomenon
> H.-M. syndrome

Hertzog
> H. lens spatula
> H. pliable probe

Hess
> H. diplopia screen
> H. eyelid operation
> H. forceps
> H. ptosis operation
> H. screen test
> H. spoon

Hess-Barraquer forceps
Hessburg
> H. corneal shield
> H. eye shield
> H. intraocular lens glide
> H. lacrimal needle
> H. lens
> H. lens forceps
> H. lens-inserting forceps
> H. subpalpebral lavage system

Hessburg-Barron
> H.-B. disposable vacuum trephine
> H.-B. suction trephine

Hess-Horwitz forceps
Hess-Lee screen
heterochromia
> atrophic h.
> binocular h.
> congenital iris h.
> Fuchs h.
> h. iridis
> h. of iris
> iris h.
> monocular h.
> simple h.
> sympathetic h.

heterochromic
> h. cataract
> h. Fuchs cyclitis

h. iridocyclitis
h. uveitis
heterogeneity
optical h.
heterogeneous
h. cell
h. donor material
heterogenous keratoplasty
heterokeratoplasty
heterometropia
heteronymous
h. diplopia
h. hemianopsia
h. image
h. parallax
h. quadrantanopia
heterophoralgia
heterophoria method
heterophoric position
**heterophthalmia, heterophthalmos,
heterophthalmus**
heteropsia
heteroptics
heteroscope
heteroscopy
heterotopia
cerebral h.
diabetic macular h.
heterotropia, heterotropy
circadian h.
comitant h.
concomitant h.
h. maculae
noncomitant h.
paralytic h.
heterotropic deviation
Hetrazan
Hexadrol Phosphate
hexafluoride
h. gas
sulfur h. (SF6)
hexagonal keratotomy
hexahydrate
trisodium phosphonoformate h.
hexametaphosphate
sodium h.
hexamethonium chloride
hexamidine
Hexon illumination system
hex procedure

hexylcaine
**Heyer-Schulte Medical Optic Center
specular microscope**
Heyner
H. curette
H. dilator
H. double cannula
H. double needle
H. expressor
H. forceps
HFA
Humphrey Field Analyzer 750
Hg
mercury
HGM
H. argon green laser
H. intravitreal laser
H. ophthalmic laser
HHH
hyperornithinemia, hyperammonemia,
and homocitrullinuria
HHH syndrome
**Hibiclens antiseptic/antimicrobial skin
cleanser**
Hidex glass lens
Hiff
H. operation
H. ptosis
high
h. altitude cerebral edema (HACE)
h. altitude retinopathy (HAR)
h. convex
h. hyperopia
h. intensity illuminator
h. myopia
h. prevalence
h. viscosity
high-add bifocal
high-altitude illness
**high-contrast distance visual acuity
(HCDVA)**
higher visual function test
high-frequency ultrasound biomicroscope
high-gain
h.-g. artifact
h.-g. digital ultrasound
highlighter
Esenbach H.
**Highlight spectral indirect
ophthalmoscope**

NOTES

H

219

High-Lite glass
highly active antiretroviral therapy
(HAART)
high-magnification (HM)
high-pass
    h.-p. resolution perimetry (HRP)
    h.-p. resolution perimetry global
      deviation (HRP-GD)
    h.-p. resolution perimetry local
      deviation (HRP-LD)
high-tension
    h.-t. glaucoma (HTG)
    h.-t. suturing technique
high-vacuum phacoemulsification
Hildreth
    H. cautery
    H. electrocautery
Hill
    H. operation
    H. procedure
    H. retractor
Hillis
    H. refractor
    H. retractor
Hilton
    H. self-retaining infusion cannula
    H. sutureless infusion cannula
hinged corneal flap
Hippel
    H. disease
    H. operation
Hippel-Lindau syndrome
hippocampal gyrus herniation
hippocampus
Hippos
HIRCAL grid
Hirji-Callandar grid
Hirschberg
    H. magnet
    H. method
    H. reflex
    H. reflex assessment
    H. test
Hirschman
    H. iris hook
    H. lens forceps
    H. lens-inserting forceps
    H. microiris hook
    H. spatula
    H. speculum
Hismanal
histiocytic
    h. disorder
    h. lymphoma
    h. tumor
Histoacryl
    H. glue
    H. glue patch

histolyticum
    Clostridium h.
histopathologic effect
Histoplasma
    H. capsulatum
    H. duboisii
histoplasmic choroiditis
histoplasmosis
    h. maculopathy
    ocular h.
    presumed ocular h.
    h. syndrome
history
    neuroophthalmologic case h.
    past ocular h. (POH)
histo spot
HIV
    human immunodeficiency virus
HIV-specific antibody
Hl
    latent hyperopia
HLA
    human leukocyte antigen
    HLA match
HLA-A29 antigen
HLA-B27
    H.-B. antigen
    H.-B. syndrome
HLA-B15 antigen
HLA-B27-associated uveitis
HLA-B5 antigen
HLA-B7 antigen
HLA-DR4 antigen
HM
    hand motion
    high-magnification
Hm
    manifest hyperopia
h/ma
    hemorrhage and microaneurysm
H-magnetic resonance spectroscopy
HM/3ft
    hand motion at 3 feet
HMS Liquifilm
HMV
    hand-motion vision
Hoaglund sign
hockey-end temple
Hodapp-Parrish-Anderson (HPA)
    H.-P.-A. visual field staging system
hoe
    Huang epithelial LASEK h.
    LASEK epithelial micro h.
    Rhein LASIK epithelial
      detaching h.
    Sloane micro h.
Hoffberger Program
Hoffer
    H. forward-cutting knife cannula

H. optical center marker
H. optic zone marker
Hoffer-Colenbrander formula
Hoffer-Laseridge intraocular lens
Hoffman/Buratto LASIK marker
Hoffman irrigation cannula
Hofmann
H. elbow
H. T-incision marker
Hofmann-Thornton globe fixation ring
Hogan operation
holder
Alabama-Green needle h.
Arruga needle h.
baby Barraquer needle h.
Barraquer curved h.
Barraquer needle h.
Belin double-ended needle h.
Birks Mark II micro cross-
action h.
Birks Mark II micro lock-type
needle h.
Bodkin thread h.
Boyce needle h.
Boynton needle h.
Castroviejo-Barraquer needle h.
Castroviejo blade h.
Castroviejo-Kalt needle h.
Castroviejo needle h.
Clerf needle h.
Cohen needle h.
Corboy needle h.
Crile needle h.
Dean knife h.
Derf needle h.
Ellis needle h.
eye h.
French needle h.
Gifford needle h.
goniotomy needle h.
Green needle h.
Grieshaber needle h.
Halsey needle h.
Ilg microneedle h.
Ilg needle h.
I-tech cannula h.
I-tech needle h.
Jaffe needle h.
Kalt needle h.
Keeler-Catford microjaws needle h.
McIntyre fish-hook needle h.
McPherson needle h.

needle h.
Neumann razor blade fragment h.
Paton needle h.
Schaefer sponge h.
Stangel modified Barraquer
microsurgical needle h.
Stephenson needle h.
Stevens needle h.
Tilderquist needle h.
Troutman blade h.
Troutman needle h.
Vickers needle h.
Webster needle h.
holding clip
hole
atrophic h.
cystoid macular h.
full thickness macular h.
iatrogenic retinal h.
idiopathic macular cyst and h.
impending macular h.
lamellar h.
macular h. (MH)
operculated retinal h.
partial thickness macular h.
retinal h.
senescent macular h.
Holladay
H. contrast acuity test
H. Diagnostic Summary topography
H. formula
H. posterior capsule polisher
Hollenhorst
H. body
H. plaque
hollowing and shadowing
hollow-sphere implant
Holmes-Adie
H.-A. pupil
H.-A. tonic pupil syndrome
Holmgren
H. color test
H. method
H. skein
H. wool skein test
Holmium
H. laser sclerostomy
holmium
h. laser
h. YAG laser sclerectomy
**Holofax Oxford retroillumination
cataract camera**

NOTES

H

Holth
>
> H. forceps
> H. iridencleisis
> H. operation
> H. scleral punch
> H. sclerectomy

Holthouse-Batten superficial choroiditis
Holt-Oram syndrome
Holzknecht unit
Homatrocel
homatropine
>
> h. hydrobromide
> Isopto H.
> h. refraction

Homén syndrome
Homer
>
> H. law
> H. muscle
> H. ptosis
> H. pupil
> H. syndrome

Homer-Wright rosette
hominis
>
> *Cardiobacterium h.*
> *Staphylococcus h.*

homocitrullinuria
>
> hyperornithinemia, hyperammonemia,
> and h. (HHH)

homocystinuria
homogeneous donor material
homogenous keratoplasty
homokeratoplasty
**homologous penetrating central limbo
keratoplasty**
homonomous quadrantanopia
homonymous
>
> h. crescent
> h. diplopia
> h. field defect
> h. hemianopic scotoma
> h. hemianopsia
> h. hemiopic hypoplasia
> h. image
> h. parallax
> h. quadrantanopsia

homoplastic keratomileusis
homotropic antibody
Honan
>
> H. balloon
> H. cuff
> H. manometer

honey bee lens
honeycomb
>
> h. dystrophy
> h. macula

hook
>
> Amenabar discission h.
> anchor h.
> angled discission h.

ASSI fixation h.
Azar lens-manipulating h.
Behler LASIK enhancement h.
Behler LASIK retreatment h.
Berens scleral h.
Birks Mark II h.
boat h.
Bonn microiris h.
Catalano muscle h.
corneal h.
Crawford h.
Culler muscle h.
discission h.
Drews-Sato suture-pickup h.
El-Naggar recession muscle h.
El-Naggar resection double h.
expressor h.
h. expressor
Fenzel angled manipulating h.
Fenzel insertion h.
Fenzel lens-manipulating h.
Fink oblique muscle h.
fixation h.
flat h.
Frazier dura h.
Fukasaku small pupil snapper h.
Gass muscle h.
Gass retinal detachment h.
Graefe strabismus h.
Graether button h.
Graether mushroom h.
Green muscle h.
Green strabismus h.
Guthrie fixation h.
Hardesty tendon h.
Hardesty tenotomy h.
Hebra h.
Helveston h.
Hirschman iris h.
Hirschman microiris h.
Hunkeler ball-point h.
iris h.
Jaeger h.
Jaffe iris h.
Jaffe lens-manipulating h.
Jaffe microiris h.
Jameson muscle h.
Katena boat h.
Kennerdell muscle h.
Kennerdell nerve h.
Kirby muscle h.
Knapp iris h.
Kratz K push-pull iris h.
Kuglen manipulating h.
Laqua black line retinal h.
Lewicky lens manipulating h.
Maidera-Stern suture h.
Manson double-ended strabismus h.
Maumenee iris h.

McIntyre irrigating h.
McReynolds lid-retracting h.
muscle h.
Nugent h.
oblique muscle h.
Ochsner h.
O'Connor flat h.
O'Connor muscle h.
O'Connor sharp h.
O'Connor tenotomy h.
ophthalmic h.
Osher h.
Praeger iris h.
push-and-pull h.
Rentsch boat h.
retinal detachment h.
Russian four-pronged fixation h.
scleral h.
Scobee oblique muscle h.
sharp h.
Sheets microiris h.
Shepard microiris h.
Shepard reversed iris h.
Sinskey lens h.
Sinskey lens-manipulating h.
Sinskey microiris h.
Sinskey microlens h.
skin h.
Smith expressor h.
Smith lid h.
spatula h.
h. spatula
squint h.
Stamler side-port fixation h.
Stevens tenotomy h.
St. Martin-Franceschetti cataract h.
strabismus h.
suture pickup h.
Tennant anchor lens-insertion h.
Tennant lens-manipulating h.
tenotomy h.
Tomas iris h.
Tomas suture h.
Trujillo LASIK enhancement h.
Tsuneoka irrigating h.
twist fixation h.
Tyrell iris h.
Visitec angled lens h.
Visitec corneal suture
  manipulating h.
Visitec micro double-iris h.
Visitec microiris h.

Visitec straight lens h.
von Graefe muscle h.
von Graefe strabismus h.
Wiener corneal h.
Wiener scleral h.
Wilson recession h.
Y h.
hook-shaped cataract
hook-type implant
**Hooper Visual Organization Test
  (HVOT)**
Hoopes corneal marker
hop eye
Hopkins rod lens telescope
Horay operation
hordeolum
external h.
h. externum
internal h.
h. internum
h. meibomianum
horizontal
h. band pallor
h. cell
h. deviation
h. diplopia
h. gaze
h. gaze center
h. hemianopsia
h. mattress suture
h. meridian
h. nystagmus
h. plane
h. prism bar
h. raphe
h. retinal disparity
h. strabismus
h. tropia
horn
cutaneous h.
lateral h.
medial h.
Horner
H. law
H. muscle
H. ptosis
H. pupil
H. syndrome
Horner-Bernard syndrome
Horner-Trantas
H.-T. dot
H.-T. spot

NOTES

H

223

horopter
Vieth-Mueller h.
horopteric
horror fusionis
horseshoe tear
Horton syndrome
Horvath operation
Hosford
H. expressor
H. lacrimal dilator
H. spud
Hoskins
H. beaked Colibri forceps
H. fine straight forceps
H. fixation forceps
H. lens
H. miniaturized micro straight
forceps
H. razor blade fragment
H. razor fragment blade
H. straight microiris forceps
H. suture forceps
Hoskins-Barkan goniotomy infant lens
Hoskins-Castroviejo corneal scissors
**Hoskins-Dallas intraocular lens-inserting
forceps**
Hoskins-Drake implant
Hoskins-Luntz forceps
Hoskins-Skeleton
H.-S. fine forceps
H.-S. micro-grooved broad-tipped
forceps
Hoskins-Westcott tenotomy scissors
hospital
King Khaled Eye Specialist H.
(KKESH)
Wills Eye H.
host
h. incision
h. tissue forceps
h. trephination
host-graft junction
hot
h. eye
h. spot
HOTV test
Hotz
H. entropion
H. entropion operation
Hotz-Anagnostakis operation
Hough drape
hour (h)
House
H. lacrimal dilator
H. miniature forceps
H. myringotomy knife
House-Bellucci alligator scissors
House-Dieter nipper

Houser
H. cul-de-sac irrigator T-tube
H. cul-de-sac irrigator tube
House-Urban-Pentax camera
Hovius
H. canal
H. circle
H. membrane
H. plexus
Howard abrader
Howard-Dolman apparatus
Howell phoria card
Hoya
H. AR-570 autorefractor
H. HDR objective refractometer
H. MRM objective refractometer
Ho:YAG laser
Hoyt-Spencer triad
HPA
Hodapp-Parrish-Anderson
HPA visual field staging system
H.P. Acthar Gel
HPCRT
HPMPC Peripheral CMV Retinitis Trial
HPMC
hydroxypropyl methylcellulose
**HPMPC Peripheral CMV Retinitis
Trial (HPCRT)**
HR
hypertensive retinopathy
HRA
Heidelberg retina angiogram
HRP
high-pass resolution perimetry
HRP-GD
high-pass resolution perimetry global
deviation
HRP-LD
high-pass resolution perimetry local
deviation
HRQOL
Health-Related Quality of Life
HRR plate
HRT
Heidelberg retina tomograph
HRT-II
Heidelberg retina tomograph II
Hruby
H. contact lens
H. implant
HS
Hartmann-Shack
Pilopine HS
HSCAS
hemodynamically significant carotid
artery stenosis
HSM-IOL
heparin surface-modified intraocular lens

HSV
> herpes simplex virus
>> HSV endotheliitis
>> HSV epithelial keratitis
>> footprints of HSV
>> HSV ocular disease
>> HSV stromal disease
>> HSV trophic keratopathy

HT
> hypertropia

Ht
> total hyperopia

HTG
> high-tension glaucoma

Huang
>> H. epithelial LASEK hoe
>> H. LASEK trephine
>> H. LASIK cannula

Hubbard corneoscleral forceps
Huco diamond knife
Hudson line
Hudson-Stähli
>> H.-S. line
>> H.-S. line of corneal pigmentation

hue
>> 28 H. de Roth test
>> 90 h. discrimination test
>> palpebral conjunctival h. (PCH)
>> salmon patch h.
>> 100 h. test

Hueck ligament
Huey scissors
Hughes
>> H. classification of chemical injury
>> H. implant
>> H. modification of Burch technique
>> H. operation
>> H. tarsoconjunctival flap

human
>> h. allograft tissue
>> h. immunodeficiency virus (HIV)
>> h. leucocyte antigen match
>> h. leukocyte antigen (HLA)
>> h. T-lymphotropic virus

humanized anti-Tac monoclonal antibody
Hummelsheim
>> H. operation
>> H. procedure

humor
>> aqueous h.
>> h. aquosus

>> h. cristallinus
>> crystalline h.
>> ocular h.
>> plasmoid aqueous h.
>> vitreous h.

humoral immunity
Humorsol Ophthalmic
Humphrey
>> H. ATLAS Eclipse corneal topography system
>> H. automatic refractor
>> H. B-scan
>> H. Field Analyzer 750 (HFA)
>> H. 24-2 glaucoma hemifield test
>> H. Instruments vision analyzer
>> H. Instruments vision analyzer overrefraction system
>> H. lens analyzer
>> H. Mastervue corneal topography system
>> H. model 2000 optical coherence tomography
>> H. perimeter
>> H. retina imager
>> H. ultrasonic pachometer
>> H. 992 videokeratographer
>> H. visual field (HVF)
>> H. visual field analyzer

Humphriss binocular balance
Hünermann disease
Hunkeler
>> H. ball-point hook
>> H. frown incision marker
>> H. lens

Hunt
>> H. chalazion forceps
>> H. chalazion scissors

Hunter-Hurler syndrome
Hunter syndrome
Hunt-Transley operation
Hurler
>> H. disease
>> H. syndrome

Hurler-Scheie
>> H.-S. compound
>> H.-S. syndrome

hurricane keratopathy
Huschke valve
Hutchinson
>> H. facies
>> H. patch
>> H. pupil

NOTES

H

Hutchinson *(continued)*
    H. sign
    H. Summer prurigo
    H. syndrome
    H. triad
Hutchinson-Tays central guttate
   choroiditis
HUV
    hypocomplementemic urticarial vasculitis
Huygenian eyepiece
HVF
    Humphrey visual field
HVOT
    Hooper Visual Organization Test
Hy
    hypermetropia
hyaline
    h. artery
    h. body
    h. degeneration
    h. fungus
    h. mass
    h. material
    h. membrane
    h. plaque
hyalinosis cutis et mucosae
hyalitis
    h. of anterior membrane
    asteroid h.
    h. punctata
    punctate h.
    h. suppurativa
    suppurative h.
Hyall
hyalohyphomycosis
hyaloid
    h. artery
    h. asteroid
    h. body
    h. canal
    h. clouding
    h. corpuscle
    h. face
    h. fossa
    h. membrane detachment
    posterior h.
    h. posterior membrane
    h. system
hyaloidal fibrovascular proliferation
hyaloidea
    fossa h.
    membrana h.
    stella lentis h.
hyaloideocapsular ligament
hyaloideoretinal degeneration
hyaloideus
    canalis h.
hyaloiditis
hyaloidotomy

hyalomucoid
hyalonyxis
hyalosis
    asteroid h.
    punctate h.
hyaluronate
    h. sodium
    h. sodium with chondroitin
hyaluronic acid
hyaluronidase
Hybriwix probe system
Hyde
    H. astigmatism ruler
    H. corneal forceps
    H. double-curved forceps
    H. irrigating/aspirating unit
    H. irrigator/aspirator unit
Hydeltrasol
Hyde-Osher keratometric ruler
Hydracon contact lens
Hydrasoft contact lens
Hydrate Injection
hydration
    stromal h.
hydraulic retinal reattachment
hydroa vacciniforme
hydroblepharon
hydrobromide
    homatropine h.
    hydroxyamphetamine h.
HydroBrush keratome
Hydrocare preserved saline
hydrochloride (HCl)
    apraclonidine h.
    benoxinate h.
    betaxolol h.
    carteolol h.
    ciprofloxacin h.
    cocaine h.
    cyclopentolate h.
    dapiprazole h.
    diphenhydramine h.
    dorzolamide h.
    hydromorphone h.
    levobetaxolol h.
    levobunolol h.
    levocabastine h.
    lidocaine h.
    lignocaine h.
    meperidine h.
    naloxone h.
    Neo-Synephrine H.
    oxybuprocaine h.
    oxymorphone h.
    papaverine h.
    phenacaine h.
    phencyclidine h.
    phenmetrazine h.
    phenoxybenzamine h.

phenylephrine h.
phenylpropanolamine h.
piperocaine h.
procaine h.
proparacaine h.
protriptyline h.
quinacrine h.
tetracaine h.
tetrahydrozoline h.
thioridazine h.
thymoxamine h.
trifluoperazine h.
trifluperidol h.
tyramine h.
hydrochlorothiazide
hydrocodone
hydrocortisone
h. acetate
bacitracin, neomycin, polymyxin B, and h.
chloramphenicol, polymyxin B, and h.
Chloromycetin H.
neomycin, polymyxin B, and h.
oxytetracycline and h.
h. suspension
Hydrocortone Phosphate
Hydrocurve II lens
hydrodelamination
hydrodelineation
hydrodiascope
hydrodissection
h. cannula
cortical cleaving h.
Kellan h.
multiquadrant h.
hydrodissector
cortical cleaving h.
Pearce nucleus h.
hydrodissector/rotator
5195 nucleus h.
HydroDIURIL
HydroEye SoftGels
hydrogel
h. contact lens
h. disk intraocular lens
extended wear h.
Hydrokeratome Mark I
hydrolysis
Koch nucleus h.
h. of solution
hydrometric chamber

hydromorphone hydrochloride
Hydron
American H.
H. lens
Hydronol
hydrophila
Aeromonas h.
hydrophilic contact lens
hydrophobic contact lens
hydrophthalmia, hydrophthalmos, hydrophthalmus
anterior h.
posterior h.
total h.
hydropic degeneration
hydrops
corneal h.
h. of iris
hydroquinone
Hydrosight lens
hydrostatic gradient
Hydroview
H. foldable IOL
H. lens
hydroxide
calcium h.
potassium h. (KOH)
sodium h.
hydroxocobalamin
hydroxyamphetamine
h. hydrobromide
h. and tropicamide
hydroxyapatite (HA)
h. ocular implant
h. orbital implant
h. spherical enucleation implant
hydroxychloroquine
h. retinopathy
h. sulfate
h. toxicity
hydroxyethyl cellulose
hydroxyethylmethacrylate (HEMA)
hydroxymethylprogesterone
hydroxypropyl
h. cellulose
h. methylcellulose (HPMC)
hydroxyquinoline
halogenated h.
hydroxystilbamidine isethionate
hydroxysultaine
cocoamidopropyl h.
hydroxyzine pamoate

NOTES

H

Hy-Flow
hyfrecator
hygroblepharic
hygroma
    perioptic h.
Hygroton
hyicus
    Staphylococcus h.
Hylan
    H. biopolymer fluid
    H. biopolymer gel-fluid
Hylashield
Hymenolepis nana
hyoscine
    Isopto H.
    scopolamine h.
hyoscyamine
hyperactive immune recovery
hyperactivity
    sympathetic h.
hyperacuity
hyperacusis
hyperacute conjunctivitis
hyperbaric oxygen therapy (HBO)
hyperbolic glasses
hypercalcemic
hypercupremia
hyperdeviation
    alternate h.
    dissociated h.
hyperemia
    ciliary h.
    conjunctival h.
    rebound conjunctival h.
hyperemic
hyperesophoria
hyperesthesia
    optic h.
    h. optica
hypereuryopia
hyperexophoria
hyperfluorescence
    choroidal h.
    stippled h.
hyperfluorescent
    h. hemorrhage
    h. window defect
hypergammaglobulinemia
hypergranulation tissue
hyperhomocysteinemia
hyperintense foci image
hyperkalemic periodic paralysis
hyperkeratotic
    h. dermatitis
    h. disorder
    h. plaque
hypermaturation

hypermature
    h. cataract
    h. lens
hypermetrope
hypermetropia (*var. of* hyperopia) **(Hy)**
hypermetropic astigmatism
hyperope
hyperophthalmopathic syndrome
hyperopia, hypermetropia (H)
    absolute h.
    axial h.
    correction of h.
    curvature h.
    facultative h.
    high h.
    index h.
    h. index
    latent h. (Hl)
    manifest h. (Hm)
    refractive h.
    relative h.
    total h. (Ht)
hyperopic (H)
    h. ablation
    h. astigmatism (AsH)
    h. automated lamellar keratoplasty
    (HALK)
    h. keratomileusis
    h. LASIK
    h. shift
hyperopization
hyperornithinemia
hyperornithinemia, hyperammonemia,
   and homocitrullinuria (HHH)
hyperosmotics
hyperphoria (H)
    circumduction h.
    left h.
    right h.
hyperplasia
    actinic h.
    benign reactive lymphoid h.
    epithelial h.
    goblet cell h.
    iris epithelial h.
    lymphoid h.
    pseudoepitheliomatous h.
    pseudosarcomatous endothelial h.
    reactive lymphoid h. (RLH)
    retinal epithelial pigment h.
hyperplastic primary vitreous
hyperpresbyopia
hyperreflective tissue
Hypersal
hypersecretion glaucoma
hypersensitivity
    h. reaction
    staphylococcal h.
hyperteloric

hypertelorism
    canthal h.
    ocular h.
    orbital h.
hypertension
    adrenal h.
    arterial h.
    essential h.
    idiopathic intracranial h. (IIH)
    intracranial h.
    malignant h.
    ocular h. (OHT)
    h. period
hypertensive
    h. encephalopathy
    h. iridocyclitis
    h. neuroretinopathy
    h. oculopathy
    h. retinitis
    h. retinopathy (HR)
hyperthermia
    malignant h.
    microwave h.
hyperthyroidism
    Graves h.
    ophthalmic h.
hyperthyroid stare
hypertonia oculi
hypertonic
    h. drops
    h. osmotherapy
    h. saline
    h. solution
hypertrophic
    h. dendriform epithelial lesion
    h. interstitial neuropathy
    h. rhinitis
hypertrophy
    epithelial h.
    follicular h.
    gelatinous-appearing limbal h.
    giant papillary h. (GPH)
    papillary conjunctival h.
    pigment epithelial h.
    retinal pigment epithelial h.
    RP h.
hypertropia (HT)
    alternating h.
    constant h.
    dissociated double h. (DDHT)
    double dissociated h.
    flick h.

    left h. (LHT)
    right h.
hyperviscosity syndrome
hypervitaminosis D
hypesthesia
    infraorbital h.
hyphema
    black-ball h.
    eight-ball h.
    layered h.
    microscopic h.
    postoperative h.
    postsurgical h.
    spontaneous h.
    total h.
    traumatic h.
    uveitis glaucoma h. (UGH)
hypnagogic hallucination
hypnopompic hallucination
hypocalcemic cataract
Hypoclear
hypocomplementemic urticarial vasculitis (HUV)
hypocyclosis
hypoesophoria
hypoesthesia
    corneal h.
hypoexophoria
hypofluorescent streak
hypogammaglobulinemia
hypoglobus
hypoglycemic cataract
hypointense foci image
hypointensity
hypokalemic periodic paralysis
hypometric saccade
hypoorbitism
hypophoria
hypophyseal artery
hypopigmentation
    oculocutaneous h.
hypoplasia
    bow-tie h.
    chiasmal h.
    hemiopic h.
    homonymous hemiopic h.
    macular h.
    optic disk h.
    optic nerve h.
    segmental h.
    thymic h.

NOTES

H

hypoplastic
    h. disk
    h. ocular nerve
hypopyon
    h. keratitis
    keratoiritis h.
    recurrent h.
    sterile h.
    h. ulcer
hyposcleral
HypoTears
    H. PF Solution
    H. Select lubricant eye drops
hypotelorism
    ocular h.
    orbital h.
hypotension
    intracranial h.
    spontaneous intracranial h.
hypotensive retinopathy
hypothalami
    pars optica h.
hypothalamic glioma
hypothalamic-pituitary-thyroid axis
hypothalamus
hypothesis
    Knudson h.
    Lyon h.
    h. testing
hypothyroidism
hypotonia oculi

hypotonic solution
hypotonus
hypotony
    bilateral h.
    essential h.
    h. maculopathy
    ocular h.
    persistent postdrainage h. (PPH)
    h. syndrome
hypotropia
    alternating h.
    constant h.
hypoxia
    orbital h.
    retinal h.
hypoxic
    h. corneal stress
    h. eyeball syndrome
hypsiconchous
Hyrexin-50 Injection
hysteric
    h. amaurosis
    h. amblyopia
    h. field
hysterical
    h. amblyopia
    h. blindness
    h. constricted field
    h. nystagmus
    h. visual field defect
Hyzine-50

I
luminous intensity
I&A
irrigating/aspirating
irrigation and aspiration
Simcoe I&A system
I/A
irrigation/aspiration
I/A cannula
I/A machine
steerable I/A
IAH
immune adherence hemagglutination
Ialo photocoagulator
ianthinopsia
iatrogenic
i. keratoconus
i. limbal stem cell deficiency
i. retinal break
i. retinal hole
i. retinal tear
ICAM-1 antigen
ICaps
ICaps Lutein & Zeaxanthin
Formula
ICaps ocular vitamins
ICaps Plus
ICaps TR dietary supplement
ICCE
intracapsular cataract extraction
ICD
intercanthal distance
ICE
iridocorneal endothelial
ICE syndrome
ice
i. ball
i. pack test
ICG
indocyanine green
ICG angiography
ICGA
indocyanine green angiography
IC-Green
I.-G. kit
I-Chlor
ichthyosis
congenital i.
i. cornea
ICK
infectious crystalline keratopathy
ICL
implantable contact lens
ICP
intracranial pressure

IC-PC
internal carotid-posterior communicating
IC-PC aneurysm
IC-PC artery aneurysm
ICRS
intrastromal corneal ring segment
ICSC
idiopathic central serous
chorioretinopathy
icteric
icterus
scleral i.
IDDM
insulin-dependent diabetes mellitus
identical point
identification acuity
idiocy
amaurotic familial i. (AFI)
idiopathic
i. acquired retinal telangiectasia
i. arteritis of Takayasu
i. central serous chorioretinopathy
(ICSC)
i. congenital esotropia
i. corneal endotheliopathy
i. demyelinating optic neuritis
i. epiretinal membrane (IERM)
i. facial palsy
i. inflammatory pseudotumor
i. intracranial hypertension (IIH)
i. juxtafoveal retinal telangiectasis
i. lipid keratopathy
i. macular cyst and hole
i. myositis
i. nongranulomatous optic neuritis
i. orbital inflammation
i. orbital inflammatory syndrome
(IOIS)
i. perifoveal telangiectasis (IPT)
i. perioptic neuritis
i. polypoidal choroidal vasculopathy
(IPCV)
i. preretinal membrane
i. pseudotumor cerebri
i. retinal vasculitis
i. retinal vasculitis, aneurysms and
neuroretinitis (IRVAN)
i. scleritis
i. sclerosing inflammation of the
orbit
i. vitreitis
i. vitreomacular traction syndrome
idioretinal light
idoxuridine (IDU)
I-Drops

IDU
idoxuridine
IEBI
intereye blink interval
IERM
idiopathic epiretinal membrane
I-Gent
ignipuncture
I-Homatrine
IIH
idiopathic intracranial hypertension
IK
interstitial keratitis
Ikeda microcapsulorrhexis forceps
I-knife
Alcon I.-k.
IL-1
Interleukin 1
ILC
Integrated Light Control
Ilg
I. capsule forceps
I. curved microtying forceps
I. insertion forceps
I. lens loupe
I. microneedle holder
I. needle
I. needle holder
I. probe
I. push/pull
Iliff
I. approach
I. exenteration
I. lacrimal probe
I. lacrimal trephine
I. operation
Iliff-Haus operation
Iliff-House sclerectomy
Iliff-Park speculum
Iliff-Wright fascia needle
I-Liqui Tears
illacrimation
illaqueation
Illiterate
I. E
I. E chart
I. eye chart
illness
high-altitude i.
illuminance
illuminated
i. near card (INC)
i. suction needle
illumination
axial i.
background i.
central i.
coaxial i.
contact i.

critical i.
dark-field i.
dark-ground i.
diffuse i.
direct i.
erect i.
focal i.
Ganzfeld i.
incoherent i.
indirect i.
Köhler i.
lateral i.
Macbeth i.
maximal i.
narrow-slit i.
oblique i.
photopic i.
sclerotic scatter i.
slit i.
tangential i.
vertical i.
illuminator
high intensity i.
Luxo surgical i.
OPMI VISU 200 BrightFlex i.
Synergetics endo i.
illusion
frequency doubling i.
Hermann grid i.
Kuhnt i.
i. of movement
oculogravic i.
oculogyral i.
optical i.
passive i.
illusory visual spread
ILM
internal limiting membrane
ILM maculorrhexis
Ilotycin Ophthalmic
image
accidental i.
aerial i.
i. analysis
astigmatic i.
catatropic i.
Clear I. III
i. degradation
digitized video fundus i.
direct i.
i. displacement
false i.
foveal i.
ghost i.
heteronymous i.
homonymous i.
hyperintense foci i.
hypointense foci i.
incidental i.

inversion of i.
inverted i.
i. jump
i. of mires
mirror i.
negative i.
ocular i.
optical i.
Placido disk i.
i. plane
i. point
pseudostereo i.
Purkinje i.
Purkinje-Sanson mirror i.
real i.
retinal i.
Sanson i.
Scheimpflug slit i.
spectacular i.
specular i.
stigmatic i.
true i.
unequal retinal i.
videooculographic i.
virtual i.
visual i.
IMAGEnet
I. image digitizing system
I. 2000 series digital imaging
system
imager
Digital fundus i.
Digital slit-lamp i.
Humphrey retina i.
Photoshop 6.0 digitized i.
IMAGE Software
image-space focus
imaging
cine-magnetic resonance i.
color Doppler i.
diffusion-weighted imaging/magnetic
resonance i. (DWI/MRI)
digital nonmydriatic fundus i.
laser light i.
magnetic resonance i. (MRI)
off-axis i.
on-axis i.
orbitocranial i.
posterior visual pathway i.
stereoscopic i.
i. technology

imbalance
binocular i.
central vestibular i.
Imbert-Fick principle
imbrication
retinal i.
immature cataract
immediate elevation
immersion
i. lens
i. method
imminens
glaucoma i.
immitis
Coccidioides i.
coccidioidomycosis i.
immune
i. adherence hemagglutination (IAH)
i. complex
i. mechanism
i. reaction
i. recovery uveitis
i. recovery vitritis
i. recovery vitritis syndrome
i. response
i. stromal keratitis (ISK)
i. system
i. Wessely ring
immunity
adaptive i.
cell-mediated i.
humoral i.
immunoadsorption therapy
immunochromatography analysis
immunodiagnostic method
immunodominant antibody
immunofluorescence
anticomplement i.
immunofluorescent
i. assay
i. staining
immunogenic inflammation
immunohistochemical technique
immunologic
i. memory
i. reaction
immunological conjunctivitis
immunology
ocular i.
immunomodulatory therapy
immunoperoxidase staining

NOTES

**immunoreactive adrenomedullin
   concentration**
immunosuppressant-induced head tremor
immunosuppressive drug
impact resistance
impaired vergence eye movement
impairment
    adduction i.
    cortical visual i.
    sensation i.
    visual i. (VI)
impatency
    congenital i.
impending macular hole
impetigo contagiosa
Impex diamond radial keratotomy knife
**Impex/Lerner foldable lens removing
   set**
impingement
implant
    ACIOL i.
    acorn-shaped eye i.
    acrylic hydroxyapatite i.
    acrylic lens i.
    Ahmed valve i.
    Allen-Braley i.
    Allen-ePTFE ocular i.
    Allen orbital i.
    Alpar i.
    Alumina i.
    aluminum oxide i.
    anterior chamber intraocular lens i.
    Arroyo i.
    Arruga i.
    Arruga-Moura-Brazil i.
    Baerveldt glaucoma i.
    Baerveldt seton i.
    Barkan infant i.
    Barraquer i.
    Berens conical i.
    Berens pyramidal i.
    Berens-Rosa scleral i.
    Binkhorst collar stud lens i.
    Binkhorst four-loop iris-fixated i.
    Binkhorst two-loop intraocular
      lens i.
    Bio-Eye ocular i.
    Biomatrix ocular i.
    Bionic eye microdetector
      subretinal i.
    Boberg-Ans lens i.
    Bonaccolto monoplex orbital i.
    Boyd orbital i.
    Brawner orbital i.
    Brown-Dohlman Silastic corneal i.
    build-up i.
    Bunker i.
    Cardona focalizing fundus lens i.
    Cardona goniofocalizing i.

    Castroviejo acrylic i.
    CE/IOL i.
    Choyce Mark VIII i.
    Cogan-Boberg-Ans lens i.
    conical i.
    conus shell-type eye i.
    conventional shell i.
    Cooper i.
    Copeland i.
    corneal i.
    cosmetic contact shell i.
    Cryo-Barrages vitreous i.
    CrystaLens model AT-45 i.
    curlback shell i.
    Cutler i.
    Dannheim eye i.
    45-degree bent reform i.
    Dermostat i.
    Doherty sphere i.
    encircling i.
    enophthalmos wedge i.
    i. entry
    Epstein collar stud acrylic i.
    i. extrusion
    Federov four-loop iris clip lens i.
    Federov type I, II lens i.
    Ferguson i.
    filtering i.
    Fine magnetic i.
    four-loop iris clip i.
    four-loop iris fixated i.
    Fox sphere i.
    Frey tunneled i.
    front build-up i.
    full-dimpled Lucite i.
    Garcia-Novito eye i.
    Gelfilm retinal i.
    glass sphere i.
    Gold eyelid load i.
    Goldmann three-mirror i.
    Gold-Mules i.
    gold sphere i.
    gonioscopic i.
    grooved silicone i.
    Guist sphere i.
    Haik i.
    hemisphere eye i.
    Herrick silicone lacrimal i.
    hollow-sphere i.
    hook-type i.
    Hoskins-Drake i.
    Hruby i.
    Hughes i.
    hydroxyapatite ocular i.
    hydroxyapatite orbital i.
    hydroxyapatite spherical
      enucleation i.
    intracanalicular collagen i.
    intracorneal i.

intraocular lens i.
intraorbital i.
intravitreal ganciclovir i.
Iovision i.
Iowa orbital i.
Ivalon sponge i.
Jordan i.
keratolens i.
King orbital i.
Koeppe gonioscopic i.
Krupin i.
Krupin-Denver long-valve i.
Kryptok i.
Landegger orbital i.
Lemoine orbital i.
i. lens
lens i.
Levitt i.
Lincoff scleral sponge i.
Lovac fundus contact lens i.
Lovac six-mirror gonioscopic
  lens i.
Lucite sphere i.
Lyda-Ivalon-Lucite i.
i. magnet
magnetic i.
McCannel i.
McGhan i.
MedDev i.
Medical Optics PC11NB intraocular
  lens i.
Medical Workshop intraocular
  lens i.
Medicornea Kratz intraocular
  lens i.
Medpor MCOI i.
Melauskas acrylic i.
Melauskas orbital i.
meridional i.
methylmethacrylate i.
i. migration
Molteno i.
motility i.
Mueller i.
Muhlberger orbital i.
Mules i.
Nocito eye i.
Oculo-Plastik ePTFE ocular i.
O'Malley self-adhering lens i.
Ophtec occlusion i.
optic i.
orbital floor i.

pars plana seton i.
peanut i.
piggyback i.
i. placement
plastic sphere i.
Platina intraocular lens i.
Plexiglas i.
pneumatically stented i. (PSI)
polyethylene i.
porous orbital i.
posterior chamber lens i. (PCLI)
posterior tube shunt i.
Precision Cosmet intraocular lens i.
primary lens i.
pseudophake i.
Radin-Rosenthal eye i.
Rayner-Choyce i.
retinal Gelfilm i.
reverse-shape i.
Ridley anterior chamber lens i.
Ridley Mark II lens i.
Rodin orbital i.
Rosa-Berens orbital i.
Ruedemann eye i.
Ruiz plano fundus lens i.
Schepens hollow hemisphere i.
Schocket tube i.
scleral i.
secondary lens i.
segmental i.
semishell i.
Severin i.
Shearing posterior chamber
  intraocular lens i.
shelf-type i.
shell i.
Sichi orbital i.
Silastic scleral buckler i.
silicone mesh i.
i. sleeve
sleeve i.
sling for i.
Smith orbital floor i.
Snellen conventional reform i.
solid silicone with Supramid
  mesh i.
sphere i.
spherical i.
i. sponge
sponge i.
Stone i.
Stone-Jordan i.

NOTES

implant *(continued)*
 Strampelli lens i.
 subperiosteal i.
 SupraFOIL i.
 Supramid-Allen i.
 Supramid lens i.
 surface i.
 tantalum mesh i.
 Teflon i.
 temporary intracanalicular
  collagen i.
 Tennant i.
 Tensilon i.
 i. tire
 tire i.
 Troncoso gonioscopic lens i.
 Troutman i.
 tunneled i.
 two-staged Baerveldt glaucoma i.
 Ultex lens i.
 Universal i.
 unpegged hydroxyapatite i.
 Uribe orbital i.
 VA magnetic orbital i.
 Varigray i.
 Varilux lens i.
 Vitallium i.
 Vitrasert intravitreal i.
 Volk conoid lens i.
 Walter Reed i.
 Wheeler eye sphere i.
 wire mesh i.
implantable
 i. contact lens (ICL)
 i. miniaturized telescope (IMT)
implantation
 Ahmed glaucoma valve i.
 in-the-bag i.
 intraocular lens i.
 i. of lens
 multifocal intraocular lens i.
 PHEMA KPro i.
 radon seed i.
implanted Artisan letter
implanter
 Geuder i.
Implens intraocular lens
impletion
implicit time
impression
 basilar i.
 i. cytology
 i. débridement
 i. tonometer
imprint
improvement
 no i.
 pinhole no i. (PHNI)

Imre
 I. keratoplasty
 I. lateral canthoplasty
 I. lateral canthoplasty operation
 I. sliding flap
 I. treatment
IMT
 implantable miniaturized telescope
Imuran
in
 base in (BI)
 in situ DNA nick end labeling
 in situ DNA nick end-labeling
  staining
inactive trachoma
INAD
 infantile neuroaxonal dystrophy
inadequacy
 blink i.
Inamura
 I. race chopper
 I. small incision capsulorrhexis
  forceps
I-Naphline Ophthalmic
inattention
 visual i.
inborn error
INC
 illuminated near card
Inc.
 Autoclave Testing Service, I.
 Integrated Orbital Implants, I.
 Richmond Products I.
incandescent lamp
incarceration
 iris i.
incidence
 angle of i.
 plane of i.
incident
 i. angle
 flux i.
 i. point
 ray i.
 i. ray of light
incidental
 i. color
 i. image
incipient cataract
incision
 Abex-Turner i.
 Agnew-Verhoeff i.
 arcuate i.
 buttonhole i.
 centrifugal i.
 centripetal i.
 chevron i.
 chord i.
 clear corneal step i.

clear corneal tunnel i.
conjunctival i.
corneal i.
corneoscleral i.
corridor i.
cutdown i.
gray-line i.
grooved i.
host i.
i. into eyelid
lateral canthal i.
limbal relaxing i. (LRI)
Lynch medial canthal i.
nasal buttonhole i.
posterior i.
relaxing i.
scleral-limbal-corneal i.
scleral tunnel i.
i. spreader
stab i.
sub-2 i.
subciliary i.
Swan i.
temporal self-sealing clear
  corneal i.
i. terminus
trap i.
trapezoid single-plane clear
  corneal i.
i. viewing instrument
von Noorden i.
incisura, pl. **incisurae**
  i. ethmoidalis ossis frontalis
  i. lacrimalis
  i. maxillae
  i. supraorbitalis
incisure
  ethmoidal i.
  frontal i.
  lacrimal i.
  supraorbital i.
inclinometer
inclusion
  i. blennorrhea
  i. body
  i. conjunctivitis
  Cowdry type A intranuclear i.
  i. cyst
  epithelial i.
  intranuclear i.
  mascara particle i.

incoherent illumination
incomitance
incomitant
  i. esodeviation
  i. vertical deviation
  i. vertical strabismus
incomplete
  i. achromatopsia
  i. hemianopsia
  i. pupil-sparing oculomotor nerve
    paresis
incongruent nystagmus
incongruous
  i. field defect
  i. hemianopsia
incontinentia pigmenti
increased
  i. tension (T+)
  i. vertical fusional amplitude
incrementally
increment threshold spectral sensitivity
incycloduction
incyclophoria
incyclotropia
incyclovergence
indapamide
indentation
  i. gonioscopy
  i. operation
  prominent i.
  scleral i.
  i. tonometer
  i. tonometry
independence
  actual degree of i.
independent event
index, pl. **indices, indexes**
  i. amblyopia
  i. ametropia
  i. case
  i. hyperopia
  hyperopia i.
  i. myopia
  myopia i.
  Ophthalmic Confidence I. (OCI)
  recession i. (RI)
  i. of refraction (IR, n)
  resistive i.
  surface asymmetry i. (SAI)
  surface regularity i. (SRI)
  visual field i.

NOTES

indicator
Berens-Tolman ocular hypertension i.
i. yellow
indinavir sulfate
indirect
i. argon laser drainage
i. choroidal rupture
i. fluorescent antibody
i. illumination
i. lens
i. ophthalmoscope
i. ophthalmoscopic laser photocoagulation
i. ophthalmoscopy
i. pupillary reaction
i. vision
Indocin ophthalmic solution
indocyanine
i. green (ICG)
i. green angiography (ICGA)
i. green dye
indolent
i. ulceration
i. ulceration of the cornea
indoltheticum
Flavobacterium i.
indomethacin toxicity keratopathy
induced
i. anisophoria
i. prism
induction
industrial spectacles
inelastic
I-Neocort
inert material for intraocular lens
infant
I. Aphakia Treatment Study
i. Karickhoff laser lens
retinopapillitis of premature i.'s
i. three-mirror laser lens
infantile
i. cataract
i. esotropia
i. glaucoma
i. neuroaxonal dystrophy (INAD)
i. nystagmus
i. optic atrophy
i. poikiloderma subgroup 1-2-3
i. purulent conjunctivitis
i. Refsum disease
i. strabismus syndrome
infarct
choroidal i.
nerve fiber layer i.
infarction
cerebral i.
eye i.
lateral medullary i.

orbital i.
paramedian thalamopeduncular i.
retinochoroidal i.
infarctive necrosis
infection
anaerobic ocular i.
bacterial i.
chlamydial i.
extended wear i.
eyelid molluscum contagiosum i.
fungal i.
graft i.
herpetic ocular i.
mycotic i.
ocular cryptococcal i.
Serratia marcescens i.
trematode i.
vaccinia i.
infectiosus
conjunctivitis necroticans i.
infectious
i. conjunctivitis
i. corneal ulcer
i. crystalline keratopathy (ICK)
i. dacryoadenitis
i. disease
i. endophthalmitis
i. epithelial keratitis
i. ophthalmoplegia
i. retinochoroiditis
infective myositis
Infectrol
inferior
i. altitudinal defect
i. arcuate bundle
arcus palpebralis i.
arteriola macularis i.
arteriola nasalis retinae i.
arteriola temporalis retinae i.
i. canaliculus
i. conjunctival fornix
i. conus
i. cornea
fissura orbitalis i.
i. fornix reformation
glandula lacrimalis i.
i. lacrimal gland
i. longitudinal fasciculus
i. macula
i. macular arteriole
i. meatus nasi
musculus tarsalis i.
i. nasal artery
i. nasal quadrant
i. nasal vein
i. oblique
i. oblique extraocular muscle
i. oblique overaction (IOOA)
i. oblique palsy

i. olivary nucleus
i. ophthalmic vein
i. orbital fissure
i. orbital rim
i. orbital septum
i. palpebral vein
i. pole
i. punctum
i. rectus (IR)
i. rectus extraocular muscle
i. retinal arcade
i. salivary nucleus
i. steepening
i. symblepharon
i. tarsal muscle
i. tarsus
i. tarsus palpebra
i. temporal arcade
i. temporal artery
i. temporal quadrant
i. temporal vein
vena ophthalmica i.
venula macularis i.
venula nasalis retinae i.
venula temporalis retinae i.
i. zone of retina
i. zygomatic foramen

inferiores
venae palpebrales i.

inferioris
pars orbitalis gyri frontalis i.

inferiorly
eye rotated i.

inferonasal artery

inferonasally

inferotemporal
i. arcade
i. artery

inferotemporally

infiltrate
anular i.
bacterial infectious corneal i.
central stromal i.
i. in cornea
corneal punctate i.
crystalline i.
inflammatory cellular i.
leukemic i.
patchy anterior stromal i.
plasmacytoid i.
ring i.

ring-shaped stromal i.
stromal anular i.
stromal ring i.
subepithelial punctate corneal i.
white stromal i.
wreath pattern stromal i.

infiltration
branching i.
choroidal i.
dermal amyloid i.
inflammatory cell i.
linear i.
lymphocytic i.
lymphoid i.
mononuclear cell i.
perivascular neutrophil i.
radial i.
sarcoidosis i.

infiltrative
i. keratitis
i. optic neuropathy

Infinitech
I. fiber optics
I. laser probe

infinite distance

infirmary
eye i.
Massachusetts Eye & Ear I.

Inflamase
I. Forte
I. Forte Ophthalmic
I. Mild
I. Mild Ophthalmic

inflamed pinguecula

inflammation
acute sterile i.
anterior chamber i.
anterior segment i.
ciliary body i.
corneal nerve i.
i. of eyelid
idiopathic orbital i.
immunogenic i.
ocular i.
vitreous i.

inflammatory
i. cell
i. cell infiltration
i. cellular infiltrate
i. changes of retina
i. dacryoadenitis
i. ectropion

NOTES

inflammatory *(continued)*
    i. glaucoma
    i. mediator
    i. meibomian gland disease
    i. myopathy
    i. optic neuritis
    i. optic neuropathy
    i. pseudotumor
    i. retinopathy
    i. syndrome
    i. target site of eye
inflow
    aqueous i.
influence of an Artisan lens
influenzae
    Haemophilus i.
influenza virus
infolding
    macular translocation with
      macular i.
    macular translocation with scleral i.
    (MTSI)
    scleral i.
information
    spatial i.
infraciliary
infraduct
infraduction
infraepitrochlear nerve
infranasal
infranuclear
    i. disorder
    i. ophthalmoplegia
    i. pathway
infraorbital
    i. anesthesia
    i. artery
    i. canal
    i. foramen
    i. groove
    i. hypesthesia
    i. margin
    i. margin of maxilla
    i. nerve
    i. region
    i. sulcus of maxilla
    i. suture
infraorbitale
    foramen i.
infraorbitalis
    nervus i.
    sutura i.
infrapalpebralis
    sulcus i.
infrapalpebral sulcus
infrared
    i. cataract
    i. heater
    i. image analysis

    i. oculography
    i. optometer
    i. pupillometry
    i. radiation
    i. slit lamp
infratentorial arteriovenous malformation
infratrochlear nerve
infravergence
infraversion
infundibular cyst
infusion
    i. cannula
    detachment i.
    i. light pipe
    i. suction cutter vitreous cutter
    Vented Gas Forced I. (VGFI)
ingrowth
    epithelial i.
    fibroblastic i.
    stromal i.
inhalation anesthetic
inhibition
    intraoperative miosis i.
    lateral i.
    paradoxic levator i.
inhibitional
    i. palsy
    i. palsy of contralateral antagonist
inhibitor
    Batimastat matrix
      metalloproteinase i.
    carbonic anhydrase i. (CAI)
    plasminogen activator i. (PAI)
inion
initial trabeculectomy
injection
    antiangiogenesis i.
    anti-VEGF i.
    botulinum i.
    ciliary i.
    circumcorneal i.
    conjunctival ciliary i.
    Cytoxan I.
    episcleral i.
    Hydrate I.
    Hyrexin-50 I.
    intracameral air i.
    intralesional triamcinolone i.
    intraocular gas i.
    intravitreal i.
    juxtascleral i.
    i. molding
    Neosar I.
    Osmitrol i.
    peribulbar i.
    periocular i.
    posterior sub-Tenon i.
    Predcor-TBA I.
    retrobulbar alcohol i.

retrobulbar corticosteroid i.
silicone oil i.
subconjunctival i.
sub-Tenon corticosteroid i.
Toradol I.
Ureaphil I.
Van Lint i.
injector
automatic twin syringe i.
Dyonics syringe i.
injector-aspirator
double-barreled i.-a.
injury
chemical i.
concussion i.
contrecoup i.
coup i.
cow horn-related ocular i.
dehydration i.
eye i.
gestational i.
Hughes classification of chemical i.
levator i.
microwave radiation i.
ocular i.
optic nerve i.
penetrating i.
radiation i.
shearing i.
ultraviolet-induced i.
in-lab lens casting technology
inlay
corneal i.
inner
i. canthus
i. limiting membrane
i. molecular layer of the retina
i. nuclear layer
i. nuclear layer of retina
i. plexiform layer
i. punctate choroidopathy
i. segment
innervate
innervation
Hering law of equal i.
Hering law of equivalent i.
Hering law of simultaneous i.
levator i.
reciprocal i.
regeneration of i.
Sherrington law of reciprocal i.

innocens
diabetes i.
innominate steal syndrome
Innovar
INNOVA System 920
Innovatome microkeratome
InnoVit
I. 1800 probe
I. vitrectomy probe
INO
internuclear ophthalmoplegia
inoculum
inositus
diabetes i.
input
nerve i.
i. nerve
supranuclear i.
inserter
AC tube i.
AMO PhacoFlex lens and i.
Fine III i.
Lens-Eze i.
insertion
tendinous i.
tensor i.
Insight
I. 4000 endoscope
I. K-3000 Automated Keratome
insipidus
diabetes i.
insonification
ultrasonic i.
inspired gas
instability
tear film i.
instillation
institute
American National Standards I. (ANSI)
Dartmouth Eye I.
Wilmer Eye I.
Wilmer Ophthalmological I.
instrument
Accurate Surgical and Scientific I.'s (ASSI)
Alcon Surgical i.
American Hydron i.
Argyll Robertson i.
Ascon i.
Biophysic Ophthascan S i.
Birks Mark II i.

NOTES

instrument *(continued)*
    Carl Zeiss i.
    Daisy irrigation/aspiration i.
    Donnenfeld striae removal i.
    DORC backflush i.
    Eckardt Heme-Stopper i.
    fixation i.
    Grieshaber ultrasharp
      microsurgery i.
    guillotine vitrectomy i.
    incision viewing i.
    IOLAB titanium i.
    IOLMaster optical i.
    Karl Ilg i.
    Kerato-Kontours i.
    Mastel Precision surgical i.
    matte black i.
    optical centering i.
    Rank-Taylor-Hobson-Talysurf i.
    Retinomax refractometry i.
    Rizzuti-Bonaccolto i.
    Rizzuti-Fleischer i.
    Rizzuti-Kayser-Fleischer i.
    Rizzuti-Lowe i.
    Rizzuti-Maxwell i.
    Rizzuti-Soemmering i.
    Rumex titanium i.
    Sonomed 1500 A-scan i.
    Sutcliffe laser shield and
      retracting i.
    Sutherland rotatable microsurgery i.
    Thomas Kapsule i.
    topographic scanning/indocyanine
      green angiography combination i.
    UTAS 2000 electroretinography i.
    vitrectomy i.
instrument/apparatus
    Squid i./a.
instrumentation
insufficiency
    accommodation i.
    accommodative i. (AI)
    convergence i. (CI)
    cortical visual i.
    divergence i.
    dynamic accommodation i.
    i. of externi
    i. of eyelid
    i. of eyelid closure
    muscular i.
    static accommodation i.
    vertebrobasilar artery i.
insular scotoma
insulin-deficient diabetes
**insulin-dependent diabetes mellitus
  (IDDM)**
insulin resistance
Intacs
    I. corneal ring segment

    KeraVision I.
    I. ring
intact
    i. anterior hyaloid face
    extraocular movement i. (EOMI)
integrated
    I. Light Control (ILC)
    I. Orbital Implants, Inc.
Integre 532 delivery system
integrity
    break in retinal i.
intensity
    luminous i. (I)
    i. profile
    radiant i.
    unit of luminous i.
interaction
    bipolar horizontal i.
    contour i.
    drug i.
    electrostatic i.
    Fas i.
    FasL i.
    spatial i.
intercalary staphyloma
intercanthal distance (ICD)
intercanthic
intercellular space
intercept
    corneal i.
interciliary fiber
intercilium
intereye blink interval (IEBI)
interface
    graft-host i.
    i. haze
    i. opacity
    parallel i.
    i. phenomena
    vitreomacular i.
    vitreoretinal i.
interfasciale
    spatium i.
interfascial space
interference
    i. filter
    i. fringe
    i. visual acuity test
Interferenzfilter 675FS20-12.5 filter
interferometer
    electron i.
    Fizeau-Tolansky i.
    Zeiss IOL Master laser i.
interferometry
    electron i.
    laser i.
    partial coherence i. (PCI)
interferon
    i. alfa-2a

i. alfa-2b
i. beta-1a
interior eye tumor
interlacing of collagen lamellae
interlamellar space
Interleukin 1 (IL-1)
intermedia
uveitis i.
intermediate
i. posterior curve (IPC)
i. uveitis
Intermedics
I. intraocular tonometer
I. lens
I. Phaco I/A unit
Pharmacia I.
intermedius
i. nerve
nervus i.
Staphylococcus i.
intermittent
i. angle-closure glaucoma
i. deviation
i. esotropia (E(T))
i. exotropia (X(T))
i. strabismus
i. tropia
intermuscular
i. membrane
i. septum
interna
axis oculi i.
folliculitis i.
membrana granulosa i.
membrana limitans i.
ophthalmoplegia i.
internal
i. axis of eye
i. capsule syndrome
i. carotid artery
i. carotid-posterior communicating (IC-PC)
i. carotid-posterior communicating artery aneurysm
i. hordeolum
i. lacrimal fistula
i. limiting membrane (ILM)
i. limiting membrane of the retina
i. nucleus hydrodelineation needle
i. ophthalmopathy
i. ophthalmoplegia
i. ostium

i. palsy
i. rectus muscle
i. reflectivity
i. squint
i. strabismus
International Study Group for Behçet Disease
internuclear
i. ophthalmoparesis
i. ophthalmoplegia (INO)
i. paralysis
internuclearis
ophthalmoplegia i.
internum
hordeolum i.
internus
axis bulbi i.
interobserver
interosseous wiring
interpalpebral
i. fissure
i. stromal disease
i. zone
interpeduncular fossa
interphotoreceptor retinoid-binding protein (IRBP)
interplexiform cell
interpolation
interpupillary distance (IPD)
interrogans
Leptospira i.
interrupted nylon suture
Intersol
Interspace YAG laser lens
interstitial
i. keratitis (IK)
i. neovascularization
i. nucleus of Cajal
interthalamic commissure
intervaginale
spatium i.
intervaginal space of optic nerve
interval
focal i.
intereye blink i. (IEBI)
Sturm i.
i. of Sturm
interwave-guided multipass
interweaving
collagen fibril i.
Interzeag bowl perimeter

NOTES

in-the-bag
  i.-t.-b. implantation
  i.-t.-b. lens
intorsion
intort
intortor muscle
intoxication amaurosis
intraaxonal
intracameral
  i. air injection
  i. anesthesia
  i. lidocaine
  i. suture
intracanalicular
  i. anatomy
  i. collagen implant
  i. optic nerve
intracanicular
intracapsular
  i. cataract extraction (ICCE)
  i. extraction of cataract
  i. ligament
intracavernous carotid artery
intracorneal
  i. cyst
  i. implant
  i. ring
intracranial
  i. anatomy
  i. aneurysm
  i. glioma
  i. granuloma
  i. hypertension
  i. hypotension
  i. mass
  i. optic nerve
  i. optic nerve decompression
  i. pressure (ICP)
intracytoplasmic inclusion body
intradermal nevus
intraepithelial
  i. cyst
  i. dyskeratosis
  i. epithelioma
  i. microcyst
  i. neoplasia
  i. neoplasm
  i. plexus
intralacrimal papilloma
intralamellar
  i. autopatch
  i. pocket procedure
intralenticular hemorrhage
intralesional triamcinolone injection
intraluminal suture
intramarginal sulcus
intramedullary segment
intranasal endoscopic
  dacryocystorhinostomy

intranuclear
  i. eosinophilic inclusion body
  i. inclusion
intraocular (IO)
  i. administration
  i. air
  i. anatomy
  i. anesthetic agent
  i. cataract extraction
  i. cilia
  i. coccidioidomycosis
  i. cysticercus
  i. distance
  i. fistula
  i. fluid
  i. forceps
  i. foreign body (IOFB)
  i. foreign body trauma
  i. gas
  i. gas bubble
  i. gas injection
  i. hemorrhage
  i. involvement
  i. lens (IOL)
  i. lens dialer
  i. lens dislocation
  i. lens exchange
  i. lens glide
  i. lens implant
  i. lens implantation
  i. lens power (IOLP)
  i. lidocaine
  i. lymphoma
  i. melanoma
  Miostat i.
  i. muscle (IOM)
  i. myelination of retinal nerve
    fiber
  i. optic nerve
  i. optic neuritis
  i. penetration
  i. pressure (IOP)
  i. pressure spike
  i. retinoblastoma
  i. silicone oil tamponade
  i. tension
  i. tuberculosis
intraoperative
  i. adjustable suture surgery
  i. bleeding
  i. blood loss
  i. B-scan echogram
  i. miosis inhibition
  i. suture adjustment (ISA)
IntraOptics lensometer
intraorbital
  i. air
  i. anatomy
  i. anesthesia

i. foreign body
i. hemorrhage
i. implant
i. margin of orbit
i. nerve dysfunction
intraosseous optic nerve
intrapapillary drusen
intraretinal
i. bleeding
i. fleck
i. hemorrhage
i. lipid deposit
i. microvascular abnormality
(IRMA)
intrascleral
i. nerve loop
i. plexus
intrasellar tumor
intrasheath tenotomy
intrastromal
i. corneal ring
i. corneal ring segment (ICRS)
i. laser
intratemporal segment
intravenous (IV)
i. fluorescein
i. fluorescein angiography (IVFA)
I. Immunoglobulin Therapy in
Optic Neuritis
i. thyrotropin-releasing hormone test
intraventricular hemorrhage (IVH)
intravitreal
i. antibiotic
i. fibrin
i. ganciclovir implant
i. hemorrhage
i. injection
i. TPA
intrinsic
i. light
i. ocular muscle
i. sympathomimetic activity
introducer
Carter sphere i.
silicone i.
sphere i.
Weaver trocar i.
Intron A
intrusion
saccadic i.
intubation
lacrimal i.

monocanalicular i.
O'Donoghue silicone i.
Silastic i.
silicone nasolacrimal i.
in-tumbling fashion
intumescent cataract
invasion
epithelial i.
invasive adenoma
inventory
Color Screening I.
Multiple Sclerosis Quality of
Life I. (MSQLI)
inversa
retinitis pigmentosa i.
inverse
i. astigmatism
i. ocular bobbing
inversion of image
inversus
blepharophimosis i.
canthus i.
epicanthal i.
epicanthus i.
situs i.
inverted image
Inverter vitrectomy system
investigation
neuroophthalmological i.
scientific i.
invisible bifocal
involutional
i. blepharoptosis
i. laxity
i. lower eyelid entropion
i. senile ectropion
i. senile entropion
i. senile ptosis
i. stenosis
involvement
intraocular i.
inward rectifier
IO
intraocular
IO muscle
Iocare
I. balanced salt solution
I. titanium needle
iodide
echothiophate i.
Metubine I.

NOTES

iodide *(continued)*
    Phospholine I.
    potassium i.
iodochlorhydroxyquin
iodopsin
iodoquinol
IOFB
    intraocular foreign body
IOFB-caused defect
IOIS
    idiopathic orbital inflammatory syndrome
IOL
    intraocular lens
        accommodative IOL
        AcrySof Natural IOL
        AcrySof single-piece IOL
        anterior chamber IOL
        Artisan iris-fixated phakic IOL
        CeeOn Edge foldable IOL
        ClariFlex foldable IOL
        C-loop IOL
        Collamer 3-piece IOL
        CV232 square-round-edge IOL
        disk IOL
        Hydroview foldable IOL
        Kearney side-notch IOL
        light-adjustable IOL
        MemoryLens IOL
        Morcher iris diaphragm IOL, type 67G
        Sensar OptiEdge foldable acrylic IOL
        silicone toric IOL
        Staar toric IOL
        Tecnis foldable IOL
IOLAB
    I. 108 B lens
    I. I&A photocoagulator
    I. intraocular lens
    I. irrigating/aspirating photocoagulator
    I. irrigating/aspirating unit
    I. irrigating needle
    I. taper-cut needle
    I. taper-point needle
    I. titanium instrument
    I. titanium needle
IOLMaster optical instrument
IOLP
    intraocular lens power
IOM
    intraocular muscle
ION
    ischemic optic neuropathy
ionizing radiation
ion laser
IOOA
    inferior oblique overaction

IOP
    intraocular pressure
        foldable IOP
Iopidine
Ioptex
    I. laser intraocular lens
    I. TabOptic lens
Iovision implant
Iowa
    I. orbital implant
    I. State fixation forceps
I/P
    iris and pupil
I-Paracaine
I-Parescein
IPC
    intermediate posterior curve
IPCV
    idiopathic polypoidal choroidal vasculopathy
IPD
    interpupillary distance
IPE
    iris pigment epithelium
I-Pentolate
I-Phrine Ophthalmic Solution
I-Picamide
I-Pilocarpine
I-Pilopine
I-Pred
I-Prednicet
ipsilateral
    i. antagonist
    i. centrocecal scotoma
    i. iris
    i. proptosis
IPT
    idiopathic perifoveal telangiectasis
IR
    index of refraction
    inferior rectus
IRBP
    interphotoreceptor retinoid-binding protein
Irene lens
I-Rescein
iridal
iridalgia
iridauxesis
iridectasis
iridectome
iridectomesodialysis
iridectomize
iridectomy
    argon laser i.
    basal i.
    Bethke i.
    buttonhole i.
    Castroviejo i.

central i.
Chandler i.
complete i. (CI)
Elschnig central i.
laser i.
i. operation
optic i.
optical i.
patent i.
peripheral i. (PI)
preliminary i.
preparatory i.
pupil-to-root i.
i. scissors
sector i.
stenopeic i.
superior sector i.
therapeutic i.
total i.
iridectopia
iridectropium
iridemia
iridencleisis
Holth i.
i. operation
iridentropium
irideremia
irides (*pl. of* iris)
iridescent
i. spot
i. vision
iridesis
iridiagnosis
iridial
i. angle
i. fold
i. muscle
iridic, iridian
iridica
stella lentis i.
iridis
angulus i.
atresia i.
coloboma i.
ectopia i.
ectropion i.
epithelium pigmentosum i.
facies anterior i.
facies posterior i.
granuloma i.
herpes i.
heterochromia i.

ligamentum pectinatum i.
margo ciliaris i.
margo pupillaris i.
melanosis i.
plicae i.
rubeosis i.
i. rubeosis
sinus circularis i.
spatia anguli i.
sphincter i.
vitiligo i.
xanthelasmatosis i.
xanthomatosis i.
iridization
iridoavulsion
iridocapsular intraocular lens
iridocapsulitis
iridocapsulotomy scissors
iridocele
iridochoroiditis
iridociliary
i. process contact
i. sulcus
iridocoloboma
iridoconstrictor
iridocorneal
i. angle
i. endothelial (ICE)
i. endothelial syndrome
i. mesodermal dysgenesis
i. synechia
i. touch
iridocornealis
angular i.
angulus i.
ligamentum pectinatum anguli i.
spatia anguli i.
iridocorneosclerectomy
iridocyclectomy
iridocyclitis
Fuchs heterochromic i.
granulomatous i.
herpes simplex i.
herpes zoster i.
heterochromic i.
hypertensive i.
i. masquerade syndrome
nongranulomatous i.
posttraumatic i.
i. septica
varicella i.

NOTES

iridocyclochoroidectomy
  Peyman i.
iridocyclochoroiditis
iridocycloretraction
iridocystectomy
iridodesis
iridodiagnosis
iridodialysis
  i. operation
  i. spatula
iridodiastasis
iridodilator
iridodonesis
iridoendothelial syndrome
iridogoniocyclectomy
iridogoniodysgenesis
iridokeratitis
iridokinesis, iridokinesia
iridokinetic
iridolenticular contact
iridoleptynsis
iridology
iridolysis
iridomalacia
iridomesodialysis
iridomotor
iridoncosis
iridoncus
iridoparalysis
iridopathy
iridoperiphakitis
iridoplasty
  argon laser peripheral i. (ALPI)
  laser i.
iridoplegia
  i. accommodation
  complete i.
  i. reflex
  sympathetic i.
iridoptosis
iridopupillary
iridorrhexis
iridoschisis
iridoschisma
iridosclerotomy
iridosteresis
iridotasis operation
iridotomy
  Abraham i.
  Castroviejo radial i.
  laser i. (LPI)
  i. lens
  i. operation
  prophylactic laser i.
  radial i.
  i. scissors
iridovitreosynechiae
iridozonular contact
I-Rinse

IRIS
  I. LIO500
  I. Medical OcuLight green laser system
  I. Medical OcuLight infrared laser system
  I. Medical OcuLight SLx
  I. OcuLight SLx indirect ophthalmoscope delivery system
  I. Oculight SLx MicroPulse laser
iris, pl. **irides**
  angle of i.
  i. architecture
  arterial circle of greater i.
  arterial circle of lesser i.
  i. atrophy
  i. bipolar forceps
  i. bombé
  i. capture
  i. chafing
  ciliary margin of i.
  circle of greater i.
  circle of lesser i.
  i. collarette
  i. coloboma
  coloboma of i.
  i. concavity
  congenital cleft of i.
  i. contraction reflex
  cosmetic i.
  i. crypt
  i. cyst
  i. dehiscence
  detached i.
  i. diameter
  i. diastasis
  i. dilator
  i. ectasia
  ectropion irides
  embryonal epithelial cyst of i.
  i. epithelial hyperplasia
  i. eye
  Florentine i.
  i. freckle
  i. frill
  greater ring of i.
  hernia of i.
  i. heterochromia
  heterochromia of i.
  i. hook
  i. hook cannula
  hydrops of i.
  i. incarceration
  ipsilateral i.
  ischemic necrosis of i.
  i. knife needle
  leiomyoma of i.
  lesser ring of i.
  major arterial circle of i.

malignant melanoma of the i.
i. melanoma
melanoma of i.
i. microscissors
neovascularization of the i. (NVI)
i. neovascularization
i. nervus
i. neurofibroma
i. nodule
notch of i.
i. pearl
pectinate ligament of i.
i. pigment dusting
pigmented epithelium of i.
pigmented layer of i.
i. pigment epithelium (IPE)
i. pit
plateau i.
i. process
i. prolapse
prolapse of i.
i. and pupil (I/P)
pupillae muscle of i.
pupillary margin of i.
i. repositor
i. retraction syndrome of Campbell
retroflexion of i.
i. ring
ring of i.
i. roll
i. root
i. scissors
shredded i.
i. spatula
i. sphincter
i. sphincter muscle
i. sphincter tear
i. strand
stroma of i.
i. stroma
i. support
i. suture
i. sweep
i. synechia
torn i.
transfixion of i.
i. transillumination defect (ITD)
tremulous i.
i. tuck
umbrella i.
iris-block glaucoma
iris-claw intraocular lens

Iriscorder
iris-fixated lens
iris-fixation technique
iris-lens diaphragm
iris-nevus syndrome
Iri-Sol
irisopsia
iris-supported lens
iritic
iritides
iritis
    i. blenorrhagique à rechutes
    i. catamenialis
    diabetic i.
    Doyne guttate i.
    fibrinous i.
    follicular i.
    i. glaucomatosa
    gouty i.
    hemorrhagic i.
    i. nodosa
    nodular i.
    nongranulomatous i.
    i. obturans
    i. papulosa
    plastic i.
    postoperative i.
    purulent i.
    quiet i.
    i. recidivans staphylococcal allergica
    i. roseata
    serous i.
    spongy i.
    sympathetic i.
    syphilitic i.
    tuberculous i.
    uratic i.
iritoectomy
iritomy
IRMA
    intraretinal microvascular abnormality
iron
    i. deposit
    i. deposition
    i. Fleischer ring
    i. line
    Pineda LASIK Flap I.
iron-ferry line
iron-Hudson-Stähli line
iron-leaking bleb
iron-Stocker line
irotomy

NOTES

irradiation
    i. cataract
    gamma i.
    heavy ion i.
    ^{90}Sr-plaque i.
irregular
    i. astigmatism
    i. nystagmus
    i. pupil
irregularity
    corneal i.
    flap i.
    surface i.
irreversible amblyopia
Irrigate eye wash
irrigating
    i. anterior chamber vectis
    i. C-hook extractor
    i. cortex extractor
    i. cystitome
    i. grasping forceps with curved shaft
    i. IOL positioner
    i. J-hook cannula
    i. pupil expander
    i. scissors with straight shaft
    i. solution
    i. vectis loop
irrigating/aspirating (I&A)
    i. cannula
    i. vectis
irrigation
    dilation and i. (D&I)
irrigation/aspiration (I/A)
    i. cannula
    i. system
    i. unit
irrigator
    anterior chamber i.
    Birch-Harman i.
    Bishop-Harman anterior chamber i.
    cul-de-sac i.
    DeVilbiss i.
    Dougherty i.
    Fink cul-de-sac i.
    Fox i.
    Gibson i.
    Hartstein i.
    LASIK flap i.
    olive-tip i.
    Randolph i.
    Sylva anterior chamber i.
    Vidaurri i.
irritation
    ocular i.
irritative
    i. hallucination
    i. miosis

IRVAN
    idiopathic retinal vasculitis, aneurysms and neuroretinitis
    IRVAN syndrome
Irvine
    I. irrigating/aspirating unit
    I. operation
    I. probe-pointed scissors
Irvine-Gass syndrome
Irving operation
ISA
    intraoperative suture adjustment
I-scan
ischemia
    carotid i.
    choroidal i.
    foveal i.
    limbal i.
    i. of optic nerve
    i. retinae
    retinal i.
    transient vertebrobasilar i.
ischemic
    i. atherosclerosis
    i. bleb
    i. chiasmal syndrome
    i. choroidal atrophy
    i. disk
    i. edema
    i. episode
    i. maculopathy
    i. necrosis
    i. necrosis of chorioid
    i. necrosis of ciliary body
    i. necrosis of iris
    i. ocular syndrome
    i. oculomotor palsy
    i. optic atrophy
    i. optic neuropathy (ION)
    i. papillitis
    i. papillopathy
    i. retina
    i. retinal whitening
    i. retinopathy
I-Scrub
iseikonia
iseikonic lens
isethionate
    dibromopropamidine i.
    hydroxystilbamidine i.
    pentamidine i.
    propamidine i.
Ishihara
    I. I-Temp cautery
    I. IV slit lamp
    I. pseudoisochromatic plate
    I. test
    I. test for color blindness

ISK
> immune stromal keratitis

island
> central i.
> isolated i.
> Traquair i.

Ismotic
isobutyl 2-cyanoacrylate
Isocaine
isochromatic plate
isocoria
isoflurophate
isoiconia
isoiconic lens
I-Sol
isolated
> i. fixed dilated pupil
> i. island
> i. oculomotor nerve dysfunction

isomerase
> retinal i.
> retinene i.

isomerization
isometropia
isophoria
isopia
isopropyl
> unoprostone i.

isopter
> nasal i.
> sloping i.

Isopto
> I. Atropine
> I. Carbachol
> I. Carbachol Ophthalmic
> I. Carpine
> I. Carpine Ophthalmic
> I. Cetamide
> I. Cetamide Ophthalmic
> I. Cetapred
> I. Cetapred ophthalmic
> I. Eserine
> I. Frin
> I. Homatropine
> I. Homatropine Ophthalmic
> I. Hyoscine
> I. Hyoscine Ophthalmic
> I. P-ES
> I. Plain
> I. Plain Solution
> I. Prednisolone
> I. Sterofrin

> I. Tears
> I. Tears Solution

isoscope
isosorbide
isothiocyanate
> fluorescein i.

isotonic solution
isotope scan
isotretinoin
ISPAN intraocular gas
israelii
> *Actinomyces i.*

I-Sulfacet
I-Sulfalone
itching
> ocular i.

ITD
> iris transillumination defect

I-tech
> I.-t. cannula
> I.-t. cannula holder
> I.-t. cannula tray
> I.-t. Castroviejo bladebreaker
> I.-t. intraocular foreign body forceps
> I.-t. needle holder
> I.-t. splinter forceps
> I.-t. tying forceps

item
> 25-I. Visual Function Questionnaire (VFQ-25)

I-Temp cautery
Ito procedure
itraconazole
I-Tropine
IV
> intravenous
> CR IV
> > trochlear nerve
> Madurai Intraocular Lens Study IV
> IV retinal fluorescein angiography
> IV slit lamp

Ivalon sponge implant
ivermectin
IVEX system
IVFA
> intravenous fluorescein angiography

IVH
> intraventricular hemorrhage

IVISC
IVISC+

NOTES

Iwanoff
   I. cyst
   I. retinal edema

I-Wash
I-White
Ixodes dammini

J

joule
  J loop
jack-in-the-box phenomenon
Jacko Low Vision Interaction
  Assessment (JLVIA)
Jackson
  J. cross cylinder
  J. lacrimal intubation set
Jacob
  J. capsule fragment forceps
  J. membrane
  J. ulcer
Jacobson
  J. hemostatic forceps
  J. retinitis
Jacob-Swann
  J.-S. gonioscope
  J.-S. gonioscopic prism
Jacoby
  border tissue of J.
Jacod-Negri syndrome
Jacod syndrome
Jacquart angle
Jadassohn
  nevus sebaceus of J.
Jadassohn-Lewandowsky syndrome
Jadassohn-type anetoderma
Jaeger
  J. acuity
  J. acuity card
  J. grading system
  J. hook
  J. keratome
  J. lid plate
  J. notation
  J. retractor
  J. test type
  J. visual test
Jaesche-Arlt operation
Jaesche operation
Jaffe
  J. capsulorrhexis forceps
  J. Cilco lens
  J. intraocular spatula
  J. iris hook
  J. laser blepharoplasty and facial
    resurfacing set
  J. lens-manipulating hook
  J. lens spatula
  J. lid retractor
  J. lid retractor set
  J. lid speculum
  J. microiris hook

  J. needle holder
  J. suturing forceps
Jaffe-Bechert nucleus rotator
Jaffe-Givner lid retractor
Jaffe/Maltzman IOL manipulator
Jahnke syndrome
Jaime lacrimal operation
Jamaican optic neuropathy
jamb
  sphenoid door j.
Jameson
  J. calipers
  J. muscle forceps
  J. muscle hook
  J. operation
Janelli clip
Jannetta procedure
Jansen-Middleton septotomy forceps
Jansky-Bielschowsky
  J.-B. disease
  J.-B. syndrome
Jardon eye shield
Jarisch-Herxheimer reaction
Jarrett side port manipulator
Javal
  J. keratometer
  J. ophthalmometer
  J. rule
Javal-Schiotz ophthalmometer
jaw
  end-gripping forceps with
    standard j.
  j. muscle pain
  j. winking
jaw-winking
  j.-w. phenomenon
  j.-w. syndrome
JCAHPO
  Joint Commission on Allied Health
  Personnel in Ophthalmology
JC virus
Jedmed A-scan
Jedmed/DGH A-scan
Jellinek sign
jelly bump
Jendrassik sign
Jenning test
Jensen
  J. capsule polisher cannula
  J. capsule scratcher
  J. choroiditis juxtapapillaris
  J. disease
  J. intraocular lens forceps
  J. jerk nystagmus
  J. juxtapapillary choroiditis

Jensen (*continued*)
  J. lens-inserting forceps
  J. operation
  J. polisher/scratcher
  J. retinitis
  J. transposition procedure
Jensen-Thomas irrigating/aspirating cannula
jequirity ophthalmia
jerk
  macro square-wave j.'s
  j. nystagmus
  quick adducting-retraction j.
  square-wave j.'s
Jervey
  J. capsule fragment forceps
  J. iris forceps
Jeune syndrome
jeweler's
  j. bipolar forceps
  j. tweezers
J-loop
  J.-l. PC lens
  J.-l. posterior chamber intraocular lens
JLVIA
  Jacko Low Vision Interaction Assessment
JNCL
  juvenile neuronal ceroid lipofuscinosis
JOAG
  juvenile open-angle glaucoma
Joal lens
Joffroy sign
John
  J. Green calipers
  J. Weiss forceps
Johnson
  J. double cannula
  J. erysiphake
  J. evisceration knife
  J. hydrodelineation cannula
  J. hydrodissection cannula
  J. operation
  J. syndrome
Johnson-Bell erysiphake
Johnson-Tooke corneal knife
Johnston
  J. axis marker and spatula
  J. fixation ring
  J. LASIK Flap Applanator
  J. LASIK spatula
Joint
  J. Commission on Allied Health Personnel in Ophthalmology (JCAHPO)
  J. Review Committee for Ophthalmic Medical Personnel (JRCOMP)

Jones
  J. dye test
  J. forceps
  J. I, II test
  J. keratome
  J. operation
  J. punctum dilator
  J. Pyrex tube
  J. repair
  J. tear duct tube
  J. towel clamp
  J. tube procedure
Jordan implant
Joseph
  J. device
  J. periosteal elevator
Josephberg probe
Joubert syndrome
joule (J)
Jr.
  Optelec Spectrum Jr.
JRCOMP
  Joint Review Committee for Ophthalmic Medical Personnel
J-shaped
  J.-s. irrigating/aspirating cannula
  J.-s. sella
JSM-54 IOLV microscope
JSM-6400 scanning electron microscope
Judd forceps
Judson-Smith manipulator
jump
  image j.
junction
  basal j.
  corneoscleral j.
  craniocervical j.
  host-graft j.
  mucocutaneous j.
  myoneural j.
  parietooccipital-temporal j.
  sclerocorneal j.
  scotoma j.
  j. scotoma
junctional
  j. bay
  j. nevus
  j. scotoma
  j. scotoma of Traquair
  j. zone
Jung-Schaffer intraocular lens
Just
  J. Tears
  J. Tears Solution
juvenile
  j. arcus
  j. corneal epithelial dystrophy
  j. developmental cataract
  j. diabetes

j. diabetes mellitus
j. glaucoma
j. iris xanthogranuloma
j. macular degeneration
j. melanoma
j. neuronal ceroid lipofuscinosis (JNCL)
j. nevoxanthoendothelioma
j. open-angle glaucoma (JOAG)
j. optic atrophy
j. pilocytic astrocytoma
j. reflex
j. systemic granulomatosis
j. xanthogranuloma (JXG)
j. X-linked retinoschisis (JXRS)
juvenile-onset high pressure glaucoma
juvenilis
angiopathia retinae j.
arcus j.
juxtacanicular

juxtafoveal
j. choroidal neovascularization
j. microaneurysm
juxtalimbal suture
juxtapapillaris
Jensen choroiditis j.
retinochoroiditis j.
juxtapapillary
j. endophytic capillary hemangioma
j. leakage
j. nerve fiber layer
j. perfusion
j. retina
juxtaposition
juxtapupillary choroiditis
juxtascleral injection
JXG
juvenile xanthogranuloma
JXRS
juvenile X-linked retinoschisis

NOTES

K

    corneal curvature
    kelvin
    phylloquinone
        K readings
        K Sol preservation solution

K-1

    Canon Auto Keratometer K-1

Kainair

Kaiser speculum

Kalt

    K. corneal needle
    K. forceps
    K. needle holder
    K. needle holder clamp
    K. spoon

Kamdar microscissors

Kamerling Capsular 90 lens

Kammann adjustable aspirating speculum

Kamppeter anomaloscope

kanamycin

Kandori

    flecked retina of K.

Kanizsa figure

Kansas fragment lens forceps

Kaplan-Meier estimation technique

Kaposi

    K. sarcoma
    xeroderma of K.

kappa

    k. angle
    K. SP lens finishing system

Kara

    K. cataract-aspirating cannula
    K. cataract needle
    K. erysiphake

Karakashian-Barraquer scissors

Karickhoff

    K. double cannula
    K. laser lens

Karl Ilg instrument

KARNS

    Krypton-Argon Regression of Neovascularization Study

Kasabach-Merritt syndrome

Katena

    K. boat hook
    K. capsulorrhexis forceps
    K. depth gauge
    K. double-edged sapphire blade
    K. iris spatula
    K. MicroFinger tip irrigating chopper
    K. product

    K. quick switch I/A system
    K. soft IOL cutter
    K. speculum
    K. trephine

katophoria

katotropia

Katzen flap unzipper

Katzin

    K. operation
    K. scissors
    K. trephine

Katzin-Barraquer forceps

Kaufman

    K. medium
    K. type II retractor
    K. type II vitrector
    K. vitreophage

Kaufman-Capella cryopreservation technique

Kawai capsulorrhexis forceps

Kawasaki disease

Kayser-Fleischer cornea ring

KCS

    keratoconjunctivitis sicca

Kearney

    K. side-notch IOL
    K. side-notch lens

Kearns-Sayre syndrome (KSS)

Keeler

    K. cryoextractor
    K. cryophake
    K. cryophake unit
    K. cryosurgical unit
    K. extended round tip forceps
    K. intraocular foreign body grasping forceps
    K. intravitreal scissors
    K. lancet tip
    K. micro round tip
    K. microscissors
    K. micro spear tip
    K. ophthalmoscope
    K. panoramic lens
    K. panoramic loupe
    K. pantoscope
    K. prism
    K. Pulsair tonometer
    K. puncture tip
    K. razor tip
    K. retinoscope
    K. retractable blade
    K. ruby knife
    K. specular microscope
    K. Tearscope
    K. triple facet tip

K

Keeler *(continued)*
    K. ultrasonic cataract removal
      lancet
Keeler-Amoils
    K.-A. curved cataract probe
    K.-A. freeze
    K.-A. glaucoma probe
    K.-A. long-shank retinal probe
    K.-A. microcurved cataract probe
    K.-A. Ophthalmic Cryosystem
    K.-A. ophthalmic curved cataract
      probe
    K.-A. ophthalmic long-shank probe
    K.-A. ophthalmic Machemer retinal
      probe
    K.-A. ophthalmic microcurved
      cataract probe
    K.-A. ophthalmic retinal probe
    K.-A. ophthalmic straight cataract
      probe
    K.-A. ophthalmic vitreous probe
    K.-A. straight cataract probe
Keeler-Catford
    K.-C. microjaws needle holder
    K.-C. needle holder with microjaws
Keeler-Fison tissue retractor
Keeler-Keislar lacrimal cannula
Keeler-Konan Specular microscope
Keeler-Meyer diamond knife
Keeler-Pierse eye speculum
Keeler-Rodger iris retractor
Keflex
Kehrer-Adie syndrome
Keith-Wagener (KW)
    K.-W. change
    K.-W. retinopathy
Keith-Wagener-Barker classification
Keizer-Lancaster
    K.-L. eye speculum
    K.-L. lid retractor
Kellan
    K. capsular sparing system
    K. hydrodissection
    K. sutureless incision blade
Kelly-Descemet membrane punch
Kelly hemostat
Kelman
    K. air cystitome
    K. aspirator
    K. cryoextractor
    K. cryophake
    K. cryosurgical unit
    K. cyclodialysis cannula
    K. flexible tripod lens
    K. iris retractor
    K. irrigating/aspirating unit
    K. irrigating handpiece
    K. knife
    K. Multiflex II lens

    K. Omnifit II intraocular lens
    K. operation
    K. PC 27LB CapSul lens
    K. phacoemulsification (KPE)
    K. phacoemulsification unit
    K. Quadriflex anterior chamber
      intraocular lens
    K. tip
Kelman-Cavitron
    K.-C. I/A unit
    K.-C. irrigating/aspirating unit
Kelman-Mackool flare tip
Kelman-McPherson
    K.-M. corneal forceps
    K.-M. lens-holding forceps
    K.-M. suturing forceps
    K.-M. tying forceps
kelvin (K)
Kenacort
Kenaject-40
Kenalog
Kenalog-10, -40
Kennedy syndrome
Kennerdell
    K. muscle hook
    K. nerve hook
Keracor laser
KeraCorneoScope
Keradiscs
Kerascan
keratalgia
keratan sulfate
keratectasia
keratectomy
    Castroviejo k.
    deep lamellar k.
    excimer laser photorefractive k.
    excimer laser phototherapeutic k.
    laser-assisted subepithelial k.
      (LASEK)
    laser-scrape photorefractive k.
    no-touch transepithelial
      photorefractive k.
    k. operation
    photoastigmatic refractive k.
      (PARK)
    photorefractive astigmatic k.
    phototherapeutic k. (PTK)
    k. scissors
    superficial lamellar k.
    surface photorefractive k.
    tracker-assisted photorefractive k.
      (T-PRK)
keratic precipitate (KP)
keratinization
    canthal k.
keratin layer
keratinoid degeneration
keratitic precipitate

keratitis
    Acanthamoeba k.
    acne rosacea k.
    actinic k.
    aerosol k.
    alphabet k.
    amebic k.
    ameboid k.
    anular k.
    arborescent k.
    artificial silk k.
    avascular k.
    bacterial k.
    band k.
    k. band
    k. bandelette
    band-shaped k.
    k. bullosa
    candidal k.
    catarrhal ulcerative k.
    chronic superficial k.
    classic dendritic k.
    Cogan interstitial k.
    confocal microscopy identification
      of *Acanthamoeba* k.
    contact lens-related microbial k.
    corneal k.
    Corynebacterium k.
    Cryptococcus laurentii k.
    deep punctate k.
    deep pustular k.
    dendriform k.
    dendrite k.
    dendritic herpes zoster k.
    desiccation k.
    diffuse deep k.
    diffuse lamellar k.
    Dimmer nummular k.
    disciform herpes simplex k.
    k. disciformis
    epithelial diffuse k.
    epithelial punctate k.
    exfoliative k.
    exposure k.
    farinaceous epithelial k.
    fascicular k.
    filament k.
    filamentary k. (FK)
    k. filamentosa
    Fuchs k.
    fungal k.
    furrow k.

    geographic k.
    gonococcal k.
    gram-positive bacterial k.
    herpes simplex k.
    herpes zoster k.
    herpetic fungal k.
    herpetic stromal k.
    HSV epithelial k.
    hypopyon k.
    immune stromal k. (ISK)
    infectious epithelial k.
    infiltrative k.
    interstitial k. (IK)
    lagophthalmic k.
    lamellar keratectomy for
      nontuberculous mycobacterial k.
    lattice k.
    k. lesion
    letter-shaped k.
    k. linearis migrans
    luetic interstitial k.
    Lyme disease k.
    Lymphogranuloma venereum k.
    marginal k.
    metaherpetic k.
    microbial k.
    mixed bacterial-fungal k.
    mixed fungal k.
    k. molluscum contagiosum
    Moraxella k.
    mumps k.
    Mycobacterium k.
    mycotic k.
    necrogranulomatous k.
    necrotizing interstitial k.
    necrotizing stromal k.
    necrotizing ulcerative k.
    neuroparalytic k.
    neurotrophic k.
    Nocardia k.
    non-*Acanthamoeba* amebic k.
    nontuberculous mycobacterial k.
    nonulcerative interstitial k.
    nummular k.
    k. nummularis
    onchocercal sclerosing k.
    oyster shuckers' k.
    paddy k.
    parenchymatous k.
    pediatric presumed microbial k.
    k. periodica fugax
    peripheral ulcerative k. (PUK)

K

NOTES

keratitis *(continued)*
 k. petrificans
 phlyctenular k.
 polymorphic superficial k.
 k. post vaccinulosa
 presumed microbial k.
 protozoan k.
 pseudodendritic k.
 k. punctata
 k. punctata leprosa
 k. punctata profunda
 k. punctata subepithelialis
 punctate epithelial k.
 purulent k.
 k. pustuliformis profunda
 pyknotic k.
 radiation k.
 k. ramificata superficialis
 reaper's k.
 red coral k.
 reticular k.
 ribbon-like k.
 ring k.
 k. rosacea
 rosacea k.
 rubeola k.
 sands of Sahara k.
 Schmidt k.
 sclerosing k.
 scrofulous k.
 secondary k.
 serpiginous k.
 k. sicca
 stellate k.
 striate k.
 stromal k.
 subepithelial k.
 superficial linear k.
 superficial punctate k. (SPK)
 suppurative k.
 syphilitic k.
 Thygeson superficial punctate k.
 trachomatous k.
 trophic k.
 tuberculous k.
 ulcerative k.
 k. urica
 k. vaccinia
 vaccinial k.
 varicella k.
 vascular k.
 vasculonebulous k.
 vesicular k.
 viral k.
 vulnificus k.
 xerotic k.
 zonular k.
keratitis-ichthyosis-deafness (KID)

keratoacanthoma
 eruptive k.
keratocele
keratocentesis operation
keratoconjunctivitis
 adenoviral k.
 allergic k.
 atopic eczema k.
 bilateral k.
 epidemic k. (EKC)
 epizootic k.
 flash k.
 granulomatous k.
 herpes follicular k.
 herpes simplex k.
 herpes zoster k.
 herpetic k.
 limbic vernal k.
 microsporidial k.
 phlyctenular k.
 shipyard k.
 k. sicca (KCS)
 staphylococcal allergic k.
 superior limbic k. (SLK)
 Theodore k.
 ultraviolet k.
 vernal k. (VKC)
 viral k.
 welder's k.
keratoconus
 anterior k.
 Collaborative Longitudinal
  Evaluation of K. (CLEK)
 k. contact lens
 k. cornea
 k. dystrophy
 k. fruste
 iatrogenic k.
 posterior k.
 Sato k.
keratocyte
keratoderma
 k. blennorrhagica
 Gomborg-Nielsen k.
 palmoplantar k.
 punctate k.
keratodermatocele
keratoectasia
keratoepithelin
keratoepitheliomileusis
keratoepitheliopathy
 diabetic k.
keratoepithelioplasty
keratoglobus cornea
Keratograph corneal topography system
keratographer
 Keravue k.

keratography
    lamellar stromal k.
    video k.
keratohelcosis
keratohemia
keratohyaline granule
keratoid
keratoiridocyclitis
keratoiridoscope
keratoiritis hypopyon
Kerato-Kontours instrument
keratokyphosis
keratolens implant
keratolenticuloplasty
keratoleptynsis
keratoleukoma
keratolimbal allograft (KLA)
Keratolux fixation device
keratolysis
keratoma, pl. **keratomas, keratomata**
    solar k.
keratomalacia
keratome
    Accutome black diamond clear
      cornea k.
    Agnew k.
    Bard-Parker k.
    Beaver k.
    Berens partial k.
    Castroviejo angled k.
    Castroviejo electro k.
    K. II Coherent-Schwind excimer
      laser
    Czermak k.
    Draeger modified k.
    K. excimer laser system
    Feather k.
    filamentary k.
    Fuchs lancet-type k.
    Grieshaber k.
    k. guard
    Guyton-Lundsgaard k.
    Hansen k.
    HydroBrush k.
    Insight K-3000 Automated K.
    Jaeger k.
    Jones k.
    Kirby k.
    Lancaster k.
    Martinez k.
    McReynolds k.
    Rowland k.

    SatinSlit k.
    Storz k.
    Tri-Beeled trapezoidal k.
    UltraShaper K.
    UniShaper K.
    Wiener k.
keratometer
    Bausch & Lomb manual k.
    Canon auto refraction k.
    Haag-Streit k.
    Helmholtz k.
    Javal k.
    manual k.
    Marco manual k.
    k. mires
    Osher surgical k.
    10 SL/O Zeiss k.
    Storz k.
    Terry k.
    Topcon k.
keratometric
    k. astigmatism
    k. flattening
    k. power (KP)
    k. readings
keratometry
    extended-range k.
    surgical k.
keratomileusis (KM)
    automated laser k. (ALK)
    autoshaped lamellar k.
    Barraquer k.
    bilateral simultaneous laser in
      situ k.
    epithelial laser-assisted
      intrastromal k. (E-LASIK)
    homoplastic k.
    hyperopic k.
    laser-assisted intrastromal k.
      (LASIK)
    laser-assisted in situ k.
    laser epithelial k. (LASEK)
    laser intrastromal k.
    laser in situ k. (LASIK)
    laser subepithelial k. (LASEK)
    myopic k. (MKM)
    k. operation
    topographically guided therapeutic
      laser in situ k.
keratomycosis
keratoneuritis
    pathognomonic radial k.

K

NOTES

keratonosis
keratonyxis
keratopathy
    aphakic bullous k. (ABK)
    band k.
    band-shaped k.
    Bietti k.
    bullous k.
    calcific band k.
    central striate k.
    chloroquine k.
    chronic actinic k.
    climatic droplet k.
    climatic proteoglycan stromal k.
    contact lens-induced k.
    crystalline k.
    dendritic k.
    discrete colliquative k.
    elastotic band k.
    epithelial infectious crystalline k.
    exposure k.
    filamentary k.
    fine punctate k.
    Fuchs aphakic k.
    HSV trophic k.
    hurricane k.
    idiopathic lipid k.
    indomethacin toxicity k.
    infectious crystalline k. (ICK)
    Labrador k.
    lamellar k.
    linear k.
    lipid k.
    Nama k.
    neuroparalytic k.
    neurotrophic k.
    pearl diver's k.
    phenothiazine k.
    plaque k.
    postinfectious epithelial k.
    pseudophakic bullous k. (PBK)
    punctate epithelial k. (PEK)
    spheroidal k.
    striate k.
    superficial punctate k.
    Thygeson superficial punctate k.
    trigeminal neuropathic k.
    trophic k.
    ultraviolet k.
    urate band k.
    uveitic band k.
    vesicular k.
    vortex k.
keratophakia
keratophakic keratoplasty
keratopigmentation
keratoplasty
    allopathic k.
    Arroyo k.

    Arruga k.
    autogenous k.
    autologous ipsilateral rotating
      penetrating k.
    automated lamellar therapeutic k.
      (ALTK)
    conductive k. (CK)
    deep lamellar endothelial k.
      (DLEK)
    Elschnig k.
    endothelial lamellar k. (ELK)
    epikeratophakic k.
    Filatov k.
    fluid lamellar k.
    full-thickness k.
    heterogenous k.
    homogenous k.
    homologous penetrating central
      limbo k.
    hyperopic automated lamellar k.
      (HALK)
    Imre k.
    keratophakic k.
    lamellar refractive k.
    laser thermal k. (LTK)
    layered k.
    manual lamellar k.
    Morax k.
    noncontact laser thermal k.
    nonpenetrating k.
    k. operation
    optic k.
    optical k.
    partial k.
    Paufique k.
    penetrating k. (PK, PKP)
    perforating k.
    photorefractive k. (PRK)
    posterior lamellar k.
    punctate epithelial k.
    refractive k.
    repeat penetrating k.
    k. scissors
    Sourdille k.
    superficial lamellar limbo k.
    surface lamellar k.
    tectonic k.
    thermal k. (TKP)
    total k.
keratoplasty-Excimer
    automated lamellar k.-E. (ALK-E)
keratoprosthesis
    Eckardt temporary k.
    Lander wide-field temporary k.
    PHEMA core-and-skirt k.
    temporary k. (TKP)
keratorefractive
    k. procedure
    k. surgery

keratorrhexis
keratorus
keratoscleritis
keratoscope
    Klein k.
    Polack k.
    wire-loop k.
keratoscopy
keratosis
    actinic k.
    eyelid k.
    k. follicularis
    k. follicularis spinulosa decalvans
    seborrheic k.
    senescent k.
    senile k.
    solar k.
keratostomy
keratotome
keratotomy
    Analysis of Radial K. (ARK)
    arcuate transverse k.
    astigmatic k. (AK)
    delimiting k.
    full-arc depth-dependent
      astigmatic k.
    hexagonal k.
    laser k.
    k. operation
    partial depth astigmatic k. (PDAK)
    Prospective Evaluation of
      Radial K. (PERK)
    radial k. (RK)
    refractive k.
    Ruiz trapezoidal k.
    trapezoidal k.
keratotorus
keratouveitis
    herpes simplex k.
    stromal k.
Keratron
    K. corneal topographer
    K. Scout topography system
    K. videokeratoscope
KeraVision
    K. Intac
    K. ring
Keravue keratographer
kerectasis
kerectomy
Kerlone Oral
Kermix antibody

keroid
kerotome
Kerrison
    K. forceps
    K. mastoid rongeur
Kershner
    K. butterfly capsulorrhexis forceps
    K. LASIK flap forceps
    K. LRI marker
    K. One-Step Micro capsulorrhexis
      forceps
    K. reversible eyelid speculum
Kestenbaum
    K. capillary count
    K. procedure
    K. rule
    K. sign
ketoconazole
ketorolac
    k. tromethamine
    k. tromethamine ophthalmic solution
ketosis-prone diabetes
ketosis-resistant diabetes
ketotifen
    k. fumarate
    k. fumarate ophthalmic solution
Keuch Pupil Dilator
Kevorkian-Younge forceps
keyhole
    k. bridge
    k. field
    lacrimal k.
    k. pupil
    k. vision
Key operation
Keystone view stereopsis test
Khodadoust line
Khosia cautery
Khouri Hydrodissection Cannula
kibisitome cystitome
KID
    keratitis-ichthyosis-deafness
      KID syndrome
Kids, Computers & Vision brochure
Kikuchi-Fujimoto disease
killer cell
Kiloh-Nevin syndrome
Kilp lens
Kimmelstiel-Wilson
    K.-W. disease
    K.-W. syndrome
Kimura platinum spatula

K

NOTES

kindergarten eye chart
kinematogram
    random-dot k.
kinematography
    random-dot k.
kinescope
kinetic
    k. echography
    k. perimeter
    k. perimetry
    k. strabismus
    k. ultrasound
    k. visual field testing
King
    K. clamp
    K. corneal trephine
    K. Khaled Eye Specialist Hospital (KKESH)
    K. operation
    K. orbital implant
kingae
    Cardiobacterium hominis, Eikenella corrodens and *Kingella k. Kingella k.*
Kingella kingae
King-Prince
    K.-P. knife
    K.-P. muscle forceps
Kirby
    K. angulated iris spatula
    K. capsule forceps
    K. cataract knife
    K. corneoscleral forceps
    K. cylindrical zonal separator
    K. flat zonal separator
    K. hook expressor
    K. intracapsular lens expressor
    K. intracapsular lens loupe
    K. intracapsular lens spoon
    K. intraocular lens loupe
    K. intraocular lens scoop
    K. iris forceps
    K. keratome
    K. lens
    K. lens dislocator
    K. lid retractor
    K. muscle hook
    K. operation
    K. refractor
    K. scissors
    K. tissue forceps
Kirby-Bauer
    K.-B. disk-diffusion method
    K.-B. disk sensitivity test
Kirisawa uveitis
Kirschner wire
Kirsch test
Kishi lens
kissing suprachoroidal hemorrhage

kit
    Bergland-Warshawski phaco/cortex k.
    IC-Green k.
    Lacrimedics occlusion starter k.
    Lobob GP Starter K.
    Massachusetts Vision K. (MVK)
    Optimum rigid gas permeable starter k.
    Refrax corneal repair k.
    Shearing cortex suction k.
    sterile indocyanine green k.
    Tearscope Plus tear film k.
Kjer
    K. disease
    K. dominant optic atrophy
KKESH
    King Khaled Eye Specialist Hospital
KLA
    keratolimbal allograft
Klebsiella
    K. oxytoca
    K. pneumoniae
***Klebsiella* endophthalmitis**
Kleen
    Velva K.
Klein
    K. curved cannula
    K. keratoscope
    K. punch
Klein-Tolentino ring
Klieg eye
Klippel-Feil anomaly
Kloepfer syndrome
Kloti vitreous cutter
Klumpke paralysis
Klyce/Wilson scale
KM
    keratomileusis
Knapp
    K. blade
    K. cataract knife
    K. eye speculum
    K. forceps
    K. iris hook
    K. iris probe
    K. iris repositor
    K. iris scissors
    K. iris spatula
    K. knife needle
    K. lacrimal sac retractor
    K. law
    K. lens loop
    K. lens spoon
    K. operation
    K. procedure
    K. refractor
    K. rule
    K. scoop

K. strabismus scissors
K. streak
K. stria
Knapp-Culler speculum
Knapp-Imre operation
Knapp-Wheeler-Reese operation
Knies sign
knife, pl. **knives**
  Accutome LRI diamond k.
  Accutome side-port diamond k.
  Agnew canaliculus k.
  Alcon A-OK crescent k.
  Alcon A-OK ShortCut k.
  Alcon A-OK slit k.
  ASICO multiangled diamond k.
  Bard-Parker k.
  Barkan goniotomy k.
  Barraquer keratoplasty k.
  Beard k.
  Beaver goniotomy needle k.
  Beaver Xstar k.
  Beer canaliculus k.
  Beer cataract k.
  Berens cataract k.
  Berens glaucoma k.
  Berens keratoplasty k.
  Berens ptosis k.
  Bishop-Harman k.
  blade k.
  bladebreaker k.
  BRVO k.
  52.00 BRVO k.
  Castroviejo discission k.
  Castroviejo twin k.
  cataract k.
  Celita elite k.
  Celita sapphire k.
  central retinal vein occlusion k.
  clear cornea angled CVD
    diamond k.
  ClearCut dual-bevel line k.
  ClearCut SatinSlit k.
  Clearpath corneal diamond k.
  corneal k.
  crescent CVD diamond k.
  CRVO k.
  52.20 CRVO k.
  Cusick goniotomy k.
  CVD diamond k.
  Dean iris k.
  Desmarres k.
  Deutschman cataract k.

  Diamatrix trapezoidal diamond k.
  diamond blade k.
  diamond-dusted k.
  diamond laser k.
  diamond phaco k.
  Diamontek k.
  discission k.
  dissector k.
  DORC illuminated diamond k.
  3D stainless steel k.
  Duredge k.
  EdgeAhead crescent k.
  EdgeAhead microsurgical k.
  EdgeAhead phaco slit k.
  Elschnig cataract k.
  Elschnig corneal k.
  Elschnig pterygium k.
  Feaster Accura diamond k.
  Feaster radial keratotomy k.
  Feather clear cornea k.
  Foucault k.
  Gill corneal k.
  Gill-Fine corneal k.
  Gill-Hess k.
  Gills pop-up arcuate diamond k.
  Gills-Welsh k.
  Goldmann serrated k.
  goniopuncture k.
  goniotomy k.
  Graefe cataract k.
  Graefe cystitome k.
  Green cataract k.
  Green corneal k.
  Grieshaber ruby k.
  Grieshaber ultrasharp k.
  k. guard
  Guyton-Lundsgaard cataract k.
  Haab scleral resection k.
  House myringotomy k.
  Huco diamond k.
  Impex diamond radial
    keratotomy k.
  Johnson evisceration k.
  Johnson-Tooke corneal k.
  Keeler-Meyer diamond k.
  Keeler ruby k.
  Kelman k.
  King-Prince k.
  Kirby cataract k.
  Knapp cataract k.
  KOI diamond k.
  Lancaster k.

K

NOTES

knife *(continued)*
  Laseredge microsurgical k.
  Lowell glaucoma k.
  Lundsgaard k.
  Martinez k.
  Maumenee goniotomy k.
  McPherson-Wheeler k.
  McPherson-Ziegler k.
  McReynolds pterygium k.
  Meyer Swiss diamond lancet k.
  Meyer Swiss diamond mini-angled k.
  Meyer Swiss diamond wedge k.
  micrometer k.
  microsurgical k.
  Multi-System incision k.
  Myocure k.
  One-Step limbal relaxing incision diamond k.
  One-Step LRI diamond k.
  Optima diamond k.
  Parker discission k.
  Paton corneal k.
  Paufique graft k.
  Paufique keratoplasty k.
  Phaco-4 diamond step k.
  preset diamond k.
  ptosis k.
  pulsed electron avalanche k. (PEAK)
  Quantum enhancement k.
  radial keratotomy k.
  razor blade k.
  Reese ptosis k.
  Rhein Advantage II diamond limbal-relaxing incision k.
  Rhein clear corneal diamond k.
  Rhein 3-D angled trapezoid diamond k.
  Rizzuti-Spizziri cannula k.
  ruby diamond k.
  sapphire k.
  SatinCrescent implant k.
  SatinShortCut implant k.
  SatinSlit implant k.
  Sato corneal k.
  scarifier k.
  Scheie goniopuncture k.
  Scheie goniotomy k.
  scleral resection k.
  self-fixating sideport diamond k.
  Sharpoint microsurgical k.
  Sharpoint slit k.
  ShortCut A-OK small-incision k.
  Shorti LRI diamond k.
  Sichel k.
  side-port fixation k.
  slit blade k.
  Smith k.
  Smith-Fisher k.
  Smith-Green cataract k.
  Spizziri cannula k.
  spoon k.
  Stealth DBO free-hand diamond k.
  Step-Knife diamond blade k.
  stiletto k.
  stitch-removing k.
  Storz cataract k.
  Storz-Duredge steel cataract k.
  Swan discission k.
  swift-cut phaco incision k.
  Thornton triple micrometer k.
  Tooke corneal k.
  Tooke cornea-splitting k.
  Tooke-Johnson corneal k.
  trapezoid angled CVD diamond k.
  Troutman corneal k.
  Troutman-Tooke corneal k.
  Unicat diamond k.
  Universal Pathfinder k.
  V-lancet k.
  von Graefe cataract k.
  Wallace-Maloney fixation diamond k.
  wave-edge k.
  Weber k.
  Weck k.
  Wheeler discission k.
  Wilder cystitome k.
  Zaldivar k.
  ZAP diamond k.
  Ziegler k.
knife/dissector
  Morlet lamellar k.
knife-edged lens
knife-needle
knives (*pl. of* knife)
Knolle
  K. anterior chamber irrigating cannula
  K. capsule polisher
  K. capsule scraper
  K. capsule scratcher
  K. lens cortex spatula
  K. lens nucleus spatula
  K. lens speculum
Knolle-Kelman cannulated cystitome
Knolle-Pearce irrigating lens loop
Knolle-Shepard lens-holding forceps
Knolle-Volker lens-holding forceps
Knoll refraction technique
knot
  bow-tie k.
  cowhitch k.
  partial throw surgeon's k.
  Tripier operation throw square k.

knuckle
    k. of choroid
    k. of loose vitreous
Knudson hypothesis
Koby
    K. cataract
    K. cataract forceps
    superficial reticular degeneration
      of K.
Koch
    K. chopper
    K. LRI marker
    K. nucleus hydrolysis
    K. nucleus manipulator
    K. phaco manipulator
Kocher sign
Koch-Minami chopper
Koch-Salz nucleus splitter
Koch-Weeks
    K.-W. bacillus
    K.-W. conjunctivitis
Kodak Surecell Chlamydia test
Koebner phenomenon
Koeller illumination system
Koenen tumor
Koeppe
    K. diagnostic lens
    K. disease
    K. goniolens
    K. gonioscopic implant
    K. gonioscopy
    K. nodule
    K. syndrome
Koerber-Salus-Elschnig syndrome
Koffler operation
KOH
    potassium hydroxide
    KOH smear
Köhler illumination
KOI diamond knife
Kollmorgen element
Kollner
    K. law
    K. rule
Kolmer crystalloid structure
Kolmogorov-Smirnov test
Konan
    K. fixed-frame method
    K. Noncon ROBO-CA SP-8000
      noncontact specular microscope
    K. Sp-5500 contact specular
      microscope

    K. SP8000 noncontact specular
      microscope
Konig bar chart
Konoto tetrad
Koo foldable IOL cutter
Kooijman eye model
Koplik stigma
Korb contact lens
Kornmehl
    K. LASIK system
    K. press
koroscope
koroscopy
Kowa
    K. fluorescein system
    K. FM-500
    K. FM-500 laser flare meter
    K. fundus
    K. hand-held slit lamp
    K. laser flare-cell photometer
    K. laser flare photometer
    K. Optimed slit lamp
    K. PRO II retinal camera
    K. RC-XV fundus camera
Koyter muscle
Kozlowski degeneration
KP
    keratic precipitate
    keratometric power
KPE
    Kelman phacoemulsification
K-plus
    Retinomax K-p. 2
KR-8000PA SUPRA
  autokeratorefractometer
Krabbe disease
Kraff
    K. capsule polisher
    K. capsule polisher curette
    K. cortex cannula
    K. fixation forceps
    K. hyperopic fixation ring
    K. intraocular utility forceps
    K. lens-holding forceps
    K. lens-inserting forceps
    K. LRI marker
    K. nucleus lens loupe
    K. nucleus splitter
    K. suturing forceps
    K. tying forceps
Kraff-Utrata
    K.-U. capsulorrhexis

K

NOTES

Kraff-Utrata *(continued)*
    K.-U. capsulorrhexis forceps
    K.-U. intraocular utility forceps
Kraft forceps
Krahn exophthalmometry
Krakau tonometer
Kramp scissors
Krasnov lens
Kratz
    K. angled cystitome
    K. aspirating speculum
    K. capsule polisher
    K. capsule scraper
    K. capsule scratcher
    K. diamond-dusted needle
    K. elliptical-style lens
    K. K push-pull iris hook
    K. lens-inserting forceps
    K. lens needle
    K. polisher/scratcher
    K. posterior chamber intraocular lens
    K. "soft" J-loop intraocular lens
Kratz-Barraquer wire eye speculum
Kratz-Jensen
    K.-J. polisher/scratcher
    K.-J. scratcher
Kratz-Johnson lens
Kratz-Sinskey
    K.-S. intraocular lens
    K.-S. loop configuration
Kraupa operation
Krause
    K. lacrimal gland
    K. syndrome
    transverse suture of K.
    K. valve
K-reading
Kreibig operation
Kreiger-Spitznas vibrating scissors
Kreiker
    K. blepharochalasis
    K. operation
Kremer
    K. corneal fixation forceps
    K. excimer laser
    K. two-point fixation forceps
Krieberg operation
Krieger wide-field fundus lens
Krill
    K. disease
    K. disk
Krimsky
    K. measurement
    K. method
    K. prism test
Krimsky-Prince accommodation rule
Kronfeld
    K. electrode

    K. refractor
    K. retractor
    K. suturing forceps
Krönlein
    K. operation
    K. procedure
Krönlein-Berke operation
KR 7000-P cycloplegic refractor
Krukenberg
    K. corneal spindle
    K. pigment spindle
    K. pigment spindle forceps
    K. sponge
Krumeich-Barraquer
    K.-B. lasitome
    K.-B. microkeratome
Krupin
    K. device
    K. eye disk
    K. implant
    K. valve
Krupin-Denver
    K.-D. long-valve implant
    K.-D. valve
krusei
    Candida k.
Kruskal-Wallis test
Krwawicz cataract extractor
Krymed Cryopexy unit
Kryptok
    K. bifocal
    K. implant
    K. lens
krypton
    k. photocoagulation
    k. red laser
Krypton-Argon Regression of Neovascularization Study (KARNS)
K-Sol medium
K-Sponge II
KSS
    Kearns-Sayre syndrome
K-tome microkeratome
Kufs syndrome
Kuglein
    K. irrigating lens manipulator
    K. push/pull
    K. refractor
    K. retractor
Kuglen
    K. lens manipulator
    K. manipulating hook
    K. nucleus manipulator
Kuhnt
    K. corneal scarifier
    K. dacryostomy
    K. eyelid operation
    K. fixation forceps
    K. illusion

K. meniscus
K. postcentral vein
K. space
K. tarsectomy
Kuhnt-Helmbold operation
Kuhnt-Junius
   K.-J. disease
   K.-J. macular degeneration
   K.-J. maculopathy
   K.-J. repair
Kuhnt-Szymanowski
   K.-S. operation
   K.-S. procedure
Kuhnt-Thorpe operation
Kuler panoramic lens
Kulvin-Kalt forceps

Kuppuswamy scale
Kurova Shursite lens series
Kurtzke Expanded Disability Status Scale
Kveim
   K. antigen
   K. test
KW
  Keith-Wagener
  KW change
KWB classification
Kwitko
   K. conjunctival spreader
   K. operation
Kynex
Kyrle disease

K

NOTES

LA
Dexone L.
L&A
light and accommodation
L.A.
Dexasone L.A.
Solurex L.A.
labeling
in situ DNA nick end l.
terminal deoxynucleotidyl
transferase-mediated dUTP-
digoxigenin nick-end l. (TUNEL)
Labrador keratopathy
Labtician oval sleeve
labyrinthine nystagmus
LaCarrere operation
lacerate
l. anterior foramen
l. middle foramen
l. posterior foramen
laceration
canalicular l.
central stellate l.
complex l.
conjunctival l.
corneal l.
corneoscleral l.
eyebrow l.
full-thickness corneal l.
lid margin l.
partial-thickness corneal l.
tarsal l.
lacertus musculi recti lateralis bulbi
lachrymal (*var. of* lacrimal)
lacquer crack
Lacramore
LacriCATH lacrimal duct catheter
Lacrigel
Lacril Ophthalmic Solution
Lacri-Lube
L.-L. NP
L.-L. SOP
lacrimal, lachrymal
l. abscess
l. acinar lobule
l. angle duct anomaly
l. anterior crest
l. apparatus
l. artery
l. awl
l. balloon catheter
l. bay
l. calculus
l. canal
l. canaliculus

l. caruncle
l. caruncula
l. conjunctivitis
l. dilator
l. drainage
l. duct
l. ductal cyst
l. duct anlage
duct T-tube l.
l. duct T-tube
l. fistula
l. fold
l. fornix
l. gland
l. gland acinus
l. gland cyst
l. gland epithelial tumor
l. gland fossa
l. gland gallium uptake
l. gland repair
l. groove
l. incisure
l. intubation
l. intubation probe
l. irrigating cannula
l. irrigation test
l. keyhole
l. lake
l. lens
l. nerve
l. notch
l. nucleus aplasia
l. osteotome
l. outflow
l. papilla
l. point
l. posterior crest
l. power
l. probing
l. process
l. pump failure
l. punctal stenosis
l. punctum
l. reflex
l. sac
l. sac bur
l. sac chisel
l. sac diverticulum
l. sac fossa
l. sac gouge
l. sac hemangiopericytoma
l. sac retractor
l. sac rongeur
l. scintillography
l. sound

L

lacrimal *(continued)*
    l. stent
    l. sulcus
    l. sulcus of lacrimal bone
    l. sulcus of maxilla
    l. surgery
    l. syringe
    l. system
    l. testing
    l. transit time
    l. trephine
    l. tubercle
    l. vein
lacrimale
    os l.
    punctum l.
lacrimales
    ductus l.
lacrimalis
    ampulla canaliculi l.
    ampulla ductus l.
    apparatus l.
    avulsion of caruncula l.
    canaliculus l.
    caruncula l.
    fistula l.
    fornix sacci l.
    Förster sacci l.
    fossa glandulae l.
    fossa sacci l.
    glandula l.
    hamulus l.
    incisura l.
    lacus l.
    nervus l.
    pars orbitalis glandulae l.
    pars palpebralis glandulae l.
    plica l.
    rivus l.
    sacculus l.
    saccus l.
    vena l.
lacrimarum
    stillicidium l.
lacrimation
    l. disorder
    excessive l.
    gustatory l.
    l. reflex
lacrimator
lacrimatory
Lacrimedics occlusion starter kit
lacrimo-auriculo-dento-digital syndrome
lacrimoconchalis
    sutura l.
lacrimoconchal suture
lacrimoethmoidal suture
lacrimomaxillaris
    sutura l.

lacrimomaxillary suture
lacrimonasal duct
lacrimotome
lacrimotomy
lacrimoturbinal suture
Lacrisert
Lacrivial
Lacrivisc unit dose
Lacrytest strips
lactate
    ammonium l.
    l. dehydrogenase
    Squalamine l.
lacteal cataract
lactoferrin test
Lactoplate
lacuna, pl. lacunae
    Blessig l.
    vitreous l.
lacunata
    Moraxella l.
lacus lacrimalis
LADARTracker Closed-Loop Tracking System
LADARVision
    L. excimer laser system
    L. Platform
LADARWave CustomCornea Wavefront System
Ladd-Franklin theory
LaForce knife spud
lag
    adduction l.
    dilation l.
    lid l.
Lagleyze
    L. needle
    L. operation
Lagleyze-Trantas operation
lagophthalmia, lagophthalmos, lagophthalmus
    blink out l.
    l. conjunctivitis
    nocturnal l.
    spastic l.
lagophthalmic keratitis
Lagrange
    L. operation
    L. sclerectomy scissors
    L. test
Laird spatula
laissez-faire lid operation
lake
    lacrimal l.
    tear l.
LAL
    laser-adjustable lens
Lalonde hook forceps

LAM-B
  lipoarabinomannan-B
lambda
  l. angle
  L. phacoemulsification technique
  L. Physik EMG 103 laser
lambert
  L. chalazion forceps
  foot l.
  L. hook forceps
Lambert-Eaton myasthenic syndrome
Lambert-Heiman scissors
lamella, pl. **lamellae**
  collagen l.
  corneal l.
  corneoscleral l.
  l. of Fuchs
  interlacing of collagen lamellae
  Rabl l.
lamellar
  l. calcification
  l. channel
  l. corneal graft
  l. corneal transplant
  l. developmental cataract
  l. groove
  l. haptic
  l. hole
  l. keratectomy for nontuberculous
   mycobacterial keratitis
  l. keratopathy
  l. patch graft
  l. refractive keratoplasty
  l. separation of lens
  l. stromal keratography
  l. zonular perinuclear cataract
lamellation
lamina, pl. **laminae**
  anterior limiting l.
  basal l.
  basalis choroideae l.
  basalis corporis ciliaris l.
  Bowman l.
  l. choriocapillaris
  l. choroidocapillaris
  l. cribrosa
  l. cribrosa sclerae
  l. densa
  l. dot
  l. elastica anterior
  l. elastica posterior
  episcleral l.

  l. fusca
  l. fusca sclerae
  l. limitans anterior corneae
  l. limitans posterior corneae
  limiting l.
  l. lucida
  orbital l.
  l. orbitalis ossis ethmoidalis
  l. papyracea
  posterior limiting l.
  l. superficialis musculi
  suprachoroid l.
  l. suprachoroidea
  l. vasculosa choroideae
  l. vitrea
  vitreal l.
  vitreous l.
laminar flow
laminated
  l. acellular mass
  l. spectacle lens
laminin
laminin-P1
  serum l.-P1
lamp
  Bausch-Lomb-Thorpe slit l.
  biomicroscope slit l.
  Birch l.
  Birch-Hirschfeld l.
  Burton l.
  Campbell slit l.
  Canon RO-4000 slit l.
  Canon RO-5000 slit l.
  carbon arc l.
  Coburn-Rodenstock slit l.
  Coherent LaserLink slit l.
  Duke-Elder l.
  Eldridge-Green l.
  fluorescent l.
  gas discharge l.
  Gullstrand slit l.
  Haag-Streit Biomicroscope 900
   slit l.
  Hague cataract l.
  Heine HSL 100 hand-held slit l.
  incandescent l.
  infrared slit l.
  Ishihara IV slit l.
  IV slit l.
  Kowa hand-held slit l.
  Kowa Optimed slit l.
  Marco slit l.

NOTES

lamp *(continued)*
    Nikon zoom photo slit l.
    Nitra l.
    Posner slit l.
    Reichert slit l.
    Rodenstock slit l.
    Specular reflex slit l.
    Thorpe slit l.
    Topcon SL-7E photo slip l.
    Topcon SL-E Series slit l.
    Topcon SL-1E slit l.
    tungsten-halogen l.
    Universal slit l.
    VG slit l.
    V-slit l.
    Wood l.
    Zeiss carbon arc slit l.
    Zeiss-Comberg slit l.

Lancaster
    L. Cross
    L. eye magnet
    L. eye speculum
    L. keratome
    L. knife
    L. lid speculum
    L. operation
    L. red-green projector
    L. red-green test
    L. screen test

Lancaster-O'Connor speculum
Lancaster-Regan
    L.-R. dial 1, 2 chart
    L.-R. test

lance
    Rolf l.

Lancereaux diabetes
lancet
    Keeler ultrasonic cataract
      removal l.
    Meyer Swiss diamond knife l.
    suture l.
    l. suture
    Swan l.
    ultrasonic cataract-removal l.

Lanchner operation
lancing pain
Landegger orbital implant
Landers
    L. biconcave lens
    L. contact lens
    L. irrigating vitrectomy ring
    L. sew-on lens
    L. subretinal aspiration cannula
    L. vitrectomy ring

Landers-Foulks temporary
  keratoprosthesis lens
Lander wide-field temporary
  keratoprosthesis

Landolt
    L. body
    L. broken ring
    L. broken-ring chart
    L. broken-ring test
    L. operation

Landolt-C
    L.-C. acuity chart
    L.-C. ring
    L.-C. test

Landry ascending paralysis
Landström muscle
Lane needle
Lang
    L. speculum
    L. stereo test
    L. stereotest

Lange
    L. blade
    L. fold

Langenbeck operation
Langer-Giedion trichorhinophalangeal
  syndrome
Langerhans granule
Langerman
    L. bi-directional phaco chopper
    L. diamond knife system

lanolin
lantern test
LaPlace law
Laqua black line retinal hook
Larcher sign
Largactil
large
    l. kappa angle
    l. physiologic cup
    l. pupil diameter

large-angled forceps
large-cell lymphoma
Larsen syndrome
larva, pl. **larvae**
    ocular l.

larval conjunctivitis
laryngeal and ocular granulation tissue
  in children from the Indian
  subcontinent (LOGIC)
Lasag
    L. Micropter II laser
    L. Microruptor

Laschal precision suture tome
lase
LASEK
    laser-assisted subepithelial keratectomy
    laser epithelial keratomileusis
    laser subepithelial keratomileusis
    LASEK alcohol well
    LASEK alcohol well and epithelial
      trephine
    LASEK bow dissector

LASEK epithelial detaching spatula
LASEK epithelial flap repositioning
spatula
LASEK epithelial micro hoe

laser

l. activity
Aesculap argon ophthalmic l.
Aesculap excimer l.
Aesculap-Meditec excimer l.
Allergan Humphrey l.
AMO YAG 100 l.
Apex Plus excimer l.
ArF excimer l.
argon blue l.
argon-fluoride excimer l.
argon green l.
argon-pumped tunable dye l.
Atlas-Elite l.
Atlas ophthalmic l.
Autonomous Technologies l.
l. biomicroscopy
Biophysic Medical YAG l.
blue-green argon l.
Britt argon/krypton l.
Britt argon pulsed l.
Britt BL-12 l.
Britt krypton l.
l. burn
l. burst
candela l.
carbon dioxide l.
Cardona l.
Carl Zeiss YAG l.
l. cavity
l. cell and flare meter (LCFM)
Cilco argon l.
Cilco Frigitronics l.
Cilco Hoffer Laseridge l.
Cilco krypton l.
Cilco/Lasertek A/K l.
Cilco/Lasertek argon l.
Cilco/Lasertek krypton l.
Cilco YAG l.
Coherent 7910 l.
Coherent 900, 920 argon l.
Coherent 920 argon/dye l.
Coherent dye l.
Coherent EPIC l.
Coherent krypton l.
Coherent Medical YAG l.
Coherent Novus Omni
multiwavelength l.

Coherent radiation argon/krypton l.
Coherent radiation argon model
800 l.
Coherent Schwind Keraton 2 l.
Coherent Selecta 7000 l.
confocal scanning l. (CSL)
continuous l.
continuous-wave argon l.
continuous-wave diode l.
Cool Touch l.
Cooper 2000, 2500 l.
Cooper Laser Sonics l.
CooperVision argon l.
CooperVision YAG l.
CO_2 Sharplan l.
l. cyclotherapy
Derma-K l.
diode l.
l. Doppler flowmeter
l. Doppler signal
l. Doppler velocimeter
l. Doppler velocimetry
dye yellow l.
EC-5000 excimer l.
Epic l.
l. epithelial keratomileusis (LASEK)
l. equipment
erbium l.
Er:YAG l.
Evergreen Lasertek l.
ExciMed UV200 excimer l.
ExciMed UV200LA l.
excimer l.
excimer l., 193193-nm
Feather Touch CO_2 l.
l. flare-cell meter
l. flare-cell photometry
l. flare photometry
flashlamp-pumped microsecond
pulse-dye l.
GentleLASE l.
Gish micro YAG l.
green l.
helium-ion aiming l.
helium-neon aiming l.
HeNe l.
HGM argon green l.
HGM intravitreal l.
HGM ophthalmic l.
holmium l.
Ho:YAG l.
l. interferometry

L

NOTES

laser *(continued)*

intrastromal l.
l. intrastromal keratomileusis
ion l.
l. iridectomy
l. iridoplasty
l. iridotomy (LPI)
IRIS Oculight SLx MicroPulse l.
Keracor l.
Keratome II Coherent-Schwind
  excimer l.
l. keratotomy
Kremer excimer l.
krypton red l.
Lambda Physik EMG 103 l.
Lasag Micropter II l.
Laserex Era 4106 YAG l.
LaserHarmonic l.
laser interferometer l.
Lasertek l.
Lazex excimer l.
l. lens
l. light imaging
liquid organic dye l.
LPK-80 II argon l.
Lumonics l.
l. manipulation
MC-7000 multi-wavelength l.
MC-7000 ophthalmic l.
Meditec MEL-60 excimer l.
MEL 60. 80 excimer l.
MEL 70 flying spot l.
MEL 60 scanning l.
Merrimac l.
Microlase transpupillary diode l.
MicroProbe ophthalmic l.
mode-locked Nd:YAG l.
molectron l.
Nanolas Nd:YAG l.
Nd:YAG l.
Nd:YLF l.
neodymium:YAG l.
neodymium:yttrium aluminum
  garnet l. (Nd:YAG)
neodymium:yttrium lithium
  fluoride l. (Nd:YLF)
neodymium:yttrium-lithium-fluoride
  photodisruptive l.
Nidek EC-1000 excimer l.
Nidek Laser System l.
193-nm excimer l.
OcuLight SL diode l.
OcuLight SLx ophthalmic l.
oculocutaneous l.
OmniMed argon-fluoride excimer l.
Ophthalas argon l.
Ophthalas argon/krypton l.
Ophthalas krypton l.
Opmilas 144 surgical l.

l. optometer
orange dye l.
l. panretinal photocoagulation
PC EDO ophthalmic office l.
l. photocoagulator
photodisrupting l.
Photon l.
PhotoPoint l.
photovaporation l.
photovaporizing l.
Prima KTP/532 l.
Pulsion FS L.
Q-switched Er:YAG l.
Q-switched Nd:YAG l.
Q-switched neodymium:YAG l.
Q-switched ruby l.
l. refractometry
l. reversal of presbyopia
l. ridge
ruby l.
scanning excimer l.
Sharplan argon l.
l. in situ keratomileusis (LASIK)
l. speckle flowgraphy
Star excimer l.
l. subepithelial keratomileusis
  (LASEK)
Summit Apex Plus excimer l.
Summit OmniMed excimer l.
Summit SVS Apex l.
Summit UV 200 Excimed l.
l. surgery
Takata l.
Technolas 217 excimer l.
TEMOO mode beam l.
THC:YAG l.
l. therapy
l. thermal keratoplasty (LTK)
l. thermokeratoplasty
l. tomography scanner (LTS)
T-PRK l.
l. trabeculoplasty
tracker-assisted PRK l.
transpupillary l.
l. transscleral cyclophotocoagulation
l. tube
tunable dye l.
twenty/twenty argon-fluoride
  excimer l.
UltraPulse l.
URAM E2 compact MicroProbe l.
Veinlaser Captured-Pulse l.
Visulas 532 l.
Visulas argon C l.
Visulas argon/YAG l.
Visulas Combi 532/YAG l.
Visulas Nd:YAG l.
Visulas 690s PDT l.
Visulas YAG C, E, S l.

Visulas YAG II plus l.
VisuMed MEL60 l.
VISX 2020 excimer l.
VISX S2, S3 excimer l.
VISX Star S2 l.
VISX Star S3 ActiveTrak l.
VISX Twenty/Twenty excimer l.
VitaLase Er:YAG l.
white l.
YAG l.
yellow dye l.
yttrium-aluminum-garnet l.
Zeiss VISULAS 532s l.
Zeiss VISULAS 532, 532s l.
Zeiss VISULAS YAG II l.

laser-adjustable lens (LAL)
laser-argon device
laser-assisted
    l.-a. intrastromal keratomileusis
      (LASIK)
    l.-a. in situ keratomileusis
    l.-a. subepithelial keratectomy
      (LASEK)
lasered
Laseredge microsurgical knife
Laserex Era 4106 YAG laser
laser-filtering surgery
Laserflex
    L. coagulator
    L. lens
LaserHarmonic laser
Laseridge
    Cilco Hoffer L.
    L. Optics lens
laser-induced glaucoma
laser-ruby device
LaserScan LSX excimer laser system
laser-scrape
    l.-s. photorefractive keratectomy
    l.-s. technique
Lasertek laser
lash
    l. abrasion of cornea
    brow, lids, l.'s (BLL)
    l. margin
    misdirected l.
LASIK
    laser-assisted intrastromal keratomileusis
    laser in situ keratomileusis
    LASIK aspiration spoon
    LASIK Banaji irrigating cannula
    bilateral simultaneous LASIK

    bitoric LASIK
    LASIK Burrato irrigating cannula
    Dishler Excimer Laser System for
      LASIK
    epithelial LASIK
    LASIK eye guard
    LASIK flap irrigator
    LASIK flap manipulator
    LASIK Guell irrigating cannula
    hyperopic LASIK
    LASIK Pettigrove irrigating cannula
    LASIK spear
    topographically guided therapeutic
      LASIK
    wavefront-guided LASIK
lasing
Lasiodiplodia theobromae
lasitome
    Krumeich-Barraquer l.
lasso
    lens l.
LAT
    latency associated transcript
    limbal autograft transplantation
lata
    Tenon fascia l.
latanoprost timolol maleate ophthalmic
  solution
late
    l. endothelial failure
    l. phase detachment
    l. postoperative suture adjustment
      (LPSA)
latency associated transcript (LAT)
latent
    l. angle-closure glaucoma
    l. deviation
    l. diabetes
    l. endophthalmitis
    l. hyperopia (Hl)
    l. nystagmus
    l. squint
    l. strabismus
late-onset
    l.-o. corneal haze
    l.-o. esotropia
    l.-o. myope
    l.-o. myopia
late-phase reaction
lateral
    l. aberration
    l. angle

NOTES

L

277

lateral *(continued)*
    l. canthal incision
    l. canthal tendon
    l. canthotomy
    l. canthus
    l. commissure of eyelid
    l. gaze
    l. geniculate body (LGB)
    l. geniculate body lesion (LGB lesion, LGB lesion)
    l. geniculate nucleus (LGN)
    l. hemianopsia
    l. horn
    l. illumination
    l. inhibition
    l. margin of orbit
    l. medullary infarction
    l. medullary syndrome
    l. nystagmus
    l. oblique conus
    l. orbital decompression
    l. orbital tubercle
    l. orbitotomy
    l. orbit tubercle
    l. palpebral ligament
    l. palpebral raphe
    l. palpebral tubercle
    l. phoria
    l. rectus (L.R.)
    l. rectus extraocular muscle
    l. rectus palsy
    l. rectus recession
lateralis
    angulus oculi l.
    commissura palpebrarum l.
    raphe palpebralis l.
laterodeviation
lateroduction
lateropulsion
laterotorsion
lathe-cut contact lens
lathe lens
lathing
    corneal l.
    l. procedure
lattice
    l. corneal dystrophy
    l. corneal dystrophy type IIIA (LCDIIIA)
    l. degeneration of retina
    l. dystrophy of cornea
    l. keratitis
    l. retinal degeneration
Lauber disease
laughing gas
Laurence-Biedl syndrome
Laurence-Moon-Bardet-Biedl syndrome
Laurence-Moon-Biedl syndrome
Laurence-Moon syndrome

laurentii
    Cryptococcus l.
Lauth canal
lavage
Lavoptik eye wash
law
    Alexander l.
    Angström l.
    Beer l.
    Bernoulli l.
    Bunsen-Roscoe l.
    Descartes l.
    Desmarres l.
    Donders l.
    Ewald l.
    Ferry-Porter l.
    Flouren l.
    Friedenwald l.
    Giraud-Teulon l.
    Gullstrand l.
    Hering l.
    Homer l.
    Horner l.
    Knapp l.
    Kollner l.
    LaPlace l.
    Listing l.
    Pascal l.
    Plateau-Talbot l.
    Poiseuille l.
    Prentice l.
    reciprocity l.
    l. of refraction
    Riccò l.
    Roscoe-Bunsen l.
    Sherrington l.
    Snell l.
    Stefan l.
    Talbot l.
    Weber l.
    Wundt-Lamansky l.
Lawford syndrome
Lawton corneal scissors
laxity
    involutional l.
    lid l.
    lower lid l.
Layden infant lens
layer
    aqueous tear l.
    bacillary l.
    basal l.
    Bowman l.
    Bruch l.
    choriocapillary l.
    columnar l.
    cuticular l.
    epithelial basement l.
    fibrin l.

ganglion cell l.
grading of retinal nerve fiber l.
Haller l.
Henle fiber l.
inner nuclear l.
inner plexiform l.
juxtapapillary nerve fiber l.
keratin l.
limiting l.
lipid tear l.
molecular external l.
molecular inner l.
molecular internal l.
molecular outer l.
mucin l.
mucous tear l.
nerve fiber l. (NFL)
nerve fiber bundle l.
nuclear external l.
nuclear inner l.
nuclear internal l.
nuclear outer l.
oil l.
outer nuclear l.
outer plexiform l. (OPL)
peripapillary nerve fiber l.
pigment l.
plexiform external l.
plexiform inner l.
plexiform internal l.
plexiform outer l.
posterior collagenous l. (PCL)
retinal ganglion cell l.
retinal nerve fiber l. (RNFL)
retinochoroidal l.
l. of rods and cones
Sattler l.
suprachoroid l.
tear l.
layered
l. hyphema
l. keratoplasty
Lazex excimer laser
lazy eye
LC-6 Daily Contact Lens Cleaner
L-Caine
LCAT
limbal-conjunctival autograft
transplantation
LC-65 Daily Contact Lens Cleaner
LCDIIIA
lattice corneal dystrophy type IIIA

LCDVA
low-contrast distance visual acuity
LCFM
laser cell and flare meter
L-cone excitation
LCSLC
Low-Contrast Sloan Letter Chart
LD
local deviation
LD+2
L/D
light/dark
L/D ratio
LDD
light-dark discrimination
LE
left eye
Le
Le Grand-Geblewics phenomenon
Le Grand-Gullstrand eye model
lead
l. encephalopathy
l. incrustation of cornea
lead-filled mallet
Leahey
L. chalazion forceps
L. operation
leak
eyelash-induced l.
glue patch l.
macular l.
point l.
leakage
corneal l.
juxtapapillary l.
microaneurysmal l.
parafoveal microvascular l.
progressive fluorescein l.
leaking filtering bleb
least diffusion circle
Lea Symbol chart
leaves of capsule
Lebensohn
L. reading chart
L. visual acuity chart
Leber
amaurosis congenita of L.
L. cell
L. congenital amaurosis
L. corpuscle
L. disease
L. hereditary optic atrophy

L

NOTES

Leber *(continued)*
  L. hereditary optic atrophy reverse
    dot-blot assay
  L. hereditary optic neuropathy
    (LHON)
  L. idiopathic stellate retinopathy
  L. lymphangiectasia hemorrhagica
  L. miliary aneurysm
  L. plus syndrome
LEC
  lens epithelial cell
lecithin-cholesterol acyltransferase
  deficiency
Lecythophora mutabilis
LED
  light-emitting diode
LED-illuminated ring
Lefler-Wadsworth-Sidbury foveal
  dystrophy
left
  l. deorsumvergence
  l. esotropia
  l. exotropia
  l. eye (LE, OS)
  l. gaze
  l. hyperphoria
  l. hypertropia (LHT)
  l. inferior oblique recession
  l. inferior rectus muscle
  l. superior oblique tuck
  l. superior rectus muscle
  l. sursumvergence
left-beating nystagmus
left-handed cornea scissors
left-to-right shunting
Legacy
  L. cataract surgical system
  L. Series 2000 Cavitron/Kelman
    phacoemulsifier aspirator
legal blindness
legally blind
Leigh
  L. capsule forceps
  L. disease
  L. encephalopathy
leiomyoma
  l. of iris
  l. of uveal tract
Leishman classification
Leishman-Donovan body
leishmaniasis
  American l.
Leishmania tropica
Leiske lens
Leitz microscope
Leland refractor
lema
lemniscus, pl. **lemnisci**
  optic l.

Lemoine
  L. orbital implant
  L. serrefine
Lemoine-Searcy fixation anchor loupe
lemon-drop nodule
Lempert rongeur
Lempert-Storz
  L.-S. lens
  L.-S. loupe
Lems lens
Lenercept
length
  axial l. (AL)
  chord l.
  eye axial l.
  focal l.
  primary focal l.
  secondary focal l.
  temple l.
lens, pl. **lenses**
  l. aberration
  Abraham iridectomy laser l.
  Abraham peripheral button
    iridotomy l.
  Abraham YAG laser l.
  accommodation of crystalline l.
  Accugel l.
  achromatic spectacle l.
  Achroplan nonapplanating 40x
    immersion objective l.
  acrylic intraocular l.
  AcrySof foldable intraocular l.
  AcrySof MA60 l.
  AcrySof Natural intraocular l.
  Acuvue Bifocal contact l.
  Acuvue brand toric contact l.
  Acuvue 1-Day disposable l.
  Acuvue disposable contact l.
  Acuvue Etafilcon A l.
  Acuvue Toric contact l.
  Acuvue 2-week UV-blocking
    disposable l.
  adherent l.
  Airy cylindric l.
  Alan-Thorpe l.
  Alcon AcrySof SA30AL single-
    piece l.
  Alcon MA30BA optic Acrysof l.
  Alges bifocal contact l.
  Alien WildEyes l.
  Allen-Thorpe l.
  Allergan AMO Array S155 l.
  all-Perspex CQ l.
  all-Perspex Kelman Omnifit l.
  all-PMMA intraocular l.
  l. alone
  Amenabar l.
  American Medical Optics Baron l.
  amnifocal l.

AMO Array foldable intraocular l.
AMO Array multifocal ultraviolet-absorbing silicone posterior chamber intraocular l.
AMO Ioptex Model ACR 360 foldable acrylic l.
AMO Phacoflex II foldable intraocular l.
amorphic l.
Amsoft l.
anastigmatic l.
angle-fixated l.
angle-supported l.
aniseikonic l.
Anis staple l.
anterior chamber intraocular l. (ACIOL)
anterior pole of the l.
anular bifocal contact l.
AO l.
AO-XT 166 l.
aphakic l.
aplanatic l.
apochromatic l.
Appolonio l.
Aquaflex contact l.
Aquasight l.
Arlt l.
Array multifocal intraocular l.
Arruga l.
artificial l.
Artisan myopia l.
aspherical ophthalmoscopic l.
aspheric cataract l.
aspheric contact l.
aspheric spectacle l.
aspheric-viewing l.
aspiration of l.
astigmatic l.
auxiliary l.
l. axis
axis of cylindric l. (x)
Azar l.
back surface toric contact l.
Bagolini l.
Baikoff l.
ballasted contact l.
bandage soft contact l.
Barkan gonioscopic l.
Barkan goniotomy l.
Baron l.
Barraquer l.

baseball l.
Bausch & Lomb Optima l.
Bausch & Lomb Surgical L161U l.
Bayadi l.
8.4 BC disposable l.
Bechert 7-mm l.
Beebe l.
beveled-edge l.
bicentric spectacle l.
biconcave contact l.
biconvex l.
bicurve contact l.
bicylindrical l.
Bietti l.
bifocal contact l.
bifocal intracorneal l.
bifocal spectacle l.
Binkhorst four-loop iris-fixated l.
Binkhorst-Fyodorov l.
Binkhorst intraocular l.
Binkhorst iridocapsular l.
Binkhorst two-loop l.
Biom l.
Biomedics contact l.
biomicroscopic indirect l.
Bi-Soft l.
bispherical l.
bitoric contact l.
l. blank
Bloodshot WildEyes l.
blooming of l.
blooming spectacle l.
Boberg-Ans l.
Boston 7 contact l.
Boston Envision contact l.
Boston EO, ES contact l.
Boston II, IV contact l.
Boston RXD contact l.
Boston XO contact l.
Bowling l.
Boys-Smith laser l.
Brücke l.
Burian-Allen contact l.
Byrne expulsive hemorrhage l.
Calendar monthly disposable contact l.
l. capsule
Cardona fiberoptic diagnostic l.
Carl Zeiss l.
cast resin l.

L

NOTES

lens *(continued)*
cataract extraction with
intraocular l. (CE/IOL)
CeeOn foldable l.
CeeOn heparin surface-modified l.
CeeOn intraocular l.
cellulose acetate butyrate contact l.
Centra-Flex l.
central posterior curve of
contact l.
central retinal l.
central thickness of contact l.
Charles hand-held infusion l.
Charles intraocular l.
Charles irrigating contact l.
chemically treated spectacle l.
Chiroflex C11UB l.
Choyce intraocular l.
Choyce Mark VIII l.
CibaSoft Visitint contact l.
Cibathin l.
Cilco MonoFlex multi-piece PMMA
intraocular l.
Cilco-Simcoe II l.
CIMA*flex* 411 foldable silicone l.
ClariFlex OptiEdge foldable
intraocular l.
clariVit central mag l.
clariVit wide angle l.
Clayman intraocular l.
Clayman posterior chamber l.
L. clear
clear crystalline l.
ClearView contact l.
l. clip
C-loop intraocular l.
C-loop posterior chamber l.
coating for spectacle l.
Coburn intraocular l.
collagen bandage l.
Collamer 3-piece intraocular l.
coloboma of l.
Comberg contact l.
ComfortKone l.
L. Comfort Ultrasound Cleaning
and Disinfecting System
composition of spectacle l.
compound l.
concave spectacle l.
concavoconcave l.
concavoconvex l.
condensing l.
conoid l.
constructional ability contact l.
contact l. (CL)
contact bandage l.
contact low-vacuum l.
convergent l.
converging meniscus l.

convexoconcave l.
convexoconvex l.
convex plano l.
convex spectacle l.
Cooper Clear DW contact l.
Cooper Toric contact l.
CooperVision PMMA-ACL Flex l.
Copeland radial panchamber
intraocular l.
Copeland radial panchamber UV l.
coquille plano l.
corneal contact l.
corrected spectacle l.
cortical substance of l.
Cosmetica hand-painted contact l.
cosmetic shell contact l.
coupling of progressive power l.
CR-39 l.
crocodile l.
Crookes l.
crossed l.
crown glass l.
l. crystallina
crystalline l.
CSI Toric contact l.
curvature of l.
curve of spectacle l.
cylinder spectacle l.
cylindrical l. (C, cyl.)
Dailies contact l.
daily-wear contact l. (DWCL)
Darin l.
1 day Acuvue contact l.
decentered l.
l. decentration
diagnostic contact l.
diagnostic fiberoptic l.
66-diopter iridectomy laser l.
direct gonioscopic l.
disk intraocular l.
dislocated l.
l. dislocation
dispersing l.
disposable contact l.
distance between lenses (DBL)
distortion of l.
divergent l.
diverging meniscus l.
dot-like l.
double concave l.
double convex l.
Doubra l.
l. dressing
Drews l.
L. Drops lubricating and rewetting
drops
dual l.
Dulaney l.
Durasoft 2 ColorBlends l.

Durasoft 3 Optifit Toric
Colorblends contact l.
Durasoft 2 Optifit Toric for light
eyes contact l.
Dura-T l.
E Clips prescription computer l.
Edge III hydrogel contact l.
edging of spectacle l.
El Bayadi-Kajiura l.
Emcee l.
Emery l.
Encore monthly disposable
contact l.
EndoView Sapphire L.
l. epithelial cell (LEC)
l. epithelium
Epstein collar stud acrylic l.
l. equator
equator of crystalline l.
ERG-Jet disposable contact l.
Eschenbach Optik l.
etafilcon A l.
l. exchange
executive spectacle l.
exfoliation of l.
l. exfoliation glaucoma
l. expressor
extended wear contact l. (EWCL)
eye l.
EZ.1 multifocal contact l.
EZVUE violet haptic intraocular l.
Falcon l.
Feaster Dualens l.
Fechtner intraocular l.
Federov type I, II intraocular l.
l. fiber
fiberoptic diagnostic l.
field l.
first definite apical clearance l.
(FDACL)
flat contact l.
flat-edge l.
Flexlens l.
Flexner-Worst iris claw l.
l. flexure effect
flint-glass l.
fluid contact l.
fluidless contact l.
Fluorex 300, 500 contact l.
F/M base curve contact l.
Focus DAILIES Toric contact l.
Focus Night & Day contact l.

foldable disk intraocular l.
foldable plate-haptic silicone
intraocular l.
FormFlex l.
four-loop l.
four-mirror goniolens l.
Franklin-style bifocal lenses
Frelex l.
Frenzel l.
Frequency 38 monthly disposable
contact l.
L. Fresh
FreshLook ColorBlends l.
Fresnel l.
Friedman hand-held Hruby l.
Friedman-Hruby l.
front surface toric contact l.
fundus contact l.
fundus focalizing l.
fundus laser l.
fused bifocal l.
fused multifocal l.
Galin intraocular implant l.
gas-permeable contact l. (GPCL)
Gel Flex l.
generating spectacle l.
Genesis l.
Gentex PDQ polycarbonate l.
Gill intraocular implant l.
Gilmore intraocular implant l.
glass l.
l. glide
glued-on hard contact l.
Goldmann diagnostic contact l.
Goldmann fundus contact l.
Goldmann macular contact l.
Goldmann multi-mirror l.
Goldmann three-mirror contact
diagnostic l.
goniofocalizing l.
goniolens l.
gonioscopic l.
Gould intraocular implant l.
Gray photochromic l.
Gridley intraocular l.
Gullstrand l.
hand-held Hruby l.
hand-held infusion l.
haptic plate l.
hard contact l. (HCL)
hardened spectacle l.
hardening of l.

L

NOTES

lens *(continued)*

Hart pediatric three-mirror l.
heparin surface-modified
intraocular l. (HSM-IOL)
Hessburg l.
Hidex glass l.
Hoffer-Laseridge intraocular l.
honey bee l.
Hoskins l.
Hoskins-Barkan goniotomy infant l.
Hruby contact l.
Hunkeler l.
Hydracon contact l.
Hydrasoft contact l.
Hydrocurve II l.
hydrogel contact l.
hydrogel disk intraocular l.
Hydron l.
hydrophilic contact l.
hydrophobic contact l.
Hydrosight l.
Hydroview l.
hypermature l.
immersion l.
l. implant
implant l.
implantable contact l. (ICL)
implantation of l.
Implens intraocular l.
indirect l.
inert material for intraocular l.
infant Karickhoff laser l.
infant three-mirror laser l.
influence of an Artisan l.
Intermedics l.
Interspace YAG laser l.
in-the-bag l.
intraocular l. (IOL)
IOLAB 108 B l.
IOLAB intraocular l.
Ioptex laser intraocular l.
Ioptex TabOptic l.
Irene l.
iridocapsular intraocular l.
iridotomy l.
iris-claw intraocular l.
iris-fixated l.
iris-supported l.
iseikonic l.
isoiconic l.
Jaffe Cilco l.
J-loop PC l.
J-loop posterior chamber
intraocular l.
Joal l.
Jung-Schaffer intraocular l.
Kamerling Capsular 90 l.
Karickhoff laser l.
Kearney side-notch l.

Keeler panoramic l.
Kelman flexible tripod l.
Kelman Multiflex II l.
Kelman Omnifit II intraocular l.
Kelman PC 27LB CapSul l.
Kelman Quadriflex anterior
chamber intraocular l.
keratoconus contact l.
Kilp l.
Kirby l.
Kishi l.
knife-edged l.
Koeppe diagnostic l.
Krasnov l.
Kratz elliptical-style l.
Kratz-Johnson l.
Kratz posterior chamber
intraocular l.
Kratz-Sinskey intraocular l.
Kratz "soft" J-loop intraocular l.
Krieger wide-field fundus l.
Kryptok l.
Kuler panoramic l.
lacrimal l.
lamellar separation of l.
laminated spectacle l.
Landers biconcave l.
Landers contact l.
Landers-Foulks temporary
keratoprosthesis l.
Landers sew-on l.
laser l.
laser-adjustable l. (LAL)
Laserflex l.
Laseridge Optics l.
l. lasso
lathe l.
lathe-cut contact l.
Layden infant l.
Leiske l.
Lempert-Storz l.
Lems l.
lenticular-cut contact l.
lenticular spectacle l.
Lewis l.
Lieb-Guerry l.
Lindstrom Centrex l.
Liteflex l.
l. localizer
long-wearing contact l.
l. loop
loose l.
lotrafilcon A l.
l. loupe
Lovac gonioscopic l.
l. lubricant
luxated l.
luxation of l.
Lynell intraocular l.

Machemer flat l.
Machemer infusion contact l.
Machemer magnifying vitrectomy l.
macular contact l.
magnifying l.
Mainster-HM retinal laser l.
Mainster retinal laser l.
Mainster-S retinal laser l.
Mainster Ultra Field PRP laser l.
Mainster-WF retinal laser l.
Mainster wide field l.
Mandelkorn suture laser lysis l.
l. manipulator
March laser l.
Mark II Magni-Focuser l.
Mark IX l.
L. Mate
mature l.
McCannel l.
McGhan 3M intraocular l.
McLean prismatic fundus laser l.
Medallion l.
Medical Optics PC11NB
   intraocular l.
Medical Workshop intraocular l.
Meditec bandage contact l.
meniscus concave l.
Meso contact l.
meter l.
microbevel edge l.
microthin contact l.
mid-coquille l.
MiniQuad XL l.
minus spectacle l.
4-Mirror Gonio l.
modified C-loop intraocular l.
modified C-loop UV l.
modified J-loop intraocular l.
modified J-loop UV l.
mold-injected l.
Momose l.
multicurve contact l.
Multiflex anterior chamber l.
multifocal spectacle l.
Multi-Optics l.
NEC MobilePro 800 Volk L.
negative meniscus l.
Neolens l.
New Orleans l.
NewVues sterile contact l.
Nike Max Rx prescription sun l.
Nikon aspheric l.

Nokrome bifocal l.
noncontact l.
Nova Aid l.
Nova Curve broad C-loop posterior
   chamber l.
Nova Curve Omnicurve l.
Nova Soft II l.
nuclear sclerosis of l.
nucleus of l.
l. nucleus
Nuvita l.
objective l.
occupational l.
Oculaid l.
ocular l.
O'Malley-Pearce-Luma l.
Omnifit intraocular l.
one-piece multifocal l.
one-piece plate haptic silicone
   intraocular l.
one-plane l.
on-eye performance of l.
L. Opacification Classification
   System (LOCS)
L. Opacities Case-Control Study
L. Opacity Classification System II
L. Opacity Classification System
   III
open l.
Ophtec Co. l.
ophthalmic progressive-power l.
optical center of spectacle l.
optical contact l.
Optical Radiation l.
optical zone of contact l.
optics of intraocular l.
Optiflex l.
Optima contact l.
Opti-Vu l.
Opt-Visor l.
Optycryl 60 contact l.
Opus III contact l.
orbital l.
ORC intraocular l.
Orthogon l.
orthoscopic l.
O'Shea l.
Osher gonio/posterior pole l.
Osher pan-fundus l.
Osher surgical gonio/posterior
   pole l.

L

NOTES

lens *(continued)*

overall diameter of contact l. (OAD)

Lenses and Overnight Orthokeratology (LOOK)

panchamber UV l.

Pannu intraocular l.

Pannu type II l.

PanoView Optics l.

Paraperm O2 contact l.

l. particle glaucoma

PBII blue loop l.

Pearce posterior chamber intraocular l.

pediatric Karickhoff laser l.

pediatric three-mirror laser l.

Percepta progressive l.

peripheral curve on contact l.

periscopic concave l.

periscopic convex l.

Permaflex l.

Permalens l.

Perspex CQ-Shearing-Simcoe-Sinskey l.

Petrus single-mirror laser l.

Peyman-Green vitrectomy l.

Peyman-Tennant-Green l.

Peyman wide-field l.

PhacoFlex II SI30NB intraocular l.

Phakic 6 l.

Phakic intraocular l.

Pharmacia intraocular l.

Pharmacia Visco J-loop l.

photobrown lenses

photochromic l.

photogray l.

photosensitive l.

photosun l.

piggyback contact l.

piggyback intraocular l.

pigmentary deposits on l.

l. pit

placode l.

l. placode

l. plane

planoconcave l.

planoconvex nonridge l.

Plano T l.

plastic l.

plate-haptic intraocular l.

plate-haptic silicone l.

Platina clip l.

L. Plus

L. Plus-Allergan

L. Plus daily cleaner

L. Plus Oxysept

L. Plus Oxysept System

L. Plus rewetting drops

L. Plus saline

plus spectacle l.

L. Plus Sterile Saline Solution

PMMA custom-made calibration contact l.

polarizing l.

polycarbonate l.

Polycon I, II contact l.

Polymacon l.

polymethylmethacrylate contact l.

positive meniscus l.

Posner diagnostic l.

posterior chamber intraocular l. (PCIOL, PC-IOL)

posterior pole of l.

posterior surface of l.

l. power

l. power calculation

Precision Cosmet l.

presbyopic intraocular l.

press-on Fresnel l.

primary l.

prismatic contact l.

prismatic effect by l.

prismatic gonioscopic l.

prismatic gonioscopy l.

prismatic goniotomy l.

prismatic spectacle l.

progressive addition l.

progressive additional lenses

progressive multifocal l.

progressive spectacles lenses

prolonged-wear contact l.

prosthetic l.

protective l.

l. protein glaucoma

punctal l.

pupillary l.

PureVision extended-wear contact l.

QuadPediatric fundus l.

radius of l.

Rayner l.

Red Reflex Lens Systems l.

refractive contact l.

l. removal

retroscopic l.

Revolution l.

RGP contact l.

ridge l.

Ridley l.

rigid contact l.

rigid gas-permeable contact l.

Ritch contact l.

Ritch nylon suture laser l.

Ritch trabeculoplasty laser l.

RLX l.

Rodenstock panfundus l.

rudiment l.

Ruiz fundus contact l.

Ruiz fundus laser l.

safety l.
SaturEyes contact l.
Saturn II contact lenses
Sauflon PW l.
Schachar l.
Schlegel l.
scleral contact l.
scratch-resistant spectacle l.
secondary curve on contact l.
secondary intraocular l.
segmental l.
self-stabilizing vitrectomy l.
semifinished contact l.
semiscleral contact l.
Sensar acrylic intraocular l.
Sensar OptiEdge intraocular l.
Severin l.
sew-on l.
Shearing planar posterior chamber
   intraocular l.
Sheets l.
short C-loop l.
Signet Optical l.
silicone acrylate contact l.
silicone elastomer l.
silicone intraocular l.
Silsoft contact l.
Simcoe II PC l.
simple plus l.
l. simulation sales tool
single-cut contact l.
Sinskey intraocular l.
l. size
slab-off l.
Slant haptic single-piece
   intraocular l.
SlimFit ovoid intraocular l.
SlimFit small-incision ovoid l.
Snellen soft contact l.
Soflens 66 l.
Soflens contact l.
SoFlex series l.
soft contact l. (SCL)
soft intraocular l.
SoftSITE high add aspheric
   multifocal contact l.
Sola Optical USA Spectralite high
   index l.
Soper cone l.
Sovereign bifocal l.
special spectacle l.
spectacle l.

Spectralite Transitions l.
spherical equivalent l.
spherocylindric l.
spherocylindrical l.
spin-cast l.
l. sponge
spontaneous extrusion of l.
l. spoon
Staar AA 4207 l.
Staar implantable contact l.
Staar intraocular l.
Staar toric l.
Staar 4203VF l.
Staar 4207VF l.
Stableflex anterior chamber l.
l. star
star l.
steep contact l.
stigmatic l.
Stokes l.
Storz CAPSULORBLUE
   intraocular l.
Strampelli l.
Style S2 clear-loop l.
styrene contact l.
subluxated l.
subluxation of l.
subluxed l.
substance of l.
Super Field NC slit lamp l.
Surefit AC 85J l.
Surevue contact l.
Surgidev PC BUV 20-24
   intraocular l.
Sussman l.
Sutherland l.
suture of l.
T l.
Tano double mirror peripheral
   vitrectomy l.
Tecnis foldable intraocular l.
telescopic l.
Tennant Anchorflex AC l.
therapeutic contact l.
thick l.
thin l.
Thorpe four-mirror goniolaser l.
Thorpe four-mirror vitreous fundus
   laser l.
three-mirror contact l.
three-piece acrylic intraocular l.
three-piece silicone intraocular l.

L

NOTES

lens *(continued)*
 tight contact l.
 Tillyer bifocal l.
 tilting l.
 tinted contact l.
 tinting of spectacle l.
 Tolentino prism l.
 Tolentino vitrectomy l.
 Topcon aspheric l.
 toric contact l.
 toric intraocular l.
 Toric-Optima series l.
 toric spectacle l.
 toroidal contact l.
 Touchlite zoom l.
 transsclerally sutured posterior
  chamber l. (TS-SPCL)
 trial case and l.
 trial contact l.
 tricurve contact lenses
 trifocal l.
 Trokel l.
 Trokel-Peyman laser l.
 truncated contact l.
 Trupower aspherical l.
 TruVision l.
 two-plane l.
 Ultex l.
 Ultra mag l.
 Ultra view SP slit lamp l.
 Ultravue l.
 uncut spectacle l.
 Uniplanar style PC II l.
 Univis l.
 Univision low-vision microscopic l.
 Urrets-Zavalia retinal surgical l.
 Uvex l.
 UV Nova Curve l.
 Varigray l.
 Varilux Pangamic thin plastic l.
 l. vault
 vaulting of contact l.
 vergence of l.
 l. vesicle
 Viscolens l.
 Vision Tech l.
 Visitec Company l.
 Volk aspheric l.
 Volk coronoid l.
 Volk High Resolution aspherical l.
 Volk 3 Mirror ANF+ l.
 Volk 3 Mirror gonio fundus
  laser l.
 Volk Quadraspheric l.
 Volk SuperField aspherical l.
 Volk SuperField NC l.
 Volk SuperMacula 2.2 focal
  laser l.
 Volk SuperQuad 160 contact l.

 Volk SuperQuad 160 panretinal l.
 Volk Transequator l.
 Wang l.
 Weber-Elschnig l.
 Wesley-Jessen l.
 L. Wet
 whorl l.
 Wild l.
 WildEyes costume contact l.
 Wise iridotomy laser l.
 Wise iridotomy-sphincterotomy
  laser l.
 with contact lenses (c̄cl)
 Wood l.
 Woods Concept l.
 working l.
 Worst Claw l.
 Worst goniotomy l.
 Worst Medallion l.
 Worst Platina iris-fixated l.
 X chrom contact l.
 Yannuzzi fundus laser l.
 l. to yield
 Youens l.
 Y-sutures of crystalline l.
 Zeiss l.
 Zeiss-Gullstrand l.
 zero power lenses
 l. zone
 l. zonule
LensCheck Advanced Logic lensometer
lensectomy
 Charles l.
 clear l.
 coal-mining l.
LENSender
 Bausch & Lomb L.
Lensept
lenses *(pl. of* lens)
Lens-Eze inserter
lens-holding forceps
lens-induced
 l.-i. secondary open-angle glaucoma
 l.-i. UGH syndrome
 l.-i. uveitis
lens-iris diaphragm
lens-maker formula
Lensmeter
 L. 701
 Badal L.
 Nagel L.
 Zeiss LA 110 projection L.
lensometer
 Allergan Humphrey l.
 AO Reichert Instruments l.
 Carl Zeiss l.
 Coburn l.
 Hardy l.
 IntraOptics l.

LensCheck Advanced Logic l.
Marco l.
Reichert Lenschek advanced
   logic l.
Topcon LM P5 digital l.
lensometry
lensopathy
lens-plus-eye system
Lensrins
lens-sparing vitrectomy
lens-threading forceps
Lens-Wet
lenta
   ophthalmia l.
lentectomize
lentectomy
lenticle
lenticonus
   anterior l.
   posterior l.
lenticula
lenticular
   l. astigmatism
   l. bowl
   l. cataract
   l. contact lens
   l. degeneration
   l. fibroxanthomatous nodule
   l. fossa
   l. fossa of vitreous body
   l. ganglion
   l. glaucoma
   l. myopia
   l. nucleus
   l. opacity
   l. ring
   l. spectacle lens
   l. vesicle
lenticular-cut contact lens
lenticule
   epikeratoplasty l.
lenticuli (*pl. of* lenticulus)
lenticulocapsular
lenticulo-optic
lenticulostriate
lenticulothalamic
lenticulus, pl. **lenticuli**
lentiform
   l. nodule
   nucleus l.
lentigines, electrocardiogram
abnormalities, ocular hypertelorism,

pulmonary stenosis, abnormal
genitalia, retardation of growth, and
deafness (LEOPARD)
lentiglobus
lentis
   apparatus suspensorius l.
   l. articularis
   axis l.
   caligo l.
   capsula l.
   cellulae l.
   chalcosis l.
   coloboma l.
   cortex l.
   ectopia l.
   epithelium l.
   equator l.
   equatorial l.
   facies anterior l.
   facies posterior l.
   fibrae l.
   gerontoxon l.
   nucleus l.
   polus anterior l.
   polus posterior l.
   radius of l.
   siderosis l.
   spontaneous ectopia l.
   substantia corticalis l.
   tunica vasculosa l.
   vortex l.
Lenz syndrome
leonine appearance
LEOPARD
   lentigines, electrocardiogram
   abnormalities, ocular hypertelorism,
   pulmonary stenosis, abnormal genitalia,
   retardation of growth, and deafness
   LEOPARD syndrome
leopard
   l. fundus
   l. retina
Lepper-Trier formula
leprae
   Mycobacterium l.
leprosa
   keratitis punctata l.
leptomeningeal metastasis
Leptospira interrogans
leptospiral uveitis
leptospirosis
   ocular l.

L

NOTES

leptotrichosis conjunctivae
lesion
acquired abducens nerve l.
acquired III nerve l.
amelanotic l.
Archer l.
basal ganglia l.
bilateral occipital lobe l.
boomerang-shaped l.
brainstem l.
branching l.
bull's eye macular l.
cerebellar l.
cerebellopontine angle l.
cerebral hemisphere l.
cervical l.
chiasm l.
chiasmal l.
chorioretinal l.
choroidal l.
concentric l.
congenital abducens nerve l.
congenital III nerve l.
conjunctival melanotic l.
cornea guttate l.
corneal punctate l.
corpus callosum l.
CPA l.
cracked windshield stromal l.
dendriform corneal l.
dendriform epithelial l.
dendritic epithelial l.
diencephalic l.
epibulbar l.
extrastriate cortex l.
facial nerve l.
frontal lobe unilateral cerebral
hemisphere l.
frontoparietal bilateral cerebral
hemisphere l.
geographic l.
hamartomatous l.
hemorrhagic disciform l.
herpetoid l.
hypertrophic dendriform epithelial l.
keratitis l.
lateral geniculate body l. (LGB
lesion, LGB lesion)
LGB l.
lateral geniculate body lesion
linear streak l.
lipocytic l.
lymphoepithelial l.
lytic l.
malignant pituitary l.
medial longitudinal fasciculus l.
(MLF lesion)
medulla l.
melanocytic conjunctival l.

melanotic l.
mesencephalic l.
mesencephalon l.
microcystic l.
MLF l.
medial longitudinal fasciculus
lesion
neural l.
occipital lobe unilateral cerebral
hemisphere l.
oculomotor nerve l.
optic chiasmal l.
optic nerve l.
optic radiation l.
optic tract l.
orange-red l.
l. of orbit
orbital l.
osseous l.
parasellar l.
parietal lobe bilateral cerebral
hemisphere l.
parietal lobe unilateral cerebral
hemisphere l.
periventricular l.
phototoxic l.
pigmented l.
pons l.
pontine l.
precancerous l.
preganglionic l.
pseudocancerous l.
punched-out l.
recurrent corneal l. (RCL)
retinal l.
retrobulbar compressive l.
retrogeniculate l.
satellite l.
sonolucent l.
space-occupying l.
subarachnoid oculomotor nerve l.
sunburst-type l.
supranuclear l.
suprasellar l.
temporal lobe unilateral cerebral
hemisphere l.
trochlear nerve l.
unifocal optic nerve l.
unilateral l.
VZV disciform l.
waxy l.
weeping eczematous l.
white laser l.
lesser
l. ring of iris
l. wing of sphenoid
Lester
L. fixation forceps
L. IOL manipulator

L. Jones operation
L. Jones tube
L. lens dialer
L. lens manipulator
Lester-Burch speculum
lethal midline granuloma
letter
l. blindness
implanted Artisan l.
Sloan l.'s
Snellen l.'s
test l.
l. test
letterbox technique
Letterer-Siwe syndrome
letter-shaped keratitis
leucitis
leukemia
leukemic
l. cell
l. infiltrate
l. infiltration of the optic disk
l. retinitis
l. retinopathy
Leukeran
leukocoria (*var. of* leukokoria)
leukocyte function associated antigen-1 (LFA-1)
leukocytoclastic vasculitis
leukoderma
periorbital l.
leukodystrophy
metachromatic l.
leukokoria, leukocoria
leukoma, pl. **leukomata**
acromegaloid features, cutis verticis gyrata, corneal l. (ACL)
l. adherens
adherent l.
l. corneae
corneal l.
leukomatous corneal opacity
leukopathia, leukopathy
congenital l.
leukopsin
leukoscope
leukotomy
transorbital l.
Leustatin
Levaquin
levator
l. aponeurosis defect

l. aponeurosis disinsertion
l. aponeurosis repair
l. function testing
l. injury
l. innervation
l. muscle of upper eyelid
l. palpebrae superioris
l. palpebrae superioris muscle
l. ptosis
l. resection
l. tendon
l. trochlear muscle
level
Brems Astigmatism Marker with L.
level-dependent
blood oxygenation l.-d. (BOLD)
leventinese
malattia l.
Levine spud
Levitt implant
levobetaxolol hydrochloride
levobunolol
l. HCl
l. hydrochloride
levocabastine
l. HCl
l. hydrochloride
levoclination
levocycloduction
levocycloversion
levodopa
levodopa-carbidopa
levoduction
levo-epinephrine
levofloxacin ophthalmic solution
levotorsion
levoversion
Lewicky
L. formed cystitome
L. lens manipulating hook
L. needle
L. self-retaining chamber maintainer
L. threaded infusion cannula
Lewis
L. lens
L. lens loupe
L. scoop
Lewy body
Lexan
Lexer operation
Lexipafant

L

NOTES

LFA-1
    leukocyte function associated antigen-1
LGB
    lateral geniculate body
        LGB lesion
            lateral geniculate body lesion
LGN
    lateral geniculate nucleus
LHON
    Leber hereditary optic neuropathy
LHT
    left hypertropia
library temple
lichenification
    eyelid l.
lichenified lid
Lichtenberg corneal trephine
LICO
    L. disposable penlight
    L. Hertel exophthalmometer
lid
    l. agglutination
    l. block
    Celsus l.
    l. closure reaction
    l. closure reflex
    l. crease
    l. crusting
    l. droop
    droopy l.
    l. ectropion
    l. edema
    l. eversion
    l. everter
    l. fissure
    l. forceps
    granular l.
    l. imbrication syndrome
    l. lag
    l. laxity
    lichenified l.
    l. loading
    lower l. (LL)
    l. margin
    l. margin laceration
    l. notching
    l. nystagmus
    l. plate
    l. retraction
    l. scrub
    l. scurf
    l. speculum
    l. thrush
    tonic l.
    l. trephine
    upper l. (UL)
    l. vesicle
    L. Wipes-SPF
LidFix speculum

lidocaine
    l. hydrochloride
    intracameral l.
    intraocular l.
    l. with epinephrine
Lidoject
Lidoject-1 with epinephrine
lids, lashes, lacrimals, lymphatics (LLLL)
lid-triggered synkinesia
Lieberman
    L. aspirating speculum
    L. fragmentor
    L. K-Wire speculum
    L. lens-holding forceps
    L. MicroFinger manipulator
    L. micro-ring lens forceps
    L. phaco crusher
    L. wire aspirating speculum with V-shape blade
Lieberman-Pollock double corneal forceps
Lieberman-type
    L.-t. speculum, reversible thin solid blade
    L.-t. speculum, thin solid blade
    L.-t. speculum with Kratz open wire blade
Lieb-Guerry lens
Liebreich symptom
Lieppman cystitome
LIF
    local intraarterial fibrinolysis
life
    Health-Related Quality of L. (HRQOL)
    Low Vision Quality of L. (LVQOL)
life-belt cataract
Li-Fraumeni syndrome
lift
    SOOF l.
    suborbicularis oculi fat l.
lifter
    Weinstein fixation ring and flap l.
ligament
    canthal l.
    check l.
    ciliary l.
    cribriform l.
    Hueck l.
    hyaloideocapsular l.
    intracapsular l.
    lateral palpebral l.
    Lockwood l.
    medial canthal l.
    medial palpebral l.
    palpebral l.
    pectinate l.

pectineal l.
suspensory l.
Weigert l.
Whitnall l.
Wieger l.
Zinn l.
ligamentum
l. circulare corneae
l. pectinatum anguli iridocornealis
l. pectinatum iridis
light
l. and accommodation (L&A)
l. adaptation
l. argon laser burn
autokinesis visible l.
axial ray of l.
Barkan l.
L. Blade laser workstation
blur anatomy point source of l.
central l.
l. coagulation
cobalt blue l.
coherent l.
convergent l.
dichromatic l.
l. difference
l. differential threshold
l. discrimination
divergent l.
emergent ray of l.
ether theory of l.
fixation l.
flashes of l.
idioretinal l.
incident ray of l.
intrinsic l.
Lumiwand l.
marginal ray of l.
l. microscope
l. microscopy
minimum l.
monochromatic red HeNe laser l.
near reaction to l.
oblique ray of l.
ophthalmoscopy with reflected l.
l. optometer reflex
paraxial ray of l.
perception of l. (PL)
l. perception (LP)
l. perception only (LPO)
peripheral ray of l.
pipe l.

l. pipe pick
polarized l.
polychromatic l.
l. projection
l. projection test
pupils equal, react to l. (PERL)
ray of l.
l. reaction
reflected l.
l. reflex ring
refracted l.
l. response of pupil
l. scatter
l. scattering
l. sensation
l. sense
l. sensitivity
Serdarevic Circle of L.
l. stimulus
l. toxicity
l. transmission
transmitted l.
ultraviolet l.
unit of l.
white l.
Young theory of l.
light-activated drug
light-adapted eye
light-adjustable IOL
LightBlade
Novatec L.
light/dark (L/D)
l./d. amplitude ratio
light-dark discrimination (LDD)
lighted flute needle
light-emitting diode (LED)
Lighthouse
L. Distance Visual Acuity Test
L. ET-DRS acuity chart
L. Low Vision Service
lighting
paraxial l.
light-near dissociation
lightning
l. cataract
l. eye movement
L. high speed cutter
L. high-speed vitrectomy handpiece
l. streak
light-optometer
light-peak to dark-trough ratio
light-stress test

NOTES

ligneous
l. conjunctivitis
lignocaine hydrochloride
lilacinus
Paecilomyces l.
limbal
l. allograft
l. approach
l. arcade
l. autografting
l. autograft transplantation (LAT)
l. bleeding
l. cell allografting
l. choristoma
l. compression
l. conjunctiva
l. conjunctivitis
l. dermoid
l. follicle
l. girdle
l. girdle of Vogt
l. groove
l. guttering
l. ischemia
l. luteus retinae
l. neurofibroma
l. palisades of Vogt
l. papillae
l. parallel orientation
l. relaxing incision (LRI)
l. stem cell
l. stem-cell deficiency
l. stem-cell transplantation
l. stroma
l. tissue
l. vasculitis
l. zone
limbal-based flap
limbal-conjunctival autograft transplantation (LCAT)
limbal-conjunctivitis autograft
limbi (*pl. of* limbus)
limbic vernal keratoconjunctivitis
limbitis
Limbitrol
limbus, pl. **limbi**
balding the l.
blue l.
circumferential vascular plexus of the l.
congenital dermoid of l.
conjunctival l.
l. of cornea
corneal inferior l.
corneoscleral l.
cystoid cicatrix of l.
l. girdle
l. guttering
l. mass

l. palpebrales anteriores
l. palpebrales posteriores
l. parallel orientation straddling tattoo mark
l. of perception
l. of sclera
limbus-based conjunctival flap
limit
Rayleigh l.
limitation
eccentric l.
limited gallium scan
limiting
l. angle
l. lamina
l. lamina anterior
l. layer
l. membrane
Lincoff
L. balloon
L. balloon catheter
L. lens sponge
L. operation
L. scleral sponge implant
Lindane Shampoo
Lindau disease
Lindau-von Hippel disease
Linde cryogenic probe
Lindner
L. operation
L. sclerotomy
L. spatula
Lindsay operation
Lindstrom
L. arcuate incision marker
L. astigmatic marker
L. Centrex lens
L. LASIK spatula
L. lens-insertion forceps
L. small incision marker
L. Star
L. Star nucleus manipulator
Lindstrom-Casebeer algorithm
Lindstrom-Chu aspirating speculum
line
absorption l.
A Maddox l.
angular l.
Arlt l.
atopic l.
blue l.
Brücke l.
chatter l.
corneal iron l.
CVD black diamond keratome l.
datum l.
l. of direction
distance between nasal l.'s (DBL)
Donders l.

Egger l.
Ehrlich-Türck l.
endothelial rejection l.
epithelial iron l.
face l.
Ferry l.
fingerprint l.
l. of fixation
flat demarcation l.
Fraunhofer l.
gray l.
Helmholtz l.
Hudson l.
Hudson-Stähli l.
iron l.
iron-ferry l.
iron-Hudson-Stähli l.
iron-Stocker l.
Khodadoust l.
mare's hair l.
mare's tail l.
Morgan l.
Paton l.
pigment demarcation l.
principal l.
pupillary l.
rejection l.
retinal stress l.
Sampaoelesi l.
Schwalbe l. (SL)
l. of sight
Snellen l.
Stähli pigment l.
Stocker l.
stromal l.
superficial corneal l.
l. test
triradiate l.
Turk l.
l. of vision
visual l.
l. of visual acuity
Vogt l.
Zentmyer l.
Zöllner l.
linea, pl. **lineae**
l. corneae senilis
l. visus
linear
l. endotheliitis
l. infiltration
l. keratopathy

l. scar
l. scarring
l. sebaceous nevus sequence
l. streak lesion
l. subcutaneous atrophy
l. vision
l. visual acuity test
linkage analysis
Linn-Graefe iris forceps
lint-free sponge
LIO500
IRIS L.
Lions
L. Doheny Eye and Tissue Transplant Bank
L. Low Vision Center
lip
anterior l.
scleral l.
lipemia retinalis
lipemic
l. retina
l. retinopathy
lipid
l. accumulation
l. cell
l. degeneration
l. deposit
l. exudate
l. keratopathy
l. tear layer
lipoarabinomannan-B (LAM-B)
lipoatrophic diabetes
lipocytic lesion
lipodermoid
conjunctival l.
lipofuscinosis
ceroid l.
juvenile neuronal ceroid l. (JNCL)
neuronal ceroid l.
lipoides
arcus lipoides
lipoidosis corneae
lipoma
orbital l.
lipomatosis
ptosis l.
lipoplethoric diabetes
Lipo-Tears Forte
lippa
lippitude, lippitudo
Lipschütz inclusion body

L

NOTES

lipuric diabetes
liquefaciens
    Serratia l.
liquefaction
    contraction and l.
    vitreal l.
liquid
    l. organic dye laser
    l. perfluorocarbon
    L. Pred
    l. vitreous-aspirating cannula
liquified vitreous
Liquifilm
    Albalon L.
    Betagan L.
    Bleph-10 L.
    L. Forte
    L. Forte Solution
    Herplex L.
    HMS L.
    Prefrin Z L.
    P.V. Carpine L.
    L. Rewetting Solution
    L. Tears
    L. Tears Solution
    L. Wetting
liquor
    l. corneae
    Morgagni l.
Lisch
    L. corneal dystrophy
    L. nodule
    L. spot
Lisinopril
lissamine
    l. green
    l. green stain
Lister
    L. forceps
    L. scissors
Listeria
Listing
    L. law
    L. plane
    L. primary position
    L. reduced eye
    L. schematic eye
    L. torsion
Lite
    Angiofluor L.
Liteflex lens
Lite-Pred
literal alexia
lithiasis
    l. conjunctivae
    conjunctival l.
    l. conjunctivitis
lithotriptor
    candela laser l.

Littauer
    L. cilia forceps
    L. dissecting scissors
Littler dissecting scissors
Littmann Galilean magnification changer
Live/Dead Kit stain
Livernois
    L. lens-holding forceps
    L. pickup and folding forceps
living-related conjunctival limbal allograft (lr-CLAL)
Livingston peribulbar wedge
Living Water Eye Lotion
Livostin
LKP
    maximum depth LKP (MD-LKP)
LL
    lower lid
LLLL
    lids, lashes, lacrimals, lymphatics
Llobera fixation forceps
Lloyd stereocampimeter
LMX1B **gene**
loading
    lid l.
loafer temple
Loa loa
lobe
    frontal l.
    occipital l.
    palpebral l.
    parietal l.
    temporal l.
    temporoparietal l.
Lobob
    L. GP Starter Kit
    L. Hard Contact Lens Wetting Solution
    Optimum by L.
    L. Rigid Hard Contact Lens Soaking Solution
lobule
    lacrimal acinar l.
lobulus, pl. lobuli
    coloboma lobuli
local
    l. anesthetic
    l. deviation (LD)
    l. intraarterial fibrinolysis (LIF)
    l. outgrowth
    l. tic
    l. tonic pupil
localization
    Comberg l.
    spatial l.
localized
    l. albinism
    l. amyloidosis

localizer
 Berman l.
 lens l.
 Roper-Hall l.
 Wildgen-Reck l.
location anomaly
locator
 Berman foreign body l.
 Bronson-Turner foreign body l.
 foreign body l.
 Roper-Hall l.
 Sweet l.
 Wildgen-Reck l.
loci (*pl. of* locus)
lock
 Luer cannula l.
Lockwood
 L. ligament
 L. light reflex
 superior tendon of L.
 L. tendon
LOCS
 Lens Opacification Classification System
Loctoplate
locus, pl. **loci**
 l. of fixation
 gene l.
 GLCIA l.
 preferred retinal l. (PRL)
 retinoblastoma l.
 trained retinal l.
lodoxamide
 l. tromethamine
 l. tromethamine ophthalmic solution
Loewi
 L. reaction
 L. sign
Löfgren syndrome
logadectomy
logarithmic Minimum Angle of
 Resolution (logMAR)
LOGIC
 laryngeal and ocular granulation tissue in
 children from the Indian subcontinent
 LOGIC syndrome
logistic discriminant analysis
logMAR
 logarithmic Minimum Angle of
 Resolution
 logMAR chart
log unit
Löhlein operation

Lombart
 L. radioscope
 L. tonometer
lomustine
Londermann
 L. corneal trephine
 L. operation
long
 l. ciliary nerve
 l. posterior ciliary artery
 l. root of ciliary ganglion
 l. sight
long-acting gas
longi
 nervi ciliares l.
longitudinal
 l. aberration
 l. axis
 l. axis of Fick
 l. ciliary muscle
 l. fasciculus
 l. fiber
 L. Optic Neuritis Study (LONS)
 L. Study of Ocular Complications
 of AIDS (LSOCA)
long-scale contrast
long/short occluder
longsightedness
long-term comparative study
long-wearing contact lens
LONS
 Longitudinal Optic Neuritis Study
LOOK
 Lenses and Overnight Orthokeratology
Look
 L. capsule polisher
 L. cortex extractor
 L. cystitome
 L. I/A coaxial cannula
 L. irrigating lens loop
 L. irrigating vectis
 L. micropuncture device
 L. retrobulbar needle
 L. suture
looking
 forced choice preferential l.
loop
 Axenfeld nerve l.
 C l.
 Clayman-Knolle irrigating lens l.
 closed l.
 congenital prepapillary vascular l.

L

NOTES

297

loop *(continued)*
>expressor l.
>flexible l.
>Flynn lens l.
>haptic l.
>intrascleral nerve l.
>irrigating vectis l.
>J l.
>Knapp lens l.
>Knolle-Pearce irrigating lens l.
>lens l.
>Look irrigating lens l.
>Meyer-Archambault l.
>Meyer temporal l.
>modified J l.
>nerve l.
>nylon l.
>open l.
>Pearce-Knolle irrigating lens l.
>prepapillary arterial l.
>prepapillary vascular l.
>temporal l.
>two-angled polypropylene l.
>vascular l.
>venous l.

loose
>l. contact lens
>l. lens

loperamide
Lopez-Enriquez
>L.-E. operation
>L.-E. scleral trephine

loratadine
Lordan chalazion forceps
lorgnette occluder
Loring ophthalmoscope
loss
>axonal l.
>blood l.
>central field l. (CFL)
>chiasmal visual field l.
>field l.
>functional visual l.
>glaucomatous visual field l.
>hearing l.
>hemisensory l.
>intraoperative blood l.
>migrainous vision l.
>nasal field l.
>nonorganic visual l.
>nonphysiologic visual field l.
>progressive hearing l.
>retrochiasmal visual field l.
>scintillating vision l.
>scotopic sensitivity l.
>sudden visual l.
>transient visual l.
>unilateral hearing l.

>vascular optical disk swelling without visual l.
>vision l.
>l. of vision
>vitreous l.
>l. of vitreous

lost rectus muscle
Lotemax ophthalmic suspension
loteprednol
>l. etabonate
>l. etabonate ophthalmic solution
>l. etabonate ophthalmic suspension

lotion
>Living Water Eye L.

Lotman Visometer
lotrafilcon A lens
Lo-Trau side-cutting needle
Lotze local sign
louchettes
loupe
>Amenabar lens l.
>angled lens l.
>angled nucleus removal l.
>Arlt lens l.
>Atwood l.
>Beebe l.
>Berens lens l.
>binocular l.
>Callahan lens l.
>Castroviejo lens l.
>Elschnig-Weber l.
>FormFlex lens l.
>Gullstrand l.
>Ilg lens l.
>Keeler panoramic l.
>Kirby intracapsular lens l.
>Kirby intraocular lens l.
>Kraff nucleus lens l.
>Lemoine-Searcy fixation anchor l.
>Lempert-Storz l.
>lens l.
>Lewis lens l.
>magnifying l.
>Mark II Magni-Focuser l.
>New Orleans lens l.
>nucleus delivery l.
>nucleus removal l.
>Ocular Gamboscope l.
>operating l.
>Opt-Visor l.
>panoramic l.
>Simcoe l.
>Simcoe double-end lens l.
>Simcoe II PC nucleus delivery l.
>Simcoe nucleus lens l.
>Snellen lens l.
>Troutman lens l.
>Visitec nucleus removal l.
>Weber-Elschnig lens l.

Wilder lens l.
Zeiss-Gullstrand l.
Zeiss operating field l.
Lovac
  L. fundus contact lens implant
  L. gonioscope
  L. gonioscopic lens
  L. six-mirror gonioscopic lens
    implant
low
  l. contrast
  l. convex
  l. myopia
  l. profile R-K marker
  l. total spherical aberration
  l. vision
  L. Vision Functional Status
    Evaluation (LVFSE)
  L. Vision Quality of Life
    (LVQOL)
  L. Vision Quality of Life
    Questionnaire (LVQOLQ)
low-contrast
  l.-c. distance visual acuity
    (LCDVA)
  L.-c. Sloan Letter Chart (LCSLC)
Lowe
  L. oculocerebrorenal syndrome
  L. ring
Lowell glaucoma knife
Löwenstein-Jensen medium
Löwenstein operation
lower
  l. canaliculus
  l. eyelid
  l. eyelid spacer
  l. hemianopsia
  l. lid (LL)
  l. lid laxity
  l. lid retractor
  l. lid sling procedure
  l. punctum
  l. retina
Lowe-Terrey-MacLachlan syndrome
low-pressure glaucoma
Lowry assay
low-tension glaucoma
low-vision
  l.-v. aid
  l.-v. enhancement system (LVES)
loxophthalmus

LP
  light perception
LPI
  laser iridotomy
LPK-80 II argon laser
LPO
  light perception only
LPSA
  late postoperative suture adjustment
L.R.
  lateral rectus
    Visine L.R.
lr-CLAL
  living-related conjunctival limbal
    allograft
LRI
  limbal relaxing incision
    LRI diamond blade
LSK
  L. One disposable Microkeratome
  L. One standard microkeratome
LSM-2100C eye bank specular
microscope
LSOCA
  Longitudinal Study of Ocular
  Complications of AIDS
L.T. Jones tear duct tube
LTK
  laser thermal keratoplasty
    noncontact LTK
LTS
  laser tomography scanner
Lube-free petrolatum, mineral oil
lubricant
lubricant
  lens l.
  Lube-free petrolatum, mineral oil l.
  silicone l.
lubricating drops
lubrication
  surface l.
Lubricoat
Lubrifair
LubriTears
  L. Lubricant Eye Ointment
  L. Solution
Lucae dressing forceps
lucency, pl. **lucencies**
lucida
  camera l.
  lamina l.

L

NOTES

lucidum
> tapetum l.

Lucite
> L. frame
> L. sphere implant

Luedde
> L. exophthalmometer
> L. transparent rule

Luer
> L. cannula lock
> L. connection
> L. syringe tip
> L. tube

Luer-Lok
> L.-L. syringe
> Yale L.-L.

luetic
> l. chorioretinitis
> l. interstitial keratitis
> l. neuropathy

lugdunensis
> *Staphylococcus l.*

lumbricoides
> *Ascaris l.*

lumen, pl. **lumina, lumens**
> capillary l.

Lu-Mendez
> L.-M. LRI guide
> L.-M. LRI guide and fixation ring

Lumigan ophthalmic solution
lumina (*pl. of* lumen)
luminance
> background l.
> l. rivalry
> l. setting
> l. size threshold perimetry

luminosity curve
luminous
> l. flux
> l. intensity (I)
> l. retinoscope

lumirhodopsin
Lumiwand light
Lumonics laser
lunata
> *Curvularia l.*
> plica l.

Lundsgaard
> L. knife
> L. rasp
> L. sclerotome

Lundsgaard-Burch
> L.-B. corneal rasp
> L.-B. sclerotome

Luneau retinoscopy rack
Luntz-Dodick punch
lupus
> l. chiasmatis

> l. erythematosus cell test
> l. oculopathy

Lurocoat
luster
> binocular l.
> corneal l.
> polychromatic l.

lusterless
lustrous central yellow point
lutea
> macula l.

lutein
> Ocuvite L.

lutetium
> motexafin l.
> l. texaphyrin (lu-tex)

luteum
> punctum l.

lu-tex
> lutetium texaphyrin

Lu type corneal LASIK marker
luxated lens
luxation
> l. of eyeball
> l. of globe
> l. of lens
> superior oblique muscle and
> trochlear l.

Luxo surgical illuminator
lux setting
luxurians
> ectropion l.

luxury perfusion
LVES
> low-vision enhancement system
> head-mounted video magnifier
> LVES

LVFSE
> Low Vision Functional Status Evaluation

LVQOL
> Low Vision Quality of Life

LVQOLQ
> Low Vision Quality of Life
> Questionnaire

LX
> Millennium LX
> LX needle

Lyda-Ivalon-Lucite implant
Lyle syndrome
Lyme disease keratitis
lymphangioma
> conjunctival l.
> eyelid l.

lymphatic
> l. drainage
> l. sinusoid chorioid

lymphatics
> lids, lashes, lacrimals, l. (LLLL)

lymphaticus
    nodulus l.
lymphoblastic lymphoma
lymphocytic
    l. choriomeningitis virus
    l. infiltration
lymphoepithelial lesion
lymphoepithelioma
Lymphogranuloma
    L. venereum conjunctivitis
    L. venereum keratitis
lymphoid
    l. follicle
    l. hyperplasia
    l. infiltration
    l. pseudotumor
    l. tumor
lymphoma
    anterior chamber l.
    histiocytic l.
    intraocular l.
    large-cell l.
    lymphoblastic l.
    MALT l.
        mucosa-associated lymphoid tissue
          lymphoma
    mucosa-associated lymphoid
      tissue l. (MALT lymphoma)
    non-Hodgkin l.
    oculocerebral l.
    orbital l.

    porcupine l.
    primary central nervous system l.
      (PCNSL)
    primary ocular l.
    reticulum cell l.
    signet-ring l.
    T-cell l.
    well-differentiated small-cell l.
      (WDSCL)
    zone B-cell l.
lymphomatosis
    ocular l.
lymphophagocytosis
lymphoproliferative tumor
Lynch
    L. approach
    L. medial canthal incision
Lynell intraocular lens
Lyon hypothesis
lysed
lysis
    cell l.
    l. of restricting strand
    symblepharon l.
lysosomal storage disease
lysozyme
    serum l.
Lythgoe effect
lytic lesion
Lytico-Bodig syndrome

L

NOTES

M
　　myopia
　　myopic
　　　M band
　　　M cell
　　　M cone excitation
3M
　　　3M small aperture Steri-Drape
　　　3M Steri-Drape drape
M4-400 freedom blade
MAC
　　monitored anesthesia care
Macbeth
　　　M. ColorChecker
　　　M. illumination
MacCallan
　　　M. classification
　　　M. classification of trachoma
Macewen sign
Machado-Joseph disease
Machat
　　　M. adjustable aspirating wire
　　　　speculum
　　　M. double-ended marker
　　　M. superior flap LASIK marker
**Machat-type adjustable aspirating
　LASIK speculum**
Mach band
Machek-Blaskovics operation
Machek-Brunswick operation
Machek-Gifford operation
Machek ptosis operation
Machemer
　　　M. calipers
　　　M. diamond-dust-coated foreign
　　　　body forceps
　　　M. flat lens
　　　M. infusion contact lens
　　　M. magnifying vitrectomy lens
　　　M. vitreous cutter
machine
　　　Catalyst m.
　　　CooperVision I/A m.
　　　Euro Precision Technology
　　　　submicron lathe m.
　　　I/A m.
　　　SITE irrigation/aspiration m.
　　　Stat Scrub handwasher m.
　　　Visual-Tech m.
Mackay-Marg
　　　M.-M. electronic tonometer
　　　M.-M. principle
Mack-Brunswick operation
Mackool system
MacRae flap flipper/retreatment spatula

macroaneurysm
　　　arterial m.
　　　retinal arterial m.
macroblepharia
macrocornea
macrocupping
　　　pseudoglaucomatous m.
macrocyst
macrocytic anemia
macrodisc
　　　congenital m.
macroerosion
macromovement
macroperforation
**macrophage migration inhibitory factor
　(MMIF)**
macrophthalmia
macrophthalmic
macrophthalmous
macropia
macropsia
macroptic
macroreticular dystrophy
macrosaccadic oscillation
macro square-wave jerks
macrostereognosis
macrovessel
MACRT
　　　Monoclonal Antibody CMV Retinitis
　　　　Trial
macula, pl. maculae
　　　m. adherens
　　　maculae ceruleae
　　　cherry-red spot in m.
　　　m. corneae
　　　dragged m.
　　　ectopia maculae
　　　false m.
　　　m. flava retinae
　　　graying of m.
　　　Henle layer of the m.
　　　heterotropia maculae
　　　honeycomb m.
　　　inferior m.
　　　m. lutea
　　　m. lutea pigment
　　　m. lutea retinae
　　　parafoveal m.
　　　superonasal m.
　　　temporal m.
　　　vitelliform degeneration of m.
**macula-off rhegmatogenous retinal
　detachment**
**macula-on rhegmatogenous retinal
　detachment**

M

macular, maculate
- m. aplasia
- m. area
- m. arteriole
- m. arteriole occlusion
- m. binocular vision
- m. branch retinal vein occlusion (MBRVO)
- m. choroiditis
- m. cluster
- m. CMV
- m. coloboma
- m. computerized psychophysical test (MCPT)
- m. contact lens
- m. corneal dystrophy
- m. cytomegalovirus
- m. detachment
- m. disciform degeneration
- m. disease
- m. displacement
- m. dragging
- m. drusen
- m. dysplasia
- m. ectopia
- m. edema
- m. epiretinal membrane
- m. evasion
- m. graying
- m. heredodegeneration
- m. hole (MH)
- m. hole formation
- m. hole surgery
- m. hypoplasia
- m. leak
- m. neuroretinopathy
- m. ocular histoplasmosis syndrome
- m. OHS
- m. photocoagulation
- M. Photocoagulation Study (MPS)
- m. photostress
- m. pseudohole (MPH)
- m. pucker
- m. puckering
- m. retinoblastoma
- m. retinopathy
- m. sparing
- m. splitting
- m. star
- m. stereopsis
- m. suppression
- m. surface wrinkling
- m. telangiectasia
- m. traction
- m. translocation
- m. translocation with macular infolding

- m. translocation with scleral infolding (MTSI)
- m. venule

MaculaRx Plus nutritional supplement
maculary fasciculus
maculate (*var. of* macular)
macule
maculocerebral
maculopapillary bundle
maculopapular bundle
maculopathy
- age-related m. (ARM)
- atrophic degenerative m.
- bull's eye m.
- cellophane m.
- cystoid m.
- diabetic m.
- dry senile degenerative m.
- exudative senile m.
- familial pseudoinflammatory m.
- Groenouw type II m.
- heredity m.
- histoplasmosis m.
- hypotony m.
- ischemic m.
- Kuhnt-Junius m.
- myopic m.
- niacin m.
- nicotinic acid m.
- operating microscope-induced phototoxic m.
- photic m.
- phototoxic m.
- pigment epithelial detachment m.
- serous detachment m.
- solar m.
- Sorsby m.
- Stargardt m.
- toxic m.
- unilateral acute idiopathic m.
- vitelliform m.

maculorrhexis
- ILM m.

maculosa
- atrophia striata et m.

MaculoScope
maculovesicular
MacVicar double-end strabismus retractor
madarosis
Maddox
- M. LASIK spatula
- M. prism
- M. rod
- M. rod method
- M. rod occluder
- M. rod test
- M. wing test

Madribon

madurae
    Actinomadura m.
Madurai Intraocular Lens Study IV
Maeder-Danis dystrophy
mafilcon A
Magendie
    M. sign
    M. symptom
Magendie-Hertwig
    M.-H. sign
    M.-H. syndrome
Magitot keratoplasty operation
magnae
    facies orbitalis alae m.
magnet
    Bronson-Magnion eye m.
    eye m.
    Gruening m.
    Haab m.
    hand-held eye m.
    Hirschberg m.
    implant m.
    Lancaster eye m.
    m. operation
    original Sweet eye m.
    rare earth intraocular m.
    Schumann giant type eye m.
    Storz-Atlas hand eye m.
    Storz Microvit m.
    Sweet original m.
magnetic
    m. extraction
    m. field-search coil test
    m. implant
    m. operation
    m. resonance angiography (MRA)
    m. resonance imaging (MRI)
    m. resonance imaging scan
    m. resonance spectroscopy (MRS)
magnification
    relative spectacle m.
magnifier
    Circline m.
    hand-held m.
    model 1559 m.
    Optelec Passport m.
    projection m.
    spectacle m.
    stand m.
magnifying
    m. glasses
    m. lens

    m. loupe
    m. power
magnitude of ptosis
magnocellular
    m. cell
    m. visual pathway
Magnus operation
Maguire-Harvey vitreous cutter
Maidera-Stern suture hook
Maier
    sinus of M.
    M. sinus
main fiber
Mainster
    M. retinal laser lens
    M. Ultra Field PRP laser lens
    M. wide field lens
Mainster-HM retinal laser lens
Mainster-S retinal laser lens
Mainster-WF retinal laser lens
maintained
    central, steady and m. (CSM)
    good, central, m. (GCM)
    good, central, not m. (GCNM)
maintainer
    anterior chamber m. (ACM)
    Blumenthal anterior chamber m.
    Fary anterior chamber m.
    Lewicky self-retaining chamber m.
    Mendez-Freeman pediatric A.C. m.
Majewsky operation
major
    m. amblyoscope
    m. amblyoscope test
    anulus iridis m.
    m. arcade
    m. arterial circle of iris
    m. basic protein (MBP)
    circulus arteriosus iridis m.
    erythema multiforme m.
    m. histocompatibility antigen
    m. histocompatibility complex
    (MHC)
    m. meridian
majoris
    facies orbitalis alae m.
Maklakoff tonometer
malalignment
malattia leventinese
Malbec operation
Malbran operation
mal del Meleda

M

NOTES

maleate
>chlorpheniramine m.
>naphazoline and pheniramine m.
>pilocarpine and timolol m.
>timolol m.

malformation
>Arnold-Chiari m.
>arteriovenous m.
>Chiari m.
>congenital brain m.
>dural arteriovenous m.
>infratentorial arteriovenous m.
>orbital arteriovenous m.
>retinal arteriovenous m.
>retinal vascular m.
>supratentorial arteriovenous m.

Malherbe calcifying epithelioma
malignant
>m. choroidal melanoma
>m. ciliary epithelioma
>m. dyskeratosis
>m. epithelial tumor
>m. exophthalmos
>m. glaucoma
>m. granular cell tumor metastatic
>m. hypertension
>m. hyperthermia
>m. melanoma of the choroid
>m. melanoma of the iris
>m. mesenchymoma
>m. myopia
>m. neurilemoma
>m. pituitary lesion
>m. schwannoma
>m. scleritis

Malis
>M. bipolar coagulating/cutting
>system
>M. forceps

Mallazine eye drops
mallet
>lead-filled m.

Maloney nucleus rotator
malprojection
MALT
>mucosa-associated lymphoid tissue
>MALT lymphoma

maltophilia
>*Stenotrophomonas m.*

Man
>Mendelian Inheritance in M.
>(MIM)

management
>medical m.

Manche
>M. irrigation cannula
>M. LASIK forceps
>M. LASIK speculum

Manche-type LASIK irrigating cannula

Mandelkorn suture laser lysis lens
maneuver
>Carlo Traverso m. (CTM)
>doll's eye m.
>doll's head m.
>Hallpike m.
>notch-and-roll m.
>Nylen-Barany m.
>oculocephalic m.
>Valsalva m.
>wall push m.

manganese superoxide dismutase
Manhattan
>M. Eye & Ear probe
>M. Eye & Ear spatula
>M. Eye & Ear suturing forceps

manifest
>m. deviation
>m. hyperopia (Hm)
>m. latent nystagmus
>m. refraction (MR)
>m. strabismus

manifestation
>neuroophthalmic m.
>neurovisual m.

manipulation
>laser m.
>pharmacologic m.
>physical m.

manipulator
>Akahoshi nucleus m.
>angled m.
>Batlle ICL m.
>button-tip m.
>Drysdale nucleus m.
>Friedman Phaco/IOL m.
>Grieshaber three-function m.
>Grieshaber two-function m.
>Guimaraes ICL m.
>Guimaraes implantable contact
>lens m.
>Jaffe/Maltzman IOL m.
>Jarrett side port m.
>Judson-Smith m.
>Koch nucleus m.
>Koch phaco m.
>Kuglein irrigating lens m.
>Kuglen lens m.
>Kuglen nucleus m.
>LASIK flap m.
>lens m.
>Lester IOL m.
>Lester lens m.
>Lieberman MicroFinger m.
>Lindstrom Star nucleus m.
>McIntyre irrigating iris m.
>Rappazzo intraocular m.
>Sharvelle side-port nucleus m.
>Sinskey IOL m.

Visitec m.
Wan side-port nucleus m.
manner
McLean m.
Mannis
M. probe
M. suture
mannitol
mannosidosis
Mann sign
Mann-Whitney U test
manometer
Honan m.
Tycos m.
manometry
manoptoscope
Manson-Aebli corneal section scissors
Manson double-ended strabismus hook
Mantel-Haenszel method
Mantoux test
manual
m. keratometer
m. kinetic perimetry
m. lamellar keratoplasty
m. vitrectomy
Manz gland
MAO
Montana Academy of Ophthalmology
map
axial curvature m.
corneal m.
m. dystrophy
elevation topography m.
m. pattern
rasterstereography-based
elevation m.
wave aberration m.
map-dot corneal dystrophy
map-dot-fingerprint (MDF)
m.-d.-f. corneal epithelial dystrophy
mapping
axial curvature m.
deletion m.
glaucomatous damage detection by
retinal thickness m.
Orbscan pachymetry m.
placido-based axial curvature m.
visually evoked potential m.
mapropsia
MAR
melanoma-associated retinopathy
MAR syndrome

marbleization
Marcaine
M. HCl
M. HCl with epinephrine
marcescens
Serratia m.
March
M. laser lens
M. laser sclerostomy needle
Marco
M. chart projector
M. lensometer
M. manual keratometer
M. perimeter
M. prism exophthalmometer
M. radius gauge
M. refractor
M. slit lamp
M. SurgiScope
Marcus
M. Gunn (MG)
M. Gunn dot
M. Gunn jaw-winking phenomenon
M. Gunn jaw-winking syndrome
M. Gunn pupil
M. Gunn pupillary sign
M. Gunn relative afferent defect
M. Gunn test
mare's
m. hair line
m. tail line
Marfan
M. sign
M. syndrome
margin
ciliary m.
eyelid m.
fimbriated m.
infraorbital m.
lash m.
lid m.
orbital m.
palpebral m.
pupillary m.
marginal
m. blepharitis
m. catarrhal ulcer
m. chalazion forceps
m. conjunctiva
m. corneal degeneration
m. corneal ulcer
m. crystalline dystrophy

NOTES

M

marginal *(continued)*
    m. degeneration of cornea
    m. entropion
    m. furrow
    m. furrow degeneration
    m. keratitis
    m. melt
    m. myotomy
    m. ray of light
    m. reflex distance (MRD)
    m. ring ulcer of cornea
    m. tear strip
marginalis
    blepharitis m.
marginoplasty
margo
    m. ciliaris iridis
    m. infraorbitalis orbitae
    m. lacrimalis maxillae
    m. lateralis orbitae
    m. medialis orbitae
    m. orbitalis
    m. palpebra
    m. pupillaris iridis
    m. supraorbitalis orbitae
    m. supraorbitalis ossis frontalis
Marie ataxia
Marinesco-Sjögren-Garland syndrome
Marinesco-Sjögren syndrome
Mariotte
    blind spot of M.
    M. blind spot
    M. experiment
    M. scotoma
Maritima
    succus cineraria M.
mark
    M. II Magni-Focuser lens
    M. II Magni-Focuser loupe
    M. IX lens
    limbus parallel orientation
      straddling tattoo m.
    Nichamin fixation right with 10-
      degree m.'s
marker
    Akura PDAK m.
    Amsler scleral m.
    Anis radial m.
    Anis suture placement m.
    Arrowsmith corneal m.
    ASSI triple m.
    astigmatic m.
    Berkeley optic zone m.
    biprong muscle m.
    Bores axis m.
    Bores optic zone m.
    Bores radial m.
    Castroviejo corneal transplant m.
    Castroviejo scleral m.

Chayet type corneal LASIK m.
corneal transplant m.
Deblasio LASIK m.
Dell astigmatism m.
Desmarres m.
Dulaney LASIK M.
Ellis astigmatism m.
Feldman RK optical center m.
Fine Toric/LRI m.
Fink biprong m.
Fink muscle m.
Friedlander incision m.
Fukuyama LRI m.
Gass scleral m.
Geggel corneal transplant m.
Gonin m.
Gonin-Amsler m.
Grandon T-incision m.
Green corneal m.
Green-Kenyon corneal m.
Hoffer optical center m.
Hoffer optic zone m.
Hoffman/Buratto LASIK m.
Hofmann T-incision m.
Hoopes corneal m.
Hunkeler frown incision m.
Kershner LRI m.
Koch LRI m.
Kraff LRI m.
Lindstrom arcuate incision m.
Lindstrom astigmatic m.
Lindstrom small incision m.
low profile R-K m.
Lu type corneal LASIK m.
Machat double-ended m.
Machat superior flap LASIK m.
Matos laser axis m.
McDonald optic zone m.
Mendez hexagon m.
Mendez type corneal LASIK m.
microsatellite m.
Neuhann glaucoma m.
Neumann-Shepard corneal m.
Neumann-Shepard oval optical
    center m.
Nordan-Ruiz trapezoidal m.
O'Brien m.
O'Connor m.
ocular m.
optical zone m.
Osher-Neumann corneal m.
Perone LASIK m.
Phillips gravity pivot axis m.
polymorphic microsatellite m.
Price Radial M.
Probst Smiley LASIK m.
radial keratotomy m.
RK m.
Ruiz-Nordan trapezoidal m.

scleral m.
Shepard optical center m.
Simcoe corneal m.
Soll suture and incision m.
Spivack axis m.
Storz radial incision m.
Thornton optical center m.
Thorton optic zone m.
Thurmond pachymetry m.
USC m.
Visitec RK zone m.
Zaldivar LRI m.
m.'s for zone
marking pen
Markwell
method of M.
Marlex mesh
Marlin Salt System II
Marlow test
Marmor
pattern dystrophy of pigment
epithelium of Byers and M.
Marner cataract
Marquez-Gomez
M.-G. conjunctival graft
M.-G. operation
Marshall syndrome
Marsh disease
Martegiani
area M.
Martinez
M. corneal transplant centering ring
M. corneal trephine blade
M. disposable corneal trephine
M. dissector
M. keratome
M. knife
Martin Surefit lens pusher
mascara particle inclusion
Masciuli silicone sponge
masked diabetes
Masket
M. capsulorrhexis forceps
M. Phaco spatula
mask-like facies
masque biliaire
masquerade
m. syndrome
m. technique
mass
choroidal m.
cicatricial m.

coalescent m.
gelatinous m.
hyaline m.
intracranial m.
laminated acellular m.
limbus m.
mulberry-shaped m.
mycelial m.
ochre m.
ovoid m.
subfoveal m.
subretinal m.
yellow-white choroidal m.
Massachusetts
M. Eye & Ear Infirmary
M. Vision Kit (MVK)
M. XII vitrectomy system (MVS)
massage
Crigler m.
ocular m.
Masselon
M. glasses
M. spectacles
massive
m. granuloma of sclera
m. osteolysis of Gorham
m. periretinal proliferation (MPP)
m. vitreous retraction (MVR)
Masson trichrome stain
mast
m. cell
m. cell stabilizer
Mastel
M. compass-guided arcuate
keratotomy system
M. diamond compass
M. Finish for application to
microkeratome head
M. Precision surgical instrument
M. trifaceted diamond blade
master-dominant eye
master eye
Masuda-Kitahara disease
match
HLA m.
human leucocyte antigen m.
mate
Lens M.
Soft M.
material
alloplastic donor m.
autogenous donor m.

NOTES

309

material *(continued)*
    coating m.
    contrast m.
    cyanographic contrast m.
    donor m.
    fibrillar m.
    gallium citrate contrast m.
    gelatinous m.
    heterogeneous donor m.
    homogeneous donor m.
    hyaline m.
    m.'s primary dye
    M.'s Testing System
    viscoelastic m.
Matos laser axis marker
M.A.T. postoperative comfort device
matrix, pl. **matrices**
    acellular m.
    extracellular m. (ECM)
    glycocalyx m.
    m. metalloproteinase (MMP)
    stromal m.
matte
    m. black forceps
    m. black instrument
matter
    particulate m.
    periaqueductal gray m.
Mattis corneal scissors
mattress suture
maturation
    delayed visual m.
    preinjury visual m.
mature
    m. cataphoria
    m. cataract
    m. lens
maturity-onset diabetes
Mauksch-Maumenee-Goldberg operation
Mauksch operation
Maumenee
    M. capsule forceps
    M. corneal forceps
    M. erysiphake
    M. goniotomy knife
    M. goniotomy knife cannula
    M. iris hook
    M. knife goniotomy cannula
    M. Suregrip forceps
    M. vitreous-aspirating needle
    M. vitreous sweep spatula
Maumenee-Colibri corneal forceps
Maumenee-Goldberg operation
Maumenee-Park eye speculum
Maunoir iris scissors
Maurer spot
Maurice corneal depot technique
mauritaniensis
    Acanthamoeba m.

Mauthner test
Max
    M. Fine forceps
    M. Fine scissors
Maxidex
maxilla, pl. **maxillae**
    incisura maxillae
    infraorbital margin of m.
    infraorbital sulcus of m.
    lacrimal sulcus of m.
    margo lacrimalis maxillae
    processus zygomaticus maxillae
    sulcus infraorbitalis maxillae
    zygomaticoorbital process of the m.
maxillaris
    nervus m.
maxillary
    m. bone
    m. nerve
    m. osteomyelitis
    m. sinusitis
maximal illumination
maximum
    m. depth LKP (MD-LKP)
    m. tolerated medical therapy
Maxitrol
MaxiVision
    M. dietary supplement
    M. Ocular Formula
    M. Whole Body Formula
Maxwell
    M. ring
    M. spot
Maxwell-Lyons sign
Mayo
    M. Clinic
    M. scissors
    M. stand
May sign
Mazzotti reaction
MBP
    major basic protein
M-brace corneal trephine
MBRVO
    macular branch retinal vein occlusion
MC-7000
    M. multi-wavelength laser
    M. ophthalmic laser
McCannel
    M. implant
    M. lens
    M. ocular pressure reducer
    M. suture
    M. suture technique
McCarey-Kaufman
    M.-K. preserved donor tissue
    M.-K. transport medium
McCarthy reflex
McClure iris scissors

McCollough effect
McCool capsule retractor
McCullough suturing forceps
McCune-Albright syndrome
McDonald
    M. expressor
    M. lens-folding forceps
    M. optic zone marker
    M. soft IOL folding forceps
McGannon
    M. refractor
    M. retractor
McGavic operation
McGhan
    M. implant
    M. 3M intraocular lens
McGregor conjunctival forceps
McGuire
    M. conformer
    M. corneal scissors
    M. I/A system
    M. marginal chalazion forceps
    M. operation
McIntyre
    M. anterior chamber cannula
    M. coaxial cannula
    M. coaxial irrigating/aspirating
    system
    M. fish-hook needle holder
    M. I/A needle
    M. I/A system
    M. III nucleus removal system
    M. infusion set
    M. irrigating/aspirating unit
    M. irrigating hook
    M. irrigating iris manipulator
    M. irrigation/aspiration needle
    M. irrigation/aspiration system
    M. nylon cannula connector
    M. reverse cystitome
    M. spatula
    M. truncated cone
McIntyre-Binkhorst irrigating cannula
McKee speculum
McKinney
    M. eye speculum
    M. fixation ring
McLaughlin operation
McLean
    M. capsule forceps
    M. capsulotomy scissors
    M. classification of melanoma

    M. fashion
    M. manner
    M. muscle recession forceps
    M. operation
    M. prismatic fundus laser lens
    M. suture
    M. technique
    M. tonometer
McMonnies questionnaire
McNeill-Goldman
    M.-G. blepharostat
    M.-G. ring
McNemar test
mCNV
    myopic choroidal neovascularization
MCP
    multifocal choroiditis with panuveitis
MCP-1
    monocyte chemotactic protein-1
McPherson
    M. angled forceps
    M. bent forceps
    M. corneal forceps
    M. corneal section scissors
    M. irrigating forceps
    M. microiris forceps
    M. microsuture forceps
    M. needle holder
    M. spatula
    M. speculum
    M. suturing forceps
    M. trabeculotome
    M. tying iris forceps
McPherson-Castroviejo corneal section scissors
McPherson-Vannas microiris scissors
McPherson-Westcott
    M.-W. conjunctival scissors
    M.-W. stitch scissors
McPherson-Wheeler
    M.-W. blade
    M.-W. knife
McPherson-Ziegler knife
MCPT
    macular computerized psychophysical test
McQueen vitreous forceps
McReynolds
    M. keratome
    M. lid-retracting hook
    M. operation
    M. pterygium knife

M

NOTES

McReynolds *(continued)*
    M. pterygium scissors
    M. pterygium transplant
    M. spatula
    M. technique
MD
    mean deviation
MDF
    map-dot-fingerprint
    MDF corneal dystrophy
MD-LKP
    maximum depth LKP
meals
    before m. (a.c.)
mean
    m. acuity
    m. corneal power
    m. deviation (MD)
    m. episcleral heat dose
    M.'s sign
    m. spherical equivalent (MSE)
measure
    Doppler flowmetry m.
    Geneva lens m.
measurement
    A m.
    B m.
    box m.
    C m.
    color-contrast sensitivity m.
    criterion-free m.
    digital fitting m.
    direct m.
    diurnal intraocular pressure m.
    entopic foveal avascular zone m.
    glare disability m.
    Krimsky m.
    one-eye m.
    postocclusion m.
    prism cover m.
    psychophysical m.
    Rushton ocular m.
    Stenstrom ocular m.
    white-to-white m.
mechanical
    m. acquired ptosis
    m. ectropion
    m. epithelial brush
    m. lid retraction
    m. strabismus
    m. vitrector
mechanics
    fluid m.
mechanism
    m. of action
    cAMP mediated m.
    cholinergic m.
    fixation m.
    Hering after-image m.

    immune m.
    oculogyric m.
    primary m.
    pursuit m.
    secondary m.
    trigger m.
mechanized scissors
Mecholyl test
Mectizan
MED
    minimal effective diameter
Medallion lens
Medcast epoxy resin
MedDev implant
media *(pl. of* medium)
medial
    m. angle
    m. angle of eye
    m. arteriole of retina
    m. canthal ligament
    m. canthal repair
    m. canthal tendon
    m. canthus
    m. commissure of eyelid
    m. ectropion
    m. horn
    m. longitudinal fasciculus (MLF)
    m. longitudinal fasciculus lesion
     (MLF lesion)
    m. palpebral ligament
    m. rectus (MR)
    m. rectus extraocular muscle
    m. rectus function
    m. rectus palsy
    m. rectus transposition
    m. superior temporal (MST)
    m. superior temporal visual area
    m. venulae of retina
    m. vestibular nucleus (MVN)
medialis
    angulus oculi m.
    commissura palpebrarum m.
    venula retinae m.
mediaometer
mediator
    inflammatory m.
medical
    m. adenomectomy
    m. management
    m. ophthalmoscopy
    M. Optics PC11NB intraocular lens
    M. Optics PC11NB intraocular lens
     implant
    m. tattooing
    M. Workshop intraocular lens
    M. Workshop intraocular lens
     implant
medicamentosa
    conjunctivitis m.

medication
    psychotropic m.
Medicornea Kratz intraocular lens implant
Medi-Duct ocular fluid management system
Meditec
    M. bandage contact lens
    M. MEL-60 excimer laser
Mediterranean anemia
medium, pl. **media**
    anaerobic m.
    chondroitin sulfate m.
    media clearing
    contrast m.
    corneal storage m.
    culture m.
    dextran m.
    dioptric m.
    gram-negative m.
    Kaufman m.
    K-Sol m.
    Löwenstein-Jensen m.
    McCarey-Kaufman transport m.
    M-K m.
    ocular m.
    media opacity
    opaque m.
    Optisol m.
    Page m.
    refracting m.
    refractive m.
    Sabouraud m.
MedJet microkeratome
Med-Logics ML Microkeratome
Medmont M600 perimeter
medocromil sodium ophthalmic solution
MedOne
    M. Ducournau fine gripping forceps
    M. ILM forceps
Medpor MCOI implant
Medrol
medroxyprogesterone acetate
medrysone
medulla lesion
medullary
    m. cystic disease
    m. optic disease
    m. ray
medullated nerve fiber
medulloblastoma tumor

medulloepithelioma
    adult m.
    embryonal m.
    orbital m.
Meek operation
Meesman
    M. epithelial corneal dystrophy
    M. juvenile epithelial dystrophy
megadose
megalocornea
megalopapilla
megalophthalmia
megalophthalmus
    anterior m.
megalopia
megalopsia, megalopia
meglumine antimonate
megophthalmus
meibomian
    m. blepharitis
    m. conjunctivitis
    m. cyst
    m. disease
    m. duct
    m. gland carcinoma
    m. gland dysfunction (MGD)
    m. gland expressor
    m. gland obstruction
    m. gland orifice metaplasia
    m. sebaceous gland
    m. secretion
    m. sty
meibomianitis
    acne rosacea m.
meibomianum
    hordeolum m.
meibomitis
meibum oleic acid
Meige syndrome
MEL
    M. 60, 80 excimer laser
    M. 70 flying spot laser
    M. 60 scanning laser
melanin
melaninogenicus
    Bacteroides m.
melanocyte
    uveal m.
melanocytic
    m. conjunctival lesion
    m. hamartoma

M

NOTES

melanocytic *(continued)*
    m. iris tumor
    m. nevus
melanocytoma
melanocytosis
    congenital ocular m.
    congenital oculodermal m.
    ocular m.
    oculodermal m.
melanokeratosis
    striate m.
melanoma
    amelanotic choroidal m.
    cavitary uveal m.
    choroidal amelanotic m.
    ciliary body m.
    ciliochoroidal m.
    conjunctival m.
    cutaneous m.
    m. of eyelid
    intraocular m.
    iris m.
    m. of iris
    juvenile m.
    malignant choroidal m.
    McLean classification of m.
    metastatic m.
    nodular m.
    ocular m.
    orbital m.
    pagetoid m.
    posterior uveal m.
    ring m.
    spindle A, B m.
    spindle cell m.
    tapioca iris m.
    uveal m.
melanoma-associated
    m.-a. retinopathy (MAR)
    m.-a. retinopathy syndrome
melanomalytic glaucoma
melanosis
    acquired m.
    m. bulbi
    diabetic m.
    m. iridis
    ocular m.
    m. oculi
    oculodermal m.
    presenile m.
    primary acquired m. (PAM)
    m. sclerae
melanosome
    giant m.
melanotic
    m. lesion
    m. sarcoma
    m. schwannoma

Melauskas
    M. acrylic implant
    M. orbital implant
Meleda
    mal del M.
Melkersson-Rosenthal syndrome
Melkersson syndrome
Mellaril
Meller
    M. operation
    M. refractor
Mellinger speculum
mellitus
    adult-onset diabetes m. (AODM)
    diabetes m. (DM)
    gestational diabetes m.
    insulin-dependent diabetes m.
     (IDDM)
    juvenile diabetes m.
    non-insulin-dependent diabetes m.
melt
    corneal m.
    corneoscleral m.
    marginal m.
    sterile m.
    stromal m.
melting
    corneal m.
    scleral m.
    stromal m.
MEM
    Monocular Estimate Method
    MEM retinoscopy
Memantine
membrana, pl. **membranae**
    m. capsularis lentis posterior
    m. choriocapillaris
    m. epipapillaris
    m. fusca
    m. granulosa externa
    m. granulosa interna
    m. hyaloidea
    m. limitans externa
    m. limitans interna
    m. nictitans
    m. pupillaris
    m. ruyschiana
    m. vitrea
membranacea
    cataracta congenita m.
membrane
    amniotic m.
    anterior basal m.
    anterior hyaloid m. (AHM)
    Barkan m.
    basement m. (BM)
    bilaminar m.
    Biopore m.
    Bowman m.

Bruch m.
choroidal neovascular m. (CNVM)
conjunctival m.
connective tissue m.
contraction of cyclitic m.
cyclitic m.
Demours m.
Descemet m.
diabetic m.
Duddell m.
endothelial cell basement m.
epimacular m.
epipapillary m.
epiretinal m. (ERM)
epithelial basement m.
external limiting m.
fibroglial m.
fibroproliferative m.
fibrovascular m.
Fresnel m.
glassy m.
gliotic m.
Haller m.
Henle m.
Hovius m.
hyaline m.
hyalitis of anterior m.
hyaloid posterior m.
idiopathic epiretinal m. (IERM)
idiopathic preretinal m.
inner limiting m.
intermuscular m.
internal limiting m. (ILM)
Jacob m.
limiting m.
m. lipid cell
macular epiretinal m.
mucous m.
neovascular m.
nictitating m.
occult choroidal neovascular m.
ochre m.
onion skin-like m.
outer limiting m.
panretinal m.
m. peeler-cutter
m. peeling
periorbital m.
pigmented preretinal m.
posterior hyaloid m. (PHM)
preretinal m.
pupillary m.

purpurogenous m.
reduplication of Descemet m.
Reichert m.
retrocorneal m.
Ruysch m.
ruyschian m.
secondary m.
serous m.
stripping m.
subfoveal neovascular m.
subretinal m. (SRM)
subretinal neovascular m. (SRNVM)
tarsal m.
Tenon m.
trabecular m.
vitreal m.
vitreous m.
Wachendorf m.
wrinkling m.
Zinn m.

membranectomy
**membranoproliferative glomerulonephritis
  type II**
membranotomy
membranous
    m. cataract
    m. conjunctivitis
    m. rhinitis
memory
    immunologic m.
    visual m.
MemoryLens
    M. IOL
    Mentor ORC M.
Mendelian Inheritance in Man (MIM)
Mendez
    M. astigmatism dial
    M. cystitome
    M. degree gauge
    M. hexagon marker
    M. multi-purpose LASIK forceps
    M. type corneal LASIK marker
Mendez-Freeman
    M.-F. pediatric A.C. maintainer
    M.-F. silicone oil cannula
**Mendez-Goldbaum Tri-Port subtenon
  anesthesia cannula**
meningeal
    m. carcinomatosis
    m. cell
    m. hemangiopericytoma

M

NOTES

meningioma
    angioblastic m.
    fibroblastic m.
    nerve sheath m.
    ocular m.
    optic nerve sheath m. (ONSM)
    orbital m.
    perioptic sheath m.
    psammomatous m. (PM)
    sphenoid wing m.
    suprasellar m.
meningitidis
    Neisseria m.
meningitis
    carcinomatous m.
    cryptococcal m.
    gummatous m.
meningocele
meningococcosis
meningococcus conjunctivitis
meningocutaneous angiomatosis
meningoencephalocele
meningosepticum
    Flavobacterium m.
meniscus, pl. menisci
    m. concave lens
    converging m.
    diverging m.
    m. floater
    Kuhnt m.
    negative m.
    periscopic m.
    positive m.
    tear of m.
Mentanium vitreoretinal instrument set
Mentor
    M. B-VAT II BVS contour circles distance stereoacuity test
    M. B-VAT II BVS random dot E distance stereoacuity test
    M. B-VAT II monitor
    M. B-VAT II video acuity tester
    M. curved eraser
    M. Exeter ophthalmoscope
    M. fine-focus microscope
    M. ORC MemoryLens
    M. precut drain
    M. wet-field cautery
    M. wet-field electrocautery
    M. wet-field eraser
Mentor-Maumenee Suregrip forceps
meperidine hydrochloride
mepivacaine HCl
Mepron
mercurialentis
mercuric oxide
mercury (Hg)
    m. bag

    millimeters of m. (mmHg, mm Hg)
    m. pressure
Meretoja syndrome
meridian
    m. of cornea
    corneal m.
    equatorial m.
    m. of eyeball
    horizontal m.
    major m.
    steepest m.
    vertical m.
meridiani bulbi oculi
meridianus
meridional
    m. aberration
    m. amblyopia
    m. balance
    m. ciliary muscle fiber
    m. fold
    m. implant
    m. refractometer
Merkel cell neoplasm
Mermoud nonpenetrating glaucoma forceps
Merocel
    M. lint-free sponge
    M. surgical spear
meropia
Merrimac laser
Mersilene suture
mesangial cell
mesencephalic
    m. lesion
    m. lid retraction
mesencephalon lesion
mesenchymal
    m. dysgenesis
    m. ridge
    m. tumor
mesenchyme
    hemocytic m.
    neurogenic m.
    orbital m.
mesenchymoma
    malignant m.
mesh
    Marlex m.
    tantalum m.
meshwork
    trabecular m. (TM)
mesiris
mesoblastic tissue
mesochoroidea
Meso contact lens
mesocornea
mesoderm
    paraxial m.
mesodermal dysgenesis

mesodermalis
    primary dysgenesis m.
mesophryon
mesopia
mesopic perimetry
mesoretina
mesoridazine
mesoropter
mesylate
    nelfinavir m.
metabolic
    m. coma
    m. syndrome cataract
metachromatic leukodystrophy
metacontrast
metaherpetic
    m. keratitis
    m. ulcer
    m. ulceration of the cornea
metakeratitis
metalloproteinase
    matrix m. (MMP)
metallosis
    toxic retinal m.
metallothionein gene
metameric color
metamorphopsia
    cerebral m.
    m. varians
metaplasia
    conjunctival m.
    meibomian gland orifice m.
    squamous m.
metaplastic epithelial cell
metarhodopsin
metastasis, pl. **metastases**
    chiasmal m.
    choroidal m.
    hematogenous m.
    hematopoietic m.
    leptomeningeal m.
    orbital m.
    pyogenic m.
    m. of tumor
    tumor m.
    uveal m.
metastatic
    m. carcinoma
    m. choroidal tumor
    m. choroiditis
    m. endophthalmitis
    malignant granular cell tumor m.

    m. melanoma
    m. ophthalmia
    m. retinitis
Metcher speculum
Metenier sign
meter
    m. angle
    foot candle m.
    Guyton-Minkowski potential
     acuity m.
    Kowa FM-500 laser flare m.
    laser cell and flare m. (LCFM)
    laser flare-cell m.
    m. lens
    potential acuity m. (PAM)
    straylight m.
    van den Berg stray-light m.
    Vuero m.
meter-candle
methacholine chloride
methacrylate
    heparin surface-modified
     polymethyl m.
    methyl m.
    passivated polymethyl m.
MethaSite
methazolamide
methicillin
methicillin-resistant *Staphylococcus aureus* (MRSA)
method
    Barraquer m.
    Bio-Optics Bambi fixed-frame m.
    confrontation m.
    Con-Lish polishing m.
    contact m.
    corners m.
    Crawford m.
    Credé m.
    Cuignet m.
    direct m.
    divide-and-conquer m.
    dot m.
    gradient m.
    grid m.
    heterophoria m.
    Hirschberg m.
    Holmgren m.
    immersion m.
    immunodiagnostic m.
    Kirby-Bauer disk-diffusion m.
    Konan fixed-frame m.

M

NOTES

method *(continued)*
Krimsky m.
Maddox rod m.
Mantel-Haenszel m.
m. of Markwell
Mishima-Hedbys m.
modified band lid m.
Monocular Estimate M. (MEM)
Mueller m.
optical density m.
PCR-SSOP m.
push-up m.
rag-wheel m.
m. of the sphere
Sweet m.
twirling m.
VISX contoured ablation m.
von Graefe prism dissociation m.
Westergren m.
Wheeler m.
Wolfe m.
Methopto
methosulfate
trimethidium m.
methotrexate
methoxsalen
Methulose
methyl
m. cyanoacrylate glue
m. methacrylate
m. propylparaben
methylcellulose
hydroxypropyl m. (HPMC)
**methylenetetrahydrofolate reductase
(MTHFR)**
methylergonovine
methylmethacrylate implant
methylparaben
methylpentynol
methylphenidate
cocaine m.
methyl-phenyl-tetrahydropyridine (MPTP)
methylprednisolone
methylsulfate
neostigmine m.
methysergide
Metico forceps
Meticorten
metilprednisona
Metimyd Ophthalmic
metipranolol
metoprolol
Metreton
metric
m. ophthalmoscope
m. ophthalmoscopy
metrizamide
MetroGel
metronidazole

metronoscope
Metubine Iodide
Metycaine
MEWDS
multiple evanescent white-dot syndrome
Meyer
M. Swiss diamond knife lancet
M. Swiss diamond lancet knife
M. Swiss diamond mini-angled
knife
M. Swiss diamond wedge knife
M. temporal loop
Meyer-Archambault loop
Meyer-Schwickerath
M.-S. coagulator
M.-S. light coagulation
M.-S. operation
Meyhoeffer
M. chalazion
M. chalazion curette
Meynert
M. commissure
superior commissura of M.
MFC
multifocal choroiditis
MFE
multifocal electroretinography
MG
Marcus Gunn
MG pupil
MGD
meibomian gland dysfunction
MGUS
monoclonal gammopathy of
undetermined significance
MH
macular hole
MHC
major histocompatibility complex
MHC gene
mica spectacles
micelles in vitreous
Michaelson
M. counter pressure
M. operation
Michel
M. pick
M. spur
miconazole
Micra double-edged diamond blade
micro
m. Colibri forceps
m. eye movement
M. One pneumatonometer
M. punctum plug
m. round-tip needle
m. Westcott scissors
microadenoma

microaneurysm
>   capillary m.
>   hemorrhage and m. (h/ma)
>   juxtafoveal m.

microaneurysmal leakage
microangiography
microangiopathy
>   circumpapillary telangiectatic m.
>   occlusive m.
>   retinal m.

microanisocoria
microbevel edge lens
microbial keratitis
microbiallergic conjunctivitis
microbiologic experience
microblepharia, microblepharism,
>   **microblepharon, microblephary**

Microcap scalpel
microcautery unit
microcirculation
>   retinal m.

microcoria
microcornea
microcyst
>   Blessig-Iwanoff m.
>   epithelial m.
>   intraepithelial m.
>   punctate epithelial m.

microcystic
>   m. corneal dystrophy
>   m. edema
>   m. epithelial dystrophy
>   m. lesion

microdots
microembolism, pl. **microemboli**
>   retinal m.

microendoscope
>   ophthalmic laser m. (OLM)

microendoscopic test card
microforceps
>   Anis m. model 2-848
>   Birks-Mathelone m.
>   Colibri m.
>   Sparta m.

Microfuge tube
Micro-Glide corneal suture
microgonioscope
microhemagglutination test
microhook
>   Visitec m.

microhyphema
>   traumatic m.

microhypopyon
microinfarct
>   retinal m.

microinfarction
microjaw
>   Keeler-Catford needle holder
>   with m.'s

**Microjet-based cutting and debriding
device**
microkeratome
>   ALTK system m.
>   Amadeus m.
>   Automated Corneal Shaper m.
>   Barraquer m.
>   Barraquer-Carriazo m.
>   BD K-3000 m.
>   Carriazo-Barraquer m.
>   Carriazo-Pendular m.
>   Chiron ACS m.
>   Chiron Hansatome m.
>   Corneal Shaper m.
>   femtosend pulse intrastromal
>   laser m.
>   FlapMaker disposable m.
>   Hansatome m.
>   Innovatome m.
>   Krumeich-Barraquer m.
>   K-tome m.
>   LSK One disposable M.
>   LSK One standard m.
>   MedJet m.
>   Med-Logics ML M.
>   MK-2000 m.
>   ML M.
>   Moria automated M2 m.
>   Moria Model One m.
>   ONE disposable m.
>   Ruiz m.
>   SCMD m.
>   SKBM m.
>   Summit Krumeich-Barraquer m.
>   (SKBM)
>   Supratome m.

microKnife
>   Ultrasharp round blade m. AU
>   681-21-3

microlaser
>   Diode m.

Microlase transpupillary diode laser
microloop curette polisher
microlymphocytotoxicity technique

NOTES

micromanipulator
  self-centering m.
Micromatic ophthalmometer
micromegalopsia
micromesh sheeting
micrometer
  diamond m.
  m. disk
  m. knife
  Tolman m.
  ultrasonic m.
micromovement
  m. of eye
  retinal m.
micronystagmus
micropannus
microperforation
microperimeter
microperimetry
microphakia
microphotography
microphthalmia, microphthalmos,
  microphthalmus
  colobomatous m.
  cystic m.
microphthalmos
  posterior m.
microphthalmoscope
microphthalmus (*var. of* microphthalmia)
micropia
micropick
  vitreoretinal m.
micropigmentation system
micropins
  Pischel m.
microplate fixation
micropoint
  m. needle
  m. suture
MicroProbe
  Endo Optiks M.
  M. integrated laser endoscope
  M. integrated laser and endoscope
  system
  M. ophthalmic laser
microproliferation
micropsia
  cerebral m.
  convergence-accommodative m.
  psychogenic m.
  retinal m.
microptic
micropuncture
  anterior stromal m.
Microputor II (MR2)
Micro-Reflux Test (MRT)
microruptor
  Lasag M.
microsaccades

microsatellite marker
microscalpel
  Oasis feather m.
microscissors
  DORC microforceps and m.
  iris m.
  Kamdar m.
  Keeler m.
  Twisk m.
microscope
  binocular m.
  Binocular Indirect Ophthalmic M.
    (BIOM)
  Bio-Optics specular m.
  Bitumi monobjective m.
  Cohan-Barraquer m.
  confocal laser scanning m.
  ConfoScan 2.0 slit corneal
    confocal m.
  CooperVision m.
  corneal m.
  Czapski m.
  electron m.
  EM-1000 specular m.
  Fiberlite m.
  Galilean m.
  Heyer-Schulte Medical Optic Center
    specular m.
  JSM-54 IOLV m.
  JSM-6400 scanning electron m.
  Keeler-Konan Specular m.
  Keeler specular m.
  Konan Noncon ROBO-CA SP-8000
    noncontact specular m.
  Konan Sp-5500 contact specular m.
  Konan SP8000 noncontact
    specular m.
  Leitz m.
  light m.
  LSM-2100C eye bank specular m.
  Mentor fine-focus m.
  Moller m.
  Nikon NS-1 slit-lamp m.
  Olympus Vanox VH-2 m.
  OM 2000 operation m.
  operating m.
  OPMI pico i m.
  OPMI PRO magis m.
  OPMI VISU 200 m.
  Optiphot m.
  PRO CEM-4 m.
  Project Research Ophthalmic
    specular m.
  Pro-Koester wide-field SCM m.
  Reichert Zetopan M.
  scanning slit confocal m.
  slit-lamp m.
  SMZ-10A zoom stereo m.
  specular m.

Storz m.
tandem scanning confocal m.
Tomey ConfoScan confocal m.
Topcon SP-1000 noncontact
  specular m.
transmission electron m.
video specular m.
Weck m.
white light tandem-scanning
  confocal m.
Wild operating m.
Zeiss-Barraquer cine m.
Zeiss-Barraquer surgical m.
Zeiss OM-3 operating m.
Zeiss OpMi-6 FR m.
microscopic hyphema
microscopy
confocal m.
fluorescence m.
fundus m.
light m.
specular m.
transmission electron m.
microscotometry
MicroSeal
M. ophthalmic handpiece
Storz M.
microserrated Tano asymmetrical
peeling forceps
MicroShape Keratome System
Micro-Sharp blade
microspatula
Birks Mark II m.
microspectroscope
Microsphaeropsis olivacea
microspherometer
microspherophakia
microsponge
Alcon m.
M. Teardrop sponge
microsporidia
microsporidial keratoconjunctivitis
microstrabismic amblyopia
microstrabismus
microsurgery
microsurgical knife
microthin contact lens
MicroTip phaco tip
microtome
Microtonometer
Computon M.
MicroTrac Direct Specimen Test

microtrauma
microtremor
ocular m.
superior oblique m.
unilateral m.
microtropia
microtropic syndrome
microtubule
microvascular
m. abnormality
m. decompression
microvasculopathy
retinal m.
microvillus, pl. microvilli
Microvit
M. probe
M. probe system
Storz Premiere M.
M. vitrector
microvitrector
microvitreoretinal (MVR)
m. blade
m. spatula
microwave
m. hyperthermia
m. plaque thermotherapy
m. radiation injury
midbrain
m. corectopia
m. disease
m. pseudo-sixth
m. ptosis
mid-coquille lens
middle
m. cerebral artery
m. temporal visual area
midfacial fracture
midget system
midline
m. granuloma
m. position
m. position of gaze
midperiphery
midsightedness
midstromal
Mietens syndrome
migraine
basilar m.
m. equivalent
m. headache
hemiplegic m.
ocular m.

NOTES

migraine *(continued)*
    ophthalmic m.
    m. ophthalmoplegia
    ophthalmoplegic m.
    retinal m.
    transformed m.
migrainous
    m. hallucination
    m. ophthalmoplegia
    m. vision loss
migrans
    erythema chronicum m.
    keratitis linearis m.
    ocular larva m.
    visceral larva m. (VLM)
migrating epithelium
migration
    bleb m.
    epithelial m.
    implant m.
    pigmentary m.
    m. theory
migratory ophthalmia
Mikamo double-eyelid operation
Mikulicz disease
Mikulicz-Radecki syndrome
Mikulicz-Sjögren syndrome
mild
    m. blurring
    m. chromic suture
    GenTeal M.
    Inflamase M.
    m. periocular hemorrhage
    Pred M.
milia
    eyelid m.
miliary
    m. aneurysm
    m. tuberculosis chorioretinitis
milk-alkali syndrome
milky cataract
Millard-Gubler syndrome
Millennium
    M. CX, LX microsurgical system
    M. LX
    M. Transconjunctival Standard
      Vitrectomy 25 System
    M. TVS25 System
    M. vitreous cutter
Miller-Fisher
    M.-F. syndrome
    M.-F. variant
Miller-Nadler glare tester
Miller syndrome
Milles syndrome
millet seed nodule
Millex filter
millimeters of mercury (mmHg, mm Hg)

Millipore filter
Milli-Q water purification system
Milroy Artificial Tears
MIM
    Mendelian Inheritance in Man
    MIM card
mimicking
    finger m.
Minardi phaco chopper
mind blindness
miner's
    m. blindness
    m. disease
    m. nystagmus
miniature
    m. blade
    m. forceps
minicircular capsulorrhexis
Mini-Drops eye therapy
mini-excimer
    Compak-200 m.-e.
miniflap
    scleral m.
mini-keratoplasty
    Castroviejo m.-k.
    m.-k. stitch scissors
minimal
    m. amplitude nystagmus
    m. brain dysfunction
    m. effective diameter (MED)
    m. pigment oculocutaneous albinism
minimum
    m. deviation
    m. light
    m. light threshold
    m. perceptible acuity
    m. separable acuity
    m. separable angle
    m. visible angle
    m. visual angle
miniophthalmic drape
miniplate
    titanium m.
    Vitallium m.
MiniQuad XL lens
Mini-tip culturette
mini-trabulectomy
Minocin
minocycline
Minolta
    M. illuminance meter TL-1
    M. LS 110 spot photometer
minor
    anulus iridis m.
    circulus arteriosus iridis m.
Minsky
    M. circle
    M. intramarginal splitting
    M. operation

minus
    m. carrier
    m. carrier contact lens
    m. cyclophoria
    m. cylinder
    m. spectacle lens
Miocel
Miochol-E
Miochol solution
miosis
    congenital m.
    irritative m.
    paralytic m.
    pupil m.
    pupillary m.
    senescent m.
    senile m.
    spastic m.
    spinal m.
    traumatic pupillary m.
Miostat intraocular
miotic
    m. alkaloid
    m. pupil
    m. therapy
Mira
    M. AGL-400
    M. cautery
    M. diathermy
    M. diathermy unit
    M. electrocautery
    M. encircling element
    M. endovitreal cryopencil
    M. photocoagulator
    M. silicone rod
Miracon
MiraFlow
    M. Daily Cleaner
    M. Extra-Strength
MiraSept System
MiraSol
mires
    image of m.
    keratometer m.
    m. of ophthalmometer
mirror
    m. area
    m. coating
    concave m.
    contact lens training m.
    convex m.
    4-M. Gonio lens

    m. haploscope
    head m.
    m. image
    power of m.
    m. rocking test
misalignment
    convergent m.
misdirected lash
misdirection
    aqueous m.
    facial nerve m.
    oculomotor nerve m.
    m. phenomenon
Mishima-Hedbys method
M.I.S. multi-port illumination system
mist
    Nature's Tears all natural soothing
        eye m.
misty vision
Mitchell viscoelastic removal I/A tip
mitochondrial
    m. disease
    m. myopathy
mitomycin C (MMC)
mitosis
    epithelial m.
mitotic
Mitsubishi HL7955 CRT screen
Mittendorf dot
MityVac simple hand pump
Mitzuo phenomenon
mivacurium
mixed
    m. astigmatism
    m. bacterial-fungal keratitis
    m. cataract
    m. esotropia
    m. fungal keratitis
    m. strabismus
    m. tumor
mixing
    color m.
mixture
    Neo-Synephrine cocaine m.
    Richardson methylene blue/aure
        II m.
Miyajima LASIK calipers
Miyake
    M. photography
    M. technique
    M. view

M

NOTES

Miyoshi chopper
mizoribine (MZR)
Mizuo-Nakamura
    M.-N. effect
    M.-N. phenomenon
MK-2000
    MK-2000 keratome system
    MK-2000 microkeratome
MK IV ophthalmoscope
MKM
    myopic keratomileusis
M-K medium
MLF
    medial longitudinal fasciculus
    MLF lesion
ML Microkeratome
MMC
    mitomycin C
    adjunctive MMC
mmHg, mm Hg
    millimeters of mercury
MMIF
    macrophage migration inhibitory factor
MMP
    matrix metalloproteinase
Möbius
    M. disease
    M. sign
    M. syndrome
Möbius-von Graefe-Stellway sign
MOBS
    modified binary search
mode
    m. of action
    free running m.
    function of Zernike m.
    pulse m.
model
    M. A-Scan DGH 500e
    Bohr m.
    m. eye
    Floater eye m.
    Gullstrand six-surface eye m.
    M. 201-20 high-flow 0.20-mm
      filter Luer lock fitting
    Kooijman eye m.
    Le Grand-Gullstrand eye m.
    m. 1559 magnifier
    reduced eye m.
    m. 177-33 viscocanalostomy
      cannula
    von Helmholtz eye m.
mode-locked Nd:YAG laser
moderate
    m. amblyopia
    GenTeal M.
    m. myopia
modification
    ApopTag m.

    Deller m.
    Smith m.
    Van Herick m.
modified
    m. band lid method
    m. binary search (MOBS)
    M. Clinical Technique test
    M. Clinical Technique vision
      screening
    m. C-loop intraocular lens
    m. C-loop UV lens
    m. corncrib (inverted T) procedure
    M. Dandy Criteria
    m. J loop
    m. J-loop intraocular lens
    m. J-loop UV lens
    m. monovision
    m. Van Lint anesthesia
    m. Van Lint block
    m. Wies procedure
Modular One pneumatonometer
modulation transfer function
Moehle
    M. cannula
    M. corneal forceps
Mohs microsurgical resection
Moiré fringe
Moistair Humidifying Chamber
moistened fine mesh gauze dressing
moisture
    m. chamber
    M. Eyes
    M. Eyes PM
    M. Eyes PM eye ointment
    M. ophthalmic drops
molded
    m. frame
    m. pressing
molding
    cast m.
    compression m.
    injection m.
mold-injected lens
molectron laser
molecular
    m. dissociation theory
    m. external layer
    m. inner layer
    m. internal layer
    m. outer layer
Moll
    M. gland
    M. gland cystadenoma
Moller microscope
Mollon-Reffin minimal test
molluscum
    m. conjunctivitis
    m. contagiosum
    m. virus

Molteno
    M. episcleral explant
    M. implant
    M. shunt tube
Momose lens
Monakow
    M. fiber
    M. syndrome
Monarch
    M. II intraocular lens delivery system
    M. II IOL delivery system
Moncrieff
    M. cannula
    M. discission
    M. operation
mongolian
    m. fold
    m. spot
mongoloid slant
moniliaceous filamentous fungus
moniliforme
    Fusarium m.
monitor
    Mentor B-VAT II m.
    Proview eye pressure m.
monitored anesthesia care (MAC)
monoblepsia
monocanalicular intubation
monochroic
monochromasia
monochromasy, monochromacy
    blue cone m.
    rod m.
monochromat
    atypical m.
    cone m.
    rod m.
monochromatic
    m. aberration
    m. cone
    m. eye
    m. ray
    m. red HeNe laser light
monochromatism
    blue cone m.
    cone m.
    rod m.
    X-linked blue cone m.
monocle
monoclonal
    m. antibody

    M. Antibody CMV Retinitis Trial (MACRT)
    m. gammopathy of undetermined significance (MGUS)
monocular
    m. aphakia
    m. bandage
    m. bobbing movement
    m. confrontation visual field test
    m. dazzle
    m. depth perception
    m. diplopia
    m. dressing
    m. electrooculogram
    M. Estimate Method (MEM)
    m. field defect
    m. fixation
    m. glaucoma
    m. heterochromia
    m. indirect ophthalmoscope
    m. nystagmus
    m. occlusion
    m. oscillopsia
    m. patch
    m. strabismus
    m. telescope
    m. temporal crescent
    m. vision
monocular-estimate-method dynamic retinoscopy
monoculus
monocyte chemotactic protein-1 (MCP-1)
monodiplopia
monofilament nylon suture
monofixational phoria
monofixation syndrome
monograph
    Gullstrand m.
monolateral strabismus
monolayered endothelium
mononuclear
    m. cell infiltration
    m. reaction
    m. response
monophosphate
    adenosine m. (AMP)
    cyclic adenosine m. (cAMP)
    cyclic guanidine m.
    cyclic guanosine m. (cGMP)
monophthalmica
    polyopia m.
monophthalmos

M

NOTES

monopia
monostearate
    glyceryl m.
monotherapy
monovision
    modified m.
montage
    retinal m.
Montana Academy of Ophthalmology (MAO)
month
    3-m. postoperative refractive cylinder
Moody fixation forceps
moon blindness
Moore
    M. lens forceps
    M. lens-inserting forceps
    M. lightning streak
Mooren
    M. corneal ulcer
    M. ulceration
Moore-Troutman corneal scissors
Moore-Wilson hyperopic conformer
Moran
    M. operation
    M. proptosis
Morax
    M. keratoplasty
    M. operation
Morax-Axenfeld conjunctivitis
Moraxella
    M. bovis
    M. catarrhalis
    M. keratitis
    M. lacunata
    M. nonliquefaciens
morbillorum
    Gemella *m.*
Morcher
    M. iris diaphragm IOL, type 67G
    M. iris diaphragm ring
    M. iris diaphragm ring, type 50C
    M. iris diaphragm ring, type 96G
Morck
    M. cement
    M. cement bifocal
Morel-Fatio-Lalardie operation
Moretsky LASIK hinge protector fixation ring
Morgagni
    M. cataract
    M. globule
    M. liquor
    M. sphere
morgagnian
    m. cataract
    m. globule

Morgan
    M. dot
    M. line
Moria
    M. automated M2 microkeratome
    M. Model One microkeratome
    M. obturator
    M. one-piece speculum
    M. trephine
Moria-France dacryocystorhinostomy clamp
Morlet lamellar knife/dissector
morning
    m. glory disk
    m. glory optic atrophy
    m. glory optic disk anomaly
    m. glory retinal detachment
    m. glory syndrome
    m. ptosis
morpheaform pattern
morphometric analysis
Morquio-Brailsford syndrome
Morquio syndrome
Morris
    M. flexible cannula
    M. vertical scissors
Morse code pattern
mosaic pattern
Mosher operation
Mosher-Toti operation
Mosler diabetes
mosquito
    m. clamp
    m. hemostatic forceps
Moss
    M. operation
    M. traction
Motais operation
motexafin lutetium
motile scotoma
motility
    artificial eye m.
    m. implant
    ocular m.
    restricted m.
motion
    m. automated perimetry
    m. detection perimetry
    m. and displacement perimetry
    hand m. (HM)
    m. parallax
    m. perception disorder
    scotoma for m.
    skew m.
    m. vision
    with m.
motoneuron
    ocular m.

motor
m. function
m. fusion
m. nerve
m. oculi
m. root
m. root of ciliary ganglion
m. tic
Visuscope m.
motor-output disability
Mot-R-Pak vitrectomy system
mottled appearance
mottling
early receptor potential m.
m. of fundus
pigment m.
retinal pigment epithelium m.
Moulton lacrimal duct tube
mounds
pearl white m.
mount
unstained wet m.
wet m.
Mount-Reback syndrome
movement
cardinal ocular m.
centripetal m.
cogwheel ocular m.
cogwheel pursuit m.
conjugate horizontal eye m.
conjugate ocular m.
corrective m.
Developmental Eye M. (DEM)
disconjugate roving eye m.
disjugate m.
disjunctive m.
drift m.
extraocular m. (EOM)
eye m.
eye-head m.
facial m.
fixational ocular m.
flick m.
following m.
fusional m.
gaze m.
hand m.
illusion of m.
impaired vergence eye m.
lightning eye m.
micro eye m.

monocular bobbing m.
nonoptic reflex eye m.
nonrapid eye m.
nystagmoid m.
ocular m.
perverted ocular m.
pursuit m.
rapid eye m. (REM)
reflex eye m.
roving eye m.
saccadic eye m.
scissors m.
slow conjugate roving eye m.
smooth-pursuit m.
synkinetic m.
torsional m.
vergence eye m. (VEM)
vermiform m.
version m.
vertical m.
voluntary eye m.
yoke m.
moxifloxacin
MPC automated intravitreal scissors
MPH
macular pseudohole
Mport lens insertion system
MPP
massive periretinal proliferation
MPS
Macular Photocoagulation Study
MPTP
methyl-phenyl-tetrahydropyridine
MP video endoscopic lens attachment
MR
manifest refraction
medial rectus
MR2
Microputor II
MRA
magnetic resonance angiography
Mr. Color test
MRD
marginal reflex distance
MRI
magnetic resonance imaging
FLAIR MRI
MRI scan
M-Rinse
MRS
magnetic resonance spectroscopy

NOTES

M

MRSA
methicillin-resistant *Staphylococcus aureus*
MRT
Micro-Reflux Test
MSE
mean spherical equivalent
MSFC
Multiple Sclerosis Functional Composite
MSQLI
Multiple Sclerosis Quality of Life Inventory
MST
medial superior temporal
MST visual area
M-TEC 2000 Surgical System
MTHFR
methylenetetrahydrofolate reductase
MTI PhotoScreener
MTL trial frame
MTSI
macular translocation with scleral infolding
MT visual area
mucin
m. layer
m. strand
m. of tear
mucin-like glycoprotein
mucinous
m. adenocarcinoma tumor
m. edema
mucocele
sinus m.
mucocutaneous
m. junction
m. lymph node syndrome
mucoepidermoid carcinoma
mucoid discharge
mucolipidosis, pl. **mucolipidoses**
m. IV
Mucomyst
mucopurulent conjunctivitis
mucormycosis
rhinoorbital m.
rhinoorbital-cerebral m.
mucosa-associated
m.-a. lymphoid tissue (MALT)
m.-a. lymphoid tissue lymphoma (MALT lymphoma)
mucosae
hyalinosis cutis et m.
mucosal
m. associated lymphoid tissue
m. neuroma
m. pemphigoid
mucotome
Castroviejo m.

mucous
m. assay
m. discharge
m. membrane
m. membrane graft
m. ophthalmia
m. tear layer
m. thread
mucous-like strand
mucus
ropy m.
m. strand
stringy m.
Mueller
M. cautery
M. cell
M. electric corneal trephine
M. electrocautery
M. electronic tonometer
M. eye shield
M. gland
M. implant
M. lacrimal sac retractor
M. method
M. muscle
M. operation
radial cells of M.
M. refractor
M. speculum
M. trigone
Muhlberger orbital implant
mulberry-shaped mass
mulberry-type papilloma
Muldoon lacrimal dilator
Mules
M. implant
M. operation
M. scoop
M. vitreous sphere
Mulibrey nanism
Müller
M. cell
M. cell footplate
M. end feet
M. fiber
M. muscle
multicore disease
multicorneal perfusion chamber
multicurve contact lens
multifactorial disease
Multiflex anterior chamber lens
multifocal
m. chorioretinal disease
m. choroiditis (MFC)
m. choroiditis with panuveitis (MCP)
m. choroidopathy syndrome
m. electroretinogram
m. electroretinography (MFE)

m. fibrosclerosis
m. hemorrhagic sarcoma
m. intraocular lens implantation
m. posterior pigment epitheliopathy
m. spectacle lens

multiforme
erythema m.
glioblastoma m.

multiincision 10-facet diamond blade
multilocular vesicle
Multilux
multinodularis
episcleritis m.

multinucleated giant epithelial cell
Multi-Optics lens
multipass
interwave-guided m.

multiplanar reconstruction
multiple
m. bottle regimen
m. evanescent white-dot syndrome (MEWDS)
m. lentigines syndrome
m. myeloma
m. ocular motor palsies
m. sclerosis
M. Sclerosis Functional Composite (MSFC)
M. Sclerosis Quality of Life Inventory (MSQLI)
m. vision

Multi-Purpose
ReNu M.-P.

multiquadrant hydrodissection
multiscope
roaming optical access m. (ROAM)

multistage correction
Multi-System incision knife
multivesicular body
mumps keratitis
Munsell color
Munson sign
mupirocin
mural cell
Murdock eye speculum
Murdock-Wiener eye speculum
Murdoon eye speculum
murine
M. Plus Ophthalmic
m. retina
M. Solution
M. sterile saline

M. Tears
M. Tears Plus

Muro
M. 128
M. Opcon
M. Opcon A
M. Tears

Murocel
M. Ophthalmic Solution

Murocoll-2 Ophthalmic
musca, pl. muscae
muscae volitantes

muscarinic cholinergic side effect
muscle
abductor m.
adductor m.
agonist m.
m. belly
bound-down m.
Bowman m.
Brücke m.
ciliary m.
circular ciliary m.
m. clamp
m. cone
congenital fibrosis of the extraocular m.'s (CFEOM)
m. contraction headache
corrugator m.
cyclorotary m.
cyclovertical m.
m. depressor
dilator m.
disinserted m.
elevator m.
external rectus m.
extraocular m. (EOM)
extrinsic m.
m. of eye
eyelid m.
m. force
m. forceps
frontalis m.
Homer m.
m. hook
Horner m.
inferior oblique extraocular m.
inferior rectus extraocular m.
inferior tarsal m.
internal rectus m.
intortor m.
intraocular m. (IOM)

NOTES

M

muscle *(continued)*
 intrinsic ocular m.
 IO m.
 iridial m.
 iris sphincter m.
 Koyter m.
 Landström m.
 lateral rectus extraocular m.
 left inferior rectus m.
 left superior rectus m.
 levator palpebrae superioris m.
 levator trochlear m.
 longitudinal ciliary m.
 lost rectus m.
 medial rectus extraocular m.
 Mueller m.
 Müller m.
 oblique m.
 ocular m.
 oculorotatory m.
 orbicularis oculi m.
 orbicularis oris m.
 orbital m.
 palpebrae superioris m.
 palsy of m.
 m. paretic nystagmus
 preseptal orbicularis m.
 pupillary dilator m.
 pupillary sphincter m.
 radial dilator m.
 recession of m.
 rectus lateralis m.
 rectus medialis m.
 resection of m.
 m. resection
 Riolan m.
 Rouget m.
 m. sheath
 sphincter m.
 superciliary m.
 superior oblique extraocular m.
 superior rectus extraocular m.
 superior tarsal m.
 tarsal m.
 temporalis m.
 m. torque
 m. transposition
 trochlear m.
 trochlea of superior oblique m.
 vertical m.
 yoke m.
 yoked m.
muscle-eye-brain disease
muscular
 m. asthenopia
 m. balance
 m. dystrophy
 m. fascia
 m. funnel

 m. insufficiency
 m. strabismus
 m. vein
musculus, pl. **musculi**
 musculi bulbi
 m. ciliaris
 m. corrugator supercilii
 m. depressor supercilii
 m. dilator pupilla
 lamina superficialis musculi
 m. levator palpebrae superioris
 m. obliquus inferior bulbi
 m. obliquus inferior oculi
 m. obliquus superior bulbi
 m. obliquus superior oculi
 musculi oculi
 m. orbicularis
 m. orbicularis oculi
 m. orbitalis
 m. procerus
 m. rectus inferior bulbi
 m. rectus inferior oculi
 m. rectus lateralis bulbi
 m. rectus lateralis oculi
 m. rectus medialis bulbi
 m. rectus medialis oculi
 m. sphincter pupilla
 m. tarsalis inferior
 m. tarsalis superior
mushroom
 corneal m.
 m. corneal graft
mustache technique
Mustarde
 M. awl
 M. graft
 M. operation
 M. rotational cheek flap
mustard gas
mutabilis
 Lecythophora m.
Mutamycin
mutation
 BIGH3 gene m.
 Gln368Stop m.
mutton-fat
 m.-f. deposit
 m.-f. keratic precipitate
mutton fat
MVB blade
MVK
 Massachusetts Vision Kit
MVN
 medial vestibular nucleus
MVR
 massive vitreous retraction
 microvitreoretinal
  MVR blade

MVS
Massachusetts XII vitrectomy system
My
myopia
Myambutol
myasthenia
focal m.
m. gravis
neonatal m.
ocular m.
pediatric m.
m. syndrome
myasthenia-like syndrome
myasthenic
m. crisis
m. nystagmus
mycelial mass
Mycitracin
mycobacteria
atypical m.
Mycobacteriaceae
mycobacterial disease
Mycobacterium
M. *africanum*
M. *avium*
M. *bovis*
M. *chelonae*
M. *chelonei*
M. *fortuitum*
M. keratitis
M. *leprae*
M. *smegmatis*
M. *tuberculosis*
Mycobutin
mycormycosis
Mycostatin
mycotic
m. infection
m. keratitis
m. snowball opacity
mycotoxicity
Mydfrin Ophthalmic Solution
Mydramide
Mydrapred
Mydriacyl
Mydriafair
mydriasis
accidental m.
alternating m.
amaurotic m.
areflexical m.
bounding m.

congenital m.
episodic unilateral m.
factitious m.
fixed m.
paralytic m.
postoperative m.
spasmodic m.
spastic m.
spinal m.
springing m.
transient unilateral m.
traumatic m.
mydriatic
m. provocative test
m. rigidity
m. test for angle-closure glaucoma
mydriatic-cycloplegic therapy
Mydrilate
myectomy
m. operation
orbicularis m.
selective facial m.
myelinated retinal nerve fiber
myelination
optic nerve m.
m. of retinal nerve
retinal nerve fiber m.
myelin disorder
myelitis
myeloidin
myeloma
multiple m.
osteosclerotic m.
myelomatosis
disseminated nonosteolytic m.
myelooptic neuropathy
myeloperoxidase
neutrophil m.
myiasis
cutaneous m.
ocular m.
MYOC
myocilin
Myochrysine
myocilin (MYOC)
myoclin gene
myoclonal
myoclonic epilepsy with ragged-red fiber
myoclonus
m. nystagmus
ocular m.

NOTES

M

myoclonus *(continued)*
    oculopalatal m.
    startle m.
    vertical m.
myoculator
Myocure
    M. blade
    M. blade scalpel
    M. knife
    M. phacoblade
myocysticercosis
myodesopsia
myodiopter
myoepithelial cell
myoepithelioma
myofibril
myogenic acquired ptosis
myoid visual cell
myokymia
    eyelid m.
    facial m.
    superior oblique m.
myoneural junction
myopathic
    m. disorder
    m. eyelid retraction
    m. ptosis
myopathy
    centronuclear m.
    congenital m.
    endocrine m.
    fingerprint body m.
    inflammatory m.
    mitochondrial m.
    nemaline m.
    ocular m.
    proximal myotonic m.
    reducing body m.
    rod m.
    systemic m.
    toxin-induced m.
    traumatic m.
    visceral m.
myope
    early-onset m.
    late-onset m.
myopia (M, My)
    abnormal nearwork-induced
      transient m.
    axial m.
    choroiditis m.
    chronic m.
    crescent m.
    curvature m.
    degenerative m.
    early-onset m.
    form-deprivation m.
    high m.
    index m.

    m. index
    late-onset m.
    lenticular m.
    low m.
    malignant m.
    moderate m.
    night m.
    nyctalopia with congenital m.
    pathologic m.
    peripheral m.
    pernicious m.
    physiologic m.
    prematurity m.
    primary m.
    prodromal m.
    progressive m.
    refractive m.
    school m.
    senile lenticular m.
    simple m.
    space m.
    transient m.
    vision deprivation m.
myopic (M)
    m. anisometropia
    m. astigmatism (AM, AsM)
    m. cave
    m. choroidal atrophy
    m. choroidal neovascularization
      (mCNV)
    m. choroidopathy
    m. conus
    m. crescent
    m. error
    m. keratomileusis (MKM)
    m. maculopathy
    m. reflex
    m. regression
    m. retinal degeneration
myorhythmia
    oculomasticatory m.
myoscope
myosin filament
myosis
myositis
    idiopathic m.
    infective m.
    orbital m.
    systemic m.
myotomy
    marginal m.
    m. operation
    Z m.
myotonia
    chondrodystrophic m.
    m. congenita
    m. dystrophica
myotonic
    m. dystrophy

m. dystrophy cataract
m. dystrophy effect
m. pupil
myringotomy blade

Mysoline
Mytrate
MZR
   mizoribine

NOTES

M

N
  nasal
n
  index of refraction
NA
  numerical aperture
NA-AION
  nonarteritic anterior ischemic optic
  neuropathy
naboctate HCl
NaCl
  sodium chloride
Nadbath
  N. akinesia
  N. facial block
Nadler superior radial scissors
nadolol
Naegeli syndrome
Naegleria
  N. cyst
  N. fowleri
Nafazair Ophthalmic
nafcillin
Naffziger
  N. operation
  N. orbital decompression
NaFl
  sodium fluorescein
NAG
  narrow-angle glaucoma
Nagahara
  N. karate chopper
  N. phaco chopper
  N. quick chopper
Nagel
  N. anomaloscope
  N. Lensmeter
  N. test
Nager syndrome
NAION
  nonarteritic anterior ischemic optic
  neuropathy
Nairobi eye
naked vision (Nv)
nalorphine
naloxone hydrochloride
Nama keratopathy
naming
  color n.
nana
  Hymenolepis n.
nanism
  Mulibrey n.
Nanolas Nd:YAG laser
nanophthalmia, nanophthalmos

NANOS
  North American Neuro-Ophthalmology
  Society
Napha-A
Napha-Forte
naphazoline
  n. and antazoline
  n. and antazoline phosphate
  n. HCl
  n. and pheniramine maleate
Naphcon
  N. Forte
  N. Ophthalmic
Naphcon-A Ophthalmic
naphthyl ethylenediamine
naproxen sodium
narrow-angle glaucoma (NAG)
narrowed arteriole
narrowing
  arteriolar n.
  n. of retinal arteriole
narrow-slit illumination
Nasahist B
nasal (N)
  n. architecture
  n. arteriole of retina
  n. border of optic disk
  n. buttonhole incision
  n. canal
  n. canthus
  n. duct
  n. field loss
  n. hemianopsia
  n. isopter
  n. periphery
  n. speculum
  n. step
  n. step defect
  n. venule of retina
  n. zone
nasalis
  commissura palpebrarum n.
nasalization
nasi
  cancrum n.
  inferior meatus n.
nasion
NAS-NRC Committee on Vision
nasoantritis
nasociliaris
  nervus n.
nasociliary
  n. nerve
  n. neuralgia

N

nasofrontalis
  vena n.
nasofrontal vein
nasojugal fold
nasolabial fold
nasolacrimal
  n. blockade
  n. canal
  n. drainage system
  n. duct (NLD)
  n. duct obstruction (NLDO)
  n. duct probe
  n. gland
  n. groove
  n. reflex
  n. sac
nasolacrimalis
  ductus n.
nasoorbital fracture
Natacyn
natamycin
National
  N. Eye Institute Visual Function
    Questionnaire (NEI-VFQ)
  N. Institute of Neurologic Diseases
    and Blindness (NINDB)
natural
  n. cornea
  N. Tears
  n. UV radiation
Naturale
  Duratears N.
  Tears N.
Nature's
  N. Tears all natural soothing eye
    mist
  N. Tears Solution
NBS
  nystagmus blockage syndrome
N-butyl-2-cyanoacrylate glue
NCCA
  noncontact corneal esthesiometer
NC-PAS
  noncontact photo-acoustic spectroscopy
NCT
  noncontact tonometer
ND-Stat
Nd:YAG
  neodymium:yttrium aluminum garnet
    laser
  Nd:YAG laser
  Nd:YAG laser cyclophotocoagulation
  Nd:YAG Photon LaserPhaco
    System
Nd:YLF
  neodymium:yttrium lithium fluoride laser
  Nd:YLF laser
Neale Reading Analysis

near
  n. acuity testing
  n. add
  at distance and at n. (D/N)
  distance and n.
  esophoria at n. (E^1)
  n. esotropia (ET′)
  n. fixation
  n. fixation position of gaze
  n. light reflex
  n. point absolute
  n. point of accommodation (NPA)
  n. point of convergence (NPC)
  n. reaction
  n. reaction to light
  n. response
  n. sight
  n. triad
  n. vision
  n. vision test
  n. vision testing
  n. visual acuity (NVA)
  n. visual point (NVP)
near-emmetropic eye
near-point
  n.-p. accommodation
  n.-p. esophoria
  n.-p. exophoria
  n.-p. phoria
  n.-p. relative
near-reflex spasm
nearsighted
nearsightedness
nebula, pl. **nebulae**
  corneal n.
nebular stromal opacity
NEC MobilePro 800 Volk Lens
necrobiotic xanthogranuloma
necrogranulomatous keratitis
necrophorum
  Fusobacterium n.
necrosis
  acute retinal n. (ARN)
  anterior segment n.
  caseous n.
  conjunctival n.
  fibrinoid n.
  infarctive n.
  ischemic n.
  perifascicular myofiber n.
  progressive outer retinal n. (PORN)
  retinal n.
  scleral n.
  stromal n.
  white retinal n.
necrotic
  n. follicle
  n. infectious conjunctivitis
  n. occlusion

necroticans
    scleritis n.
necrotizing
    n. herpetic retinopathy
    n. interstitial keratitis
    n. nocardial scleritis
    n. nodular scleritis
    n. papillitis
    n. retinitis
    n. sclerocorneal ulceration (NSU)
    n. stromal keratitis
    n. ulcerative keratitis
    n. vasculitis
nedocromil
    n. sodium
    n. sodium ophthalmic solution
needle
    ACS n.
    Agnew tattooing n.
    Agrikola tattooing n.
    Alcon CU-15 4-mil n.
    Alcon irrigating n.
    Alcon reverse cutting n.
    Alcon spatula n.
    Alcon taper cut n.
    Alcon taper point n.
    Amsler aqueous transplant n.
    aqueous transplant n.
    Atkinson retrobulbar n.
    Atkinson single-bevel blunt-tip n.
    Atkinson tip peribulbar n.
    Barraquer n.
    Barraquer-Vogt n.
    BD n.
    bent blunt n.
    bent 22-gauge n.
    blunt n.
    Bowman cataract n.
    Bowman stop n.
    Burr butterfly n.
    butterfly n.
    BV100 n.
    Calhoun n.
    Calhoun-Hagler lens n.
    Calhoun-Merz n.
    Castroviejo vitreous aspirating n.
    cataract n.
    cataract-aspirating n.
    CD-5 n.
    Charles flute n.
    Charles vacuuming n.
    Chiba eye n.

    Cibis ski n.
    CIF4 n.
    Cleasby spatulated n.
    Colorado n.
    CooperVision irrigating n.
    CooperVision spatulated n.
    corneal n.
    couching n.
    Crawford n.
    Curran knife n.
    Daily cataract n.
    Davis knife n.
    Dean knife n.
    discission n.
    Drews cataract n.
    DS-9 n.
    Ellis foreign body n.
    Elschnig extrusion n.
    Empire n.
    Ethicon BV-75-3 n.
    extended round n.
    extrusion n.
    Fisher eye n.
    flute n.
    foreign body n.
    four-sided cutting n.
    Fritz vitreous transplant n.
    30-gauge n.
    Geuder keratoplasty n.
    Girard anterior chamber n.
    Girard cataract-aspirating n.
    Girard phacofragmatome n.
    Girard-Swan knife n.
    Graefe n.
    Grieshaber ophthalmic n.
    GS-9 n.
    Gueder keratoplasty n.
    Haab knife n.
    Hessburg lacrimal n.
    Heyner double n.
    n. holder
    n. holder clamp
    Ilg n.
    Iliff-Wright fascia n.
    illuminated suction n.
    internal nucleus hydrodelineation n.
    Iocare titanium n.
    IOLAB irrigating n.
    IOLAB taper-cut n.
    IOLAB taper-point n.
    IOLAB titanium n.
    iris knife n.

N

NOTES

needle *(continued)*
  Kalt corneal n.
  Kara cataract n.
  Knapp knife n.
  Kratz diamond-dusted n.
  Kratz lens n.
  Lagleyze n.
  Lane n.
  Lewicky n.
  lighted flute n.
  Look retrobulbar n.
  Lo-Trau side-cutting n.
  LX n.
  March laser sclerostomy n.
  Maumenee vitreous-aspirating n.
  McIntyre I/A n.
  McIntyre irrigation/aspiration n.
  micropoint n.
  micro round-tip n.
  nucleus hydrolysis n.
  Oaks double n.
  peribulbar n.
  probe n.
  n. probe
  puncture n.
  puncture-tip n.
  razor n.
  razor-tip n.
  retrobulbar n.
  Reverdin suture n.
  reverse-cutting n.
  Riedel n.
  Rycroft n.
  Sabreloc n.
  Sato cataract n.
  Scheie cataract-aspirating n.
  sclerostomy n.
  Sharpoint Ultra-Guide ophthalmic n.
  side-cutting spatulated n.
  Simcoe II PC aspirating n.
  Simcoe suture n.
  SITE irrigating/aspirating n.
  SITE macrobore plus n.
  SITE Phaco I/A n.
  ski n.
  n. spatula
  spatulated n.
  spoon n.
  n. spoon
  n. spud
  spud n.
  n. stick
  Stocker n.
  Straus curved retrobulbar n.
  Subco n.
  subconjunctival n.
  Surgicraft suture n.
  suturing n.
  Swan n.

  taper-cut n.
  taper-point n.
  tattooing n.
  tax double n.
  TG-140 n.
  Thornton n.
  titanium n.
  translocation n.
  triple facet-tip n.
  ultrasonic cataract-removal lancet n.
  Universal soft tip cannulated
   sliding extrusion n.
  Viers n.
  vitreous aspirating n.
  vitreous transplant n.
  Vogt-Barraquer corneal n.
  Vogt-Barraquer eye n.
  von Graefe knife n.
  Weeks n.
  Wergeland double n.
  Wooten n.
  Worst n.
  Wright fascia n.
  Wright ophthalmic n.
  Yale Luer-Lok n.
  Ziegler iris knife-n.
needleless regional anesthesia
negative
  n. accommodation
  n. afterimage
  n. convergence
  n. eyepiece
  false n.
  n. image
  n. meniscus
  n. meniscus lens
  n. scotoma
  n. vertical divergence
  n. vertical vergence
  n. visual phenomenon
neglect dyslexia
Neher operation
Nehra-Mack operation
Neisseria
  N. gonorrhoeae
  N. meningitidis
neisserial conjunctivitis
Neitz
  N. CT-R cataract camera
  N. Instruments Company
NEI-VFQ
  National Eye Institute Visual Function
  Questionnaire
NEI Visual Acuity Impairment Survey
  study
nelfinavir mesylate
Nelson
  N. classification
  N. grading system

nemaline myopathy
nematode
Nembutal
Neocidin
Neo-Cobefrin
NeoDecadron
    N. Ophthalmic
    N. Topical
Neo-Dexair
Neo-Dexameth Ophthalmic
Neodexasone
neodymium:YAG laser
neodymium:yttrium
    n. aluminum garnet laser
      (Nd:YAG)
    n. lithium fluoride laser (Nd:YLF)
neodymium:yttrium-lithium-fluoride
    n.-l.-f. laser segmentation
    n.-l.-f. photodisruptive laser
Neo-Flow
neoformans
    Cryptococcus n.
Neofrin
Neo-Hydeltrasol
NeoKnife cautery
Neolens lens
Neolyte laser indirect ophthalmoscope
Neo-Medrol
Neomixin
neomycin
    n., polymyxin B, and
      dexamethasone
    n., polymyxin B, and gramicidin
    n., polymyxin B, and
      hydrocortisone
    n., polymyxin B, and prednisolone
    n. sulfate
Neomycin-Dex
neonatal
    n. gliosis
    n. inclusion blennorrhea
    n. inclusion conjunctivitis
    n. myasthenia
    n. onset multisystem inflammatory
      disease (NOMID)
    n. ophthalmia
neonatorum
    blennorrhea n.
    ophthalmia n.
neoplasia
    conjunctival intraepithelial n. (CIN)
    conjunctival squamous cell n.

    corneal conjunctival
      intraepithelial n.
    intraepithelial n.
neoplasm
    choroidal n.
    intraepithelial n.
    Merkel cell n.
    orbital n.
    secondary malignant n.
neoplastic angioendotheliomatosis
Neo-Polycin
Neopolydex
Neoral
Neosar Injection
Neosporin
    N. drops
    N. Ophthalmic Ointment
    N. Ophthalmic Solution
neostigmine
    n. methylsulfate
    n. test
Neo-Synephrine
    N.-S. cocaine mixture
    N.-S. Hydrochloride
    N.-S. Ophthalmic Solution
Neotal
Neo-Tears
Neotricin HC Ophthalmic Ointment
neovascular
    n. angle-closure glaucoma
    n. membrane
    n. net
    n. tuft
neovascularization
    choroidal n. (CNV)
    choroidovitreal n.
    classic choroidal n.
    corneal n.
    n. of disk (NVD)
    disk n.
    disseminated asymptomatic
      unilateral n.
    extraretinal n.
    interstitial n.
    n. of the iris (NVI)
    iris n.
    juxtafoveal choroidal n.
    myopic choroidal n. (mCNV)
    n. of new vessels elsewhere
      (NVE)
    occult choroidal n.
    peripapillary subretinal n.

NOTES

N

neovascularization *(continued)*
    preretinal n.
    n. of retina
    retinal quadrant n.
    secondary n.
    stromal n.
    subfoveal choroidal n.
    subretinal n. (SRNV)
    vitreous n.
Neovastat
nephritica
    retinitis n.
nephropathic cystinosis
Neptazane
Nernst glower
nerve
    abducens n. (CN VI)
    abducent n. (N.VI, CN VI)
    aberrant degeneration of third n.
    aberrant regeneration of n.
    aberrant reinnervation of the
      oculomotor n.
    acoustic n.
    afferent n.
    aplasia of optic n.
    atrophy of optic n.
    basal epithelial n.
    block n.
    n. block
    cavernous portion of the
      oculomotor n.
    ciliary n.
    coloboma of optic n.
    n. core
    corneal n.
    cranial n. (CN)
    n. cross section
    cupping of optic n.
    efferent n.
    eighth cranial n.
    facial n.
    n. fiber
    N. Fiber Analyzer laser
      ophthalmoscope
    n. fiber axon
    n. fiber bundle
    n. fiber bundle defect
    n. fiber bundle layer
    n. fiber layer (NFL)
    n. fiber layer analyzer
    n. fiber layer dropout
    n. fiber layer hemorrhage
    n. fiber layer infarct
    n. fiber technology
    fifth cranial n. (CN V)
    fourth cranial n. (CN IV)
    frontal n.
    ganglionic layer of optic n.
    ganglionic stratum of optic n.

    ganglion layer of optic n.
    ganglion stratum of optic n.
    greater superficial petrosal n.
    n. growth factor
    n. head angioma
    n. head drusen
    hypoplastic ocular n.
    infraepitrochlear n.
    infraorbital n.
    infratrochlear n.
    n. input
    input n.
    intermedius n.
    intervaginal space of optic n.
    intracanalicular optic n.
    intracranial optic n.
    intraocular optic n.
    intraosseous optic n.
    ischemia of optic n.
    lacrimal n.
    n. layer of retina
    long ciliary n.
    n. loop
    maxillary n.
    motor n.
    myelination of retinal n.
    nasociliary n.
    oculomotor n. (N.III)
    ophthalmic n.
    optic n. (N.II, ON)
    orbital optic n.
    output n.
    n. palsy
    peripapillary retinal n.
    peripheral oculomotor n.
    petrosal n.
    postganglionic short ciliary n.
    prechiasmal optic n.
    preganglionic oculomotor n.
    prelaminar optic n.
    regeneration of n.
    n. regeneration
    second cranial n.
    secretomotor n.
    sensory n.
    seventh cranial n. (CN VII)
    n. sheath
    n. sheath meningioma
    short ciliary n.
    sixth cranial n. (CN VI)
    supraorbital n.
    supratrochlear n.
    tentorial n.
    third cranial n. (CN III)
    trigeminal n. (NV)
    trochlear n. (CR IV, N.IV)
    tumor of optic n.
    vascular circle of optic n.
    vestibular n.

vidian n.
zygomatic n.
zygomaticofacial n.
zygomaticotemporal n.
nervea
Brücke tunica n.
tunica n.
nervi (*pl. of* nervus)
Nervocaine with epinephrine
nervous asthenopia
nervus, pl. **nervi**
nervi ciliares breves
nervi ciliares longi
n. infraorbitalis
n. intermedius
iris n.
n. lacrimalis
n. maxillaris
n. nasociliaris
n. oculomotorius
n. ophthalmicus
n. opticus
n. supraorbitalis
n. trigeminus
n. trochlearis
n. zygomaticus
Nesacaine
nests and strands of cells
net
neovascular n.
parafoveal capillary n.
Nettleship-Falls X-linked ocular albinism
Nettleship iris repositor
Nettleship-Wilder dilator
network
choriocapillaris vascular n.
Gerlach n.
peritarsal n.
trabecular n.
vascular n.
Neubauer forceps
Neuhann
N. cystitome
N. glaucoma marker
Neumann razor blade fragment holder
Neumann-Shepard
N.-S. corneal marker
N.-S. oval optical center marker
Neuprex
neural
n. crest
n. crest cell

n. ganglionic cell
n. lesion
n. retina
n. rim
n. transfer function
n. tube
neuralgia
nasociliary n.
postherpetic n.
Raeder paratrigeminal n.
supraorbital n.
trifacial n.
trigeminal n.
vidian n.
neurasthenic asthenopia
neurectomy
opticociliary n.
vidian n.
neurilemmosarcoma
neurilemoma
ameloblastic n.
eyelid n.
malignant n.
neuritic atrophy
neuritis, pl. **neuritides**
acute idiopathic demyelinating optic n.
anterior ischemic optic n.
asymptomatic optic n.
atherosclerotic ischemic n.
chronic demyelinating optic n.
idiopathic demyelinating optic n.
idiopathic nongranulomatous optic n.
idiopathic perioptic n.
inflammatory optic n.
intraocular optic n.
Intravenous Immunoglobulin Therapy in Optic N.
n. nodosa
optic demyelinating n.
orbital n.
parainfectious optic n.
paraneoplastic optic n.
perioptic n.
postocular n.
postvaccination optic n.
retrobulbar optic n.
subclinical optic n.
neuro-Behçet disease
neuroblastic

N

NOTES

neuroblastoma
olfactory n.
neurochorioretinitis
neurochoroiditis
neurodealgia
neurodeatrophia
neurodegenerative syndrome
neurodermatica
cataracta n.
neuroectodermal
neuroepithelial layer of retina
neuroepithelioma
orbital n.
neuroepithelium
neurofibroma
eyelid n.
iris n.
limbal n.
orbital n.
plexiform n.
uveal n.
Neurofibromatosis Type 1 Optic Pathway Glioma Task Force
neurofilament triplets antibody
neurogenic
n. iris atrophy
n. mesenchyme
n. tumor
neurogenic-acquired ptosis
Neuroguard pulsed wave transducer
neuroimaging
neuroleptic malignant syndrome
neurologic
n. deficit
n. disorder
n. dysfunction
n. examination
neuroloptic drug
neuroma
acoustic n.
facial n.
mucosal n.
orbital n.
plexiform n.
neuromuscular
n. blocking drug
n. disorder
n. disorder-causing drug
n. effect
n. eyelid retraction
n. ptosis
neuromyelitis optica
neuromyotonia
ocular n.
neuron
abducens internuclear n.
cholinergic n.
Golgi I, II n.
retinal n.

sympathetic n.
third order n.
neuronal ceroid lipofuscinosis
neuron-specific
n.-s. endolase (NSE)
n.-s. endolase antibody
neuroophthalmic manifestation
neuroophthalmologic
n. case history
n. diagnosis
n. examination
neuroophthalmological investigation
neuroophthalmology
neuropapillitis
neuroparalytic
n. keratitis
n. keratopathy
n. ophthalmia
neuropathic
n. disease
n. eyelid retraction
n. tonic pupil
neuropathy
anterior compressive optic n.
anterior ischemic optic n. (AION)
arteriosclerotic ischemic optic n.
arteritic anterior ischemic optic n.
autoimmune-related retinopathy and optic n. (ARRON)
autosomal-dominant hereditary optic n.
autosomal-recessive hereditary optic n.
compressive optic n.
Cuban epidemic optic n.
demyelinating optic n.
distal optic n.
dysthyroid optic n.
giant axonal n.
glaucomatous optic n.
hereditary optic n.
hypertrophic interstitial n.
infiltrative optic n.
inflammatory optic n.
ischemic optic n. (ION)
Jamaican optic n.
Leber hereditary optic n. (LHON)
luetic n.
myelooptic n.
nonarteritic anterior ischemic optic n. (NA-AION, NAION)
nutritional optic n.
onion bulb n.
optic n.
parainfectious optic n.
paraneoplastic optic n.
peripheral n.
posterior ischemic optic n. (PION)
radiation-induced optic n.

radiation optic n. (RON)
retrobulbar compressive optic n.
retrobulbar ischemic optic n.
shock optic n.
subacute myelooptic n. (SMON)
toxic optic n.
traumatic optic n. (TON)
tropical optic n.
uremic optic n.

neurophakomatosis
neuroradiologic
neuroretinal rim
neuroretinitis
cat scratch disease n.
diffuse unilateral subacute n.
  (DUSN)
idiopathic retinal vasculitis,
  aneurysms and n. (IRVAN)

neuroretinopathy
acute macular n.
hypertensive n.
macular n.

neurosecretory granule
neurosensory
n. retina
n. retinal detachment

neurosyphilis
neurotomy
opticociliary n.

neurotonic pupil
neurotransmitter
retinal n.

neurotrophic
n. keratitis
n. keratopathy

neurotropism
neurovisual manifestation
neutral
n. density filter
n. density filter test
n. point
n. zone

neutralization
neutralizer
AoDisc N.

neutrophil myeloperoxidase
nevi
Actinomyces n.
nevi (*pl. of* nevus)
nevocyte
nevoid

nevoxanthoendothelioma
juvenile n.

nevus, pl. **nevi**
basal cell n.
blue n.
choroidal n.
compound n.
conjunctival pigmented n.
cystic amelanotic n.
dermal n.
episcleral n.
epithelial n.
eyelid n.
n. flammeus
intradermal n.
junctional n.
melanocytic n.
nonpigmented n.
Ota n.
n. of Ota
n. sebaceus of Jadassohn
Spitz n.
strawberry n.
subepithelial n.
uveal n.

Nevyas
N. double sharp cystitome
N. lens forceps
N. retractor

new
N. England Eye Bank
N. Orleans Eye & Ear fixation
  forceps
N. Orleans lens
N. Orleans lens loupe
n. vessel disk
N. York erysiphake
N. York Eye & Ear Hospital
  fixation forceps

newborn
aniridia in the n.
Clinical Trial of Eye Prophylaxis
  in the N.
n. conjunctivitis

Newcastle disease virus
Newman collagen plug inserter forceps
Newsom
N. cracker model 8-07116 in
  stainless steel
N. cracker model 05-4063 in
  titanium
N. side port nucleus cracker

N

NOTES

Newton disk
newtonian aberration
NewVues sterile contact lens
Nexacryl
    N. cohesive product
    N. tissue adhesive
NFL
    nerve fiber layer
niacin maculopathy
Niamtu video imaging system
NIBOT
    noninvasive break-up time
Nichamin
    N. fixation right with 10-degree marks
    N. fixation ring
    N. hydrodissection cannula
    N. I and II nucleus quick chopper
    N. LASIK irrigating cannula
    N. triple chopper
    N. vertical chopper
nicking
    arteriolar n.
    arteriovenous n.
    AV n.
    n. of retinal vein
    retinal venous n.
Nicol prism
nicotinic acid maculopathy
nictation
nictitans
    membrana n.
nictitating
    n. membrane
    n. spasm
nictitation
Nida nicking operation
Nidek
    N. AR-2000 Objective Automatic refractor
    N. Auto Refractometer NR-1000F
    N. 3Dx stereodisk camera
    N. EC-1000 excimer laser
    EchoScan by N.
    N. EC-5000 refractive laser system
    N. Laser System laser
    N. MK-2000 Keratome System
Nieden syndrome
Niemann-Pick
    N.-P. disease
    N.-P. disease type A, B
night
    n. blindness
    N. & Day Tears Again sterile lubricant gel
    n. myopia
    n. sight
    n. vision
night-vision goggles

nigra
    cataracta n.
nigricans
    acanthosis n.
    pseudoacanthosis n.
nigroid body
nigrum
    pigmentum n.
    tapetum n.
N.II
    optic nerve
N.III
    oculomotor nerve
Nike Max Rx prescription sun lens
Nikolsky sign
Nikon
    N. aspheric lens
    N. Auto Refractometer NR-1000F
    N. FS-3 photo slit lamp biomicroscope
    N. NS-1 slit-lamp microscope
    N. Retinomax K-Plus autorefractor
    N. Retinopan fundus camera
    N. zoom photo slit lamp
NINDB
    National Institute of Neurologic Diseases and Blindness
NIPH
    no improvement with pinhole
niphablepsia
niphotyphlosis
nipper
    House-Dieter n.
NITFBUT
    noninvasive tear film breakup time
    conjunctival NITFBUT
Nitra lamp
nitrate
    cellulose n.
    Grocott-Gomori methenamine silver n.
    phenylmercuric n.
    pilocarpine n.
    silver n.
nitrocellulose filter paper
N.IV
    trochlear nerve
nivalis
    ophthalmia n.
    n. ophthalmia
Nizetic operation
Nizoral
NLD
    nasolacrimal duct
NLDO
    nasolacrimal duct obstruction
NLP
    no light perception

NM-1000 digital non-mydriatic fundus camera
193-nm excimer laser
NMG
    no Marcus Gunn
532nm Green laser photocoagulator
no
    no improvement
    no improvement with pinhole (NIPH)
    no light perception (NLP)
    no Marcus Gunn (NMG)
    No Rub Opti-Free Express multi-purpose disinfecting solution
Noble forceps
Nocardia
    N. asteroides
    N. brasiliensis
    N. caviae
    N. keratitis
nocardial endophthalmitis
nocardiosis
    ocular n.
nociceptive sensation
Nocito eye implant
N₂O cryosurgical unit

nocturnal
    n. amblyopia
    n. lagophthalmia
nodal
    n. plane
    n. point
node
    Rosenmüller n.
nodiformis
    cataracta n.
nodosa
    conjunctivitis n.
    endophthalmitis ophthalmia n.
    iritis n.
    neuritis n.
    ophthalmia n.
    periarteritis n. (PAN, PN)
    polyarteritis n.
nodular
    n. conjunctivitis
    n. corneal degeneration
    n. episcleritis
    n. fasciitis
    n. iritis
    n. melanoma

nodule
    Busacca n.
    conjunctival n.
    Dalen-Fuchs n.
    epibulbar Fordyce n.
    episcleral rheumatic n.
    Fordyce n.
    iris n.
    Koeppe n.
    lemon-drop n.
    lenticular fibroxanthomatous n.
    lentiform n.
    Lisch n.
    millet seed n.
    pseudorheumatoid n.
    rheumatic n.
    Salzmann n.
    n.'s in sparganosis
    subepidermal calcified n.
nodulus
    n. conjunctivalis
    n. lymphaticus
    n. syndrome
Nokrome
    N. bifocal
    N. bifocal lens
Nolahist
no-light-perception vision
Nolvadex
NOMID
    neonatal onset multisystem inflammatory disease
nomogram
    Casebeer-Lindstrom n.
    Harrison-Stein n.
    n. system
nonabsorbable suture
non-*Acanthamoeba* amebic keratitis
nonaccommodation
nonaccommodative
    n. esodeviation
    n. esophoria
    n. esotropia
Non-Allergenic
    N.-A. Clear Clean
    Polish Brite/Super Cleaner, N.-A.
nonarteritic
    n. anterior ischemic optic neuropathy (NA-AION, NAION)
nonaspirating ultrasonic phaco chopper tip
nonatopic allergic conjunctivitis

N

NOTES

noncaseating conjunctival granuloma
noncentral ulcer
noncicatricial entropion
noncomitant
    n. heterotropia
    n. squint
    n. strabismus
nonconcomitant strabismus
nonconfluent plaque
noncongestive glaucoma
noncontact
    n. corneal esthesiometer (NCCA)
    n. corneal pachymetry
    n. laser thermal keratoplasty
    n. lens
    n. LTK
    n. photo-acoustic spectroscopy (NC-PAS)
    n. pneumatic esthesiometer
    n. tonometer (NCT)
noncycloplegic distance static retinoscopy
nondeposited tear coating
nondominant eye
nonepithelial tumor
nonfenestrated capillary
nonfilamentous fungus
nonfixed tissue
nongranulomatous
    n. anterior uveitis
    n. choroiditis
    n. iridocyclitis
    n. iritis
non-Hodgkin lymphoma
non-insulin-dependent diabetes mellitus
noninvasive
    n. break-up time (NIBOT)
    n. corneal redox fluorometry
    n. tear film breakup time (NITFBUT)
noninvasively sectioning
nonischemic CRVO
nonleaking bleb
nonliquefaciens
    Moraxella n.
nonmechanical trephination
nonmembrane-bound vacuoles
nonmydriatic retinal photography
nonneovascular age-related macular degeneration
Nonne syndrome
nonneural ganglionic cell
nonnutrient agar
nonocular muscle group
nonoptic reflex eye movement
nonorbital childhood parameningeal embryonal rhabdomyosarcoma
nonorganic
    n. blepharospasm

    n. disorder diagnosis
    n. paresis
    n. visual loss
Nonoxynol
nonparalytic strabismus
nonpenetrant gene
nonpenetrating
    n. deep sclerectomy
    n. keratoplasty
nonperfusion
    capillary n.
    retinal capillary n.
nonphysiologic visual field loss
nonpigmented
    n. ciliary epithelium
    n. nevus
nonpreserved artificial tears
nonproliferative diabetic retinopathy (NPDR)
nonrapid eye movement
nonreflex tearing
nonrefractive accommodative esotropia
nonrhegmatogenous retinal detachment
non-Sjögren keratoconjunctivitis sicca
nonsteroidal antiinflammatory drug
nontuberculous mycobacterial keratitis
nonulcerative
    n. blepharitis
    n. interstitial keratitis
Noonan syndrome
noradrenaline
Nordan-Ruiz trapezoidal marker
norepinephrine
norfloxacin
normal
    n. distribution
    n. eye
    n. fundus
    n. retinal correspondence (NRC)
    n. tension (TN)
    n. upward corrective saccade
    n. viewing condition
normal-finger tension
normalized Zernike expansion
normal-pressure glaucoma
normal-tension glaucoma (NTG)
Norman-Wood syndrome
normocytic hypochromic anemia
normokalemic periodic paralysis
Norrie disease
North
    N. American Neuro-Ophthalmology Society (NANOS)
    N. Carolina macular dystrophy
Northern
    Tracor N.
Nosema corneum
no-stitch phacoemulsification surgery

notation
Jaeger n.
Snellen n.
standard n.
notch
cerebellar n.
n. of iris
lacrimal n.
supraorbital n.
notch-and-roll maneuver
notching
lid n.
rim n.
note blindness
Nothnagel syndrome
not invasive break-up time
**no-touch transepithelial photorefractive
keratectomy**
Nott retinoscopy
Nova
N. Aid lens
N. Curve broad C-loop posterior
chamber lens
N. Curve Omnicurve lens
Dioptron N.
N. Soft II lens
Novantrone
Novatec LightBlade
novel remedy
Novesine
Novocaine
Novus
N. Omni 2000 photocoagulator
N. 2000 ophthalmoscope
novyi
Borrelia n.
Noyes
N. forceps
N. iridectomy scissors
N. iris scissors
NP
Lacri-Lube NP
NP-3S auto chart projector
NPA
near point of accommodation
NPC
near point of convergence
NPDR
nonproliferative diabetic retinopathy
NRC
normal retinal correspondence

NR-1000F
Nidek Auto Refractometer N.
Nikon Auto Refractometer N.
NS
nuclear sclerosis
nuclear sclerotic
NS cataract
NSE
neuron-specific endolase
NSU
necrotizing sclerocorneal ulceration
NTG
normal-tension glaucoma
nubecula
Nuck
canal of N.
nuclear
n. antigen
n. arc
n. bronzing
n. change
n. cytoplasmic ratio
n. developmental cataract
n. expression
n. external layer
n. horizontal gaze paralysis
n. inner layer
n. internal layer
n. layer of the retina
n. ophthalmoplegia
n. outer layer
n. palsy
n. ring
n. sclerosis (NS)
n. sclerosis of lens
n. sclerotic (NS)
n. sclerotic cataract
n. tissue
n. zone
nuclear-fascicular trochlear nerve palsy
nucleus, pl. nuclei
accessory n.
brainstem motor n.
n. cracker
n. delivery loupe
dense brunescent n.
Edinger n.
Edinger-Westphal n.
n. expressor
geniculate n.
5195 n. hydrodissector/rotator
n. hydrolysis needle

N

NOTES

nucleus *(continued)*
>inferior olivary n.
>inferior salivary n.
>lateral geniculate n. (LGN)
>lens n.
>n. of lens
>lenticular n.
>n. lentiform
>n. lentis
>medial vestibular n. (MVN)
>oculomotor n.
>Perlia n.
>n. of posterior commissure
>pretectal n.
>pyknotic nuclei
>n. removal loupe
>rostral interstitial n.
>n. rotator
>salivary n.
>n. spatula
>superior salivary n.
>suprachiasmatic n. (SCN)
>trochlear nerve n.
>vestibular n.

nudge test

Nugent
>N. fixation forceps
>N. hook
>N. soft cataract aspirator
>N. superior rectus forceps

Nugent-Gradle scissors
Nugent-Green-Dimitry erysiphake
Nulicaine
null
>n. condition
>n. point
>n. zone

number
>Snellen n.

numerical
>n. aperture (NA)
>n. visual acuity

nummular
>n. atrophy
>n. keratitis

nummularis
>keratitis n.

Nunery classification of Graves disease, type I, II
Nurolon suture
nut
>retrocorneal n.

nutans
>spasmus n.

Nu-Tears II Solution
NutraTear
nutritional
>n. amblyopia
>n. blindness

>n. deficiency cataract
>n. optic neuropathy

Nutrivision
Nuvita lens
NuVue
NV
>trigeminal nerve

Nv
>naked vision

NVA
>near visual acuity

NVD
>neovascularization of disk

NVE
>neovascularization of new vessels elsewhere

NVI
>neovascularization of the iris

N.VI
>abducent nerve

NVP
>near visual point

nyctalope
nyctalopia with congenital myopia
Nylen-Barany maneuver
nylon
>n. frame
>n. loop
>n. 66 suture

nystagmic
nystagmiform
nystagmogram
nystagmograph
nystagmography
nystagmoid-like oscillation
nystagmoid movement
nystagmus
>acquired jerk n.
>acquired pendular n.
>ageotropic n.
>amaurosis n.
>amaurotic n.
>arthrokinetic n.
>ataxic n.
>audiokinetic n.
>aural n.
>Baer n.
>Bekhterev n.
>blockage n.
>n. blockage syndrome (NBS)
>Bruns n.
>caloric n.
>caloric-induced n.
>central vestibular n.
>centripetal n.
>cervical n.
>Cheyne n.
>circular n.
>compressive n.

congenital n.
conjugate n.
constant n.
convergence-evoked n.
convergence retraction n.
convergence-retractory n.
deviational n.
disconjugate n.
disjunctive n.
dissociated vertical n.
divergence n.
downbeat n.
drug-induced n.
elliptic n.
elliptical n.
end-gaze n.
end-point n.
end-position n.
epileptic n.
eyelid n.
fatigue n.
fixation n.
galvanic n.
gaze n.
gaze-evoked n.
gaze-paretic n.
geotropic n.
head n.
hemi-seesaw n.
horizontal n.
hysterical n.
incongruent n.
infantile n.
irregular n.
Jensen jerk n.
jerk n.
labyrinthine n.
latent n.
lateral n.
left-beating n.
lid n.
manifest latent n.
miner's n.

minimal amplitude n.
monocular n.
muscle paretic n.
myasthenic n.
myoclonus n.
oblique n.
occlusion n.
ocular n.
opticokinetic n.
optokinetic n. (OKN)
oscillating n.
paretic n.
pendular n.
periodic alternating windmill n.
peripheral vestibular n.
perverted n.
physiologic n.
positional n.
pseudocaloric n.
railroad n.
rebound n.
retraction n.
rhythmic n.
right-beating n.
rotary n.
rotation n.
rotational n.
rotatory n.
see-saw n.
sensory deprivation n.
strabismal n.
n. test
torsional n.
undulatory n.
upbeat n.
vasculopathic downbeat n.
vertical n.
vestibular n.
vibratory n.
voluntary n.
n. with demyelination

nystatin

NOTES

OAD
overall diameter of contact lens
OAG
open-angle glaucoma
Oaks
O. double needle
O. double straight cannula
OAO
ophthalmic artery occlusion
Oasis
O. Collagen Plug
O. feather microscalpel
OAV
oculoauriculovertebral
OAV dysplasia
obcecation
OBF tonometer
object
Berens test o.
o. blindness
o. displacement
o. distance
fixation o.
o. of regard
o. size
o. space
test o.
object/image
o. conjugacy
o. relationship
objective
achromatic o.
apochromatic o.
o. cross-cylinder aberroscope
o. lens
o. noninvasive technology
o. optometer
o. perimetry
o. prism-neutralized cover test
o. refractor
o. vertigo
ObjectiVision
object-space focus
obligate carrier
obligatory suppression
oblique
o. aberration
o. astigmatism
o. dysfunction
o. fiber
o. illumination
inferior o.
o. muscle
o. muscle hook
o. nystagmus

o. palsy
o. position
o. prism
o. prism device
o. ray of light
obliterans
endarteritis o.
thromboangiitis o.
obliteration
ductal orifice o.
O'Brien
O. akinesia
O. akinesia technique
O. anesthesia
O. cataract
O. fixation forceps
O. lid block
O. marker
O. spud
O. stitch scissors
O'Brien-Elschnig fixation forceps
obscura
camera o.
obscuration
transient visual o.
obscured fovea
obscure vision
observation
An O. Study on Recurrence of Amblyopia After Discontinuation of Treatment
Obstbaum
O. lens spatula
O. synechia spatula
obstruction
carotid o.
congenital nasolacrimal duct o.
meibomian gland o.
nasolacrimal duct o. (NLDO)
outflow o.
primary acquired nasolacrimal duct o. (PANDO)
silent central retinal vein o.
obstructive
o. glaucoma
o. retinal vasculitis
obturans
iritis o.
obturator
Moria o.
occipital
o. apoplexy
o. cortex
o. lobe

C

occipital (*continued*)
    o. lobe unilateral cerebral
      hemisphere lesion
occipitofrontalis
    venter frontalis musculi o.
occipitothalamica
    radiatio o.
occipitothalamic radiation
occludable
occluded pupil
occludens
    zonula o.
occluder
    black/white o.
    clip-on/tie-on o.
    eye o.
    Halberg trial clip o.
    long/short o.
    lorgnette o.
    Maddox rod o.
    Parasol punctal o.
    pinhole o.
    Plus punctal o.
    Pram o.
    red lens o.
    Rumison side port fixation o.
    single/double o.
    thumb o.
occlusion
    o. amblyopia
    branch retinal artery o. (BRAO)
    branch retinal vein o. (BRVO)
    o. of branch vein
    carotid artery o.
    central retinal artery o. (CRAO)
    central retinal vein o. (CRVO)
    choroidal vascular o.
    cilioretinal artery o.
    combined cilioretinal artery and
      central retinal vein o.'s
    macular arteriole o.
    macular branch retinal vein o.
      (MBRVO)
    monocular o.
    necrotic o.
    o. nystagmus
    ophthalmic artery o. (OAO)
    peripheral branch retinal vein o.
      (PBRVO)
    punctal o.
    o. of pupil
    retinal arterial o.
    retinal branch vein o.
    retinal central artery o.
    retinal central vein o.
    retinal vascular o.
    retinal vein o.
    o. of retinal vein
    retinal venous o.

    o. therapy
    tributary vein o.
    vascular o.
occlusive
    o. microangiopathy
    o. retinal arteritis
    o. vascular disease
occlusor
    Elastoplast eye o.
occult
    o. anular ciliary body
    o. choroidal neovascularization
    o. choroidal neovascular membrane
    o. temporal arteritis of Simmons
occupational
    o. bifocal
    o. lens
    o. ophthalmology
ochre
    o. hemorrhage
    o. mass
    o. membrane
ochronosis
    exogenous o.
    ocular o.
Ochsner
    O. cartilage forceps
    O. hook
    O. tissue/cartilage forceps
    O. tissue forceps
OCI
    Ophthalmic Confidence Index
OCLM
    oculomedin
    OCLM gene
o'clock
    1-12 o. position
O'Connor
    O. depressor
    O. flat hook
    O. iris forceps
    O. lid forceps
    O. marker
    O. muscle hook
    O. operation
    O. sharp hook
    O. sponge forceps
    O. tenotomy hook
O'Connor-Elschnig fixation forceps
O'Connor-Peter operation
OCP
    ocular cicatricial pemphigoid
OCT
    optical coherence tomography
octafluoropropane gas
Octopus
    O. 1-2-3
    O. automated perimetry
    O. 101 bowl perimeter

O. 500 EZ
O. 201 perimeter
O. 201 perimeter test
O. threshold perimetry
Ocu-Bath
Ocu-Caine
OcuCaps
    Akorn O.
Ocu-Carpine
Ocu-Chlor
OcuClear Ophthalmic
OcuClenz
OcuCoat PF Ophthalmic Solution
Ocu-Cort
Ocu-Dex
Ocudose
    Timoptic O.
Ocu-Drop
Ocufen Ophthalmic
ocufilcon
Ocufit SR
Ocuflox ophthalmic
Ocugene glaucoma genetic test
Ocugestrin
Ocu-Guard
OcuHist
Oculab Tono-Pen
Oculaid lens
ocular
    o. adnexa
    o. adnexal tumor
    o. albinism
    o. alignment
    o. angle
    o. ataxia
    o. axis
    o. ballottement
    o. barrier
    o. bartonellosis
    o. blepharospasm
    O. blood flow analyzer
    o. bobbing
    o. capsule
    o. cicatricial pemphigoid (OCP)
    o. circulation dislocated
    o. coherence tomography
    o. coloboma
    o. cone
    o. conjunctiva
    o. crisis
    o. cryptococcal infection
    o. cul-de-sac

o. cup
o. decongestant
o. dipping
o. dominance
o. dominance column
o. duction
o. dysmetria
o. echography
o. flora
o. flutter
O. Gamboscope loupe
o. gymnastics
o. hemodynamic assessment
o. hemodynamic value
o. herpes
o. histoplasmosis
o. histoplasmosis syndrome (OHS)
o. humor
o. hypertelorism
o. hypertension (OHT)
o. hypertension glaucoma
O. Hypertension Treatment Study (OHTS)
o. hypertensive glaucoma
o. hypotelorism
o. hypotony
o. image
o. immunology
o. inflammation
o. injury
o. irritation
o. ischemic syndrome (OIS)
o. itching
o. larva
o. larva migrans
o. lens
o. leptospirosis
o. lyme borreliosis
o. lymphomatosis
o. marker
o. massage
o. medium
o. melanocytosis
o. melanoma
o. melanosis
o. meningioma
O. Microcirculation View Analysis Treatment (OMVAT)
o. microtremor
o. migraine
o. motility
o. motility disorder

NOTES

ocular (*continued*)
- o. motility effect
- o. motility test
- o. motoneuron
- o. motor apraxia
- o. motor syndrome
- o. motor system
- o. movement
- o. muscle
- o. muscle palsy
- o. muscle paralysis
- o. muscle transplant
- o. myasthenia
- o. myasthenia ptosis
- o. myiasis
- o. myoclonus
- o. myopathy
- o. neuromyotonia
- o. nocardiosis
- o. nystagmus
- o. ochronosis
- o. onchocerciasis
- o. oscillation
- o. pathology
- o. pemphigus
- o. perfusion pressure (OPP)
- o. phthisis
- o. plagiocephaly
- o. pressure reducer
- o. prosthesis
- o. pseudoexfoliation syndrome
- o. refraction
- o. region
- o. rigidity
- o. rosacea
- o. saccade
- o. siderosis
- o. sign
- o. sparganosis
- o. spectrum
- o. surface
- o. surface disease (OSD)
- o. syphilis
- o. syphilitic disease
- o. tension (Tn)
- o. tilt reaction (OTR)
- o. torticollis
- o. total higher-order aberration (OTHA)
- o. toxicity
- o. toxocariasis
- o. toxoplasmosis
- o. trauma
- o. ultrasound
- o. vaccinial conjunctivitis
- O. Vergence and Accommodation Sensor (OVAS)
- o. vertigo
- o. vesicle

ocularis
- angor o.
- foveola o.
- vitrina o.

ocularist

oculentum

Oculex drug delivery system

oculi (*pl. of* oculus)

OcuLight
- O. GL/GLx green laser photocoagulator
- O. GLx green laser photocoagulator
- O. SL diode laser
- O. SLx ophthalmic laser

Oculinum

oculist

oculistics

oculoauditory syndrome

oculoauricular dysplasia

oculoauriculovertebral (OAV)
- o. dysplasia

oculobuccogenital syndrome

oculocardiac reflex

oculocephalic
- o. maneuver
- o. reflex
- o. synkinesis
- o. test
- o. vascular anomaly

oculocephalogyric reflex

oculocerebral
- o. lymphoma
- o. syndrome

oculocerebromucomycosis

oculocerebrorenal
- o. dystrophy
- o. syndrome

oculocerebrovasculometer

oculocutaneous
- o. albinism
- o. albinoidism
- o. hypopigmentation
- o. laser
- o. syndrome

oculodentodigital (ODD)
- o. dysplasia

oculodermal
- o. disorder
- o. melanocytosis
- o. melanosis

oculodigital reflex

oculofacial paralysis

oculoglandular
- o. conjunctivitis
- o. disease
- o. syndrome
- o. tularemia

oculography
    infrared o.
    photoelectric o.
    photosensor o.
oculogravic illusion
oculogyral illusion
oculogyration
oculogyria
oculogyric
    o. auricular reflex
    o. crisis
    o. mechanism
oculomandibulodyscephaly
oculomasticatory myorhythmia
oculomedin (OCLM)
oculometer
oculometroscope
oculomotor
    o. apraxia
    o. cranial nerve palsy
    o. decussation
    o. disorder
    o. nerve (N.III)
    o. nerve fascicle
    o. nerve lesion
    o. nerve misdirection
    o. nerve schwannoma
    o. nerve synkinesis
    o. nucleus
    o. paresis with cyclic spasm
    o. root
    o. root of ciliary ganglion
    o. system
oculomotorius
    nervus o.
oculomucous membrane syndrome
oculomycosis
oculonasal
Ocu-Lone
oculopalatal
    o. myoclonus
    o. myoclonus syndrome
    o. tremor
oculopathy
    hypertensive o.
    lupus o.
    pituitarigenic o.
oculopharyngeal
    o. dystrophy
    o. reflex
    o. syndrome
oculoplastics

Oculo-Plastik ePTFE ocular implant
oculoplasty corneal protector
oculoplethysmography
oculopneumoplethysmography (OPG)
oculopupillary reflex
oculoreaction
oculorenal syndrome
oculorespiratory reflex
oculorotatory muscle
oculosensory cell reflex
oculospinal
oculosporidiosis
oculosympathetic
    o. dysfunction
    o. paresis
    o. pathway
oculotoxic
oculovertebral dysplasia
oculovestibular reflex
oculozygomatic
Ocu-Lube
oculus, pl. **oculi**
    adnexa oculi
    albuginea oculi
    aqua oculi
    O. BIOM noncontact lens system
    bulbus oculi
    camera oculi
    congenital melanosis oculi
    deprimens oculi
    o. dexter (right eye)
    O. Easyloupes
    elephantiasis oculi
    endothelium oculi
    equator bulbi oculi
    fascia lata musculares oculi
    fiber orbicularis oculi
    fundus oculi
    hypertonia oculi
    hypotonia oculi
    melanosis oculi
    meridiani bulbi oculi
    motor oculi
    musculi oculi
    musculus obliquus inferior oculi
    musculus obliquus superior oculi
    musculus orbicularis oculi
    musculus rectus inferior oculi
    musculus rectus lateralis oculi
    musculus rectus medialis oculi
    pars caeca oculi

O

oculus *(continued)*
pars lacrimalis musculi orbicularis oculi
pars orbitalis musculi orbicularis oculi
pars palpebralis musculi orbicularis oculi
polus anterior bulbi oculi
polus posterior bulbi oculi
pseudotumor oculi
o. sinister (left eye)
sphincter oculi
tapetum oculi
tendo oculi
O. trial frame
trochlea musculi obliqui superioris oculi
tunica adnata oculi
tunica albuginea oculi
tunica conjunctiva bulbi oculi
tunica fibrosa oculi
tunica nervosa oculi
tunica vasculosa oculi
tutamina oculi
oculi unitas (both eyes)
oculi uterque (each eye) (OU)
vaginae oculi
vena choroideae oculi
visio o.
vitrina oculi
white tunica fibrosa oculi
OcuMax solution
Ocumeter
Ocu-Mycin
Ocu-Pentolate
Ocu-Phrin
Ocu-Pred
O.-P. A
O.-P. Forte
Ocupress
O. Ophthalmic
O. Ophthalmic Solution
Ocuscan
O. A-scan biometric ultrasound
Sonometric O.
O. 400 transducer
Ocusert
O. device
O. Pilo-20
O. Pilo-40
Ocusert-Pilo
Ocusil
OCuSoft
O. eyelid cleanser
O. scrub
Ocu-Sol
Ocu-Spor B, G
Ocusporin
Ocu-Tears PF

Ocutome
O. II fragmentation system
O. probe
O. vitrectomy unit
ocutome
Berkeley Bioengineering o.
CooperVision o.
disposable o.
Ocutricin HC
Ocu-Trol
Ocu-Tropic
Ocu-Tropine
Ocuvite
O. Extra
O. Lutein
O. Lutein Antioxidant Supplement
O. Lutein tablet
O. PreserVision vitamins
Ocu-Zoline
OCVM system
OD
right eye
ODD
oculodentodigital
ODD dysplasia
ODM
ophthalmodynamometry
O'Donoghue
O. angled DCR probe
O. silicone intubation
Odyssey phacoemulsification system
Oestrus ovis
off-axis imaging
OFF-center bipolar cell
OFF-pathway
ofloxacin ophthalmic solution
O'Gawa
O. cataract-aspirating cannula
O. suture-fixation forceps
O. two-way aspirating cannula
OGPR
OptiMed glaucoma pressure regulator
Ogston-Luc operation
Oguchi disease
Ogura
O. cartilage forceps
O. operation
O. tissue/cartilage forceps
O. tissue forceps
OHS
ocular histoplasmosis syndrome
macular OHS
OHT
ocular hypertension
OHTS
Ocular Hypertension Treatment Study
oil
o. layer
silicone o.

oily secretion
ointment (ung)
    AK-Spore H.C. Ophthalmic O.
    Akwa Tears lubricant
     ophthalmic o.
    anesthetic o.
    bland ophthalmic o.
    Cortisporin Ophthalmic O.
    Dexacine o.
    Dry Eyes lubricant o.
    LubriTears Lubricant Eye O.
    Moisture Eyes PM eye o.
    Neosporin Ophthalmic O.
    Neotricin HC Ophthalmic O.
    ophthalmic o.
    petrolatum ophthalmic o.
    Polycin-B O.
    Sty Ophthalmic O.
    Tears Naturale PM lubricant
     eye o.
    Tears Renewed O.
    Terak Ophthalmic O.
    Terramycin w/polymyxin B
     Ophthalmic O.
    ticrynafen o.
OIP
    ophthalmomyiasis interna posterior
OIS
    ocular ischemic syndrome
    OIS image digitizing system
    OIS WinStation 5000 Ophthalmic
     Imaging System
Okamura technique
Oklahoma iris wire retractor
OKN
    optokinetic nystagmus
OKT3
    orthoclone
Okuma plate
old
    o. eye
    o. sight
oleosa
    blepharitis o.
olfactory neuroblastoma
oligonucleotide primers
olivacea
    Microsphaeropsis o.
Olivella-Garrigosa photocoagulator
olive-tip
    o.-t. cannula

    o.-t. capsule polisher
    o.-t. irrigator
olivopontocerebellar atrophy (OPCA)
Olk
    O. vitreoretinal pick
    O. vitreoretinal spatula
OLM
    ophthalmic laser microendoscope
olopatadine hydrochloride ophthalmic solution
Olson
    O. calibrated cornea trephine
     system
    O. phaco chopper
    O. quick chopper
Olympus
    O. fundus camera
    O. Vanox VH-2 microscope
OM
    O. 2000 operation microscope
    O. 4 ophthalmometer
O'Malley-Heintz
    O.-H. infusion cannula
    O.-H. vitreous cutter
O'Malley-Pearce-Luma lens
O'Malley self-adhering lens implant
OMM
    ophthalmomandibulomelic
     OMM syndrome
Omnifit intraocular lens
OmniMed argon-fluoride excimer laser
Omni-Park speculum
OMP
    ophthalmic medical personnel
OMVAT
    Ocular Microcirculation View Analysis
     Treatment
ON
    optic nerve
on-axis imaging
ON-center bipolar cell
Onchocerca
    O. caecutiens
    O. volvulus
onchocercal sclerosing keratitis
onchocerciasis
    ocular o.
onchocercosis
ONE
    O. disposable microkeratome
    O. solution
one-and-a-half syndrome

NOTES

one-eye measurement
one-handed phacoemulsification
one-piece
    o.-p. bifocal
    o.-p. multifocal lens
    o.-p. plate haptic silicone
      intraocular lens
one-plane lens
one-snip
    o.-s. punctum
    o.-s. punctum operation
one-stage reconstruction of eye socket
  and eyelids
One-Step
    O.-S. limbal relaxing incision
      diamond knife
    O.-S. LRI diamond knife
on-eye
    o.-e. performance of lens
    o.-e. predicted power
Ong capsulotomy scissors
ONH
    optic nerve head
ONHD
    optic nerve head drusen
onion
    o. bulb neuropathy
    o. skin-like membrane
only
    light perception o. (LPO)
Onodi cell
ON-pathway
ONSD
    optic nerve sheath decompression
ONSF
    optic nerve sheath fenestration
ONSM
    optic nerve sheath meningioma
oozing
    transconjunctival aqueous o.
OP
    oscillatory potential
OP-05 hollow fiber filter
opaca
    cornea o.
opacification
    capsular o.
    o. cherry-red spot
    corneal o.
    cortical o.
    cyan o.
    polygonal stromal o.
    posterior capsular o.
    posterior capsule o. (PCO)
    subepithelial o.
opacified cuff
opacity
    calcium-containing o.
    Caspar ring o.

    congenital lens o.
    corneal o. (CO)
    corneal deep o.
    cortical o.
    crystalline o.
    deep corneal stromal o.
    dense o.
    disciform o.
    dust-like o.
    early lens o.
    evanescent corneal epithelial o.
    facetted avascular disciform o.
    interface o.
    lenticular o.
    leukomatous corneal o.
    media o.
    mycotic snowball o.
    nebular stromal o.
    peripheral corneal o.
    posterior subcapsular o.
    posterior supine position
      capsular o.
    pulverulent o.
    punctate corneal o.
    snowball o.
    spotty corneal o.
    striate o.
    stromal o.
    subepithelial corneal o.
    vitreous o.
    whorled corneal o.'s
opalescent cornea
OPAQUE
    O. Herrick Lacrimal Plug
opaque medium
OPCA
    olivopontocerebellar atrophy
Opcon
    O. Maximum Strength Allergy
      Drops
    Muro O.
    O. Ophthalmic
Opcon-A
OPD-Scan diagnostic system
open
    o. globe surgery
    o. lens
    o. loop
open-angle glaucoma (OAG)
open-funnel detachment
opening
    apraxia of eyelid o. (AEO)
    compulsive eye o.
    orbital o.
    o. of orbital cavity
    palpebral o.
    punctal o.
open-loop accommodation

open-sky
    o.-s. cataract wound
    o.-s. cryoextraction
    o.-s. cryoextraction operation
    o.-s. dissection
    o.-s. technique
    o.-s. trephination
    o.-s. vitrectomy
operating
    o. loupe
    o. microscope
    o. microscope-induced phototoxic
      maculopathy
operation
    ab externo filtering o.
    Adams o.
    Adler o.
    Agnew o.
    Agrikola o.
    Allen o.
    Allport o.
    Alsus o.
    Alsus-Knapp o.
    Alvis o.
    Ammon o.
    Amsler o.
    Anagnostakis o.
    Anel o.
    Angelucci o.
    anular corneal graft o.
    Argyll Robertson o.
    Arion o.
    Arlt o.
    Arlt-Jaesche o.
    Arrowhead o.
    Arroyo o.
    Arruga o.
    Arruga-Berens o.
    Badal o.
    Bangerter pterygium o.
    Bardelli lid ptosis o.
    Barkan-Cordes linear cataract o.
    Barkan double cyclodialysis o.
    Barkan goniotomy o.
    Barraquer enzymatic zonulolysis o.
    Barraquer keratomileusis o.
    Barrie-Jones
      canaliculodacryorhinostomy o.
    Barrio o.
    Basterra o.
    Beard o.
    Beard-Cutler o.

Beer o.
Benedict orbit o.
Berens sclerectomy o.
Berens-Smith o.
Berke o.
Berke-Motais o.
Bethke o.
Bielschowsky o.
Birch-Hirschfeld entropion o.
Blair o.
Blasius lid flap o.
Blaskovics canthoplasty o.
Blaskovics dacryostomy o.
Blaskovics inversion of tarsus o.
Blaskovics lid o.
Blatt o.
Böhm o.
Bonaccolto-Flieringa scleral ring o.
Bonaccolto-Flieringa vitreous o.
Bonnet enucleation o.
Bonzel o.
Borthen iridotasis o.
Bossalino blepharoplasty o.
Bowman o.
Boyd o.
Brailey o.
Bridge o.
bridge pedicle flap o.
Briggs strabismus o.
Bromley foreign body o.
Bronson foreign body removal o.
Budinger blepharoplasty o.
Burch eye evisceration o.
Burow flap o.
Buzzi o.
Byron Smith ectropion o.
Cairns o.
Calhoun-Hagler lens extraction o.
Callahan o.
Campodonico o.
Carter o.
Casanellas lacrimal o.
Casey o.
Castroviejo o.
Castroviejo-Scheie cyclodiathermy o.
cataract extraction o.
cautery o.
Celsus-Hotz o.
Celsus spasmodic entropion o.
cerclage o.
Chandler-Verhoeff o.
Chandler vitreous o.

NOTES

operation *(continued)*

Cibis o.
cinching o.
Cleasby iridectomy o.
Collin-Beard o.
Comberg foreign body o.
Conrad orbital blowout fracture o.
Cooper o.
corneal graft o.
Crawford sling o.
crescent o.
Critchett o.
Crock encircling o.
cryoextraction o.
cryotherapy o.
Csapody orbital repair o.
Cupper-Faden o.
Cusick o.
Cusick-Sarrail ptosis o.
Custodis o.
Cutler o.
Cutler-Beard o.
cyclodiathermy o.
Czermak pterygium o.
dacryoadenectomy o.
dacryocystectomy o.
dacryocystorhinostomy o.
dacryocystostomy o.
dacryocystotomy o.
Dailey o.
Dalgleish o.
Daviel o.
decompression of orbit o.
de Grandmont o.
Deiter o.
De Klair o.
de Lapersonne o.
Del Toro o.
Derby o.
Desmarres o.
de Vincentiis o.
de Wecker o.
Dianoux o.
diathermy o.
Dickey o.
Dickey-Fox o.
Dickson-Wright o.
Dieffenbach o.
dilation of punctum o.
discission of lens o.
D'ombrain o.
drainage of lacrimal gland o.
drainage of lacrimal sac o.
Duke-Elder o.
Dunnington o.
Dupuy-Dutemps o.
Durr o.
Duverger-Velter o.
Elliot o.

Elschnig canthorrhaphy o.
Ely o.
encircling of globe o.
encircling of scleral buckle o.
enucleation of eyeball o.
equilibrating o.
Erbakan inferior fornix o.
Escapini cataract o.
Esser inlay o.
Eversbusch o.
evisceration o.
Ewing o.
excision of lacrimal gland o.
excision of lacrimal sac o.
exenteration of orbital contents o.
extracapsular cataract extraction o.
Faden o.
Fanta cataract o.
Fasanella o.
Fasanella-Servat ptosis o.
fascia lata sling for ptosis o.
Fergus o.
Filatov o.
Filatov-Marzinkowsky o.
filtering o.
Fink o.
Flajani o.
Förster o.
Fould entropion o.
Fox o.
Franceschetti coreoplasty o.
Franceschetti corepraxy o.
Franceschetti deviation o.
Franceschetti keratoplasty o.
Franceschetti pupil deviation o.
Fricke o.
Friede o.
Friedenwald o.
Friedenwald-Guyton o.
Frost-Lang o.
Fuchs canthorrhaphy o.
Fuchs iris bombe transfixation o.
Fukala o.
Gayet o.
Gifford delimiting keratotomy o.
Gillies scar correction o.
Girard keratoprosthesis o.
Goldmann-Larson foreign body o.
Gomez-Marquez lacrimal o.
Gonin cautery o.
goniotomy o.
Gradle keratoplasty o.
Graefe o.
Greaves o.
Grimsdale o.
Grossmann o.
Gutzeit dacryostomy o.
Guyton ptosis o.
Halpin o.

Harman o.
Harms-Dannheim trabeculotomy o.
Hasner o.
Heine o.
Heisrath o.
Herbert o.
Hess eyelid o.
Hess ptosis o.
Hiff o.
Hill o.
Hippel o.
Hogan o.
Holth o.
Horay o.
Horvath o.
Hotz-Anagnostakis o.
Hotz entropion o.
Hughes o.
Hummelsheim o.
Hunt-Transley o.
Iliff o.
Iliff-Haus o.
Imre lateral canthoplasty o.
indentation o.
iridectomy o.
iridencleisis o.
iridodialysis o.
iridotasis o.
iridotomy o.
Irvine o.
Irving o.
Jaesche o.
Jaesche-Arlt o.
Jaime lacrimal o.
Jameson o.
Jensen o.
Johnson o.
Jones o.
Katzin o.
Kelman o.
keratectomy o.
keratocentesis o.
keratomileusis o.
keratoplasty o.
keratotomy o.
Key o.
King o.
Kirby o.
Knapp o.
Knapp-Imre o.
Knapp-Wheeler-Reese o.
Koffler o.

Kraupa o.
Kreibig o.
Kreiker o.
Krieberg o.
Krönlein o.
Krönlein-Berke o.
Kuhnt eyelid o.
Kuhnt-Helmbold o.
Kuhnt-Szymanowski o.
Kuhnt-Thorpe o.
Kwitko o.
LaCarrere o.
Lagleyze o.
Lagleyze-Trantas o.
Lagrange o.
laissez-faire lid o.
Lancaster o.
Lanchner o.
Landolt o.
Langenbeck o.
Leahey o.
Lester Jones o.
Lexer o.
Lincoff o.
Lindner o.
Lindsay o.
Löhlein o.
Londermann o.
Lopez-Enriquez o.
Löwenstein o.
Machek-Blaskovics o.
Machek-Brunswick o.
Machek-Gifford o.
Machek ptosis o.
Mack-Brunswick o.
Magitot keratoplasty o.
magnet o.
magnetic o.
Magnus o.
Majewsky o.
Malbec o.
Malbran o.
Marquez-Gomez o.
Mauksch o.
Mauksch-Maumenee-Goldberg o.
Maumenee-Goldberg o.
McGavic o.
McGuire o.
McLaughlin o.
McLean o.
McReynolds o.
Meek o.

O

NOTES

361

operation *(continued)*

Meller o.
Meyer-Schwickerath o.
Michaelson o.
Mikamo double-eyelid o.
Minsky o.
Moncrieff o.
Moran o.
Morax o.
Morel-Fatio-Lalardie o.
Mosher o.
Mosher-Toti o.
Moss o.
Motais o.
Mueller o.
Mules o.
Mustarde o.
myectomy o.
myotomy o.
Naffziger o.
Neher o.
Nehra-Mack o.
Nida nicking o.
Nizetic o.
O'Connor o.
O'Connor-Peter o.
Ogston-Luc o.
Ogura o.
one-snip punctum o.
open-sky cryoextraction o.
orbital implant o.
Pagenstecher o.
Panas o.
pars plana o.
pattern cut corneal graft o.
Paufique o.
peripheral iridectomy o.
Peters o.
Physick o.
Pico o.
plombage o.
pocket o.
Polyak o.
Poulard o.
Power o.
Preziosi o.
probing lacrimonasal duct o.
Putenney o.
Quaglino o.
Raverdino o.
Ray-Brunswick-Mack o.
Ray-McLean o.
reattachment of choroid o.
reattachment of retina o.
recession of ocular muscle o.
Redmond-Smith o.
Reese-Cleasby o.
Reese-Jones-Cooper o.
Reese ptosis o.

removal of foreign body o.
Richet o.
Rosenburg o.
Rosengren o.
Roveda o.
Rowbotham o.
Rowinski o.
Rubbrecht o.
Ruedemann o.
Rycroft o.
Saemisch o.
Safar o.
Sanders o.
Sato o.
Savin o.
Sayoc o.
Scheie o.
Schepens o.
Schimek o.
Schirmer o.
Schmalz o.
scleral buckling o.
scleral fistulectomy o.
scleral shortening o.
scleroplasty o.
sclerotomy o.
sector iridectomy o.
Selinger o.
seton o.
Shaffer o.
Shugrue o.
Sichi o.
Silva-Costa o.
Silver-Hildreth o.
slant muscle o.
Smith eyelid o.
Smith-Indian o.
Smith-Kuhnt-Szymanowski o.
Snellen ptosis o.
Soria o.
Soriano o.
Sourdille keratoplasty o.
Sourdille ptosis o.
Spaeth cystic bleb o.
Spaeth ptosis o.
Speas o.
Spencer-Watson Z-plasty o.
splitting lacrimal papilla o.
Stallard eyelid o.
Stallard flap o.
Stallard-Liegard o.
step graft o.
Stock o.
Stocker o.
Straith eyelid o.
Strampelli-Valvo o.
Streatfield o.
Streatfield-Fox o.
Streatfield-Snellen o.

Suarez-Villafranca o.
Summerskill o.
suture of cornea o.
suture of eyeball o.
suture of iris o.
suture of muscle o.
suture of sclera o.
Szymanowski o.
Szymanowski-Kuhnt o.
Tansley o.
Tasia o.
tattoo of cornea o.
Teale-Knapp o.
tenotomy o.
Terson o.
Tessier o.
Thomas o.
three-snip punctum o.
Tillett o.
Toti o.
Toti-Mosher o.
Townley-Paton o.
trabeculectomy o.
Trainor o.
Trainor-Nida o.
transfixion of iris o.
transplantation of muscle o.
Trantas o.
trap-door scleral buckle o.
Tripier o.
Troutman o.
Truc o.
Tudor-Thomas o.
tumbling technique o.
Ulloa o.
Uyemura o.
Van Milligen o.
Verhoeff o.
Verhoeff-Chandler o.
Verwey eyelid o.
Viers o.
Vogt o.
von Ammon o.
von Blaskovics-Doyen o.
von Graefe o.
von Hippel o.
Waldhauer o.
Walter Reed o.
Watzke o.
Weeker o.
Weeks o.
Weisinger o.

Wendell Hughes o.
Werb o.
West o.
Weve o.
Wharton-Jones o.
Wheeler o.
Wheeler-Reese o.
Whitnall sling o.
Wicherkiewicz eyelid o.
Wiener o.
Wies o.
Wilmer o.
Wolfe ptosis o.
Worst o.
Worth ptosis o.
Wright o.
Young o.
Ziegler o.
Zylik o.

operculated
    o. retinal hole
    o. retinal tear
    o. tear

operculum, pl. **opercula**
    free o.
    peripheral retinal o.

OPG
    oculopneumoplethysmography

Ophacet

ophryogenes
    ulerythema o.

ophryosis

Ophtec
    O. Co. lens
    O. 9.0 mm trephine
    O. occlusion implant

Ophthacet

Ophthaine

Ophthalas
    O. argon/krypton laser
    O. argon laser
    O. krypton laser

Ophthalgan Ophthalmic

ophthalmagra

ophthalmalgia

ophthalmatrophia

ophthalmectomy

ophthalmencephalon

Ophthalmetron
    Safir O.

ophthalmia
    actinic ray o.

NOTES

363

ophthalmia *(continued)*
    Brazilian o.
    catarrhal o.
    caterpillar o.
    caterpillar-hair o.
    o. eczematosa
    Egyptian o.
    electric o.
    o. electrica
    flash o.
    gonococcal o.
    gonorrheal o.
    granular o.
    o. hepatica
    jequirity o.
    o. lenta
    metastatic o.
    migratory o.
    mucous o.
    neonatal o.
    o. neonatorum
    neuroparalytic o.
    o. nivalis
    nivalis o.
    o. nodosa
    periodic o.
    phlyctenular o.
    pseudotuberculous o.
    purulent o.
    reaper's o.
    scrofulous o.
    spring o.
    strumous o.
    sympathetic o.
    transferred o.
    ultraviolet ray o.
    varicose o.
    vegetable o.
ophthalmiatrics
ophthalmic
    Absorbonac o.
    Achromycin O.
    Acular O.
    Adsorbocarpine O.
    Akarpine O.
    AK-Chlor O.
    AK-Cide O.
    AK-Con o.
    AK-Dex O.
    AK-Homatropine O.
    AK-Neo-Dex O.
    AK-Poly-Bac O.
    AK-Pred O.
    AKPro O.
    AK-Sulf O.
    AKTob O.
    AK-Tracin O.
    Albalon-A O.
    Albalon Liquifilm O.

alpha-2-adrenergic agonist agent, o.
Antazoline-V O.
o. artery
o. artery aneurysm
o. artery occlusion (OAO)
Betimol O.
Betoptic S O.
Bleph-10 O.
Blephamide O.
Carbastat O.
Carboptic O.
o. cautery
Cetamide O.
Cetapred o.
Chloroptic O.
Chloroptic-P O.
Ciloxan O.
Collyrium Fresh O.
Comfort O.
O. Confidence Index (OCI)
o. corticosteroid
o. cul-de-sac
o. cup
Cyclomydril O.
Degest 2 O.
o. disorder
o. drill
o. drug
Econopred O.
o. electrocautery
o. endoscope
Estivin II O.
o. examination
Eyesine O.
Floropryl O.
o. ganglion
Geneye O.
Genoptic S.O.P. o.
Gentacidin o.
Gentak o.
o. glucocorticoid
o. Graves disease
Herplex O.
o. hook
Humorsol O.
o. hyperthyroidism
Ilotycin O.
I-Naphline O.
Inflamase Forte O.
Inflamase Mild O.
Isopto Carbachol O.
Isopto Carpine O.
Isopto Cetamide O.
Isopto Cetapred o.
Isopto Homatropine O.
Isopto Hyoscine O.
o. laser microendoscope (OLM)
o. medical personnel (OMP)
Metimyd O.

o. migraine
O. Moldite Powder
Murine Plus O.
Murocoll-2 O.
Nafazair O.
Naphcon O.
Naphcon-A O.
NeoDecadron O.
Neo-Dexameth O.
o. nerve
OcuClear O.
Ocufen O.
Ocuflox o.
Ocupress O.
o. ointment
Opcon O.
Ophthalgan O.
Optigene O.
OptiPranolol O.
Osmoglyn O.
Paremyd O.
Phospholine Iodide O.
O. Photographers Society (OPS)
Pilagan O.
Pilocar O.
Pilopine HS O.
Piloptic O.
Pilostat O.
o. plexus
Polysporin O.
Polytrim O.
Pred Forte O.
Pred-G O.
Pred Mild O.
Profenal O.
o. progressive-power lens
Propine O.
PxEx O.
o. reaction
Sodium Sulamyd O.
o. solution
o. sponge
Sulf-10 O.
o. test
Tetrasine Extra O.
Timoptic O.
Timoptic-XE O.
TobraDex O.
Tobrex O.
Vasocidin O.
VasoClear O.
Vasocon-A O.

Vasocon Regular O.
Vasosulf O.
o. vein
o. vesicle
Vira-A O.
Viroptic O.
Visine Extra O.
Visine L.R. o.
o. vitreous surgical technique
Voltaren O.
ophthalmica
vesicula o.
zona o.
ophthalmicus
caliculus o.
herpes zoster o.
nervus o.
varicella zoster o.
zoster o.
ophthalmitic
ophthalmitis
ophthalmoblennorrhea
ophthalmocarcinoma
ophthalmocele
ophthalmocopia
ophthalmodesmitis
ophthalmodiagnosis
ophthalmodiaphanoscope
ophthalmodiastimeter
ophthalmodonesis
ophthalmodynamometer
Bailliart o.
Reichert o.
suction o.
ophthalmodynamometry (ODM)
ophthalmodynia
ophthalmoeikonometer
ophthalmofunduscope
ophthalmogram
ophthalmograph
ophthalmography
ophthalmogyric
ophthalmoleukoscope
ophthalmolith
ophthalmologic
ophthalmologist
European Contact Lens Society
of O.'s
Royal Australian College of O.'s
Royal College of O.'s (UK)
ophthalmology
American Academy of O. (AAO)

O

NOTES

ophthalmology *(continued)*
    American Board of O. (ABO)
    American Society of
      Contemporary O. (ASCO)
    Association for Research in Vision
      and O. (ARVO)
    Association of Technical Personnel
      in O. (ATPO)
    Certified Registered Nurse in O.
      (CRNO)
    Fellow of the American Academy
      of O. (FAAO)
    Joint Commission on Allied Health
      Personnel in O. (JCAHPO)
    Montana Academy of O. (MAO)
    occupational o.
ophthalmomalacia
ophthalmomandibulomelic (OMM)
    o. dysplasia
ophthalmomelanosis
ophthalmomeningea
    vena o.
ophthalmomeningeal vein
ophthalmometer
    Haag-Streit o.
    Javal o.
    Javal-Schiotz o.
    Micromatic o.
    mires of o.
    OM 4 o.
ophthalmometroscope
ophthalmometry
ophthalmomycosis
ophthalmomyiasis
    Cuterebra o.
    o. interna posterior (OIP)
ophthalmomyitis
ophthalmomyositis
ophthalmomyotomy
ophthalmoneuritis
ophthalmoneuromyelitis
ophthalmoparesis
    internuclear o.
ophthalmopathy
    dysthyroid o.
    endocrine o.
    external o.
    Graves o.
    internal o.
    thyroid o.
    thyroid-associated o. (TAO)
ophthalmophacometer
ophthalmophantom
ophthalmophlebotomy
ophthalmophthisis
ophthalmoplasty
ophthalmoplegia
    autosomal-dominant o.
    autosomal-recessive o.

    basal o.
    binocular internuclear o. (BINO)
    chronic progressive external o.
      (CPEO)
    exophthalmic o.
    o. externa
    external o.
    fascicular o.
    infectious o.
    infranuclear o.
    o. interna
    internal o.
    internuclear o. (INO)
    o. internuclearis
    migraine o.
    migrainous o.
    nuclear o.
    orbital o.
    painful o.
    Parinaud o.
    partial o.
    o. partialis
    posterior internuclear o.
    o. progressiva
    progressive external o. (PEO)
    pseudointernuclear o.
    Sauvineau o.
    sensory ataxic neuropathy with
      dysarthria and o. (SANDO)
    supranuclear o.
    thyrotoxicosis o.
    total o.
    o. totalis
    wall-eyed bilateral internuclear o.
ophthalmoplegic
    o. exophthalmos
    o. migraine
    o. muscular dystrophy
ophthalmoptosis
ophthalmoreaction
    Calmette o.
ophthalmorrhagia
ophthalmorrhea
ophthalmorrhexis
ophthalmoscope
    Alcon indirect o.
    All Pupil II indirect o.
    AO Reichert Instruments binocular
      indirect o.
    Bailliart o.
    binocular indirect o.
    Canon SLO scanning laser o.
    confocal laser scanning o.
    cordless monocular indirect o.
    demonstration o.
    direct o.
    Doran pattern stimulator o.
    Exeter o.
    Fison indirect binocular o.

Friedenwald o.
Ful-Vue o.
ghost o.
Gullstrand o.
Halberg indirect o.
halogen o.
Heidelberg retina angiograph digital scanning laser o.
Helmholtz o.
Highlight spectral indirect o.
indirect o.
Keeler o.
Loring o.
Mentor Exeter o.
metric o.
MK IV o.
monocular indirect o.
Neolyte laser indirect o.
Nerve Fiber Analyzer laser o.
Novus 2000 o.
Panoramic200 Non-Mydriatic O.
polarizing o.
Polle pod attachment for o.
Propper-Heine o.
Propper indirect o.
Reichert binocular indirect o.
Reichert Ful-Vue binocular o.
Rodenstock scanning laser o.
scanning laser o. (SLO)
Schepens binocular indirect o.
Schepens-Pomerantzeff o.
TopSS scanning laser o.
Vantage o.
Video Binocular indirect o. (VBIO)
Visuscope o.
Welch-Allyn o.
Zeiss o.
ophthalmoscopic
   o. detectability
   o. examination
ophthalmoscopy
   binocular indirect o.
   confocal laser scanning o. (cLSO)
   direct o.
   distant direct o.
   dynamic scanning laser o.
   indirect o.
   medical o.
   metric o.
   slit-lamp o.
   o. with reflected light
ophthalmospectroscope

ophthalmospectroscopy
ophthalmostasis
ophthalmostat
ophthalmostatometer
ophthalmosteresis
ophthalmosynchysis
ophthalmothermometer
ophthalmotomy
ophthalmotonometer
ophthalmotonometry
ophthalmotoxin
ophthalmotrope
ophthalmotropometer
ophthalmotropometry
ophthalmovascular
ophthalmoxerosis
ophthalmoxyster
Ophthalon suture
Ophthalsonic pachometer
Ophtha P/S
Ophthascan
   Alcon-Biophysic O. S
Ophthasonic Ultrasonic Biometer
Ophthas subjective optometer
Ophthel
Ophthetic
Ophthilon
Ophthimus
   O. High-Pass Resolution perimeter
   O. ring perimeter
Ophthochlor
Ophthocort
opiate analgesic
OPL
   outer plexiform layer
OPMI
   O. pico i microscope
   O. PRO magis microscope
   O. VISU 200 BrightFlex illuminator
   O. VISU 200 microscope
Opmilas 144 surgical laser
OPP
   ocular perfusion pressure
opponent
   o. color
   o. colors theory
Opraflex drape
OPS
   Ophthalmic Photographers Society
opsin
   cone o.

NOTES

O

opsiometer
opsoclonia
opsoclonus
    paraneoplastic o.
Optacon
Optacryl
Opt-Ease
Optec 3000 contrast sensitivity test
Optef
Optelec
    O. Passport magnifier
    O. Spectrum Jr.
Op-Temp
    O.-T. disposable cautery
    O.-T. disposable electrocautery
optesthesia
Op-Thal-Zin
Opthascan Mini-A scan
Optho
    RO O.
Opti-Bon
optic
    o. agnosia
    o. angle
    o. aphasia
    o. artery
    o. ataxia
    o. axis
    biconvex o.
    o. canal
    o. center
    o. chiasm
    o. chiasmal lesion
    o. chiasmal syndrome
    o. commissure
    o. cul-de-sac
    o. cup
    o. cup-to-disk ratio
    o. decussation
    o. demyelinating neuritis
    o. disc change
    o. disc topography
    o. disk
    o. disk anomaly
    o. disk atrophy
    o. disk cupping
    o. disk dragging
    o. disk drusen
    o. disk drusen calcification
    o. disk drusen retinopathy
    o. disk dysplasia
    o. disk edema
    o. disk hypoplasia
    o. disk pallor
    o. disk pit
    o. disk swelling
    o. disk tubercle
    o. evagination
    o. foramen

o. fundus
o. ganglion
o. groove
o. hyperesthesia
o. implant
o. iridectomy
o. keratoplasty
o. lemniscus
o. muscle recession
o. nerve (N.II, ON)
o. nerve aplasia
o. nerve atrophy
o. nerve coloboma
o. nerve cupping
o. nerve disease
o. nerve disorder
o. nerve dysfunction
o. nerve dysplasia
o. nerve fiber
o. nerve glioma
o. nerve head (ONH)
o. nerve head appearance
o. nerve head drusen (ONHD)
o. nerve hemangioblastoma
o. nerve hypoplasia
o. nerve injury
o. nerve lesion
o. nerve myelination
o. nerve pit
o. nerve sheath
o. nerve sheath decompression (ONSD)
o. nerve sheath fenestration (ONSF)
o. nerve sheath meningioma (ONSM)
o. nerve tumor
o. neuropathy
o. papilla (P)
o. papilla cavity
o. perineuritis
o. primordium
o. radiation
o. radiation lesion
o. recess
o. stalk
o. strut
o. sulcus
o. thalamus
o. tract
o. tract compression
o. tract damage
o. tract lesion
o. tract syndrome
o. vesicle
optica, pl. **opticae**
commissurae opticae
hyperesthesia o.

neuromyelitis o.
radiatio o.
Opticaid
    Spring Clip O.
optical
    o. aberration
    o. alexia
    o. allachesthesia
    American O. (AO)
    o. axis
    o. bench
    o. blur
    o. breakdown
    o. center
    o. centering instrument
    o. center of spectacle lens
    o. clarity
    o. coherence tomography (OCT)
    o. contact lens
    o. correction
    o. cross
    o. density method
    o. disk anomaly
    o. disk swelling
    o. dispenser
    o. fossa
    o. frame
    o. glass
    o. heterogeneity
    o. illusion
    o. image
    o. iridectomy
    o. keratoplasty
    o. nodal point
    o. pachymeter
    o. performance
    o. power
    o. quality
    O. Radiation lens
    o. ray tracing
    o. rehabilitation
    o. side effect
    o. system
    o. transfer function
    o. zone (OZ)
    o. zone centration
    o. zone of contact lens
    o. zone diameter
    o. zone marker
optically empty
Opticath

optici
    circulus vasculosus nervi o.
    discus nervi o.
    evulsio nervi o.
    excavatio papillae nervi o.
    radix lateralis tractus o.
    radix medialis tractus o.
    vaginae externa nervi o.
    vaginae interna nervi o.
optician
opticianry
opticist
Opti-Clean II
Opti-Clear
opticoacoustic nerve atrophy
opticocerebral syndrome
opticochiasmatic, optochiasmic
    o. arachnoiditis
opticociliary
    o. neurectomy
    o. neurotomy
    o. shunt
    o. shunt vein
    o. shunt vessel
opticocinerea
opticocochleodentate degeneration
opticofacial winking reflex
opticokinetic nystagmus
opticomyelitis
opticonasion
opticopupillary
opticopyramidal syndrome
Opticrom
optics
    Allergan Medical O. (AMO)
    American Medical O.
    confocal o.
    Fresnel o.
    gaussian o.
    geometric o.
    Infinitech fiber o.
    o. of intraocular lens
    physical o.
    physiologic o.
    reverse o.
opticum
    chiasma o.
    foramen o.
opticus
    axis o.
    canaliculus infraorbitalis o.
    canalis o.

NOTES

opticus *(continued)*
    discus o.
    nervus o.
    porus o.
    recessus o.
Opticyl
Optiflex lens
Opti-Free
    O.-F. Daily Cleaner
    O.-F. Enzymatic Cleaner
    O.-F. Express Multi-Purpose
    Solution
    O.-F. Rewetting Drops
    O.-F. Rinsing Disinfecting and
    Storage
    O.-F. Supraclens
Optigene
    O. 3
    O. Ophthalmic
Optik
Optikon 2000 placido-based corneal topography system Keratron Scout
Optima
    O. contact lens
    O. diamond knife
OptiMed
    O. device
    O. glaucoma pressure regulator
    (OGPR)
Optimine
Optimize viscoelastic
Optimmune
Optimum
    O. blade
    O. Cleaning, Disinfecting, and
    Storage Solution
    O. by Lobob
    O. by Lobob Daily Cleaner
    O. by Lobob Gas Permeable
    Cleaning/Disinfecting/Storage
    O. by Lobob Gas Permeable
    Wetting/Rewetting
    O. by Lobob Wetting and
    Rewetting Drops
    O. rigid gas permeable starter kit
Optimyd
Opti-One
    O.-O. Conditioning Solution
    O.-O. Multi-Purpose Solution
    O.-O. Rewetting Drops
Optiphot microscope
OptiPranolol Ophthalmic
Optipress
Opti-Pure System
Optique 1 Eye Drops
Optised
Opti-Soak
    O.-S. Conditioning Solution
    O.-S. Daily Cleaner

Optisoap
Opti-Soft
Optisol-GS
Optisol medium
optist
Opti-Tears
Optivar ophthalmic solution
Opti-Vu lens
Opti-Zyme enzymatic cleaner
OPTN gene
optoblast
optochiasmatic
    o. arachnoiditis
    o. tuberculoma
optochiasmic *(var. of* opticochiasmatic)
optociliary shunt vessel
optogram
optokinesis
optokinetic
    o. drum
    o. nystagmus (OKN)
    o. reflex
    o. stimulator
    o. stimulus
    o. system
    o. tape
    o. test
optomeninx
optometer
    automatic infrared o.
    infrared o.
    laser o.
    objective o.
    Ophthas subjective o.
    Vernier o.
optometric
    para o.
optometrist
optometry
    American Academy of O. (AAO)
    Fellow of the American Academy
    of O. (FAAO)
optomotor reflex
optomyometer
optophone
optostriate
optotype
    Sloan o.
    Snellen letter o.
Optrex
Optrin
Opt-Visor
    O.-V. lens
    O.-V. loupe
Optycryl 60 contact lens
Optyl frame
Opus III contact lens
OR
    overrefraction

ora (*pl. of* os)
oral
    AllerMax O.
    Banophen O.
    Belix O.
    Benadryl O.
    Cartrol O.
    Cytoxan O.
    Dimetabs O.
    Kerlone O.
    Phendry O.
    Siladryl O.
    Toradol O.
orange
    o. dye laser
    o. punctate pigmentation
orange-red lesion
Oratrol
orb
orbiculare
    Pityrosporum o.
orbiculare
    os o.
orbicularis
    alopecia o.
    o. ciliaris
    musculus o.
    o. myectomy
    o. oculi muscle
    o. oris muscle
    o. phenomenon
    o. pupillary reflex
    o. reaction
    o. sign
    o. strength
orbicular muscle of eye
orbiculoanterocapsular fiber
orbiculociliary fiber
orbiculoposterocapsular fiber
orbit
    aneurysm of o.
    o. blade
    blow-out fracture of o.
    contusion of o.
    CT scan of o.
    dermoid of o.
    emphysema of o.
    fracture of o.
    o. hamartoma
    idiopathic sclerosing inflammation
      of the o.
    intraorbital margin of o.

    lateral margin of o.
    lesion of o.
    roof of o.
    supraorbital margin of o.
orbitae
    aditus o.
    corpus adiposum o.
    exenteratio o.
    margo infraorbitalis o.
    margo lateralis o.
    margo medialis o.
    margo supraorbitalis o.
    paries interior o.
    paries lateralis o.
    paries medialis o.
    paries superior o.
orbital
    o. adipose tissue
    o. akinesia
    o. amyloidosis
    o. anesthesia
    o. aneurysm
    o. angiography
    o. angioma
    o. angiosarcoma
    o. aperture
    o. apex
    o. apex syndrome
    o. arch
    o. arch of frontal bone
    o. arteriovenous malformation
    o. axis
    o. blow-out fracture
    o. border of sphenoid bone
    o. canal
    o. cavity
    o. cellulite
    o. cellulitis
    o. conjunctiva
    o. content
    o. crest
    o. CT scan
    o. cyst
    o. decompression
    o. decompression surgery
    o. depressor
    o. dermoid
    o. dystopia
    o. echography
    o. emphysema
    o. encephalocele
    o. enlargement

NOTES

O

orbital *(continued)*

o. enucleation compressor
o. exenteration
o. extension
o. fascia
o. fasciitis
o. fat
o. fat pad
o. fat suppression
o. fibroma
o. fibromatosis
o. fibrosarcoma
o. floor
o. floor fracture
o. floor implant
o. floor prosthesis
o. ganglion
o. glioma
o. granuloma
o. hamartoma
o. height
o. hemangioendothelioma
o. hemangioma
o. hemangiopericytoma
o. hematoma
o. hemorrhage
o. hernia
o. hypertelorism
o. hypotelorism
o. hypoxia
o. implant operation
o. infarction
o. infarction syndrome
o. inferior rim
o. inflammatory pseudotumor
o. lamina
o. lens
o. lesion
o. lipoma
o. lymphoma
o. margin
o. medulloepithelioma
o. melanoma
o. meningioma
o. mesenchyme
o. metastasis
o. muscle
o. myositis
o. neoplasm
o. neuritis
o. neuroepithelioma
o. neurofibroma
o. neuroma
o. opening
o. ophthalmoplegia
o. optic nerve
o. palsy
o. pathology
o. periosteum

o. periostitis
o. pit
o. plane
o. plane of frontal bone
o. plaque brachytherapy
o. plate of ethmoid bone
o. plate of frontal bone
o. polymyositis
o. portion of eyelid
o. radiology
o. radiotherapy
o. region
o. resilience
o. rhabdomyosarcoma
o. rim fracture
o. roentgenogram
o. roof
o. schwannoma
o. section
o. septum
o. subperiosteal abscess
o. sulci of frontal bone
o. sulcus
o. superior fissure
o. tomography
o. trauma
o. tumor
o. varix
o. vasculitis
o. vein thrombosis
o. venography
o. vessel
o. wall fracture
o. width
o. wing of sphenoid bone
o. x-ray

orbitale
planum o.
septum o.

orbitales
fasciae o.

orbitalia
cribra o.

orbitalis
margo o.
musculus o.

orbitectomy
radical o.

orbitocranial
o. imaging
o. trauma

orbitography
Graves o.

orbitomalar foramen
orbitonasal
orbitonometer
orbitonometry
orbitopalpebral

orbitopathy
    congestive o.
    dysthyroid o.
    Graves o.
    thyroid o.
orbitostat
orbitotemporal
orbitotomy
    Berke-Krönlein o.
    lateral o.
Orbscan
    O. corneal topography
    O. II multidimensional diagnostic
      system
    O. II topography system
    O. pachymetry mapping
    O. topography analysis system
Orca surgical blade
ORC intraocular lens
order
    random o.
ordered array
ordering
    Dyer nomogram system of lens o.
organ
    o. culture
    o. transplantation
    vestibular o.
    o. of vision
    visual o.
organic amblyopia
organism
    coliform o.
    HACEK group o.
organized vitreous
organizer
    Richard Products fundus camera
      drug o.
organum
    o. visuale
    o. visus
orientation
    epithelial o.
    false o.
    limbal parallel o.
oriented
    radially o.
original
    o. Sweet eye magnet
    Visine O.

oris
    pars marginalis musculi
      orbicularis o.
    sphincter o.
ornithine tolerance test
orodigitofacial dysplasia
orthoclone (OKT3)
orthogonal
Orthogon lens
ortho-K
orthokeratology
    Lenses and Overnight O. (LOOK)
    o. lens wear
Ortho-Lite
orthometer
orthophoria
orthophoric
orthopia
orthoposition
orthoptic
orthoptist
    Certified O. (CO)
orthoptoscope
Ortho-Rater
orthoscope
orthoscopic
    o. lens
    o. spectacles
orthoscopy
Ortopad orthoptic patch
Or-Toptic M
OS
    left eye
os, pl. ora
    ora globule
    o. lacrimale
    o. orbiculare
    o. palatinum
    o. planum
    ora serrata retinae
    o. unguis
oscillating
    o. nystagmus
    o. vision
oscillation
    convergent-divergent pendular o.
    macrosaccadic o.
    nystagmoid-like o.
    ocular o.
    voluntary saccadic o.
oscillatory potential (OP)

O

NOTES

oscillopsia
>monocular o.
>torsional o.

OSD
>ocular surface disease

O'Shea lens

Osher
>O. foreign body forceps
>O. gonio/posterior pole lens
>O. hook
>O. pan-fundus lens
>O. surgical gonio/posterior pole lens
>O. surgical keratometer

Osher-Neumann corneal marker

Osmitrol injection

osmium
>o. tetroxide
>o. tetroxide solution

Osmoglyn Ophthalmic

osmolarity
>tear o.

osmotherapy
>hypertonic o.

osmotic
>o. cataract
>o. pressure

ossea
>bulla o.
>cataracta o.

osseous
>o. anomaly
>o. choristoma
>o. lesion
>o. metaplasia over the choroidal hemangioma
>o. system

osseus
>tarsus o.

ossis
>bulla ethmoidalis o.

ossium
>fragilitas o.

osteitis deformans

osteoma
>choroidal o.
>uveal o.

osteomyelitis
>maxillary o.

osteoporosis-pseudoglioma syndrome

osteosclerotic myeloma

osteotome
>lacrimal o.

osteotomy

ostium
>internal o.

Ota
>nevus of O.

>O. nevus
>O. nevus syndrome

OTHA
>ocular total higher-order aberration

oticus
>herpes zoster o.

Otis-Lennon School Ability Test

OTI ultrasound B & A scan

otolithic-ocular reflex

OTR
>ocular tilt reaction

OU
>both eyes
>oculi uterque (each eye)

out
>base o. (BO)
>pericyte drop o.

outcome
>refractive o.

outer
>o. canthus
>o. limiting membrane
>o. nuclear layer
>o. nuclear layer of retina
>o. plexiform layer (OPL)
>o. retinal necrosis syndrome
>o. segment

outflow
>aqueous o.
>coefficient of facility of o.
>conventional o.
>o. disorder
>facility of o.
>lacrimal o.
>o. obstruction
>parasympathetic o.
>o. resistance
>trabecular o.
>unconventional o.
>uveoscleral o.

outfolding
>scleral o.

outgrowth
>extrascleral o.
>local o.

outpouching

output nerve

Ovadendron sulphureo-ochraceum **endophthamitis**

oval
>o. cornea
>o. cup erysiphake
>o. eye
>o. eye patch

ovale
>patent foramen o. (PFO)
>*Pityrosporum* o.

oval-shaped vernal ulcer

OVAS
    Ocular Vergence and Accommodation
    Sensor
overaction
        inferior oblique o. (IOOA)
overall diameter of contact lens (OAD)
overcorrection
over-dipping
overflow diabetes
overpigmentation
overrefraction (OR)
overripe cataract
overt diabetes
overwear syndrome (OWS)
ovis
        Oestrus o.
ovoid mass
OWS
        overwear syndrome
oxidation of solution
oxide
        cocoamidopropylamine o.
        mercuric o.
oxidopamine
Oxi-Freeda
oximetry sensor
oxprenolol

Oxsoralen
oxyblepsia
oxybuprocaine hydrochloride
oxycephaly
oxycodone
oxygen
        o. flux
        o. permeability (Dk, DK)
        o. transmissibility (Dk/L)
oxymetazoline HCl
oxymorphone hydrochloride
oxyopia
oxyopter
oxyphenbutazone
oxyphenonium
Oxysept
        Lens Plus O.
oxysporum
        Fusarium o.
oxytetracycline
        o. and hydrocortisone
        o. and polymyxin B
oxytoca
        Klebsiella o.
oyster shuckers' keratitis
OZ
        optical zone

NOTES

O

P

optic papilla
pupil

P55 Pachymetric Analyzer

PA

phakic-aphakic

Pachette

DGH-500 P.
P. 2 ultrasonic pachymeter

PachKnife

Corneo-Gage P.

pachometer

Alcon ultrasound p.
corneal p.
Humphrey ultrasonic p.
Ophthalsonic p.
Packo pars plana cannula p.
Sonogage ultrasound p.
ultrasound p.

Pach-Pen

P.-P. XL pachymeter
P.-P. XL tonometer

pachyblepharon
pachyblepharosis
pachymeter

Advent p.
BVI PAXIS biometric ruler and p.
Compuscan-P p.
corneal p.
DGH 2000 AP ultrasonic p.
optical p.
Pachette 2 ultrasonic p.
Pach-Pen XL p.
Ultrasonic p.
Villasensor ultrasonic p.

pachymetry

cornea p.
corneal p.
noncontact corneal p.
ultrasonic p.

pack

Barrier Phaco Extracapsular P.

Packer

P. tunnel silicone sponge
P. Wick extrusion handpiece

Packo

P. conjunctiva forceps
P. pars plana cannula
P. pars plana cannula pachometer

Paclitaxel
PACT

prism and alternate cover test

pad

eye p.
fat p.

felt p.
orbital fat p.
Pro-Ophtha eye p.
spectacle frame p.
Telfa p.

paddle

Rosen nucleus p.
p. temple

paddy keratitis
Paecilomyces lilacinus
Page medium
Pagenstecher operation
pagetoid

p. melanoma
p. spread

PAI

plasminogen activator inhibitor

pain

atypical facial p.
boring p.
facial p.
jaw muscle p.
lancing p.
p. reaction
trigeminal p.

painful ophthalmoplegia
pak

Hedges Corneal Wetting P.

palatine bone
palatini

processus orbitalis ossis p.

palatinum

os p.

palatoethmoidalis

sutura p.

palatomaxillaris

sutura p.

palatomaxillary suture
pale

p. conjunctiva
p. optic disk

palinopsia
palisades of Vogt
palisading orbital granuloma
palladium

p. 103 ophthalmic plaque
brachytherapy
p. 103 ophthalmic plaque
radiotherapy

pallidotomy
pallidum

Treponema p.

pallidus

globus p. (GP)

Pallin lens spatula

P

Pallister-Hall syndrome
pallor
    p. of conjunctiva
    discussion p.
    disk p.
    horizontal band p.
    optic disk p.
    sector p.
    temporal artery p.
    temporal optic disk p.
Palmitate-A
palmoplantar keratoderma
palpable purpura
palpebra, pl. **palpebrae**
    inferior tarsus p.
    margo p.
    palpebrae superioris muscle
    superior tarsus p.
    tertius p.
    tunica conjunctiva p.
palpebral
    p. adipose bag
    p. aperture
    p. cartilage
    p. commissure
    p. conjunctiva
    p. conjunctival hue (PCH)
    p. fascia
    p. fissure
    p. fissure widening
    p. fold
    p. furrow
    p. gland
    p. ligament
    p. lobe
    p. margin
    p. oculogyric reflex
    p. opening
    p. raphe
    p. slant
    p. vein
palpebrale
    coloboma p.
    sebum p.
palpebrales
    venae p.
palpebralis
    epicanthus p.
palpebrarum
    dermatolysis p.
    facies anterior p.
    facies posterior p.
    pediculosis p.
    phthiriasis p.
    raphe p.
    rima p.
    tendo p.
    xanthoma p.
palpebrate

palpebration
palpebritis
palpebromandibular reflex
palpebronasal fold
palpebronasalis
    plica p.
palsy, pl. **palsies**
    abducens nerve p.
    accommodative p.
    Bell p.
    brachial plexus p.
    cerebral p.
    complete p.
    congenital abducens nerve p.
    congenital oculomotor nerve p.
    conjugate gaze p.
    cranial nerve p.
    double elevator p.
    elevator p.
    external p.
    extraocular muscle p.
    facial nerve p.
    Féréol-Graux p.
    fourth nerve p.
    gaze p.
    idiopathic facial p.
    inferior oblique p.
    inhibitional p.
    internal p.
    ischemic oculomotor p.
    lateral rectus p.
    medial rectus p.
    multiple ocular motor palsies
    p. of muscle
    nerve p.
    nuclear p.
    nuclear-fascicular trochlear nerve p.
    oblique p.
    ocular muscle p.
    oculomotor cranial nerve p.
    orbital p.
    progressive supranuclear p.
    pseudoabducens p.
    pseudobulbar p.
    saccade p.
    sector p.
    seventh cranial nerve p.
    sixth cranial nerve p.
    stem p.
    subarachnoid oculomotor nerve p.
    superior division p.
    superior oblique p.
    supranuclear ocular p.
    third cranial nerve p.
    trochlear nerve p.
    twelfth nerve p.
PAM
    potential acuity meter

primary acquired melanosis
    PAM procedure
pamoate
    hydroxyzine p.
PAN
    periarteritis nodosa
Panamax
Panas operation
pANCA
    perinuclear antineutrophil cytoplasmic
    antibody
panchamber UV lens
Pancoast
    P. superior sulcus syndrome
    P. tumor
pancreatic
    p. diabetes
    p. disease
pancuronium bromide
pancytokeratin antibody
PANDO
    primary acquired nasolacrimal duct
    obstruction
panel
    Farnsworth D-15 p.
panencephalitis
    subacute sclerosing p.
panfundus
panfunduscope
    Rodenstock p.
Panmycin
panni (*pl. of* pannus)
Pannu
    P. intraocular lens
    P. type II lens
Pannu-Kratz-Barraquer speculum
pannus, pl. panni
    allergic p.
    p. carnosus
    corneal p.
    p. crassus
    degenerative p.
    p. degenerativus
    p. eczematosus
    eczematous p.
    fibrovascular p.
    glaucomatous p.
    phlyctenular p.
    p. siccus
    p. tenuis
    p. trachomatosus
    trachomatous p.

panophthalmia
panophthalmitis
    clostridial p.
Panoptic bifocal
Panoramic
Panoramic200
    P. Non-Mydriatic Ophthalmoscope
    P. Ultra-Widefield Ophthalmic
        Imaging Device
panoramic loupe
PanoView Optics lens
panphotocoagulation
panretinal
    p. ablation
    p. argon laser photocoagulation
    p. membrane
pansinusitis
panstromal
pantachromatic
pantankyloblepharon
pantoscope
    Keeler p.
pantoscopic
    p. angle
    p. angling
    p. effect
    p. spectacles
    p. tilt
Panum
    P. fusional space
    P. fusion area
panuveitis
    granulomatous p.
    herpes p.
    multifocal choroiditis with p.
        (MCP)
papaverine hydrochloride
paper
    nitrocellulose filter p.
    Schirmer filter p.
    Whatman No. 1 qualitative-type
        filter p.
papilla, pl. papillae
    Bergmeister p.
    cobblestone p.
    conjunctival p.
    drusen of optic p.
    giant p.
    lacrimal p.
    limbal papillae
    optic p. (P)
    splitting of lacrimal p.

NOTES

papillary
p. area
p. capillary hemangioma
p. conjunctival hypertrophy
p. conjunctivitis
p. ruff
p. stasis
papilledema
asymmetric p.
chronic p.
unilateral p.
papilliform tumor
papillitis
ischemic p.
necrotizing p.
papilloma
caruncular p.
conjunctival p.
eyelid p.
intralacrimal p.
mulberry-type p.
pedunculated p.
sessile p.
squamous p.
verruca vulgaris p.
papillomacular
p. nerve fiber bundle
p. retinal fold
papillomatosis
papillopathy
diabetic p.
ischemic p.
papillophlebitis
papillopruritic dermatosis
papilloretinitis
papillovitreal
papulosa
iritis p.
papyracea
lamina p.
PAR
posterior apical radius
PAR CTS corneal topography system
parablepsia
paracentesis
anterior chamber p.
aqueous p.
paracentral
p. cell
p. defect
p. nerve fiber bundle
p. ring scotoma
p. visual field
paracentric
paracetamol
parachroma
parachromatism
parachromatopsia

Paradigm ocular blood flow analyzer
paradoxic
p. gustolacrimal reflex
p. levator excitation
p. levator inhibition
paradoxical
p. darkness reaction
p. diplopia
p. movement of eyelid
p. pupil
p. pupillary phenomenon
p. pupillary reflex
paraequilibrium
paraflocculus syndrome
parafovea
parafoveal
p. capillary net
p. cystic space
p. fluorescein
p. halo
p. macula
p. microvascular leakage
p. serous retinal elevation
parafoveolar
paraganglioma
paragraph
Gray Standardized Oral Reading P.'s
parainfectious
p. optic neuritis
p. optic neuropathy
parainfluenzae
Haemophilus p.
parallactic
parallax
binocular p.
crossed p.
direct p.
heteronymous p.
homonymous p.
motion p.
stereoscopic p.
p. test
vertical p.
parallel
p. interface
p. ray
parallelism of gaze
parallel-plate flow chamber
paralysis, pl. **paralyses**
abducens facial p.
abducens nerve p.
p. of accommodation
amaurotic pupillary p.
bulbar p.
congenital abducens facial p.
congenital abduction p.
congenital bulbar p.
congenital oculofacial p.

conjugate p.
convergence p.
divergence p.
Duchenne p.
Duchenne-Erb p.
Erb p.
Erb-Duchenne p.
facial p.
familial periodic p.
p. of gaze
hyperkalemic periodic p.
hypokalemic periodic p.
internuclear p.
Klumpke p.
Landry ascending p.
normokalemic periodic p.
nuclear horizontal gaze p.
ocular muscle p.
oculofacial p.
periodic p.
psychogenic p.
pupillary p.
sectoral iris p.
Todd p.
vagus nerve p.
Weber p.
paralytic
p. ectropion
p. heterotropia
p. miosis
p. mydriasis
p. pontine exotropia
p. strabismus
paralyticum
ectropion p.
paramacular
paramedian thalamopeduncular infarction
parameter
stereometric p.
paramethasone acetate
paramyotonia congenita
paranasal
p. sinus
p. sinusitis
paraneoplastic
p. cerebellar degeneration
p. lichen planus
p. opsoclonus
p. optic neuritis
p. optic neuropathy

p. retinopathy
p. syndrome
para optometric
Paraperm O2 contact lens
parapsilosis
　　　Candida p.
parasellar
p. lesion
p. syndrome
parasitic
p. blepharitis
p. uveitis
parasitica
blepharitis p.
Parasol punctal occluder
parastriate area
parasympathetic
p. fiber
p. nerve system
p. nervous system
p. outflow
p. pathway
parasympatholytic drug
parasympathomimetic drug
parathyroid
p. adenoma
p. disorder
paratrachoma
paraxial
p. lighting
p. mesoderm
p. ray
p. ray of light
Parcaine
PAR-C-Scan videokeratoscope
Paredrine
Parel-Crock vitreous cutter
Paremyd Ophthalmic
parenchymatosus
xerosis p.
parenchymatous
p. corneal dystrophy
p. keratitis
paresis
abducens p.
accommodation p.
complete but pupil-sparing
oculomotor nerve p.
cyclic oculomotor p.
divergence p.
incomplete pupil-sparing oculomotor
nerve p.

NOTES

P

paresis *(continued)*
    nonorganic p.
    oculosympathetic p.
    vertical gaze p.
paretic nystagmus
parfocal
paries
    p. interior orbitae
    p. lateralis orbitae
    p. medialis orbitae
    p. superior orbitae
parietal
    p. eye
    p. lobe
    p. lobe bilateral cerebral
      hemisphere lesion
    p. lobe field defect
    p. lobe unilateral cerebral
      hemisphere lesion
parietooccipital artery
parietooccipitalis
    arcus p.
parietooccipital-temporal junction
Parinaud
    P. oculoglandular conjunctivitis
    P. oculoglandular syndrome
    P. ophthalmoplegia
Parinaud-plus syndrome
PARK
    photoastigmatic refractive keratectomy
Park
    P. speculum
    P. three-step test
Parker discission knife
Parker-Heath
    P.-H. anterior chamber syringe
    P.-H. cautery
    P.-H. electrocautery
    P.-H. piggyback probe
Park-Guyton-Callahan speculum
Park-Guyton-Maumenee speculum
Park-Guyton speculum
Park-Maumenee speculum
Parks-Bielschowsky three-step head-tilt test
paromomycin
parophthalmia
parophthalmoncus
paropsia, paropsis
Parrot sign
Parry disease
pars, pl. **partes**
    p. caeca oculi
    p. caeca retinae
    p. ciliaris retinae
    p. corneoscleralis
    p. iridica retinae
    p. lacrimalis musculi orbicularis
      oculi

    p. marginalis musculi orbicularis
      oris
    p. nervosa retinae
    p. optica hypothalami
    p. optica retinae
    p. orbitalis glandulae lacrimalis
    p. orbitalis gyri frontalis inferioris
    p. orbitalis musculi orbicularis
      oculi
    p. orbitalis ossis frontalis
    p. palpebralis glandulae lacrimalis
    p. palpebralis musculi orbicularis
      oculi
    p. pigmentosa retinae
    p. plana
    p. plana approach
    p. plana Baerveldt tube insertion
      with vitrectomy
    p. plana corporis ciliaris
    p. plana operation
    p. plana seton implant
    p. planitis
    p. plicata
    p. plicata corporis ciliaris
    p. uvealis
partial
    p. albinism
    p. cataract
    p. coherence interferometry (PCI)
    p. conjunctival flap (PCF)
    p. depth astigmatic keratotomy
      (PDAK)
    p. keratoplasty
    p. ophthalmoplegia
    p. response
    p. sclerectasia
    p. thickness macular hole
    p. throw surgeon's knot
    p. vitrectomy
partialis
    ophthalmoplegia p.
partially sighted
partial-thickness
    p.-t. corneal laceration
    p.-t. trephination
participant
    healthy control p.
particulate
    p. matter
    p. retinopathy
parvocellular
    p. cell
    p. pathway
parvum
    Chrysosporium p.
PAS
    periodic acid-Schiff
    peripheral anterior synechia

Prism Adaptation Study
PAS stain
Pascal law
Pascheff conjunctivitis
pass
pupil p.
passant
boutons en p.
Passarelli one-pass capsulorrhexis forceps
passivated polymethyl methacrylate
passive
p. duction
p. forced duction test
p. illusion
Passport disposable injection system
past ocular history (POH)
past-pointing
PAT
prism adaptation test
Patanol
patch
binocular eye p.
Bitot p.
Cogan p.
cotton-wool p.
Donaldson eye p.
p. eye
glue p.
p. graft
Histoacryl glue p.
Hutchinson p.
monocular p.
Ortopad orthoptic p.
oval eye p.
salmon p.
Snugfit eye p.
venous sheath p.
wicking glue p.
patching
pressure p.
patchy
p. anterior stromal infiltrate
p. atrophy
p. window defect
patency
tear duct p.
patent
p. foramen ovale (PFO)
p. iridectomy
Paterson-Brown-Kelly syndrome
PathFinder Corneal Analysis software

pathognomonic radial keratoneuritis
pathologic
p. cupping
p. myopia
pathological astigmatism
pathology
ocular p.
orbital p.
systemic p.
pathometer attachment
pathway
afferent visual p.
anterior visual p.
cAMP final common p.
canalicular p.
infranuclear p.
magnocellular visual p.
oculosympathetic p.
parasympathetic p.
parvocellular p.
pregeniculate visual p.
retinogeniculate p.
retrochiasmal p.
sensory visual p.
supranuclear p.
sympathetic p.
visual p.
patient
primary glaucoma p.
straight-eyed p.
Paton
P. anterior chamber lens implant forceps
P. capsule forceps
P. corneal knife
P. corneal transplant forceps
P. corneal trephine
P. double spatula
P. eye shield
P. line
P. needle holder
P. single spatula
P. single speculum
P. suturing forceps
P. transplant spatula
P. transplant speculum
P. tying/stitch removal forceps
pattern
A p.
abnormal staining p.
Antoni p.
arborization p.

NOTES

pattern *(continued)*
    p. arborization
    arteriovenous p.
    AV p.
    blur p.
    classic flower petal p.
    coarse vascular p.
    comedo p.
    contiguous p.
    Contoured Ablation P. (CAP)
    p. cut corneal graft operation
    p. discrimination perimetry
    p. dystrophy
    p. dystrophy of pigment epithelium
      of Byers and Marmor
    p. electroretinogram
    flower petal p.
    Harrington-Flocks multiple p.
    map p.
    morpheaform p.
    Morse code p.
    mosaic p.
    petaloid p.
    racquet-like p.
    p. recognition
    scatter p.
    shagreen p.
    staining p.
    p. standard deviation (PSD)
    stippled p.
    umbrella-like p.
    V p.
    p. visual-evoked response (PVER)
    VISX Contoured Ablation P.
    vortex p.
    Zellballen p.
pattern-cut corneal graft
pattern-evoked electroretinogram
  (PERG)
Paufique
    P. graft knife
    P. keratoplasty
    P. keratoplasty knife
    P. operation
    P. suturing forceps
    P. synechiotomy
    P. trephine
Paul lacrimal sac retractor
Pautler infusion cannula
paving-stone degeneration
Pavlo-Colibri corneal forceps
Payne retractor
PBC
    point of basal convergence
PBII blue loop lens
PBK
    pseudophakic bullous keratopathy
PBRVO
    peripheral branch retinal vein occlusion

PBZ-SR tablet
PBZ tablet
PC
    posterior chamber
      PC EDO ophthalmic office laser
P&C
    prism and cover
      P&C test
PcB
    point of basal convergence
PCD
    posterior corneal deposit
P-cell
PCF
    partial conjunctival flap
PCH
    palpebral conjunctival hue
PCI
    partial coherence interferometry
PCIOL, PC-IOL
    posterior chamber intraocular lens
PCL
    posterior collagenous layer
PCLI
    posterior chamber lens implant
PCMD
    pellucid corneal marginal degeneration
PCNSL
    primary central nervous system
      lymphoma
PCO
    posterior capsule opacification
PCR
    polymerase chain reaction
PCR-SSOP
    polymerase chain reaction-sequence
      specific oligonucleotide probe
      PCR-SSOP method
PD
    prism diopter
    pupillary distance
      frame PD
PDAK
    partial depth astigmatic keratotomy
PDR
    proliferative diabetic retinopathy
PDS
    pigment dispersion syndrome
PDT
    photodynamic therapy
PDVR
    proliferative diabetic vitreoretinopathy
PE
    pigment epithelium
PE-400 ERG/VEP system
Peacekeeper cannula
PEAK
    pulsed electron avalanche knife

peaking
> temporal p.

peak latencies of pattern electroretinogram

peanut implant

pear cataract

Pearce
> P. coaxial irrigating/aspirating cannula
> P. nucleus hydrodissector
> P. posterior chamber intraocular lens
> P. trabeculectomy

Pearce-Knolle irrigating lens loop

pearl
> p. cyst
> p. diver's keratopathy
> Elschnig p.
> iris p.
> p. white mounds

pear-shaped pupil

Pearson chi-square test

Pease-Allen Color test

peau de chagrin

pectinate
> p. ligament
> p. ligament of iris
> p. villi

pectineal ligament

Peczon
> P. I/A cannula
> P. I/A unit
> P. I/A vectis

PED
> pigment epithelial detachment

pedal
> Vit Commander foot p.

PEDF
> pigment epithelium-derived factor
> PEDF gene

pediatric
> P. Eye Disease Investigator Group (PEDIG)
> p. Karickhoff laser lens
> p. lid speculum
> p. myasthenia
> p. ocular sarcoidosis
> p. orbital floor fracture
> p. presumed microbial keratitis
> p. three-mirror laser lens
> p. vitrectomy lens set

pedicle
> p. cone
> p. flap
> tarsoconjunctival p.

pediculated flap

pediculosis palpebrarum

pediculous blepharitis

PEDIG
> Pediatric Eye Disease Investigator Group

pedigree
> p. analysis
> p. chart

peduncular hallucination

pedunculated
> p. congenital corneal dermoid
> p. papilloma

peek sign

peeler

peeler-cutter
> Accurus p.-c. (APC)
> membrane p.-c.

peeling
> membrane p.
> spontaneous p.

pefloxacin

Pegvisomant

PEHO
> progressive encephalopathy with edema, hypsarrhythmia and optic atrophy
> PEHO syndrome

PEK
> punctate epithelial keratopathy

Pel crisis

Pel-Ebstein crisis

pellet extrusion

Pelli-Robson
> P.-R. contrast sensitivity chart
> P.-R. letter chart

pellucid
> corneal p.
> p. corneal marginal degeneration (PCMD)
> p. marginal corneal degeneration
> p. marginal retinal degeneration

pellucidum
> septum čavum p.

pemirolast
> p. potassium
> p. potassium ophthalmic solution

pemphigoid
> benign mucosal p.
> Brunsting-Perry cicatricial p.

NOTES

P

pemphigoid *(continued)*
    bullous p.
    Cibis p.
    cicatricial p.
    mucosal p.
    ocular cicatricial p. (OCP)
pemphigus
    ocular p.
pen
    Accu-Line surgical marking p.
    ASSI Accu-line surgical marking p.
    gentian violet marking p.
    marking p.
    piokutanin p.
    Rhein reusable cautery p.
    skin marking p.
    surgical marking p.
Penbritin
pencil
    astigmatism of oblique p.'s
    cataract p.
    p. cautery
    20-gauge straight bipolar p.
    glaucoma p.
    p. push-ups
    retinal detachment p.
    vitreous p.
    Wallach cryosurgical p.
pendular-jerk waveform
pendular nystagmus
penetrant gene
penetrating
    p. corneal transplant
    p. full-thickness corneal graft
    p. injury
    p. keratoplasty (PK, PKP)
    p. keratoplasty astigmatism
    p. keratoplasty button
    p. keratoplasty and glaucoma
    (PKPG)
penetration
    intraocular p.
penicillin
    acid-resistant p.
    p. G
    p. G benzathine
    synthetic p.
penicillinase
peninsula pupil
penlight
    Heine p.
    LICO disposable p.
    Welch-Allyn halogen p.
Penn-Anderson scleral fixation forceps
pentachromic
pentafilcon A
pentagonal block excision
pentamidine isethionate
Penthrane

pentigetide
pentobarbital sodium
Pentolair
pentolinium
Pentostam
Pentothal
pentoxifylline
penumbra
PEO
    progressive external ophthalmoplegia
pepper-and-salt fundus
Pepper Visual Skills for Reading Test
peptide-binding groove
Peptococcus
Peptostreptococcus
perborate
    sodium p.
Percepta progressive lens
perceptible acuity
perception
    binocular depth p.
    color p.
    contrast threshold for motion p.
    (CTMP)
    depth p.
    p. dissociation
    dissociation of visual p.
    facial p.
    form p.
    Frostig Development Test of
    Visual P.
    light p. (LP)
    p. of light (PL)
    limbus of p.
    monocular depth p.
    no light p. (NLP)
    shape p.
    simultaneous foveal p. (SFP)
    simultaneous macular p. (SMP)
    visual p.
perennial rhinoconjunctivitis
perfilcon A
perfluorocarbon
    p. coaxial I/A cannula
    p. gas
    liquid p.
perfluorodecalin
perfluorohexyloctane
Perfluoron
perfluoro-N-octane (PFO)
perfluoropropane (C_3F_3)
    p. gas (C3F8)
perforans
    scleromalacia p.
perforating keratoplasty
perforation
    corneal p.
    globe p.

performance
    clinically viable methods maximum
      optimization of visual p.
    distance visual p.
    optical p.
    predictive of visual p.
perfringens
    Clostridium p.
perfusion
    capillary p.
    juxtapapillary p.
    luxury p.
PERG
    pattern-evoked electroretinogram
Periactin
periaqueductal
    p. gray matter
    p. syndrome
periarteritis
    p. nodosa (PAN, PN)
    regional p.
peribulbar
    p. anesthesia
    p. injection
    p. needle
pericanalicular connective tissue
pericecal scotoma
pericentral
    p. rod-cone dystrophy
    p. scotoma
perichiasmal
perichoroidal, perichorioidal
    p. space
perichoroideale
    spatium p.
periconchitis
pericorneal plexus
pericyte
    p. drop out
    tissue-specific p.
peridectomy
perifascicular myofiber necrosis
perifoveal
    p. arteriole
    p. posterior vitreous detachment
      (PPVD)
perifoveolar
perihemangioma subretinal hemorrhage
perikeratic
perilenticular
perilimbal
    p. conjunctival vessel

p. stroma
p. suction
p. suction cup
p. ulceration
p. vitiligo
perilimbic circulation
perimacular vasculature
perimeter
    AccuMap multifocal objective p.
    Allergan Humphrey p.
    arc and bowl p.
    automated hemisphere p.
    Brombach p.
    Canon p.
    Cilco p.
    CooperVision imaging p.
    p. corneal reflex test
    Digilab p.
    Ferree-Rand p.
    Goldmann manual projection p.
    Henson CFS 2000 p.
    Humphrey p.
    Interzeag bowl p.
    kinetic p.
    Marco p.
    Medmont M600 p.
    Octopus 201 p.
    Octopus 101 bowl p.
    Ophthimus High-Pass Resolution p.
    Ophthimus ring p.
    Peritest p.
    projection p.
    p. projection
    Schweigger hand p.
    static p.
    Topcon p.
    Tübinger p.
perimetric
perimetry
    achromatic automated p. (AAP)
    Aimark p.
    arc p.
    automated static threshold p.
    binocular p.
    blue-yellow p.
    chromatic p.
    color p.
    computed p.
    FDT p.
    flicker p.
    frequency doubling p.
    Goldmann kinetic p.

NOTES

P

perimetry *(continued)*
    hemisphere projection p.
    high-pass resolution p. (HRP)
    kinetic p.
    luminance size threshold p.
    manual kinetic p.
    mesopic p.
    motion automated p.
    motion detection p.
    motion and displacement p.
    objective p.
    Octopus automated p.
    Octopus threshold p.
    pattern discrimination p.
    profile p.
    quantitative threshold p.
    resolution acuity p.
    ring p.
    Scanning Laser Ophthalmoscope p.
    scotopic p.
    short wavelength automated p. (SWAP)
    standard automated p. (SAP)
    static p.
    suprathreshold static p.
    tangent p.
    temporal modulation p.
    Tendency-Oriented P. (TOP)
    Tübinger p.
perineural cell
perineuritis
    optic p.
    syphilitic optic p.
perinuclear
    p. antineutrophil cytoplasmic antibody (pANCA)
    p. cataract
periocular
    p. depigmentation
    p. drug sensitivity
    p. injection
    p. surgery
period
    hypertension p.
periodic
    p. acid-Schiff (PAS)
    p. alternating gaze deviation
    p. alternating windmill nystagmus
    p. esotropia
    p. exotropia
    p. ophthalmia
    p. paralysis
    p. strabismus
periophthalmia
periophthalmic
periophthalmitis
perioptic
    p. cerebrospinal fluid
    p. hygroma

    p. neuritis
    p. sheath meningioma
    p. subarachnoid space
perioptometry
periorbit
periorbita
periorbital
    p. cellulitis
    p. edema
    p. fat atrophy
    p. hemangioma
    p. leukoderma
    p. membrane
    p. volume augmentation
periorbitis
periosteum
    orbital p.
periostitis
    orbital p.
peripapillary
    p. central serous choroidopathy
    p. choroid
    p. choroidal arterial system
    p. choroidal atrophy
    p. coloboma
    p. nerve fiber layer
    p. retinal height
    p. retinal nerve
    p. retinal nerve fiber
    p. scar
    p. sclerosis
    p. scotoma
    p. staphyloma
    p. subretinal neovascularization
periphacitis, periphakitis
peripheral
    p. anterior synechia (PAS)
    p. branch retinal vein occlusion (PBRVO)
    p. cataract
    p. chorioretinal atrophic spot
    p. chorioretinal atrophy
    p. corneal opacity
    p. corneal ulcer
    p. curve on contact lens
    p. cystoid degeneration
    p. detection test
    p. disciform degeneration
    p. endotheliitis
    p. fusion
    p. glare
    p. glioma
    p. granuloma
    p. intraretinal hemorrhage
    p. iridectomy (PI)
    p. iridectomy operation
    p. iris roll
    p. light scatter
    p. multifocal chorioretinitis (PMC)

p. myopia
p. necrotizing retinitis
p. neuropathy
p. oculomotor nerve
p. placement
p. proliferation
p. ray of light
p. retina
p. retinal ablation
p. retinal operculum
p. retinal pigment dispersion
p. retinal vascular sheathing
p. ring infiltrate
p. rod function
p. scotoma
p. tapetochoroidal degeneration
p. ulcerative keratitis (PUK)
p. uveitis
p. vestibular nystagmus
p. vision
p. visual field
p. vitreoretinal traction
peripherin/RDS gene
periphery
nasal p.
posterior pole and p. (PP&P)
periphlebitis
p. retinae
retinal p.
periphoria
periretinal edema
periscleral space
periscleritis
perisclerotic
periscopic
p. concave lens
p. convex lens
p. meniscus
p. spectacles
perisellar
peristaltic pump
peristriate visual cortex
peritarsal network
peritectomy
Peritest perimeter
peritomize
peritomy
perivascular
p. neutrophil infiltration
p. sheathing
p. stromal cell

perivasculitis
retinal p.
periventricular lesion
PERK
Prospective Evaluation of Radial
Keratotomy
PERK Study
Perkins
P. applanation tonometer
P. brailler
PERL
pupils equal, react to light
PERLA
pupils equal, reactive to light and
accommodation
Perlia nucleus
Perma-Brite
Perma-Cote
Permaflex lens
Permalens lens
permeability
oxygen p. (Dk, DK)
permeable
permethrin
pernicious
p. anemia
p. myopia
Perone
P. LASIK Flap Forceps
P. LASIK marker
peroxisomal disorder
Per-Protocol-Observed Case
Perritt double-fixation forceps
PERRLA
pupils equal, round, reactive to light and
accommodation
perseveration
visual p.
persistence of vision
persistent
p. anterior hyperplastic primary
vitreous
p. epithelial defect
p. hypertrophic primary vitreous
(PHPV)
p. postdrainage hypotony (PPH)
p. posterior hyperplastic primary
vitreous
p. primary hyperplastic vitreous
p. pupillary membrane remnant
Personna steel blade

NOTES

P

personnel
> Joint Review Committee for
> Ophthalmic Medical P. (JRCOMP)
> ophthalmic medical p. (OMP)

Perspex
> P. CQ
> P. CQ-Shearing-Simcoe-Sinskey lens
> P. CQ UV PMMA
> P. frame
> P. rod

pertussis
> *Bordetella p.*

perverted
> p. nystagmus
> p. ocular movement

P-ES
> Isopto P-ES

petaloid pattern

Peters
> P. anomaly
> P. operation
> P. pupil dilator

Petit canal

Petriellidum boydii

petrificans
> conjunctivitis p.
> keratitis p.

petrolatum ophthalmic ointment

petrosal nerve

petrous
> p. apex
> p. bone
> p. ridge

Petrus single-mirror laser lens

Pettigrove
> P. irrigation cannula
> P. LASIK set

Petzetakis-Takos syndrome

Petzval surface

PEXG
> pseudoexfoliative glaucoma

Peyman
> P. full-thickness eye-wall resection
> P. iridocyclochoroidectomy
> P. silicone oil cannula
> P. vitrectomy unit
> P. vitrector
> P. vitreophage unit
> P. wide-field lens

Peyman-Green
> P.-G. vitrectomy lens
> P.-G. vitreous forceps

Peyman-Tennant-Green lens

PF
> Acular PF
> AquaSite PF
> Ocu-Tears PF
> Visine Tears PF

P.F. Lee pediatric goniolens

PFO
> patent foramen ovale
> perfluoro-N-octane

PGC
> pontine gaze center

PGTP
> primary glaucoma triple procedure

PH
> pinhole

phacitis

phaco
> P. Cavitron irrigating/aspirating unit
> P. Emulsifier Cavitron unit
> p. quick chop
> p. sleeve
> p. trabeculectomy

Phaco-4 diamond step knife

phacoallergica
> endophthalmitis p.

phacoanaphylactic
> p. endophthalmitis
> p. uveitis

phacoanaphylactica
> endophthalmitis p.

phacoanaphylaxis

phacoantigenic endophthalmitis

phacoaspiration

phacoblade
> Myocure p.

phacocele

phaco-chop technique

phacocyst

phacocystectomy

phacocystitis

phacodonesis

phacoemulsification, phakoemulsification
> p. cautery
> choo-choo chop and flip p.
> clear corneal p.
> endocapsular p.
> endolenticular p.
> Er:YAG laser p.
> extracapsular p.
> p. handpiece
> high-vacuum p.
> Kelman p. (KPE)
> one-handed p.
> sclerocorneal p.
> small-incision p.
> two-handed p.

phacoemulsifier

phacoemulsify

phacoerysis

phacoexcavation

phacoexcavator

PhacoFlex
> P. II SI30NB intraocular lens
> Single-Stitch P.

phacofracture

phacofragmatome
phacofragmentation
phacogenetica
phacogenic, phakogenic
    p. glaucoma
    p. uveitis
phacoglaucoma
phacohymenitis
phacoid
phacoiditis
phacoidoscope
Phacojack Phaco System
phacolase
    Er:YAG p.
phacolysin
phacolysis
    calcific p.
phacolytic, phakolytic
    p. glaucoma
    p. uveitis
phacoma
phacomalacia
phacomatosis
phacometachoresis
phacometer
phacomorphic, phakomorphic
    p. glaucoma
phacopalingenesis
phacoplanesis
phacosclerosis
phacoscope
phacoscopy
phacoscotasmus
phacotmesis
phacotoxic uveitis
phagocytosed cellular debris
Phakan
phakia
phakic
    p. cystoid macular edema
    p. eye
    p. glaucoma
    P. intraocular lens
    P. 6 lens
    p. pupillary block
phakic-aphakic (PA)
phakitis
phakodonesis
phakoemulsification (var. of
  phacoemulsification)
phakofragmatome
    Girard p.

phakogenic (var. of phacogenic)
phakolytic (var. of phacolytic)
phakoma
phakomatosis
    Bourneville p.
phakomatous
    p. choristoma
    p. choristoma tumor
phakomorphic (var. of phacomorphic)
Phakonit nucleus division technique
phalangosis
phantom vision
Pharmacia
    P. corneal trephine
    P. Intermedics
    P. intraocular lens
    P. Visco J-loop lens
pharmacological
    p. blockade
    p. dilation
pharmacologic manipulation
pharyngoconjunctival fever
phase
    ascent p.
    p. difference haloscope
    ultra-late p.
PHEMA
    P. core-and-skirt keratoprosthesis
    P. KPro implantation
phemfilcon A
phenacaine hydrochloride
phenacetin
Phenazine
phenazopyridine
phencyclidine hydrochloride
Phendry Oral
phenelzine sulfate
Phenergan
phengophobia
phenindamine
pheniramine maleate and naphazoline
  HCl
phenmetrazine hydrochloride
phenobarbital sodium
phenolphthalein
phenomenon, pl. phenomena
    Alder-Reilly p.
    aqueous-influx p.
    Ascher aqueous-influx p.
    Ascher glass-rod p.
    Aubert p.
    autokinetic visible light p.

NOTES

P

phenomenon *(continued)*
    Becker p.
    Bell p.
    Bezold-Brücke p.
    Bielschowsky head-tilt p. (BHP)
    blood-influx p.
    blue field entoptic p.
    break p.
    breakup p.
    Brücke-Bartley p.
    click p.
    crowding p.
    doll's head p.
    entoptic p.
    escape p.
    extinction p.
    fatigue p.
    Fick p.
    flicker p.
    Galassi pupillary p.
    Gartner p.
    glass-rod negative p.
    glass-rod positive p.
    Gunn jaw-winking p.
    halo p.
    hemifield slide p.
    Hertwig-Magendie p.
    interface phenomena
    jack-in-the-box p.
    jaw-winking p.
    Koebner p.
    Le Grand-Geblewics p.
    Marcus Gunn jaw-winking p.
    misdirection p.
    Mitzuo p.
    Mizuo-Nakamura p.
    negative visual p.
    orbicularis p.
    paradoxical pupillary p.
    phi p.
    Piltz-Westphal p.
    positive visual p.
    prostaglandin-mediated p.
    pseudo-Graefe p.
    Pulfrich stereo p.
    Purkinje p.
    Riddoch p.
    Schlieren p.
    setting-sun p.
    shot-silk p.
    Tournay p.
    Tulio p.
    Tyndall p.
    Uhthoff p.
    Westphal p.
    Westphal-Piltz p.
Phenoptic

phenothiazine
    p. keratopathy
    p. toxicity
phenoxybenzamine hydrochloride
phenylephrine
    p. hydrochloride
    sulfacetamide p.
phenylmercuric
    p. acetate
    p. nitrate
phenylpropanolamine hydrochloride
Phenytoin
Phialophora
Philadelphia
    Wills Eye Hospital/Children's Hospital of P. (WEH/CHOP)
Phillips
    P. fixation forceps
    P. gravity pivot axis marker
phi phenomenon
phlebitis
    retinal p.
phlebophthalmotomy
phlebosclerosis
phlegmatous conjunctivitis
phlegmonous dacryocystitis
phlorhizin diabetes
phlyctenar
phlyctenular
    p. conjunctivitis
    p. keratitis
    p. keratoconjunctivitis
    p. ophthalmia
    p. pannus
phlyctenule
    conjunctival p.
    corneal p.
phlyctenulosis
    allergic p.
    conjunctival p.
    corneal p.
    tuberculous p.
PHM
    posterior hyaloid membrane
PHNI
    pinhole no improvement
phocomelia
    Roberts-SC p.
phonometer
    Tektronix digital p.
phoria
    basal p.
    decompensated p.
    far p.
    lateral p.
    monofixational p.
    near-point p.
    vertical p.
phoriascope

phorometer
phorometry
phorooptometer
Phoroptor
    P. retractor
    Ultramatic Rx Master P.
    P. vision tester
phoroscope
phorotone
phosphate
    Aralen P.
    Decadron P.
    dexamethasone sodium p.
    p. diabetes
    disodium hydrogen p.
    ganciclovir cyclic p.
    Hexadrol P.
    Hydrocortone P.
    naphazoline and antazoline p.
    potassium p.
    prednisolone sodium p.
    sodium p.
phosphate-buffered saline
phosphene
    accommodation p.
phospholine
    echothiophate p.
    P. Iodide
    P. Iodide Ophthalmic
photalgia
photerythrous
photesthesia
photic
    p. maculopathy
    p. retinal toxicity
photo
    fundus p. (FP)
    p. screening
photoablation
    excimer laser transepithelial p.
    stromal p.
    transepithelial p.
photoablative laser goniotomy (PLG)
photoastigmatic refractive keratectomy
  (PARK)
photobrown lenses
photoceptor
photochemical
    p. process
    p. visual pigment
photochemistry

photochromic
    p. lens
    p. spectacles
photocoagulation
    argon laser p.
    focal laser p.
    grid laser p. (GLP)
    indirect ophthalmoscopic laser p.
    krypton p.
    laser panretinal p.
    macular p.
    panretinal argon laser p.
    retinal laser p.
    retinal scatter p.
    scatter p.
    subthreshold subfoveal diode
     laser p. (SSDLP)
    transscleral retinal p.
    xenon arc p.
photocoagulator
    Clinitex p.
    Coherent p.
    EyeLite p.
    Ialo p.
    IOLAB I&A p.
    IOLAB irrigating/aspirating p.
    laser p.
    Mira p.
    532nm Green laser p.
    Novus Omni 2000 p.
    OcuLight GL/GLx green laser p.
    OcuLight GLx green laser p.
    Olivella-Garrigosa p.
    semiconductor GaAIAs infrared
     diode laser p.
    Ultima 2000 p.
    VIRIDIS p.
    VIRIDIS-LITE p.
    xenon arc p.
    Zeiss p.
photodisrupting laser
photodisruptor
    Aura Nd:YAG p.
photodynamic therapy (PDT)
photodynia
photodysphoria
photoelasticity
photoelectric oculography
photofrin
photogene
photogrammeter
    Raster p.

NOTES

photograph
  fundus p.
  p. reading analysis
  red free p.
  stereo optic disc p.
  stereoscopic fundus p.
photographer
  Tearscope Plus p.
photography
  central endothelial p.
  cross-polarization p.
  fluorescence retinal p.
  Miyake p.
  nonmydriatic retinal p.
  red-free p.
  Scheimpflug p.
photogray lens
photokeratitis
photo-kerato attachment
photokeratopathy
photokeratoscope
  Allergan Humphrey p.
  Allergan Medical Optics p.
  computerized p.
  CooperVision refractive surgery p.
  Corneascope nine-ring p.
  Tomey TMS-1 p.
photokeratoscopy
  digital subtraction p.
photolysis
  Dodick p.
photometer
  Bunsen grease spot p.
  flame p.
  flicker p.
  Förster p.
  Kowa laser flare p.
  Kowa laser flare-cell p.
  Minolta LS 110 spot p.
  Spectra-Pritchard 1980-PR p.
photometry
  laser flare p.
  laser flare-cell p.
photomydriasis
  Clinitex p.
photon
  P. cataract removal system
  P. laser
  P. Laser Phacolysis Probe
  P. Ocular Surgery System
photonic
photophobia
  psychogenic p.
photophobic
photophthalmia
photopia
photopic
  p. adaptation
  p. ERG

  p. eye
  p. illumination
  p. vision
photopigment
  cone p.
PhotoPoint
  P. laser
  P. laser therapy
  P. treatment
photopsia
  transient p.
photopsin
photopsy
photoptarmosis
photoptometer
  Förster p.
photoptometry
photoreception
photoreceptive
photoreceptor
  p. cell
  p. dysfunction
  p. preservation
  rod p.
  p. transplantation
  p. transplantation ineffective
    alternative
photoreceptor-bipolar synapse
photorefraction
  eccentric p.
photorefractive
  p. astigmatic keratectomy
  p. keratoplasty (PRK)
  p. surgery
photoretinitis
photoretinopathy
photoscopy
PhotoScreener
  MTI P.
  P. pediatric camera
photosensitive lens
photosensitization
photosensitizer
photosensor oculography
Photoshop 6.0 digitized imager
photostress
  macular p.
  p. recovery time (PRT)
  p. test
photosun lens
phototherapeutic keratectomy (PTK)
phototherapy
Phototome System 2700
phototonus
phototoxic
  p. lesion
  p. maculopathy
phototoxicity
phototransduction cascade

photovaporation laser
photovaporization
photovaporizing laser
PHPV
    persistent hypertrophic primary vitreous
phthalocyanine
phthiriasis palpebrarum
phthiriatica
    blepharitis p.
Phthirus pubis
phthisical eye
phthisis
    p. bulbi
    p. cornea
    essential p.
    ocular p.
phycomycosis
    cerebral p.
phylloquinone (K)
physical
    p. manipulation
    p. optics
physician
    Fellow of the Royal College
    of P.'s (FRCP)
    Randomized Trial of Aspirin and
    Cataracts in U.S. P.'s
Physick operation
physiologic
    p. anisocoria
    p. astigmatism
    p. blind spot
    p. cup
    p. excavation
    p. myopia
    p. nystagmus
    p. optics
    p. retina
    p. scotoma
physostigmine
    pilocarpine and p.
    p. and pilocarpine
    p. sulfate
phytohemagglutinin cell
PI
    peripheral iridectomy
pial
    p. arterial plexus
    p. sheath
    p. system
PIC
    punctate inner choroidopathy

pick
    Burch p.
    45-degree scissor with
      membrane p.
    Desmarres fixation p.
    fiberoptic p.
    fixation p.
    fixation/anchor p.
    light pipe p.
    Michel p.
    Olk vitreoretinal p.
    P. retinitis
    Rice p.
    scleral p.
    P. sign
    Sinskey p.
    Synergetics Awh serrated p.
    P. vision
Pickford-Nicholson analmoscope
pickup
    Shoch foreign body p.
    p. spatula suture
Pico operation
pictograph
picture chart
piebald eyelash
piece
    end p.
    preformed p.
pie-in-the-sky
    p.-i.-t.-s. defect
    p.-i.-t.-s. quadrantanopia
pie-on-the-floor
    p.-o.-t.-f. defect
    p.-o.-t.-f. quadrantanopia
Pierce
    P. coaxial irrigating/aspirating
    cannula
    P. I/A cannula
    P. I/A irrigating vectis
    P. I/A unit
    P. irrigating vectis
Pierre-Marie ataxia
Pierse
    P. corneal Colibri-type forceps
    P. eye speculum
    P. fixation forceps
Pierse-Hoskins forceps
Pierse-type Colibri forceps
piezoelectric transducer technique
piezometer

NOTES

P

395

piggyback
 p. contact lens
 p. graft
 p. implant
 p. intraocular lens
 p. probe
pigment
 p. atrophy
 p. cell
 p. change
 clumped retinal p.
 p. clumping
 p. demarcation line
 p. deposition
 p. derangement
 discoloration of p.
 p. dispersion
 p. dispersion syndrome (PDS)
 p. epithelial detachment (PED)
 p. epithelial detachment
  maculopathy
 p. epithelial dystrophy
 p. epithelial hypertrophy
 p. epitheliitis
 epitheliitis focal retinal p.
 p. epitheliopathy
 p. epithelium (PE)
 p. epithelium-derived factor (PEDF)
 p. floater
 gold tattoo p.
 p. granule
 p. layer
 p. layer ectropion
 macula lutea p.
 p. mottling
 photochemical visual p.
 placoid p.
 platinum tattoo p.
 p. precipitate
 p. seam
 silver tattoo p.
 tattoo p.
 trabecular membrane p.
 unwanted migration of p.
 visual p.
 white p.
 xanthophyll p.
pigmentary
 p. deposits on lens
 p. dilution
 p. dispersion glaucoma
 p. dispersion syndrome
 p. dropout
 p. halo
 p. migration
 p. perivenous chorioretinal
  degeneration
 p. rarefaction and clumping
 p. retinopathy

pigmentation
 clumped p.
 congenital optic disk p.
 hematogenous p.
 Hudson-Stähli line of corneal p.
 orange punctate p.
 p. rarefaction
pigmented
 p. epithelium of iris
 p. keratic precipitate
 p. layer of ciliary body
 p. layer of eyeball
 p. layer of iris
 p. layer of retina
 p. lesion
 p. line of cornea
 p. macular pucker
 p. paravenous chorioretinal atrophy
 p. paravenous retinochoroidal
  atrophy
 p. preretinal membrane
 p. stroma
 p. veil
pigmenti
 incontinentia p.
pigmento
 retinitis pigmentosa sine p.
 RP sine p.
pigmentosa
 autosomal-dominant retinitis p.
 pseudoretinitis p.
 Randomized Trial of Vitamin A
  and Vitamin E Supplementation
  for Retinitis P.
 retinitis p. (RP)
 RP10 gene variant of retinitis p.
 sector retinitis p.
 X-linked retinitis p. (XLRP)
pigmentosum
 conjunctivitis xeroderma p.
 xeroderma p.
pigmentum nigrum
pigtail
 p. fixation
 p. probe
Pilagan Ophthalmic
PilaSite
Pillat dystrophy
pillow
 Richard p.
Pilo-20
 Ocusert P.
Pilo-40
 Ocusert P.
Pilocar Ophthalmic
pilocarpine
 epinephrine and p.
 p. and epinephrine
 p. HCl

p. nitrate
p. and physostigmine
physostigmine and p.
p. test
timolol and p.
p. and timolol maleate
Pilocel
pilocytic astrocytoma
Pilofrin
Pilokair
pilomatrixoma tumor
Pilomiotin
Pilopine
P. HS
P. HS gel
P. HS Ophthalmic
Piloptic Ophthalmic
Pilopto-Carpine
Pilostat Ophthalmic
pilot application
Piltz sign
Piltz-Westphal phenomenon
pimaricin
pimelopterygium
pin
p. cushion distortion
Pischel p.
Walker micro p.
pince-nez
pineal
p. blastoma
p. eye
p. gland
pinealoblastoma
pinealoma
Pineda LASIK Flap Iron
ping-pong gaze
pinguecula, pinguicula, pl. **pingueculae**
inflamed p.
pinhole (PH)
p. accommodation
p. disk
p. and dominance test
p. goggles
p. no improvement (PHNI)
no improvement with p. (NIPH)
p. occluder
potential acuity p.
p. pupil
p. vision
pink
p. eye

p. eye disk
sharp and p. (S&P)
pinkeye conjunctivitis
Pinky ball
pinocytotic vesicle
pinpoint pupil
piokutanin pen
PION
posterior ischemic optic neuropathy
pipe
effusion light p.
flute p.
infusion light p.
p. light
piperacillin
piperazine
piperocaine hydrochloride
piqûre diabetes
piroxicam
Pischel
P. electrode
P. micropins
P. pin
P. scleral rule
pisciform cataract
pit
congenital optic nerve p.
foveal p.
Gaule p.
Herbert peripheral p.
Herbit p.
iris p.
lens p.
optic disk p.
optic nerve p.
orbital p.
temporal p.
pituitarigenic
p. oculopathy
pituitary
p. ablation
p. adenoma
apoplexy of p.
p. apoplexy
p. body
p. gland
p. tumor
Pityrosporum
P. orbiculare
P. ovale
pivot point
pixel

NOTES

P

PK
  penetrating keratoplasty
PKC
  protein kinase C
PKP
  penetrating keratoplasty
PKPG
  penetrating keratoplasty and glaucoma
PL
  perception of light
placebo eye drops
placement
  implant p.
  peripheral p.
placido
  P. disk
  P. disk image
  p. ring
placido-based axial curvature mapping
Placido-disk videokeratoscopy system
Placidyl
placode
  lens p.
  p. lens
placoid
  p. pigment
  p. pigmentation of epithelium
  p. pigment epitheliopathy
pladaroma, pladarosis
plagiocephaly
  ocular p.
plain
  p. catgut suture
  p. collagen suture
  p. gut suture
  Isopto P.
plaited frill
plana
  cornea p.
  pars p.
  trans pars p.
Planar
  P. blade
  P. Haag Streit attachment
plane
  Broca visual p.
  Daubenton p.
  equivalent refracting p.
  eye/ear p.
  Frankfort horizontal p.
  horizontal p.
  image p.
  p. of incidence
  lens p.
  Listing p.
  nodal p.
  orbital p.
  p. parallel plate
  principal p.

  p. of regard
  spectacle p.
  unity conjugacy p.'s
  vertical p.
  visual p.
planer
  USC scleral p.
plane-surface refraction
Plange spud
planitis
  cyclitis in pars p.
  pars p.
planned extracapsular cataract extraction
planner
  VISX Refractive P.
planoconcave lens
planoconvex nonridge lens
planoconvex-shaped disk
Plano T lens
planum
  p. orbitale
  os p.
  xanthoma p.
planus
  paraneoplastic lichen p.
plaque
  avascular p.
  p. brachytherapy
  brachytherapy episcleral p.
  cholesterol p.
  cobalt-60 eye p.
  delayed mucous p.
  demyelinating p.
  endothelial p.
  episcleral eye p.
  eye p.
  eyelid p.
  gold eye p.
  gray p.
  Hollenhorst p.
  hyaline p.
  hyperkeratotic p.
  p. keratopathy
  nonconfluent p.
  preretinal p.
  radioactive eye p.
  p. radiotherapy
  red scaly p.
  ruthenium p.
  ruthenium-106 ophthalmic p.
  scaly p.
  subcapsular p.
  subepithelial p.
Plaquenil
plaque-type psoriasis
plasma
  p. cell
  p. cell tumor

plasmacytoid infiltrate
plasmin
plasminogen
    p. activator inhibitor (PAI)
    tissue p.
Plasmodium
plasmoid
    p. agglutination
    p. aqueous
    p. aqueous humor
plaster shell
plastic
    p. bifocal
    p. cyclitis
    p. disposable irrigating vectis
    p. eye shield
    p. frame
    p. iritis
    p. lens
    p. prism
    p. repair of eyelid
    p. sphere implant
plate
    American Optical Hardy-Rand-
      Rittler color p.
    base p.
    depth p.
    embryonic p.
    Gelfilm p.
    Hardy-Rand-Ritter
      pseudoisochromatic p.
    Hardy-Rand-Ritter screening p.
    HRR p.
    Ishihara pseudoisochromatic p.
    isochromatic p.
    Jaeger lid p.
    lid p.
    Okuma p.
    plane parallel p.
    pseudoisochromatic color p.
    reticular p.
    scar p.
    Silastic p.
    Stahl caliper p.
    standard pseudoisochromatic p.
      (SPP)
    standard pseudoisochromatic p.'s
      part 2
    Stilling p.
    Storz lid p.
    tarsal p.

    Teflon p.
    Thayer-Martin p.
plateau
    p. iris
    p. iris configuration
    p. iris syndrome
Plateau-Talbot law
plate-haptic
    p.-h. intraocular lens
    p.-h. silicone lens
platform
    Alfonso cutting p.
    LADARVision P.
Platina
    P. clip
    P. clip lens
    P. intraocular lens implant
platinum
    p. probe spatula
    p. tattoo pigment
platysmal reflex
pleomorphic
    p. adenoma
    p. spindle cell tumor
pleoptic exercise
pleoptics
    Bangerter method of p.
    Cüppers method of p.
pleoptophor
plesiopia
plethysmographic goggles
plethysmography
plexiform
    p. external layer
    p. inner layer
    p. internal layer
    p. neurofibroma
    p. neuroma
    p. outer layer
Plexiglas
    P. frame
    P. implant
plexus, pl. plexus, plexuses
    angular aqueous sinus p.
    anular p.
    capillary p.
    ciliary ganglionic p.
    epithelial nerve p.
    Hovius p.
    intraepithelial p.
    intrascleral p.
    ophthalmic p.

NOTES

P

plexus *(continued)*
    pericorneal p.
    pial arterial p.
    scleral p.
    stroma p.
    subepithelial p.
    sympathetic carotid p.
    vascular p.
Pley extracapsular forceps
PLG
    photoablative laser goniotomy
Pliagel
plica, pl. **plicae**
    plicae ciliares
    p. ciliaris
    plicae iridis
    p. lacrimalis
    p. lunata
    p. palpebronasalis
    p. semilunaris
    p. semilunaris conjunctivae
plicata
    pars p.
plication
    retractor p.
Plitz reflex
plombage operation
plug
    arrow-shaft silicone punctal p.
    Berkeley Bioengineering brass scleral p.
    brass scleral p.
    collagen p.
    Dohlman p.
    EaglePlug tapered-shaft punctum p.
    EagleVision Freeman punctum p.
    epithelial p.
    Freeman punctum p.
    Herrick lacrimal p.
    Micro punctum p.
    Oasis Collagen P.
    OPAQUE Herrick Lacrimal P.
    punctal p.
    punctum p.
    Ready-Set punctum p.
    Sharpoint UltraPlug punctum p.
    silicone p.
    Soft Plug punctal p.
    Super punctum p.
    tapered-shaft punctum p.
    TearSaver punctum p.
    Tears Naturale silicone punctum p.
    Teflon p.
    Umbrella punctum p.
plugging
    follicular p.
plumes
    corneal ablation p.

plus
    Amvisc P.
    BSS P.
    p. cyclophoria
    p. disease
    Duramist P.
    Econopred P.
    fatter add p. (FAP)
    ICaps P.
    Lens P.
    Murine Tears P.
    P. punctal occluder
    Refresh P.
    p. spectacle lens
    Tears P.
    Unisol P.
    Wet-N-Soak P.
Plus-Allergan
    Lens P.-A.
plus-minus syndrome
PM
    psammomatous meningioma
    Moisture Eyes PM
    Refresh PM
PMC
    peripheral multifocal chorioretinitis
PMMA
    polymethylmethacrylate
    Blue core PMMA
    PMMA custom-made calibration contact lens
    Perspex CQ UV PMMA
PMP
    Pocket Multimedia Presentation
PN
    periarteritis nodosa
PNET
    primitive neuroectodermal tumor
pneumatic
    p. retinopathy
    p. retinopexy
    p. tonometer
    p. trabeculoplasty
    p. vitrectomy
pneumatically stented implant (PSI)
pneumatonograph
    Alcon applanation p.
pneumatonometer
    Micro One p.
    Modular One p.
pneumococcal
    p. bacillus
    p. conjunctivitis
    p. endophthalmitis
    p. ulcer
pneumococcus
    Streptococcus p.
    p. ulcer

Pneumocystis
>P. carinii
>P. carinii pneumonia

pneumoencephalography
pneumonia
>Pneumocystis carinii p.

pneumoniae
>Klebsiella p.
>Streptococcus p.

pneumotomography
pneumotonometer
pneumotonometry
POAG
>primary open-angle glaucoma

pocket
>corneal p.
>detachment p.
>P. Multimedia Presentation (PMP)
>p. operation
>p. red filter
>stromal p.

POH
>past ocular history

POHS
>presumed ocular histoplasmosis
>syndrome
>pseudo POHS

poikiloderma
>p. atrophicans and cataract
>p. congenitale
>infantile p. subgroup 1-2-3

point
>anterior focal p.
>axial p.
>p. of basal convergence (PBC, PcB)
>blur p.
>break p.
>cardinal p.
>central yellow p.
>congruent p.
>conjugate p.
>convergence p.
>correspondence p.
>corresponding retinal p.
>diathermy p.
>disparate retinal p.
>p. of dispersion
>p. of divergence
>eye p.
>far p.
>p. of fixation

>fixation p.
>fixed p.
>focal image p.
>identical p.
>image p.
>incident p.
>lacrimal p.
>p. leak
>lustrous central yellow p.
>near visual p. (NVP)
>neutral p.
>nodal p.
>null p.
>optical nodal p.
>pivot p.
>posterior focal p.
>principal p.
>p. of regard
>restoration p.
>retinal p.
>secondary focal p.
>p. source
>sphere end p.
>stereo-identical p.
>supraorbital p.
>p. system test type
>virtual p.
>visual p.
>yellow p.

point-of-purchase display
Poiseuille law
poisoning degenerative cataract
Polack keratoscope
Poladex
polar
>p. bear tracks
>p. cataract

Polaramine
polarimeter
>confocal scanning laser p.
>scanning laser p.

polarimetry
>scanning laser p. (SLP)

polariscope
polariscopic
polariscopy
polarization
>angle of p.

polarized light
polarizing
>p. lens
>p. ophthalmoscope

NOTES

P

401

Polaroid
 P. 3D Vectograph test
 P. filter
 P. vectograph slide
Polaron sputter coater
pole
 anterior p.
 inferior p.
 posterior p.
 superior p.
pol gene
polioencephalitis
 superior p.
poliosis
Polish Brite/Super Cleaner, Non-Allergenic
polisher
 Buedding squeegee cortex extractor and p.
 capsule p.
 Drews capsule p.
 felt disk p.
 Gills-Welsh capsule p.
 Holladay posterior capsule p.
 Knolle capsule p.
 Kraff capsule p.
 Kratz capsule p.
 Look capsule p.
 microloop curette p.
 olive-tip capsule p.
 squeegee capsule p.
 Terry silicone capsule p.
 Yaghouti LASIK p.
polisher/scratcher
 Jensen p./s.
 Kratz p./s.
 Kratz-Jensen p./s.
polishing
 diamond-bur p.
 posterior capsular p.
Polle pod attachment for ophthalmoscope
Pollock
 P. forceps
 P. punch
Polocaine
polus
 p. anterior bulbi oculi
 p. anterior lentis
 p. posterior bulbi oculi
 p. posterior lentis
Polyak operation
polyarteritis nodosa
polycarbonate lens
polychondritis
 atrophic p.
 relapsing p.

polychromatic
 p. light
 p. luster
Polycin-B Ointment
Polycon I, II contact lens
polycoria
 p. spuria
 p. vera
Polycycline
polycythemicus
 fundus p.
Polydek suture
Poly-Dex Suspension
polydimethylsiloxane
polydystrophy
 pseudo-Hurler p.
polyester suture
polyethylene
 p. glycol
 p. implant
 p. T-tube
 p. tube
polyglactin 910 suture
polyglycolate suture
polyglycolic acid suture
polygonal
 p. pigmented cell
 p. stromal opacification
polyhedral cells
polyhexamethylene biguanide
Polymacon lens
polymegethism
polymerase
 p. chain reaction (PCR)
 p. chain reaction-sequence specific oligonucleotide probe (PCR-SSOP)
polymer ring
polymethylmethacrylate (PMMA)
 p. contact lens
 p. frame
polymorphic
 p. cataract
 p. macular degeneration of Brayley
 p. microsatellite marker
 p. superficial keratitis
polymorphonuclear
 p. reaction
 p. response
polymorphous dystrophy
Polymox
Polymycin
polymyositis
 orbital p.
polymyxin
 p. B
 p. B sulfate
 p. B and Terramycin
 p. E

oxytetracycline and p. B
trimethoprim and p. B
polyopia, polyopsia
binocular p.
cerebral p.
p. monophthalmica
polyopy
polyphaga
Acanthamoeba p.
polypoidal choroidal vasculopathy
Poly-Pred Ophthalmic Suspension
polypropylene suture
polypseudophakia
Polyquad
Polysporin Ophthalmic
polystichia
polytome x-ray
Polytracin
Polytrim Ophthalmic
polyvinyl alcohol (PVA)
pons lesion
pontine
p. gaze center (PGC)
p. lesion
Pontocaine Eye
pontomesencephalic dysfunction
pool
tear p.
pooling
p. of dye
fluorescein p.
population-based cross-sectional survey
porcupine lymphoma
PORN
progressive outer retinal necrosis
~~porofocon~~
porous
p. hydroxyapatite sphere
p. orbital implant
port
Berkeley Bioengineering infusion
terminal p.
butterfly needle infusion p.
Gills-Welsh guillotine p.
3-p. pars plana vitrectomy
sclerotomy p.
self-sealing side p.
side p.
p. vitrectomy
portable PT100 noncontact tonometer
porus opticus

position
p. accommodation
p. ametropia
Bertel p.
bipolar electrode p.
cardinal p.
convergence p.
p. cyclophoria
dissociated p.
p. error
p. eyepiece
face-down p.
fusion-free p.
heterophoric p.
Listing primary p.
midline p.
oblique p.
1-12 o'clock p.
primary p.
Rhese p.
p. scotoma
secondary p.
sulcus fixated p.
tertiary p.
vertical divergence p.
positional
p. abnormality of retina
p. nystagmus
positioner
irrigating IOL p.
positive
p. accommodation
p. afterimage
p. convergence
cyclophoria p.
p. eyepiece
false p.
p. meniscus
p. meniscus lens
p. scotoma
p. spherical aberration
p. vertical divergence
p. visual phenomenon
Posner
P. diagnostic gonioprism
P. diagnostic lens
P. slit lamp
P. surgical gonioprism
Posner-Schlossman syndrome
post
p. chamber
p. chiasmal

NOTES

post *(continued)*
    p. saccadic drift
    p. scrape
postbasic stare
postcanalicular system
postcataract bleb
postconceptual age
postequatorial retina
posterior
    p. amorphous corneal dysgenesis
    p. amorphous corneal dystrophy
    p. angle
    p. apical radius (PAR)
    camera bulbi p.
    camera oculi p.
    p. capsular opacification
    p. capsular polishing
    p. capsular zonular barrier
    p. capsular zonular disruption
    p. capsule opacification (PCO)
    p. capsule opacification software
    p. capsulotomy
    p. central curve
    p. cerebral artery
    p. chamber (PC)
    p. chamber intraocular lens
      (PCIOL, PC-IOL)
    p. chamber lens implant (PCLI)
    p. chiasmatic commissure
    p. choroiditis
    p. ciliary artery
    p. ciliary vein
    p. collagenous layer (PCL)
    p. conical cornea
    p. conjunctival artery
    p. conjunctival vein
    p. corneal curvature
    p. corneal deposit (PCD)
    p. corneal depression
    p. corneal tissue
    p. discission
    p. dislocation
    p. embryotoxon
    p. epithelium of cornea
    p. explant
    p. fixation suture
    p. focal point
    p. fossa nerve decompression
    p. hyaloid
    p. hyaloid membrane (PHM)
    p. hydrophthalmia
    p. incision
    p. inferior cerebellar artery
      syndrome
    p. intermediate curve
    p. internuclear ophthalmoplegia
    p. ischemic optic neuropathy
      (PION)
    p. keratoconus

    p. lamellar disk
    p. lamellar keratoplasty
    lamina elastica p.
    p. lamina raphe
    p. lenticonus
    p. limiting lamina
    p. limiting ring
    membrana capsularis lentis p.
    p. microphthalmos
    ophthalmomyiasis interna p. (OIP)
    p. optical zone (POZ)
    p. peribulbar block
    p. peripheral curve (PPC)
    p. pigment epitheliopathy
    p. pituitary ectopia
    p. polar cataract
    p. pole
    p. pole of eye
    p. pole of eyeball
    p. pole of lens
    p. pole and periphery (PP&P)
    p. polymorphic dystrophy (of
      cornea) (PPMD)
    p. polymorphous corneal dystrophy
    p. scleritis
    p. sclerochoroiditis
    p. sclerotomy
    p. segment
    p. segment of the eye
    p. staphyloma
    p. subcapsular cataract (PSC)
    p. subcapsular opacity
    p. sub-Tenon injection
    p. supine position capsular opacity
    p. surface of lens
    p. symblepharon
    p. synechia
    p. thermal sclerostomy
    p. toric
    p. tube shunt implant
    p. uveal melanoma
    p. uveitis
    p. visual pathway imaging
    p. vitrectomy
    p. vitreous
    p. vitreous detachment (PVD)
posteriores
    limbus palpebrales p.
postganglionic
    p. fiber
    p. fiber regeneration
    p. Horner syndrome
    p. short ciliary nerve
**postgeniculate congenital homonymous
  hemianopsia**
Post-Harrington erysiphake
postherpetic
    p. headache
    p. neuralgia

posticum
    staphyloma p.
postinfectious epithelial keratopathy
postinflammatory
    p. atrophy
    p. cataract
postkeratoplasty
postlensectomy
postmarital amblyopia
postocclusion measurement
postocular neuritis
postoperative
    p. adjustment
    p. amblyopia
    p. blindness
    p. endophthalmitis
    p. flat anterior chamber
    p. hyphema
    p. iritis
    p. irregular astigmatism
    p. laser in situ keratomileusis
      visual aberration
    p. LASIK visual aberration
    p. mydriasis
postorbital
postpapilledema atrophy
postplaced suture
postsurgical hyphema
postsynaptic congenital myasthenic disorder
posttraumatic
    p. accommodative spasm
    p. headache
    p. iridocyclitis
postural exophthalmos
postvaccination optic neuritis
postvitrectomy
    p. cataract
    p. fibrin
Posurdex
potassium
    p. acetate
    p. hydroxide (KOH)
    p. iodide
    pemirolast p.
    p. phosphate
potential
    p. acuity meter (PAM)
    p. acuity pinhole
    compound muscle action p. (CMAP)
    early receptor p.

    evoked p.
    flash visual-evoked p. (fVEP)
    oscillatory p. (OP)
    receptor p.
    S p.
    p. visual acuity
    visual-evoked p. (VEP)
    visual-evoked cortical p. (VECP)
POTF
    preocular tear film
Potter-Bucky diaphragm
Potter syndrome
pouch
    Rathke p.
Poulard
    P. entropion
    P. operation
Pourcelot ratio
povidone-iodine
powder
    Ophthalmic Moldite P.
Powell wand
power
    add p.
    back vertex p. (BVP)
    bending p.
    p. calculation
    contact lens vertex p.
    dioptric p.
    equivalent p.
    front vertex p.
    intraocular lens p. (IOLP)
    keratometric p. (KP)
    lacrimal p.
    lens p.
    magnifying p.
    mean corneal p.
    p. of mirror
    on-eye predicted p.
    P. operation
    optical p.
    Prentice position p.
    radiant p.
    refractive p.
    resolving p.
    topographic simulated
      keratometric p. (TOPO)
    p. vergence
    vertex of p.
    zero optical p.
POZ
    posterior optical zone

NOTES

P

PP
    punctum proximum of convergence
p.p.
    punctum proximum
PPC
    posterior peripheral curve
PPDR
    preproliferative diabetic retinopathy
PPH
    persistent postdrainage hypotony
PPMD
    posterior polymorphic dystrophy (of
      cornea)
PP&P
    posterior pole and periphery
PPVD
    perifoveal posterior vitreous detachment
PR
    presbyopia
p.r.
    punctum remotum
practolol
Praeger iris hook
prairie conjunctivitis
Pram occluder
Prausnitz-Kustner reaction
praziquantel
prebleached dark-adapted threshold
precancerous lesion
precapillary arteriole
prechiasmal
    p. compression
    p. disorder
    p. optic nerve
    p. optic nerve compression
      syndrome
PreChopper
    Akahoshi Combo P.
    Akahoshi Phaco P.
    Akahoshi Universal P.
pre-chopping forceps
precipitate
    granulomatous keratic p.
    keratic p. (KP)
    keratitic p.
    mutton-fat keratic p.
    pigment p.
    pigmented keratic p.
    punctate keratic p.
precision
    p. astigmatism reduction
    p. astigmatism reduction procedure
    P. Cosmet intraocular lens implant
    P. Cosmet lens
    P. refractor
    p. suture tome
PreClean soak system
precorneal tear film

Pred
    P. Forte
    P. Forte Ophthalmic
    P. G SOP
    Liquid P.
    P. Mild
    P. Mild Ophthalmic
Predair
    P. A
    P. Forte
Predamide
Predate
Predcor-TBA Injection
Pred-G Ophthalmic
predictive
    p. value
    p. of visual performance
predisposing condition
Prednefrin Forte
prednisolone
    p. acetate
    p. and atropine
    chloramphenicol and p.
    p. and gentamicin
    Isopto P.
    neomycin, polymyxin B, and p.
    p. sodium phosphate
    sulfacetamide and p.
prednisone
Pred-Phosphate
Predsulfair
Predulose
preeclamptic hypertensive retinopathy
preexisting well-balanced cornea-lens
preferential-looking technique
preferred retinal locus (PRL)
Preflex for Sensitive Eyes
preformed piece
Prefrin
    P. Liquifilm Vasoconstrictor and
      Lubricant Eye Drops
    P. Ophthalmic Solution
    P. Z Liquifilm
Prefrin-A
preganglionic
    p. Horner syndrome
    p. lesion
    p. oculomotor nerve
    p. parasympathetic axon
pregeniculate visual pathway
pregnancy
    toxemic retinopathy of p.
preinjury visual maturation
prelaminar optic nerve
PRELEX
    presbyopic lens exchange
    presbyopic lens exchange procedure
preliminary iridectomy

premacular
>p. gliosis
>p. subhyaloid hemorrhage

premature presbyopia

prematurity
>cataract of p.
>cicatricial retinopathy of p.
>Cryotherapy for Retinopathy of P. (CRYO-ROP)
>Effects of Light Reduction on Retinopathy of P.
>p. myopia
>retinopathy of p. (ROP)
>p. retinopathy
>Supplemental Therapeutic Oxygen for Prethreshold Retinopathy of P.
>threshold stage III of retinopathy of p. (TS III ROP)

premelanosome

Premiere
>P. irrigation/aspiration unit
>P. SmallPort phaco system
>P. vitreous cutter

Prentice
>P. law
>P. position power
>P. rule

preocular tear film (POTF)

preoperative

preorbita

prepapillary
>p. arterial loop
>p. hemorrhage
>p. vascular loop

preparatory iridectomy

preplaced suture

preponderance
>directional p.

prepresbyopia

preproliferative diabetic retinopathy (PPDR)

preretinal
>p. gliosis
>p. hemorrhage
>p. macular fibrosis
>p. membrane
>p. neovascularization
>p. plaque

presbyope

presbyopia (PR)
>p. glasses

>laser reversal of p.
>premature p.
>surgical reversal of p. (SRP)

presbyopic
>p. intraocular lens
>p. lens exchange (PRELEX)
>p. lens exchange procedure (PRELEX)

presbytia

presbytism

preschooler
>Vision in P.'s (VIP)

prescrape

prescription verification

presenile
>p. cataract
>p. melanosis

presentation
>Pocket Multimedia P. (PMP)
>rapid serial visual p. (RSVP)

preseptal
>p. cellulitis
>p. orbicularis muscle
>p. space

Presert

preservation
>photoreceptor p.
>visual p.

Preservative-Free Moisture Eyes

preservatives in solution

preset diamond knife

press
>Kornmehl p.

pressing
>eye p.
>molded p.

press-on
>p.-o. Fresnel lens
>p.-o. prism

pressure
>p. amaurosis
>applanation p.
>p. bandage
>digital p.
>episcleral venous p. (EVP)
>exophthalmos due to p.
>eye restored to normotensive p.
>intracranial p. (ICP)
>intraocular p. (IOP)
>mercury p.
>Michaelson counter p.
>ocular perfusion p. (OPP)

NOTES

P

407

pressure *(continued)*
    osmotic p.
    p. patch dressing
    p. patching
    p. phosphene tonometer
    p. shield
    white without p.
presumed
    p. microbial keratitis
    p. ocular histoplasmosis
    p. ocular histoplasmosis syndrome
        (POHS)
**presynaptic congenital myasthenic
    disorder**
pretectal
    p. area
    p. nucleus
    p. region
    p. syndrome
prethreshold disease
prevalence
    high p.
    p. of ocular trauma
Prevost sign
Preziosi operation
prezonular space
Price
    P. Corneal Punch
    P. corneal transplant system
    P. Donor Cornea Punch set
    P. Radial Marker
Priestley-Smith retinoscope
Prima KTP/532 laser
Primaria tissue culture flask
primary
    p. acetylcholine receptor deficiency
    p. acquired melanosis (PAM)
    p. acquired nasolacrimal duct
        obstruction (PANDO)
    p. action
    p. angle-closure glaucoma
    p. anophthalmia
    p. cataract
    p. central nervous system
        lymphoma (PCNSL)
    p. color
    p. cone dysfunction
    p. demyelinating disease
    p. deviation
    p. dye test
    p. dysgenesis mesodermalis
    p. eye
    p. familial amyloidosis
    p. focal length
    p. gaze alignment
    p. glaucoma patient
    p. glaucoma triple procedure
        (PGTP)
    p. graft failure

p. infantile glaucoma
p. infantile glaucoma blepharospasm
p. lens
p. lens implant
p. line of sight
p. mechanism
p. myopia
p. ocular disease
p. ocular lymphoma
p. open-angle glaucoma (POAG)
p. optic atrophy
p. perivasculitis of retina
p. persistent hyperplastic vitreous
p. pigmentary degeneration
p. position
p. position of gaze
p. retinal fold
p. visual cortex
Primbs suturing forceps
primers
    oligonucleotide p.
**primitive neuroectodermal tumor
    (PNET)**
primordium, pl. **primordia**
    optic p.
Prince
    P. cautery
    P. electrocautery
    P. muscle clamp
    P. muscle forceps
    P. rule
principal
    p. fiber
    p. focus
    p. line
    p. line of direction
    p. optic axis
    p. plane
    p. point
    p. visual direction
principle
    Carriazo-Barraquer p.
    Fresnel p.
    Imbert-Fick p.
    Mackay-Marg p.
    Scheimpflug p.
    Scheiner p.
printers' point system
**Prio video display terminal vision
    tester**
prism
    P. Adaptation Study (PAS)
    p. adaptation test (PAT)
    Allen-Thorpe gonioscopic p.
    p. and alternate cover test (PACT)
    p. angle
    AO rotary p.
    p. apex
    apex of p.

ballast p.
p. ballast
p. ballast contact lens
bar p.
p. bar
p. base
base-down p.
base-out p.
BD p.
Becker gonioscopic p.
Berens p.
BI p.
p. and cover (P&C)
p. cover measurement
p. degree
p. diopter (PD)
diopter p.
4 p. diopter base-out test
dispersion p.
p. dissociation test
Drews inclined p.
Fresnel press-on p.
Goldmann contact lens p.
Goldmann three-mirror p.
gonioscopic p.
hand-held rotary p.
induced p.
Jacob-Swann gonioscopic p.
Keeler p.
Maddox p.
Nicol p.
oblique p.
plastic p.
press-on p.
reflecting p.
refracting angle of p.
right-angle p.
Risley rotary p.
rotary p.
scanning p.
p. segment
p. shift test
p. spectacles
square p.
temporary p.
three-mirror p.
p. vergence test
Wolff-Eisner p.

prismatic

p. contact lens
p. dioptric value
p. effect

p. effect by lens
p. fundus
p. gonioscopic lens
p. gonioscopy lens
p. goniotomy lens
p. spectacle lens
p. spectacles

prism-neutralized cover test
prismosphere
Pritikin punch
PRK
photorefractive keratoplasty
PRL
preferred retinal locus
probe

Accurus 2500 p.
Alcon vitrectomy p.
Anel p.
angled p.
Bodian lacrimal pigtail p.
Bodian mini lacrimal p.
Bowman lacrimal p.
Castroviejo lacrimal sac p.
p. cataract
Clark p.
Clinitex Charles
  endophotocoagulator p.
cryopexy p.
cryotherapy p.
curved retinal p.
Dodick photolysis p.
Ellis foreign body spud needle p.
French lacrimal p.
Frigitronics freeze-thaw cryopexy p.
Harms trabeculotomy p.
Hertzog pliable p.
Ilg p.
Iliff lacrimal p.
Infinitech laser p.
InnoVit 1800 p.
InnoVit vitrectomy p.
Josephberg p.
Keeler-Amoils curved cataract p.
Keeler-Amoils glaucoma p.
Keeler-Amoils long-shank retinal p.
Keeler-Amoils microcurved
  cataract p.
Keeler-Amoils ophthalmic curved
  cataract p.
Keeler-Amoils ophthalmic long-
  shank p.

NOTES

P

probe *(continued)*
  Keeler-Amoils ophthalmic
   Machemer retinal p.
  Keeler-Amoils ophthalmic
   microcurved cataract p.
  Keeler-Amoils ophthalmic retinal p.
  Keeler-Amoils ophthalmic straight
   cataract p.
  Keeler-Amoils ophthalmic
   vitreous p.
  Keeler-Amoils straight cataract p.
  Knapp iris p.
  lacrimal intubation p.
  Linde cryogenic p.
  Manhattan Eye & Ear p.
  Mannis p.
  Microvit p.
  nasolacrimal duct p.
  needle p.
  p. needle
  Ocutome p.
  O'Donoghue angled DCR p.
  Parker-Heath piggyback p.
  Photon Laser Phacolysis P.
  piggyback p.
  pigtail p.
  polymerase chain reaction-sequence
   specific oligonucleotide p. (PCR-
   SSOP)
  Quickert-Dryden p.
  Quickert lacrimal intubation p.
  Ritleng p.
  Rolf lacrimal p.
  Rollet lacrimal p.
  Simpson lacrimal p.
  spatula p.
  p. spatula
  straight retinal p.
  Synergetics directional laser p.
  p. syringe
  Theobald p.
  trabeculotomy p.
  Vygantas-Wilder retinal drainage p.
  Werb right-angle p.
  Williams p.
  Worst pigtail p.
  Ziegler p.
probenecid
probing
  lacrimal p.
  p. lacrimonasal duct
  p. lacrimonasal duct operation
Probst Smiley LASIK marker
procaine hydrochloride
procedure
  acuity card p.
  advancement p.
  Anderson-Kestenbaum p.
  artificial divergence p.

Baerveldt filtering p.
Bick p.
buckling p.
burst hemiflip p.
Cairns p.
Cibis liquid silicone p.
ciliary p.
collagen wick p.
Custodis nondraining p.
cyclodestructive p.
Donders p.
Faden p.
Fasanella-Servat p.
filtering p.
Girard p.
guarded filtration p.
hamular p.
Harada-Ito p.
hex p.
Hill p.
Hummelsheim p.
intralamellar pocket p.
Ito p.
Jannetta p.
Jensen transposition p.
Jones tube p.
keratorefractive p.
Kestenbaum p.
Knapp p.
Krönlein p.
Kuhnt-Szymanowski p.
lathing p.
lower lid sling p.
modified corncrib (inverted T) p.
modified Wies p.
PAM p.
precision astigmatism reduction p.
presbyopic lens exchange p.
 (PRELEX)
primary glaucoma triple p. (PGTP)
Quickert p.
Ruiz p.
Salleras p.
Sato p.
Savin p.
Sayoc p.
scleral buckling p.
scleral expansion band p.
situ keratomileuis p.
sling p.
strip p.
surgical decompression p.
tarsal strip p.
Thal p.
Toti p.
triple p.
tube-shunt p.
tuck p.
tumbling p.

uncinate p.
up-and-down staircases p.
VISX p.
Wheeler p.
Wies p.
Zaldivar anterior p. (ZAP)
PRO CEM-4 microscope
procerus
musculus p.
process
ciliary p.
disciform p.
emmetropization p.
fine iris p.
iris p.
lacrimal p.
photochemical p.
replamineform p.
Sand p.
spin-cast p.
visual p.
zygomaticoorbital p.
processus
p. ciliares
p. frontosphenoidalis ossis
zygomatici
p. orbitalis ossis palatini
p. zygomaticus maxillae
ProConcept
P. Contact Lens Cleaner
P. Wetting and Soaking Solution
Procyon digital infrared pupillometer
procyonis
Baylisascaris p.
prodromal
p. glaucoma
p. myopia
product
convolution p.
Katena p.
Nexacryl cohesive p.
SPP color deficiency testing p.
standard pseudoisochromatic plates
color deficiency testing p.
Xomed Surgical P.'s
production
reflex tear p.
Profenal Ophthalmic
professional community
profile
p. analyzer

intensity p.
p. perimetry
ProFinesse II ultrasonic handpiece
ProFree/GP weekly enzymatic cleaner
profunda
keratitis punctata p.
keratitis pustuliformis p.
prognosis
visual p.
program
Casebeer keratorefractive
planning p.
diagnostic p.
Hoffberger P.
Rabinowitz-Klyce/Maeda keratoconus
screening p.
progression
Contact Lens and Myopia P.
(CLAMP)
progressiva
ophthalmoplegia p.
progressive
p. additional lenses
p. addition lens
p. cataract
p. choroidal atrophy
p. cone degeneration
p. cone dystrophy
p. cone-rod dystrophy
p. encephalopathy with edema,
hypsarrhythmia and optic atrophy
(PEHO)
p. external ophthalmoplegia (PEO)
p. fluorescein leakage
p. foveal dystrophy
p. hearing loss
p. hemifacial atrophy
p. herpetic corneal endotheliopathy
p. macular dystrophy
p. multifocal lens
p. myopia
p. myopic degeneration
p. optic atrophy
p. outer retinal necrosis (PORN)
p. outer retinal necrosis syndrome
p. spectacles lenses
p. supranuclear palsy
p. systemic sclerosis
p. tapetochoroidal dystrophy
p. vaccinia
progressive-add bifocal

NOTES

P

project
    Cataract PPO p.
projecting staphyloma
projection
    erroneous p.
    false p.
    light p.
    p. magnifier
    perimeter p.
    p. perimeter
    retinocortical p.
    retinogeniculostriate p.
    visual p.
Project-O-Chart
    AO Reichert Instruments P.-O.-C.
    Ultramatic P.-O.-C. (UPOC)
projector
    acuity visual p.
    Eletrohome Marquee 8500 Ultra
      graphics p.
    fiberoptic light p.
    Lancaster red-green p.
    Marco chart p.
    NP-3S auto chart p.
    Topcon chart p.
    Ultramatic Project-O-Chart p.
    UPOC p.
Project Research Ophthalmic specular microscope
Pro-Koester wide-field SCM microscope
prolactin-secreting adenoma
prolapse
    iris p.
    p. of iris
    vitreous p.
Prolene suture
proliferans
    fibrous p.
    retinitis p.
proliferating retinitis
proliferation
    anterior hyaloidal fibrovascular p.
    conjunctival lymphoid p.
    epimacular p.
    epiretinal membrane p. (EMP)
    extraretinal fibrovascular p.
    fibrovascular p.
    glial p.
    hyaloidal fibrovascular p.
    massive periretinal p. (MPP)
    peripheral p.
    retinal angiomatous p.
proliferative
    p. background diabetic retinopathy
    p. choroiditis
    p. diabetic retinopathy (PDR)
    p. diabetic vitreoretinopathy
      (PDVR)
    p. lupus retinopathy

    p. retinitis
    p. sickle-cell retinopathy
prolonged-wear contact lens
promethazine
prominence
    Ammon scleral p.
prominent
    p. buckle
    p. indentation
    p. Schwalbe ring
Pro-Ophtha
    P.-O. drape
    P.-O. dressing
    P.-O. eye pad
    P.-O. sponge
    P.-O. stick
propamidine isethionate
proparacaine
    p. HCl
    p. hydrochloride
    p. ophthalmic drops
prophylactic
    p. antibiotic
    p. laser iridotomy
    p. retinopexy
prophylaxis
    Credé p.
    retinal p.
Propine Ophthalmic
propionate
    clobetasol p.
    sodium p.
Propionibacterium
    P. acnes
    P. acnes endophthalmitis
    P. propionicus
propionicus
    Propionibacterium p.
proportional fragmentation
Propper-Heine ophthalmoscope
Propper indirect ophthalmoscope
propria
    substantia p.
proprioception
proprioceptive
    p. head-turning reflex
    p. oculocephalic reflex
    p. stimulus
proptometer
proptosis
    axial p.
    ipsilateral p.
    Moran p.
    unilateral p.
proptotic
propylene glycol
propylparaben
    methyl p.
Prorex

PROSHIELD collagen corneal shield
prosopagnosia
> apperceptive p.
> associative p.
> developmental p.

prospective
> P. Evaluation of Radial Keratotomy (PERK)
> P. Evaluation of Radial Keratotomy Study
> p. study

prostaglandin analog
prostaglandin-mediated phenomenon
prosthesis, pl. **prostheses**
> ocular p.
> orbital floor p.
> shell p.
> socket p.

prosthesis-induced trachoma
prosthetic
> p. lens
> P. Orthotic Associates

prosthetophacos
prosthokeratoplasty
Prostigmin test
protan
> anomalous projection p.
> p. color blindness

protanomal
protanomalopia
protanomalous
> protanope p.

protanomaly
protanope protanomalous
protanopia
protanopic
protanopsia
protease
> serine p.

protective
> p. lens
> p. spectacles
> p. sports eye wear

protector
> Arroyo p.
> Arruga p.
> Buratto flap p.
> eye p.
> oculoplasty corneal p.
> Vinciguerra LASEK p.

protein
> antiglial fibrillary acidic p.

> bactericidal permeability-increasing p. (BPI)
> p. deposit
> eosinophil cationic p. (ECP)
> Fas liquid p.
> glial fibrillary acidic p. (GFAP)
> interphotoreceptor retinoid-binding p. (IRBP)
> p. kinase C (PKC)
> major basic p. (MBP)
> retained lens p.
> RNA III activating p. (RAP)
> silver p.

protein-1
> monocyte chemotactic p. (MCP-1)

proteinaceous
> p. aqueous exudation
> p. coating
> p. cyst

proteinolipidic film
proteolytic enzyme
Proteus
Proteus syndrome
protocol
> Yasuma p.

protometer
proton beam
ProTon portable tonometer
Protovir
protozoan
> p. keratitis
> p. uveitis

protriptyline hydrochloride
protruding eyes
protrusion
> conical p.
> corneal p.

Proview eye pressure monitor
Provisc
provocative
> p. test
> p. testing

Prowazek-Greeff body
Prowazek-Halberstaedter body
Prowazek inclusion body
proximal
> p. convergence
> p. myotonic myopathy

proximum
> punctum p. (p.p.)

proxymetacaine HCl 0.5%

NOTES

P

PRRE
pupils round, regular, and equal
PRT
photostress recovery time
prurigo
actinic p.
Hutchinson Summer p.
psammoma body
psammomatous meningioma (PM)
PSC
posterior subcapsular cataract
PSD
pattern standard deviation
Pseudallescheria boydii
pseudo
p. POHS
p. sinus dilatans
pseudoabducens palsy
pseudoacanthosis nigricans
pseudoaccommodation
pseudo-Argyll Robertson pupil
pseudobaggy eyelid
pseudoblepsia, pseudoblepsis
pseudobulbar palsy
pseudocaloric nystagmus
pseudocancerous lesion
pseudochiasmal
pseudocoloboma
pseudo-CSF signal
pseudocyst
foveal p.
pseudocystoid macular edema
pseudodendrites
Acanthamoeba keratitis p.
pseudodendritic keratitis
pseudodiphtheriticum
Corynebacterium p.
pseudodoubling
pseudodrusen
pseudoendothelial dystrophy
pseudoenophthalmos
pseudoephedrine
carbinoxamine and p.
pseudoepitheliomatous hyperplasia
pseudoesotropia
pseudoexfoliation (PXF)
p. of lens capsule
p. syndrome
pseudoexfoliative
p. capsular glaucoma
p. glaucoma (PEXG)
pseudoexophoria
pseudoexophthalmos
pseudoexotropia
pseudo-Foster Kennedy syndrome
pseudoglaucoma
pseudoglaucomatous macrocupping
pseudoglioma

pseudo-Graefe
p.-G. phenomenon
p.-G. sign
pseudohemianopsia
pseudohistoplasmosis
pseudohole
macular p. (MPH)
pseudo-Hurler polydystrophy
pseudohypoparathyroidism
pseudohypopyon
pseudoinflammatory
p. macular dystrophy
p. macular dystrophy of Sorsby
pseudointernuclear ophthalmoplegia
pseudoiritis
pseudoisochromatic
p. chart
p. color plate
p. color test
pseudomembrane
conjunctival p.
pseudomembranous
p. conjunctivitis
p. rhinitis
Pseudomonas
P. aeruginosa
P. cepacia
P. pyocyanea
P. stutzeri
pseudomycosis
pseudomyopia
pseudonystagmus
pseudooperculum
pseudopannus
pseudopapilledema
pseudopapillitis
pseudopemphigoid
pseudophacos, pseudophakos
pseudophake implant
pseudophakia
p. adiposa
p. fibrosa
pseudophakic
p. bullous keratopathy (PBK)
p. detachment
p. eye
pseudophakodonesis
pseudophakos (*var. of* pseudophacos)
pseudopit
pseudopolycoria
pseudopresumed ocular histoplasmosis syndrome (pseudo POHS)
pseudoprolactinoma
pseudoproptosis
pseudopseudohypoparathyroidism
pseudopsia
pseudopterygia
pseudopterygium
pseudoptosis

pseudoretinitis pigmentosa
pseudoretinoblastoma
pseudorheumatoid nodule
pseudorosette
pseudosarcomatous endothelial
  hyperplasia
pseudosclerosis
  spastic p.
pseudoscopic vision
pseudo-sixth
  midbrain p.-s.
pseudostereo image
pseudostrabismus
pseudotabes
  pupillotonic p.
pseudotemporal arteritis
pseudotrachoma
pseudotuberculous ophthalmia
pseudotumor
  p. cerebri (PTC)
  idiopathic inflammatory p.
  inflammatory p.
  lymphoid p.
  p. oculi
  orbital inflammatory p.
pseudovernal conjunctivitis
pseudoxanthoma
  elastic p.
  p. elasticum (PXE)
PSI
  pneumatically stented implant
psittaci
  Chlamydia p.
Psoralens
psoriasis
  plaque-type p.
psoriatic corneal abscess
psorophthalmia
psychic blindness
psychogenic
  p. micropsia
  p. paralysis
  p. photophobia
psychophysical measurement
psychophysics
  visual p.
psychosis
  black patch p.
  Wernicke-Korsakoff p.
psychotropic medication
PTC
  pseudotumor cerebri

pterion
pterygial tissue
pterygium, pl. pterygia
  active p.
  Arlt p.
  belly of p.
  cicatricial p.
  congenital p.
  conjunctival p.
  epitarsus p.
  p. scissors
  p. unguis
pterygium-induced astigmatism
pterygoid levator synkinesis
pterygomaxillary fissure
pterygopalatine ganglion
ptilosis
PTK
  phototherapeutic keratectomy
ptosis, pl. ptoses
  acquired myopathic p.
  p. adiposa
  age-related p.
  aponeurotic p.
  Berke p.
  bilateral p.
  Blaskovics-Berke p.
  botulism-induced p.
  cerebral p.
  congenital dystrophic p.
  congenital myopathic p.
  cortical p.
  p. crutch spectacles
  developmental p.
  drug-induced p.
  eyelid p.
  false p.
  fatigable p.
  p. forceps
  guarding p.
  Hiff p.
  Homer p.
  Horner p.
  involutional senile p.
  p. knife
  levator p.
  p. lipomatosis
  magnitude of p.
  mechanical acquired p.
  midbrain p.
  morning p.
  myogenic acquired p.

NOTES

P

ptosis *(continued)*
    myopathic p.
    neurogenic-acquired p.
    neuromuscular p.
    ocular myasthenia p.
    p. scissors
    senescent p.
    snake bite-induced p.
    p. sympathetica
    traumatic p.
    upside-down p.
    waking p.
ptotic
pubis
    Phthirus p.
pucker
    macular p.
    pigmented macular p.
puckering
    macular p.
puddler's cataract
puff of loose vitreous
PUK
    peripheral ulcerative keratitis
Pulfrich
    P. effect
    P. stereo phenomenon
pulpit spectacles
Pulsair tonometer
pulsatile exophthalmos
pulsating exophthalmos
pulsation
    spontaneous retinal venous p.
    venous p.
pulse
    choroidal p.
    p. mode
    radiofrequency p.
    retinal venous p.
    saccadic p.
    square-wave p.
pulsed electron avalanche knife (PEAK)
pulseless disease
pulsing
Pulsion FS Laser
pulverulenta
    cataracta centralis p.
    cataracta zonularis p.
pulverulent opacity
pump
    AE-2910 Carones LASEK p.
    AMO HPF 500 p.
    Carones LASEK p.
    frame-mounted p.
    MityVac simple hand p.
    peristaltic p.
    tear p.
    TurboStaltic p.
pump-leak system

punch
    Barron donor corneal p.
    Barron marking corneal p.
    Berens corneoscleral p.
    p. block
    bone p.
    bone-biting p.
    Carpel one-step trabeculectomy p.
    Castroviejo corneoscleral p.
    Christensen p.
    corneal p.
    corneoscleral p.
    Descemet membrane p.
    Gass corneoscleral p.
    Gass scleral p.
    Gass sclerotomy p.
    Hardy p.
    Holth scleral p.
    Kelly-Descemet membrane p.
    Klein p.
    Luntz-Dodick p.
    Pollock p.
    Price Corneal P.
    Pritikin p.
    Reiss punctal p.
    Rothman Gilbard cornea p.
    Rubin-Holth p.
    scleral p.
    sclerectomy p.
    sclerotomy p.
    Storz corneoscleral p.
    Tanne corneal p.
    Tanne guillotine-style p.
    p. trephine
    Troutman p.
    Walser corneoscleral p.
    Walton p.
punched-out
    p.-o. chorioretinal scar
    p.-o. lesion
puncta *(pl. of* punctum)
punctal
    p. cautery
    p. dilator
    p. ectropion
    p. lens
    p. occlusion
    p. opening
    p. plug
    p. stenosis
punctata
    p. albescens retinopathy
    chondrodystrophia calcificans
      congenita p.
    hyalitis p.
    keratitis p.
punctate
    p. cataract
    p. corneal epithelial defect

p. corneal opacity
p. epithelial erosion
p. epithelial keratitis
p. epithelial keratopathy (PEK)
p. epithelial keratoplasty
p. epithelial microcyst
p. hemorrhage
p. hyalitis
p. hyalosis
p. inner choroiditis
p. inner choroidopathy (PIC)
p. keratic precipitate
p. keratitis of Thygeson
p. keratoderma
p. oculocutaneous albinism
p. oculocutaneous albinoidism
p. outer retinal toxoplasmosis
p. retinitis
p. staining
punctiform
punctograph
punctoplasty
punctum, pl. **puncta**
p. aplasia
p. caecum
p. cecum
dilation of p.
p. dilator
erythematous pouting of the p.
eversion of p.
everted p.
inferior p.
lacrimal p.
p. lacrimale
lower p.
p. luteum
one-snip p.
p. piug
p. proximum (p.p.)
p. proximum of accommodation
p. proximum of convergence (PP)
p. remotum (p.r.)
p. stenosis
superior p.
three-snip p.
upper p.
punctumeter
puncture
anterior p.
p. diabetes
diathermy p.
p. needle

self-sealing scleral p.
p. wound
Ziegler p.
puncture-tip needle
Puntenney forceps
pupil (P)
Adie tonic p.
amaurotic p.
Argyll Robertson p. (ARP)
artificial p.
attention reflex of the p.
Behr p.
p. block
p. block glaucoma
blown p.
bounding p.
Bumke p.
catatonic p.
cat's eye p.
cholinergic p.
cogwheel p.
constricted p.
contraction of p.
cornpicker's p.
p. cycle induction test
diabetic Argyll Robertson p.
diffraction-limited p.
dilated p.
p. dilation
p. dilator
dilator muscle of p.
p. disorder
elliptic p.
entrance p.
p.'s equal, reactive to light and
   accommodation (PERLA)
p.'s equal, react to light (PERL)
p.'s equal, round, reactive to light
   and accommodation (PERRLA)
exclusion of pupil
exit p.
fixed dilated p.
Gunn p.
hammock p.
Holmes-Adie p.
Homer p.
Horner p.
Hutchinson p.
iris and p. (I/P)
irregular p.
isolated fixed dilated p.
keyhole p.

NOTES

P

pupil *(continued)*
    light response of p.
    local tonic p.
    Marcus Gunn p.
    MG p.
    p. miosis
    miotic p.
    myotonic p.
    neuropathic tonic p.
    neurotonic p.
    occluded p.
    occlusion of p.
    paradoxical p.
    p. pass
    pear-shaped p.
    peninsula p.
    pinhole p.
    pinpoint p.
    pseudo-Argyll Robertson p.
    reverse Marcus Gunn p.
    rigid p.
    Robertson p.
    p.'s round, regular, and equal
      (PRRE)
    Saenger p.
    scalloped p.
    seclusion of p.
    p. size
    skew p.
    sphincter muscle of p.
    p. spreader/retractor forceps
    spring p.
    square p.
    stiff p.
    p. stretching
    tadpole p.
    teardrop p.
    tonic p.
    updrawn p.
    Wernicke p.
    white p.
pupilla, pl. **pupillae**
    caligo p.
    ectopia lentis et pupillae
    pupillae muscle of iris
    musculus dilator p.
    musculus sphincter p.
    sphincter pupillae
    synizesis pupillae
    synkinesis p.
pupillaris
    membrana p.
pupillary
    p. aperture
    p. areflexia
    p. athetosis
    p. axis
    p. block

    p. block glaucoma
    p. capture
    p. center
    p. dilator muscle
    p. disorder
    p. distance (PD)
    p. effect
    p. entrapment
    p. escape
    p. floater
    p. hemiakinesia
    p. iris cyst
    p. lens
    p. light reflex
    p. line
    p. margin
    p. margin of iris
    p. membrane
    p. membrane remnant
    p. miosis
    p. near response
    p. paradoxic reflex
    p. paralysis
    p. sparing
    p. sphincter akinesis
    p. sphincter contraction
    p. sphincter muscle
    p. zone
pupilloconstrictor fiber
pupillograph
pupillography
pupillometer
    Colvard handheld infrared p.
    corneal reflection p. (CRP)
    Procyon digital infrared p.
    Pupilscan II p.
    reflex p.
pupillometry
    infrared p.
pupillomotor fiber
pupilloplasty
pupilloplegia
pupilloscope
pupilloscopy
pupillostatometer
pupillotonia
pupillotonic pseudotabes
Pupilscan II pupillometer
pupil-to-root iridectomy
Puralube
    P. Tears
    P. Tears Solution
pure
    p. alexia
    p. color
    p. cyclitis
    P. Eyes-CIBA
    P. Eyes Cleaner/Rinse

P. Eyes Disinfection/Soaking Solution
P. Eyes soaking solution
PureVision extended-wear contact lens
Purilens UV Disinfection Solution
purinergic
selective p.
Purisol
Purkinje
P. effect
P. figure
P. image
P. image tracker
P. phenomenon
P. shadow
P. shift
Purkinje-Sanson mirror image
Purlytin
purple
visual p.
purpura
palpable p.
purpurea
Digitalis p.
purpuriferous
purpuriparous
purpurogenous membrane
pursuit
cogwheel p.
p. mechanism
p. movement
saccadic p.
smooth p.
p. testing
p. tracking
Purtscher
P. angiopathic retinopathy
P. disease
Purtscher-like retinopathy
purulent
p. conjunctivitis
p. cyclitis
p. iritis
p. keratitis
p. ophthalmia
p. retinitis
p. rhinitis
push-and-pull hook
pusher
Aker lens p.
De LaVega lens p.

Martin Surefit lens p.
Visitec lens p.
push-plus refraction technique
push/pull
Ilg p./p.
Kuglein p./p.
push-up
pencil p.-u.'s
push-up method
pustular blepharitis
Putenney operation
Putterman
P. levator resection clamp
P. ptosis clamp
Putterman-Chaflin ocular asymmetry device
Putterman-Mueller blepharoptosis clamp
P.V.
P.V. Carpine
P.V. Carpine Liquifilm
PVA
polyvinyl alcohol
PVA spear
p value
PVD
posterior vitreous detachment
PVER
pattern visual-evoked response
PVR
PXE
pseudoxanthoma elasticum
PxEx Ophthalmic
PXF
pseudoexfoliation
pyknotic
p. keratitis
p. nuclei
pyocyanea
Pseudomonas p.
pyocyaneus
Bacillus p.
pyogenes
Streptococcus p.
pyogenic
p. granuloma
p. metastasis
Pyopen
pyophthalmia
pyophthalmitis
pyramidal
p. cataract
p. system

NOTES

P

Pyrex
- P. eye sphere
- P. T-tube
- P. tube

pyridoxine
pyrimethamine

13q-syndrome
q arm
Q-banding
Q-switched
    Q.-s. Er:YAG laser
    Q.-s. Nd:YAG laser
    Q.-s. neodymium:YAG laser
    Q.-s. ruby laser
Quad cutting tip
QuadPediatric fundus lens
quad-ported LASIK irrigating cannula
quadrant
    q. hemianopsia
    inferior nasal q.
    inferior temporal q.
quadrantanopia
    crossed binasal q.
    crossed bitemporal q.
    heteronymous q.
    homonomous q.
    pie-in-the-sky q.
    pie-on-the-floor q.
quadrantanopsia, quadrantanopia
    homonymous q.
    superior q.
quadrantic
    q. defect
    q. hemianopsia
    q. sclerectomy with internal drainage
    q. scotoma
quadrantopia
Quaglino operation
quality
    average retinal image q.
    optical q.
    tear q.
quantitative
    q. echography
    q. haze assessment
    q. static threshold
    q. threshold perimetry
quantity
    tear q.
Quantum enhancement knife
quaternary
    q. ammonium chloride
    q. ammonium compound
QUEST
    quick estimation by sequential testing

Questek laser tube
questionnaire
    Dry Eye q.
    25-Item Visual Function Q. (VFQ-25)
    Low Vision Quality of Life Q. (LVQOLQ)
    McMonnies q.
    National Eye Institute Visual Function Q. (NEI-VFQ)
    VF-14 q.
    Visual Activities Q.
    Visual Function Q. (VFQ)
Quevedo
    Q. fixation forceps
    Q. suturing forceps
quick
    q. adducting-retraction jerk
    Q. Care System
    q. estimation by sequential testing (QUEST)
    q. left/right component
Quickert
    Q. lacrimal intubation probe
    Q. procedure
    Q. suture
    Q. three-suture technique
Quickert-Dryden
    Q.-D. probe
    Q.-D. tube
QuickRinse automated instrument rinse system
Quickswitch irrigation/aspiration ophthalmic system
quiescent stromal scarring
quiet
    q. chamber
    deep and q. (D&Q)
    eye was q.
    q. iritis
Quiet-Vac
quinacrine hydrochloride
Quinamm
quinine
    q. amblyopia
    q. sulfate
Quire mechanical finger forceps
Quixin ophthalmic solution

Rabinowitz-Klyce/Maeda keratoconus screening program
Rabinowitz-McDonnell test
Rabl lamella
raccoon eyes
racemose
  r. aneurysm
  r. angioma
  r. hemangioma
  r. hemangiomatosis
racemosum
  staphyloma corneae r.
rack
  Luneau retinoscopy r.
racquet body
racquet-like pattern
radial
  r. astigmatism
  r. cells of Mueller
  r. dilator muscle
  r. fiber
  r. infiltration
  r. iridotomy
  r. iridotomy scissors
  r. keratotomy (RK)
  r. keratotomy knife
  r. keratotomy marker
  r. sponge
  r. transillumination defect
  r. vessel array
radially oriented
radiance
radiant
  r. absorptance
  r. emittance
  r. energy
  r. intensity
  r. and luminous flux
  r. power
  r. reflectance
radiata
  corona r.
radiatio
  r. occipitothalamica
  r. optica
radiation
  artificial UV r.
  beta r.
  r. burn
  r. cataract
  r. effect
  electromagnetic r.
  geniculocalcarine r.
  Goldmann Coherent r.
  heavy ion r.

  infrared r.
  r. injury
  ionizing r.
  r. keratitis
  natural UV r.
  occipitothalamic r.
  optic r.
  r. optic neuropathy (RON)
  r. retinopathy
  solar r.
  r. therapy
  ultraviolet r.
  visual r.
radiation-induced
  r.-i. carcinoma
  r.-i. optic neuropathy
radical
  r. astigmatism
  r. orbitectomy
radicans
  Rhus r.
radices (*pl. of* radix)
radii (*pl. of* radius)
Radin-Rosenthal eye implant
radioactive
  r. eye plaque
  r. plaque brachytherapy
radiofrequency pulse
radiogenic vasculopathy
radioimmunoassay technique
radioisotope scan
radiology
  orbital r.
radioscope
  Lombart r.
radiotherapy
  orbital r.
  palladium 103 ophthalmic plaque r.
  plaque r.
radius, pl. radii
  apical r.
  axial length/corneal r. (AL:CR)
  back optic zone r. (BOZR)
  r. of curvature
  front optic zone r. (FOZR)
  r. gauge
  r. of lens
  r. of lentis
  posterior apical r. (PAR)
radix, pl. radices
  r. lateralis tractus optici
  r. medialis tractus optici
  r. oculomotoria ganglii ciliaris
  r. sympathica ganglii ciliaris

radon
    r. ring brachytherapy
    r. seed implantation
Raeder paratrigeminal neuralgia
ragged-red fiber
rag-wheel method
railroad nystagmus
rainbow
    r. symptom
    r. syndrome
    r. vision
raindrop-shaped keratometric reflection
Rainin
    R. air injection cannula
    R. clip-bending spatula
    R. lens spatula
Raji cell assay
rake
    Trujillo LASIK enhancement r.
raking
    endoscopic r.
Raman
    R. effect
    R. spectrum
Ramsden eyepiece
ramus, pl. **rami**
    tentorii r.
Randolph
    R. cyclodialysis cannula
    R. irrigator
random-dot
    r.-d. kinematogram
    r.-d. kinematography
    r.-d. stereogram (RDS)
randomized
    A R. Trial Comparing Daily Atropine Versus Weekend Atropine
    A R. Trial Comparing Part-Time Versus Full-Time Patching for Amblyopia
    A R. Trial Comparing Part-Time Versus Minimal-Time Patching for Moderate Amblyopia
    R. Trial of Acetazolamide for Uveitis-Associated Cystoid Macular Edema
    R. Trial of Aspirin and Cataracts in U.S. Physicians
    R. Trial of Beta-Carotene and Macular Degeneration
    R. Trials of Vitamin Supplements and Eye Disease
    R. Trial of Vitamin A and Vitamin E Supplementation for Retinitis Pigmentosa
random order
Randot
    R. chart
    R. circle
    R. Dot E stereo test
    R. Stereo Smile test
range
    r. of accommodation
    r. of convergence
    vertical fusion r.
Rank-Taylor-Hobson-Talysurf instrument
RAP
    RNA III activating protein
RAPD
    relative afferent pupillary defect
raphe
    canthal r.
    horizontal r.
    lateral palpebral r.
    palpebral r.
    r. palpebralis lateralis
    r. palpebrarum
    r. plica semilunaris
    posterior lamina r.
    retinal r.
    temporal r.
rapid
    r. antibiotic susceptibility testing (RAST)
    r. eye movement (REM)
    r. serial visual presentation (RSVP)
Rappazzo intraocular manipulator
rare earth intraocular magnet
rarefaction
    pigmentation r.
rasp
    Lundsgaard r.
    Lundsgaard-Burch corneal r.
RAST
    rapid antibiotic susceptibility testing
Raster photogrammeter
rasterstereography
rasterstereography-based elevation map
rate
    aspiration flow r.
    seropositivity r.
    spontaneous eye blink r. (SEBR)
    susceptibility kill r.
    tear clearance r.
Rathke
    R. cleft cyst
    R. pouch
    R. pouch tumor
ratio
    accommodation-convergence r.
    accommodative convergence/accommodation r. (AC/A)
    AL/CR r.
    aperture r.
    Armaly cup/disk r.
    arteriovenous r.

artery-to-vein r. (A/V)
axial length/corneal radius r.
CA/C r.
convergence accommodation r.
cup-disk r.
cup-to-disk r. (C/D, CDR)
L/D r.
light/dark amplitude r.
light-peak to dark-trough r.
nuclear cytoplasmic r.
optic cup-to-disk r.
Pourcelot r.
rim-to-disk r.

Raven Progressive Matrices test
Raverdino operation
ray
convergent r.
converging r.
divergent r.
emergent r.
r. incident
r. of light
medullary r.
monochromatic r.
parallel r.
paraxial r.
r. tracing

Ray-Brunswick-Mack operation
Rayleigh
R. color matching test
R. limit
R. scattering

Ray-McLean operation
Raymond-Cestan syndrome
Raymond syndrome
Rayner-Choyce implant
Rayner lens
razor
Bard-Parker r.
r. blade
r. bladebreaker
r. blade knife
r. needle

razor-blade trephine
razor-tip needle
RBRVS
Resource-Based Relative Value Scale
RC-2 fundus camera
RCL
recurrent corneal lesion
RD
retinal detachment

RDS
random-dot stereogram
reaction
Alamar blue redox r.
anaphylactic r.
anterior chamber r.
Arthus r.
basophilic r.
Calmette conjunctival r.
Calmette ophthalmic r.
conjunctival r.
consensual r.
direct pupillary light r.
early-phase r.
eosinophilic r.
Griess r.
hemiopic pupillary r.
hypersensitivity r.
immune r.
immunologic r.
indirect pupillary r.
Jarisch-Herxheimer r.
late-phase r.
lid closure r.
light r.
Loewi r.
Mazzotti r.
mononuclear r.
near r.
ocular tilt r. (OTR)
ophthalmic r.
orbicularis r.
pain r.
paradoxical darkness r.
polymerase chain r. (PCR)
polymorphonuclear r.
Prausnitz-Kustner r.
toxic r.
vestibular pupillary r.
Weil-Felix r.
Wernicke r.

reactive lymphoid hyperplasia (RLH)
reader
bar r.
reading
r. card
r. chart
r. glasses
keratometric r.'s
r. rectangle
r. vision
Ready-Set punctum plug

NOTES

reagent
>Brücke r.
>r. strip

real
>r. focus
>r. image

reaper's
>r. keratitis
>r. ophthalmia

reasoning
>Garway-Heath r.

reattachment
>r. of choroid
>r. of choroid operation
>hydraulic retinal r.
>r. of retina
>r. of retina operation

Rebif

rebleeding

rebound
>r. conjunctival hyperemia
>r. nystagmus

receptacle
>dome r.

receptive field

receptor
>r. amblyopia
>expression of chemokine r.
>r. potential

recess
>Arlt r.
>Arlt-Jaesche r.
>canthal r.
>optic r.
>suprapineal r.
>von Arlt r.

recessed-angle glaucoma

recession
>angle r.
>bimedial r.
>r. clamp
>conjunctival r.
>r. forceps
>r. index (RI)
>lateral rectus r.
>left inferior oblique r.
>r. of muscle
>r. of ocular muscle operation
>optic muscle r.
>tendon r.
>traumatic angle r.

recession-angle glaucoma

recession-resection (R&R)

recessive dystrophic epidermolysis bullosa

recess-resect (R&R)

recessus opticus

rechutes
>iritis blenorrhagique à r.

recipient bed

reciprocal innervation

reciprocity law

Recklinghausen
>R. disease
>R. syndrome

reclination

recognition
>pattern r.

reconstruction
>r. of eyelid
>multiplanar r.
>socket r.
>V-Y advancement
> myotarsocutaneous flap for upper eyelid r.

recorder
>DVCPRO digital video r.

recovery
>fluid-attenuated inversion r. (FLAIR)
>hyperactive immune r.
>retinal r.

rectangle
>reading r.

rectangular
>r. blade
>r. two-thirds-thickness sclerotomy

rectifier
>delayed r.
>inward r.

rectus
>inferior r. (IR)
>lateral r. (L.R.)
>r. lateralis muscle
>medial r. (MR)
>r. medialis muscle
>superior r. (SR)

recurrent
>r. central retinitis
>r. choroiditis
>r. corneal erosion
>r. corneal erosion syndrome
>r. corneal lesion (RCL)
>r. epithelial erosion
>r. erosion of cornea
>r. exophthalmos
>r. hypopyon
>r. pupillary sparing

recurrentis
>*Borrelia* r.

red
>r. blindness
>r. cone degeneration
>r. coral keratitis
>r. desaturation
>r. eye
>r. filter
>r. flash stimulus

R

r. free photograph
r. glare test
r. glass test
r. lens occluder
r. reflex
R. Reflex Lens Systems lens
r. rubber catheter
ruthenium r.
r. scaly plaque
r. vision
redeepening
redetachment
retinal r.
red-eyed shunt syndrome
red-filter
r.-f. test
r.-f. therapy
red-free
r.-f. filter
r.-f. photography
red-green
r.-g. axis
r.-g. blindness
r.-g. glasses
Reditron refractometer
Redmond-Smith operation
redness
sectoral r.
reduced
r. eye
r. eye model
r. Snellen card
r. vergence
reducer
McCannel ocular pressure r.
ocular pressure r.
reducing body myopathy
reductase
aldose r.
methylenetetrahydrofolate r.
(MTHFR)
reduction
r. of aberration
contrast sensitivity r.
precision astigmatism r.
reduplicated cataract
reduplication
r. of Descemet membrane
Reed-Sternberg cell
Reeh scissors
reel aspiration cannula
reepithelialization

Reese
R. Ellsworth classification system
R. muscle forceps
R. ptosis knife
R. ptosis operation
R. syndrome
Reese-Cleasby operation
Reese-Ellsworth
R.-E. classification
R.-E. group Va, Vb disease
R.-E. group V retinoblastoma
R.-E. stage IIIA retinoblastoma
Reese-Jones-Cooper operation
refined refraction
refixation
Ref-Keratometer
Canon R-5+ Auto R.-K.
reflectance
radiant r.
reflected
r. color
r. light
reflecting
r. prism
r. retinoscope
r. surface
reflection
angle of r.
corneal r.
D-shaped keratometric r.
raindrop-shaped keratometric r.
shiny cellophane r.
specular r.
reflective scattering
reflectivity
internal r.
reflectometer
reflectometry
reflex
r. accommodation
accommodation r.
accommodative pupillary r.
acquired gustolacrimal r.
r. amaurosis
r. amblyopia
attention r.
audito oculogyric r.
auditory oculogyric r.
Bekhterev r.
Bell r.
black r.
r. blepharospasm

NOTES

reflex *(continued)*

blind spot r.
blink r.
blunted red r.
blunted retinoscopic r.
cat's eye r.
cellophane macular r.
cerebral cortex r.
cerebropupillary r.
cervicoocular r. (COR)
Charleaux oil droplet r.
choked r.
ciliary r.
ciliospinal r.
circumpapillary light r.
coaxially sighted corneal r.
cochleopupillary r.
congenital paradoxic
  gustolacrimal r.
conjunctival r.
consensual light r.
consensual pupillary r.
convergency r.
copper-wire r.
corneal light r.
corneomandibular r.
corneomental r.
corneopterygoid r.
corticopupillary r.
crescentic circumpapillary light r.
crossed r.
cutaneous pupillary r.
dazzle r.
direct-light r.
direct pupillary r.
doll's eye r.
emergency light r.
eye r.
eyeball compression r.
eyeball-heart r.
eye-closure r.
eyelid-closure r.
r. eye movement
eye-popping r.
fixation r.
foveal r.
foveolar r.
fundal r.
fundus r.
fusion r.
Gault r.
Gifford r.
Gifford-Galassi r.
golden tapetal-like fundus r.
Gunn pupillary r.
gustatolacrimal r.
Haab r.
head-turning r.
Hirschberg r.

iridoplegia r.
iris contraction r.
juvenile r.
lacrimal r.
lacrimation r.
lid closure r.
light optometer r.
Lockwood light r.
McCarthy r.
myopic r.
nasolacrimal r.
near light r.
oculocardiac r.
oculocephalic r.
oculocephalogyric r.
oculodigital r.
oculogyric auricular r.
oculopharyngeal r.
oculopupillary r.
oculorespiratory r.
oculosensory cell r.
oculovestibular r.
opticofacial winking r.
optokinetic r.
optomotor r.
orbicularis pupillary r.
otolithic-ocular r.
palpebral oculogyric r.
palpebromandibular r.
paradoxical pupillary r.
paradoxic gustolacrimal r.
platysmal r.
Plitz r.
proprioceptive head-turning r.
proprioceptive oculocephalic r.
pupillary light r.
pupillary paradoxic r.
r. pupillometer
red r.
retinal r.
reversed pupillary r.
Ruggeri r.
senile r.
shot-silk r.
silver-wire r.
skin pupillary r.
spasm of the near r.
stretch r.
supraorbital r.
synkinetic near r.
tapetal light r.
r. tear production
r. tear secretion
threat r.
trigeminal r.
r. trigeminus
trigeminus r.
utricular r.
vestibuloocular r.

visual orbicularis r.
water-silk r.
Weiss r.
Westphal-Piltz r.
Westphal pupillary r.
white fundus r.
white pupillary r.
wink r.
yellow light r.

reflux
r. of tears
r. vergence

reformation
r. of chamber
fornix r.
inferior fornix r.

Refractec ViewPoint CK System
refracted light
refractile
r. body
r. crystal
r. deposit

refracting
r. angle of prism
r. medium

refraction
angle of r.
r. angle
autorefractometer r.
cycloplegic r. (CR)
cylindric r.
direct-light r.
double r.
dynamic r.
fogged manifest r.
fogging system of r.
homatropine r.
index of r. (IR, n)
law of r.
manifest r. (MR)
ocular r.
plane-surface r.
refined r.
r. spectacles
spherical r.
static r.
unrefined r.

refractionist
refractionometer
Hartinger Coincidence r.
vertex r.
Zeiss vertex r.

refractive
r. accommodative esotropia
r. amblyopia
r. ametropia
r. anisometropia
r. astigmatism
r. contact lens
r. error
R. Error Study in Children
r. hyperopia
r. keratoplasty
r. keratotomy
r. medium
r. myopia
r. outcome
r. power
r. state
r. surgery

refractivity
refractometer
Abbe r.
Canon auto r.
Hoya HDR objective r.
Hoya MRM objective r.
meridional r.
Reditron r.
Rodenstock eye r.
Speedy-1 Auto r.
8000 Supra Series auto r.
Topcon eye r.
Topcon RM-A2300 auto r.

refractometry
laser r.
urine r.

refractor
Agrikola r.
Allergan Humphrey r.
Amoils r.
AR 1000 r.
automated r.
automatic r.
Berens r.
Brawley r.
Bronson-Turtz r.
Campbell r.
Canon r.
Castallo r.
Castroviejo r.
Coburn r.
CooperVision Diagnostic Imaging r.
Desmarres r.
Elschnig r.

NOTES

refractor *(continued)*
    Ferris-Smith r.
    Ferris-Smith-Sewall r.
    Fink r.
    Goldstein r.
    Gradle r.
    Graether r.
    Green r.
    Groenholm r.
    Hartstein r.
    Hillis r.
    Humphrey automatic r.
    Kirby r.
    Knapp r.
    Kronfeld r.
    KR 7000-P cycloplegic r.
    Kuglein r.
    Leland r.
    Marco r.
    McGannon r.
    Meller r.
    Mueller r.
    Nidek AR-2000 Objective
      Automatic r.
    objective r.
    Precision r.
    Reichert r.
    Remote Vision electronic r.
    Rizzuti r.
    Rollet r.
    Schepens r.
    SR-IV Programmed Subjective r.
    Stevenson r.
    subjective r.
    Topcon r.
    Wilmer r.
refractory
    vernal keratoconjunctivitis r.
Refrax corneal repair kit
Refresh
    R. Endura eye drops
    R. Liquigel dry eye treatment
    R. Liquigel eye drops
    R. Plus
    R. Plus lubricant eye drops
    R. Plus Ophthalmic Solution
    R. PM
    R. Tears eye drops
refringence
refringent
Refsum
    R. disease
    R. syndrome
Regan-Lancaster dial
Regan low-contrast acuity chart
regard
    area of conscious r.
    object of r.

    plane of r.
    point of r.
regeneration
    aberrant r.
    r. aberration
    r. of innervation
    nerve r.
    r. of nerve
    postganglionic fiber r.
regimen
    multiple bottle r.
region
    ciliary r.
    ethmoidal r.
    infraorbital r.
    ocular r.
    orbital r.
    pretectal r.
    retrochiasmatic r.
    scutum r.
    third framework r. (FR3)
regional
    r. block
    r. periarteritis
registry
    Australian Corneal Graft R.
regression
    myopic r.
    univariate linear r.
    univariate polytomous logistic r.
regular
    r. astigmatism
    Eye Drops R.
    Vasocon R.
regulator
    OptiMed glaucoma pressure r.
    (OGPR)
rehabilitation
    optical r.
Reichert
    R. binocular indirect
      ophthalmoscope
    R. camera
    R. Ful-Vue binocular
      ophthalmoscope
    R. Ful-Vue spot retinoscope
    R. Lenschek advanced logic
      lensometer
    R. membrane
    R. noncontact tonometer
    R. ophthalmodynamometer
    R. radius gauge
    R. refractor
    R. slit lamp
    R. Zetopan Microscope
Reichert-Jung Ultracut ultramicrotome
Reichling corneal scissors
reimplantation
Reinecke-Carroll lacrimal tube

reinforcement
scleral r.
Reinverting Operating Lens System (ROLS)
Reis-Bücklers
R.-B. disease
R.-B. ring-shaped dystrophy
R.-B. superficial corneal dystrophy
Reisinger lens-extracting forceps
Reisman sign
Reiss punctal punch
Reiter
R. conjunctivitis
R. disease
R. syndrome
rejection
allograft corneal r.
r. line
Rekoss disk
relapsing polychondritis
relapsing/remitting multiple sclerosis (RR-MS)
relationship
agonist-antagonist r.
object/image r.
relative
r. accommodation
r. afferent pupillary defect (RAPD)
r. amblyopia
r. convergence
r. divergence
first-degree r.
r. hemianopsia
r. hyperopia
near-point r.
r. scotoma
second-degree r.
r. size
r. spectacle magnification
r. strabismus
relaxing incision
releasable suture
release
r. hallucination
r. of traction for hypotony and vitreoretinopathy
relevant spatial frequency
reliable wave front sensor
Relief Ophthalmic Solution
relucency
REM
rapid eye movement

remaining visual field
remedy
novel r.
remnant
persistent pupillary membrane r.
pupillary membrane r.
remodeling
corneal stromal r.
Remote Vision electronic refractor
remotum
punctum r. (p.r.)
removal
r. of foreign body
r. of foreign body operation
lens r.
remover
Alger brush rust ring r.
Bailey foreign body r.
DMV II contact lens r.
frog cortex r.
Soft Mate protein r.
Remy separator
renal
r. coloboma syndrome
r. diabetes
r. retinitis
r. retinopathy
r. ultrasound
Renewed
Tears R.
renin-angiotensin system
rent
traumatic r.
Rentsch boat hook
ReNu
R. Effervescent enzymatic cleaner
R. Multi-Purpose
R. Rewetting Drops
R. 1 Step Enzymatic Cleaner
R. Thermal enzymatic cleaner
repair
Arlt epicanthus r.
Arlt eyelid r.
Blair epicanthus r.
blepharochalasis r.
blepharoptosis r.
Jones r.
Kuhnt-Junius r.
lacrimal gland r.
levator aponeurosis r.
medial canthal r.

NOTES

repair *(continued)*
 trichiasis r.
 Wheeler halving r.
reparative giant cell granuloma
repeat penetrating keratoplasty
repens
 Dirofilaria r.
replaceable blade
replacement
 annual r.
replacer
 Green iris r.
 Smith-Fisher iris r.
replamineform process
reposited
repositioning
repositor
 iris r.
 Knapp iris r.
 Nettleship iris r.
 Sloane flap r.
reproducibility of evaluation
rescue
 autologous stem cell r. (ASCR)
Rescula
resection
 levator r.
 Mohs microsurgical r.
 muscle r.
 r. of muscle
 Peyman full-thickness eye-wall r.
 scleral r.
 wedge r.
reserve
 base-in r.
 base-out r.
 divergence r.
 fusional r.
residual
 r. accommodation
 r. astigmatism
 r. cortex
 r. vision
resilience
 orbital r.
resin
 Medcast epoxy r.
resistance
 impact r.
 insulin r.
 outflow r.
resistive index
resistor
 Guardian scalpel with myoguard
 depth r.
Resochin
resolution
 r. acuity
 r. acuity perimetry

 logarithmic Minimum Angle of R.
 (logMAR)
Resolve/GP
resolving power
resorption
 spontaneous r.
**Resource-Based Relative Value Scale
 (RBRVS)**
response
 accommodation r.
 accommodative r.
 acquired immune r.
 allergic r.
 better visual r.
 cone r.
 consensual light r.
 consensual pupillary r.
 curve r.
 direct-light r.
 direct pupillary r.
 eosinophilic r.
 flare r.
 r. function
 immune r.
 mononuclear r.
 near r.
 partial r.
 pattern visual-evoked r. (PVER)
 polymorphonuclear r.
 pupillary near r.
 rod b-wave r.
 synkinetic near r.
 trabecular meshwork-inducible
 glucocorticoid r. (TIGR)
 vestibuloocular r. (VOR)
 visual-evoked r. (VER)
 visual-vestibulo-ocular r.
Restasis
restoration
 Berens-Smith cul-de-sac r.
 r. point
restrainer
 Gulani globe stabilizer and flap r.
restricted motility
restricting strand
restrictive syndrome
rest test
result
 false-negative r.
 false-positive r.
 visual performance r.
retained
 r. foreign body (RFB)
 r. lens protein
RetCam 120 fiberoptic fundus camera
reticle
 hand-held magnifying r.
reticular
 r. cystoid degeneration

r. dystrophy
r. haze
r. keratitis
r. plate
reticule accommodation
reticulum
r. cell
r. cell lymphoma
r. cell sarcoma
endoplasmic r.
extraconal fat r.
fat r.
rough endoplasmic r.
retina
angiomatosis of r.
arteriosclerosis of r.
artificial silicone r.
avascular peripheral r.
central fovea of r.
cerebral layer of r.
cerebral stratum of r.
cholesterol emboli of r.
coloboma of r.
concussion of the r.
congenital grouped pigmentation
   of r.
deep r.
demarcation line of r.
detached r.
detachment of r.
disciform degeneration of r.
disinserted r.
disinsertion of r.
dragged r.
dysplastic r.
external limiting membrane of r.
falciform fold of r.
fat embolism of r.
flecked r.
foveal r.
ganglionic layer of r.
ganglionic stratum of r.
ganglion layer of r.
giant cyst of r.
glioma of r.
gyrate atrophy of choroid and r.
inferior zone of r.
inflammatory changes of r.
inner molecular layer of the r.
inner nuclear layer of r.
internal limiting membrane of
   the r.

ischemic r.
juxtapapillary r.
lattice degeneration of r.
leopard r.
lipemic r.
lower r.
medial arteriole of r.
medial venulae of r.
murine r.
nasal arteriole of r.
nasal venule of r.
neovascularization of r.
nerve layer of r.
neural r.
neuroepithelial layer of r.
neurosensory r.
nuclear layer of the r.
outer nuclear layer of r.
peripheral r.
physiologic r.
pigmented layer of r.
positional abnormality of r.
postequatorial r.
primary perivasculitis of r.
reattachment of r.
rivalry of r.
sensory r.
separation of r.
shot-silk r.
R. Society classification
stiff r.
superior zone of r.
tear of r.
temporal arteriole of r.
temporal venule of r.
temporal zone of r.
tented-up r.
thrombosis in r.
tigroid r.
upper r.
vascularization elsewhere in the r.
   (VNE)
vessel abnormality of r.
watered-silk r.
yellow spot of r.
retinae
ablatio retinae
albedo r.
amotio retinae
angiomatosis r.
arteriola medialis r.
atrophia choroideae et r.

NOTES

433

retinae *(continued)*

coloboma r.
commotio r.
cyanopsia retinae
cyanosis r.
dialysis r.
ischemia r.
limbal luteus r.
macula flava r.
macula lutea r.
ora serrata r.
pars caeca r.
pars ciliaris r.
pars iridica r.
pars nervosa r.
pars optica r.
pars pigmentosa r.
periphlebitis r.
rubeosis r.
stratum cerebrale r.
striae r.
sublatio r.
torpor r.
vasa sanguinea r.
vasculitis r.
vena centralis r.
venula medialis r.

retinal

r. abiotrophy
r. abnormality
r. adaptation
r. angiography
r. angioma
r. angiomatosis
r. angiomatous proliferation
r. anlage tumor
r. aplasia
r. apoplexy
r. arterial filling
r. arterial macroaneurysm
r. arterial occlusion
r. arteriole
r. arteriovenous malformation
r. artery
r. artery aneurysm
r. asthenopia
r. astrocytic hamartoma
r. astrocytoma
r. atresia
r. axon
r. blood
r. blur spot
r. branch vein occlusion
r. break
r. burn
r. camera
r. capillaritis
r. capillary bed
r. capillary blood flow

r. capillary nonperfusion
r. central artery occlusion
r. central vein occlusion
r. circinate
r. circulation
r. clouding
r. cone
r. cone dystrophy
r. correspondence
r. cryopexy
r. cryotherapy
r. crystal
r. cyst
r. degeneration slow (RDS) gene
r. dehiscence
r. demarcation band
r. detachment (RD)
r. detachment hook
r. detachment pencil
r. detachment syringe
R. Detachment Using Optical Coherence Tomography
r. dialysis
r. disease
r. disorder
r. disparity
r. dragging
r. drusen
r. dysplasia
r. edema
r. element
r. ellipsometer
r. embolism
r. epithelial pigment hyperplasia
r. error
r. excavation
r. exudate
r. fixed fold
r. flap
r. foveola
r. ganglion
r. ganglion cell layer
r. Gelfilm implant
r. gliocyte
r. glioma
r. gliosarcoma
r. gliosis
r. hemorrhage
r. hole
r. horseshoe tear
r. hypoxia
r. ice ball
r. image
r. image size
r. imbrication
r. impact site
r. ischemia
r. isomerase
r. laser photocoagulation

r. lattice degeneration
r. lesion
r. microangiopathy
r. microcirculation
r. microembolism
r. microinfarct
r. micromovement
r. micropsia
r. microvasculopathy
r. migraine
r. montage
r. necrosis
r. necrosis syndrome
r. nerve fiber layer (RNFL)
r. nerve fiber myelination
r. neuron
r. neurotransmitter
r. periphlebitis
r. perivasculitis
r. phlebitis
r. pigmentary dystrophy
r. pigment epithelial atrophy
r. pigment epithelial defect
r. pigment epithelial hypertrophy
r. pigment epitheliitis
r. pigment epitheliopathy
r. pigment epithelium (RPE)
r. pigment epithelium dropout
r. pigment epithelium mottling
r. pigment epithelium serous
  detachment
r. point
r. probe sleeve
r. prophylaxis
r. quadrant neovascularization
r. raphe
r. recovery
r. redetachment
r. reflex
r. rivalry
r. rod
r. scatter photocoagulation
r. spike
r. staphyloma
r. stress line
r. striation
r. surgery
r. tack
r. telangiectasia
r. telangiectasis
r. thickness analysis (RTA)
r. thickness analyzer (RTA)

r. thrombosis
r. toxicity
r. translocation
r. tuft
r. vascular malformation
r. vascular occlusion
r. vasculature
r. vasculitis
r. vasculopathy
r. vein
r. vein occlusion
r. vein sheathing
r. venous beading
r. venous nicking
r. venous occlusion
r. venous pulse
r. venule
r. vessel
r. visual cell
r. whitening
r. wrinkling
r. zone
retinal-choroidal anastomosis
retinalis
  lipemia r.
retinal-slip velocity
RetinaLyze System
retinascope
retinectomy
retinene isomerase
retinex theory
retinitis
  acquired toxoplasmosis r.
  actinic r.
  AIDS-related r.
  albuminuric r.
  apoplectic r.
  azotemic r.
  candidal r.
  central angiospastic r.
  r. centralis serosa
  central serous r.
  r. circinata
  circinate r.
  CMV r.
  Coats r.
  cytomegalovirus r.
  diabetic r.
  r. disciformans
  r. exudativa
  exudative r.
  foveomacular r.

NOTES

435

retinitis *(continued)*
    Ganciclovir Implant Study for Cytomegalovirus R.
    gravid r.
    r. gravidarum
    gravidic r.
    r. haemorrhagica
    herpes simplex r.
    hypertensive r.
    Jacobson r.
    Jensen r.
    leukemic r.
    metastatic r.
    necrotizing r.
    r. nephritica
    peripheral necrotizing r.
    Pick r.
    r. pigmentosa (RP)
    r. pigmentosa GTPase regulator gene (RPGR)
    r. pigmentosa inversa
    r. pigmentosa sine pigmento
    r. proliferans
    proliferating r.
    proliferative r.
    r. punctata albescens
    punctate r.
    purulent r.
    recurrent central r.
    renal r.
    rubella r.
    r. sclopetaria
    secondary r.
    septic r.
    serous r.
    simple r.
    solar r.
    splenic r.
    r. stellata
    striate r.
    suppurative r.
    syphilitic r.
    r. syphilitica
    toxoplasmic r.
    uremic r.
    varicella-zoster r.
    Wagner r.
    X-linked r.

retinoblastoma
    bilateral sporadic r.
    calcified r.
    r. cell
    familial r.
    r. gene
    intraocular r.
    r. locus
    macular r.
    Reese-Ellsworth group V r.
    Reese-Ellsworth stage IIIA r.

    trilateral r.
    unilateral sporadic r.
retinocerebellar angiomatosis
retinochoroid
retinochoroidal
    r. atrophy
    r. coloboma
    r. infarction
    r. layer
retinochoroidectomy
retinochoroiditis
    birdshot r.
    infectious r.
    r. juxtapapillaris
    toxoplasmic r.
retinochoroidopathy
    birdshot r.
    central serous r.
retinocortical projection
retinocytoma
retinodialysis
Rétinofocomètre
retinogeniculate pathway
retinogeniculostriate projection
retinograph
retinography
retinoid
retinoma
retinomalacia
Retinomax
    R. 2 autorefractor
    R. cordless hand-held autorefractor
    R. K-plus 2
    R. K-Plus autorefractor/keratometer
    R. refractometry instrument
retinometer
    Heine Lambda 100 r.
Retinopan 45 camera
retinopapillitis of premature infants
retinopathy
    acute anular outer r.
    acute zonal occult outer r. (AZOOR)
    angiopathic r.
    arteriosclerotic r.
    background diabetic r. (BDR)
    Bietti crystalline r.
    birdshot r.
    blood-and-thunder r.
    r. of blood dyscrasia
    bull's eye r.
    cancer-associated r. (CAR)
    canthaxanthin crystalline r.
    carbon monoxide r.
    carotid occlusive disease r.
    cellophane r.
    central angiospastic r.
    central disk-shaped r.
    central serous r. (CSR)

chloroquine r.
chloroquine/hydroxychloroquine r.
circinate r.
CMV r.
compression r.
crystalline r.
cytomegalovirus r.
diabetic r. (DR)
dot-and-fleck r.
drug abuse r.
dysoric r.
dysproteinemic r.
eclamptic hypertensive r.
eclipse r.
electric r.
embolic r.
external exudative r.
exudative r.
familial exudative r. (FER)
foveomacular r.
gold dust r.
gravidic r.
r. hemorrhage
hemorrhagic r.
herpetic necrotizing r.
high altitude r. (HAR)
hydroxychloroquine r.
hypertensive r. (HR)
hypotensive r.
inflammatory r.
ischemic r.
Keith-Wagener r.
Leber idiopathic stellate r.
leukemic r.
lipemic r.
macular r.
melanoma-associated r. (MAR)
necrotizing herpetic r.
nonproliferative diabetic r. (NPDR)
optic disk drusen r.
paraneoplastic r.
particulate r.
pigmentary r.
pneumatic r.
preeclamptic hypertensive r.
r. of prematurity (ROP)
prematurity r.
preproliferative diabetic r. (PPDR)
proliferative background diabetic r.
proliferative diabetic r. (PDR)
proliferative lupus r.
proliferative sickle-cell r.

punctata albescens r.
Purtscher angiopathic r.
Purtscher-like r.
radiation r.
renal r.
rubella r.
salt-and-pepper r.
serous r.
sickle cell r.
solar r.
stellate r.
surface wrinkling r.
syphilitic r.
tamoxifen r.
tapetoretinal r.
thioridazine r.
toxic r.
traumatic r.
Valsalva r.
van Heuven anatomical
 classification of diabetic r.
vascular r.
venous stasis r. (VSR)
venous stenosis r.
vitrectomy for proliferative r.
Wisconsin Epidemiologic Study of
 Diabetic R. (WESDR)
X-linked juvenile r.
retinopexy
cyanoacrylate r.
pneumatic r.
prophylactic r.
transpupillary r.
transscleral r.
retinopiesis
retinoschisis
acquired r.
age-related degenerative r.
bullous r.
congenital r.
degenerative r.
familial foveal r. (FFR)
Goldmann-Favre r.
juvenile X-linked r. (JXRS)
senescent r.
senile r.
X-linked juvenile r.
retinoscope
Copeland streak r.
Ful-Vue spot r.
Ful-Vue streak r.
Keeler r.

NOTES

retinoscope *(continued)*
    luminous r.
    Priestley-Smith r.
    reflecting r.
    Reichert Ful-Vue spot r.
    spot r.
    streak r.
retinoscopy
    Auto Ref-keratometer ARK-900
      autorefractor and r.
    Copeland r.
    Cross r.
    cylinder r.
    dark r.
    fogging r.
    MEM r.
    monocular-estimate-method
      dynamic r.
    noncycloplegic distance static r.
    Nott r.
    static r.
    streak r.
retinosis
retinotomy
retinotopic stimulus
retinotoxic
retraction
    congenital myopathic eyelid r.
    convergence r.
    endocrine lid r.
    eyelid r.
    flap r.
    lid r.
    massive vitreous r. (MVR)
    mechanical lid r.
    mesencephalic lid r.
    myopathic eyelid r.
    neuromuscular eyelid r.
    neuropathic eyelid r.
    r. nystagmus
    spontaneous eyelid r.
    r. syndrome
    thyroid lid r.
    vitreous r.
retractor
    Agrikola lacrimal sac r.
    Alexander-Ballen r.
    Amenabar iris r.
    Amoils r.
    angled iris r.
    Arruga elevator r.
    Arruga orbital r.
    Ballen-Alexander orbital r.
    Barbie r.
    Barraquer-Krumeich-Swinger r.
    Bechert-Kratz cannulated nucleus r.
    Berens lid r.
    Blair r.
    Brawley r.

Bronson-Turtz r.
Campbell r.
Castallo r.
Castroviejo lid r.
Coleman r.
conjunctiva r.
Converse double-ended alar r.
Conway lid r.
Coston-Trent iris r.
deep blunt rake r.
Desmarres eyelid r.
Desmarres lid r.
Drews-Rosenbaum iris r.
Duane r.
Eliasoph lid r.
Elschnig r.
eyelid r.
Fasanella r.
Ferris-Smith r.
Ferris-Smith-Sewall r.
Fink lacrimal r.
Fisher lid r.
flexible translimbal iris r.
Forker r.
Fullerview iris r.
Givner lid r.
Goldstein lacrimal sac r.
Good r.
Gradle r.
Graether collar-button micro-iris r.
Great Big Barbie r.
Grieshaber flexible iris r.
Groenholm r.
Gross r.
Harrington r.
Harrison r.
Hartstein irrigating iris r.
Helveston Big Barbie tissue r.
Helveston Great Big Barbie r.
Hill r.
Hillis r.
Jaeger r.
Jaffe-Givner lid r.
Jaffe lid r.
Kaufman type II r.
Keeler-Fison tissue r.
Keeler-Rodger iris r.
Keizer-Lancaster lid r.
Kelman iris r.
Kirby lid r.
Knapp lacrimal sac r.
Kronfeld r.
Kuglein r.
lacrimal sac r.
lower lid r.
MacVicar double-end strabismus r.
McCool capsule r.
McGannon r.
Mueller lacrimal sac r.

R

Nevyas r.
Oklahoma iris wire r.
Paul lacrimal sac r.
Payne r.
Phoroptor r.
r. plication
Rizzuti iris r.
Rollet r.
Rosenbaum-Drews r.
Sanchez-Bulnes lacrimal sac r.
Sato lid r.
Schepens orbital r.
Schultz iris r.
self-adhering lid r.
self-retaining r.
Senn r.
Sewall r.
Stevens muscle hook r.
Stevenson lacrimal sac r.
Teflon iris r.
Thomas r.
Tiko pliable iris r.
Ultramatic Rx Master phoroptor r.
Vaiser-Cibis muscle r.
Vasco-Posada orbital r.
Visitec iris r.
Welsh iris r.
Wilder scleral r.
Wilmer r.
retrieval device
retriever
Utrata r.
retroauricular complex graft
retrobulbar
r. abscess
r. akinesia
r. alcohol injection
r. anesthesia
r. artery
r. compressive lesion
r. compressive optic neuropathy
r. corticosteroid injection
r. hemorrhage
r. hemorrhage glaucoma
r. ischemic optic neuropathy
r. lid block
r. needle
r. optic neuritis
r. space
retrochiasmal
r. pathway

r. visual field defect
r. visual field loss
retrochiasmatic region
retrocorneal
r. membrane
r. nut
retrodisplacement
retroequatorial sclera
retroflexion of iris
retrogeniculate lesion
retrograde transsynaptic degeneration
retrohyaloid premacular hemorrhage
retroilluminate
retroillumination
retroiridian
retrolaminar
retrolental fibroplasia (RLF)
retrolenticular
retromembranous
retroocular space
retroorbital headache
retroplacement
retropupillary
retroscopic lens
retrospective study
retrotarsal fold
Reuss
R. color chart
R. color table
Reverdin suture needle
reversal agent
reverse
r. amblyopia
r. bobbing
r. dipping
r. Marcus Gunn pupil
r. optics
r. pupillary block
reverse-cutting needle
reversed
r. astigmatism
r. ophthalmic artery flow (ROAF)
r. pupillary reflex
reverse-shape implant
reversible
r. amblyopia
r. lid speculum
Rēv-Eyes
Revilliod sign
Revolution lens
Reynold lead citrate
Rey-Osterreith Complex Figure

NOTES

RFB
 retained foreign body
RGP
 rigid gas-permeable
 RGP contact lens
rhabdoid tumor
rhabdomyosarcoma
 nonorbital childhood parameningeal
 embryonal r.
 orbital r.
**rhegmatogenous retinal detachment
 (RRD)**
Rhein
 R. Advantage II diamond limbal-
 relaxing incision knife
 R. Artisan lens-holding forceps
 R. aspiration cannula
 R. blade cleaning system
 R. capsulorrhexis cystitome forceps
 R. clear corneal diamond knife
 R. 3-D angled trapezoid diamond
 knife
 R. 3-D trapezoid diamond blade
 R. fine foldable lens-insertion
 forceps
 R. irrigation cannula
 R. LASIK epithelial detaching hoe
 R. LASIK epithelial detaching
 spatula
 R. LASIK flap elevator and
 stromal spatula
 R. LASIK flap forceps
 R. LASIK flap repositioning
 spatula
 R. reusable cautery pen
Rheofilter AR 2000 filtrator
Rhese position
rheumatic nodule
rheumatoid
 r. hyperviscosity syndrome
 r. related ulceration
 r. sclerouveitis
rheumatoid-associated nuclear antigen
rhexis
rhinitis
 acute catarrhal r.
 allergic r.
 atrophic r.
 r. caseosa
 chronic catarrhal r.
 croupous r.
 dyscrinic r.
 fibrinous r.
 gangrenous r.
 hypertrophic r.
 membranous r.
 pseudomembranous r.
 purulent r.
 scrofulous r.

 r. sicca
 syphilitic r.
 tuberculous r.
rhinocanthectomy
rhinoconjunctivitis
 perennial r.
 seasonal r.
rhinodacryolith
rhinoorbital-cerebral mucormycosis
rhinoorbital mucormycosis
rhinophyma
rhinoplasty
rhinoscleroma
rhinosporidiosis
 conjunctival r.
Rhinosporidium seeberi
rhinotomy
rhodogenesis
rhodophylactic
rhodophylaxis
rhodopsin
Rhus
 R. radicans
 R. toxicodendron
rhythmic nystagmus
rhytid
 eyelid r.
RI
 recession index
ribbon gauze dressing
ribbon-like keratitis
Riccò law
Rice pick
Richard
 R. pillow
 R. Products fundus camera drug
 organizer
**Richardson methylene blue/aure II
 mixture**
Richet operation
Richmond Products Inc.
Richner-Hanhart syndrome
Ricinus communis agglutinin
rickettsial blepharitis
Ridaura
Riddoch
 R. phenomenon
 R. syndrome
ridge
 laser r.
 r. lens
 mesenchymal r.
 petrous r.
 supraorbital r.
 synaptic r.
riding bow temple
Ridley
 R. anterior chamber lens implant

R. lens
R. Mark II lens implant
Riedel
R. needle
R. thyroiditis
Rieger
R. anomaly
R. syndrome
Rifkind sign
rifle
air r.
right
r. deorsumvergence
r. deviation
r. esotropia
r. exotropia
r. eye (OD)
r. gaze
r. gaze verticals
r. hyperphoria
r. hypertropia
r. sursumvergence
right-angle
r.-a. deflected venule
r.-a. prism
right-beating nystagmus
right-handed cornea scissors
right/left corneoscleral scissors
rigid
r. gas-permeable (RGP)
r. gas-permeable contact lens
r. pupil
rigidity
mydriatic r.
ocular r.
scleral r.
Riley-Day syndrome
Riley-Smith syndrome
rim
corneoscleral r.
inferior orbital r.
neural r.
neuroretinal r.
r. notching
orbital inferior r.
saucering of r.
superior r.
rima, pl. **rimae**
r. cornealis
r. palpebrarum
rimexolone ophthalmic suspension
rimless frame

rim-to-disk ratio
ring
r. abscess
abscess r.
anterior limiting r.
anular r.
Bloomberg SuperNumb anesthetic r.
Bonaccolto-Flieringa scleral r.
Bonaccolto scleral r.
Bores twist fixation r.
Burr corneal r.
Caspar r.
cataract mask r.
r. cataract mask eye shield
centering r.
choroidal r.
ciliary r.
Coats white r.
collagenolytic trabecular r.
collagenous trabecular r.
common tendinous r.
conjunctival r.
corneal iron r.
corneal transplant centering r.
R. D chromosome syndrome
Dell fixation r.
Döllinger tendinous r.
Donders r.
Fine crescent fixation r.
Fine-Thornton scleral fixation r.
fixation r.
fixation/anchor r.
Fleischer keratoconus r.
Fleischer-Strumpell r.
Flieringa-Kayser copper r.
Flieringa-Kayser fixation r.
Flieringa-LeGrand fixation r.
Flieringa scleral fixation r.
r. forceps
Gimbel stabilization r.
Gimbel stabilizing r.
Girard scleral-expander r.
glaucomatous r.
glial r.
Hansatome 8.5 mm suction r.
Hofmann-Thornton globe fixation r.
immune Wessely r.
r. infiltrate
Intacs r.
intracorneal r.
intrastromal corneal r.
iris r.

NOTES

R

ring *(continued)*
  r. of iris
  iron Fleischer r.
  Johnston fixation r.
  Kayser-Fleischer cornea r.
  r. keratitis
  KeraVision r.
  Klein-Tolentino r.
  Kraff hyperopic fixation r.
  Landers irrigating vitrectomy r.
  Landers vitrectomy r.
  Landolt broken r.
  Landolt-C r.
  LED-illuminated r.
  r. lens expressor
  lenticular r.
  light reflex r.
  Lowe r.
  Lu-Mendez LRI guide and
    fixation r.
  Martinez corneal transplant
    centering r.
  Maxwell r.
  McKinney fixation r.
  McNeill-Goldman r.
  r. melanoma
  Morcher iris diaphragm r.
  Morcher iris diaphragm r., type
    50C
  Morcher iris diaphragm r., type
    96G
  Moretsky LASIK hinge protector
    fixation r.
  Nichamin fixation r.
  nuclear r.
  r. perimetry
  placido r.
  28-r. Placido cone
  polymer r.
  posterior limiting r.
  prominent Schwalbe r.
  rust r.
  Saturn r.
  Schwalbe anterior border r.
  scleral expander r.
  scotoma r.
  r. scotoma
  Soemmering r.
  r. of Soemmering
  subretinal pigment r.
  suction r.
  symblepharon r.
  Tano r.
  tantalum "O" r.
  Thornton-Fine r.
  Thornton fixating r.
  Thornton limbal fixation r.
  Thorton globe fixation r.
  Tolentino r.
  r. ulcer
  r. ulcer of cornea
  Villasenor-Navarro fixation r.
  Vossius lenticular r.
  Weinstein fixation r.
  Weiss r.
  Wessely r.
  white r.
  Whitten fixation r.
  Zinn r.
Ringer lactate solution
ring-form congenital cataract
ring-like corneal dystrophy
ring-shaped
  r.-s. cataract
  r.-s. dystrophy
  r.-s. stromal infiltrate
ring-tip forceps
Riolan muscle
Ripault sign
rip-cord suture
ripe cataract
risk
  r. factor
  r. factors in ARMD
Risley rotary prism
Ritalin
Ritch
  R. contact lens
  R. nylon suture laser lens
  R. trabeculoplasty laser lens
Ritch-Krupin-Denver eye valve-insertion
  forceps
Ritleng probe
Ritter fiber
rivalry
  binocular r.
  luminance r.
  r. of retina
  retinal r.
river blindness
rivus lacrimalis
Rizzuti
  R. graft carrier spoon
  R. iris retractor
  R. lens expressor
  R. rectus forceps
  R. refractor
  R. scleral fixation forceps
Rizzuti-Bonaccolto instrument
Rizzuti-Fleischer instrument
Rizzuti-Furniss cornea-holding forceps
Rizzuti-Kayser-Fleischer instrument
Rizzuti-Lowe instrument
Rizzuti-Maxwell instrument
Rizzuti-McGuire corneal section scissors
Rizzuti-Soemmering instrument
Rizzuti-Spizziri cannula knife

RK
    radial keratotomy
      RK marker
RK-5000
    ultrasound pachymeter-KMI R.
RLF
    retrolental fibroplasia
RLH
    reactive lymphoid hyperplasia
RLX
    R. coating
    R. lens
RNA III activating protein (RAP)
RNFL
    retinal nerve fiber layer
ROAF
    reversed ophthalmic artery flow
Roaf syndrome
ROAM
    roaming optical access multiscope
roaming optical access multiscope (ROAM)
Robertson
    R. pupil
    R. sign
Roberts-SC phocomelia
Robin chalazion clamp
Robinow syndrome
Rocephin
Rochat test
Rochon-Duvigneaud
    bouquet of R.-D.
    R.-D. bouquet of cones
rod
    r. achromatopsia
    bipolar r.
    r. b-wave amplitude
    r. b-wave response
    r. cell
    r.'s and cones
    r. electroretinogram
    r. fiber
    r. function
    graceful swirling r.
    r. granule
    Maddox r.
    Mira silicone r.
    r. monochromasy
    r. monochromat
    r. monochromatism
    r. myopathy
    Perspex r.

    r. photoreceptor
    retinal r.
    scleral sponge r.
    silicone r.
    Viers r.
    r. vision
    vision r.
rod-cone
    r.-c. amplitude
    r.-c. degeneration
    r.-c. dysfunction
    r.-c. dystrophy
Rodenstock
    R. eye refractometer
    R. panfunduscope
    R. panfundus lens
    R. scanning laser ophthalmoscope
    R. slit lamp
    R. system
rodent ulcer
Rodin orbital implant
roentgenogram
    orbital r.
Rolf
    R. dilator
    R. forceps
    R. lacrimal probe
    R. lance
roll
    Fluftex gauze r.
    iris r.
    peripheral iris r.
    scleral r.
rolled-up epithelium with wavy border
roller forceps
Rollet
    R. irrigating/aspirating unit
    R. lacrimal probe
    R. refractor
    R. retractor
    R. rougine
    R. syndrome
rolling
    counter r.
    r. of eyes
ROLS
    Reinverting Operating Lens System
Romaña sign
Romberg
    R. sign
    R. syndrome

NOTES

Rommel
    R. cautery
    R. electrocautery
Rommel-Hildreth
    R.-H. cautery
    R.-H. electrocautery
Romycin
RON
    radiation optic neuropathy
Rondec
    R. Drops
    R. Filmtab
    R. Syrup
Rondec-TR
rongeur
    Belz lacrimal sac r.
    biting r.
    bone r.
    Citelli r.
    Kerrison mastoid r.
    lacrimal sac r.
    Lempert r.
    single-action r.
Ronne nasal step
roof
    r. fracture
    r. of orbit
    orbital r.
RO Optho
root
    iris r.
    motor r.
    oculomotor r.
    sensory r.
ROP
    retinopathy of prematurity
Roper alpha-chymotrypsin cannula
Roper-Hall
    R.-H. classification
    R.-H. localizer
    R.-H. locator
ropy mucus
Roquinimex
Rosa-Berens orbital implant
rosacea
    acne r.
    blepharitis r.
    blepharoconjunctivitis r.
    keratitis r.
    r. keratitis
    ocular r.
rosacea-meibomianitis
Rosai-Dorfman disease
Roscoe-Bunsen law
rose
    r. bengal
    r. bengal red solution
    r. bengal stain

roseata
    iritis r.
Rosen
    R. nucleus paddle
    R. phaco splitter
Rosenbach sign
Rosenbaum
    R. card
    R. pocket vision screener
Rosenbaum-Drews retractor
Rosenblatt scissors
Rosenburg operation
Rosengren operation
Rosenmüller
    R. body
    R. gland
    R. node
    valve of R.
    R. valve
rosette
    Flexner-Wintersteiner r.
    Homer-Wright r.
    Wintersteiner r.
Rosner tonometer
Rostaporfin
rostral
    r. interstitial medial longitudinal
      fasciculus
    r. interstitial nucleus
rotary
    r. cutting tip
    r. nystagmus
    r. prism
rotating brush
rotating-type cutter
rotation
    center of r.
    eye r.
    r. nystagmus
    suture r.
    toric intraocular lens axis r.
    wheel r.
rotational
    r. nystagmus
    r. test
rotator
    Bechert nucleus r.
    Espaillat-Deblasio nucleus r.
    Jaffe-Bechert nucleus r.
    Maloney nucleus r.
    nucleus r.
rotatory nystagmus
Roth
    R. spot
    R. spot syndrome
Roth-Bielschowsky
    R.-B. deviation
    R.-B. syndrome
Rothman Gilbard cornea punch

Rothmund syndrome
Rothmund-Thomson syndrome
rotoextractor
    Douvas r.
rotundum foramen
Rouget muscle
rough endoplasmic reticulum
rougine
    Rollet r.
round
    r. hemorrhage
    r. top bifocal
route
    canalicular r.
    external r.
    transconjunctival r.
Rovamycine
Roveda
    R. lid everter
    R. operation
roving eye movement
Rowbotham operation
Rowen spatula
Rowinski operation
Rowland keratome
Rowsey fixation cannula
royal
    R. Australian College of
      Ophthalmologists
    R. College of Ophthalmologists
      (UK)
    R. National Institute for the Blind
      (UK)
RP
    retinitis pigmentosa
    RP hypertrophy
    RP sine pigmento
RP10 gene variant of retinitis
pigmentosa
RPE
    retinal pigment epithelium
    hemorrhagic RPE
RPGR
    retinitis pigmentosa GTPase regulator
    gene
R&R
    recession-resection
    recess-resect
RRD
    rhegmatogenous retinal detachment
RR-MS
    relapsing/remitting multiple sclerosis

RSVP
    rapid serial visual presentation
RTA
    retinal thickness analysis
    retinal thickness analyzer
Rubbrecht operation
rubella
    r. cataract
    r. retinitis
    r. retinopathy
Rubenstein type LASIK irrigating
cannula
rubeola
    r. conjunctivitis
    r. keratitis
rubeosis
    iridis r.
    r. iridis
    r. iridis diabetica
    r. retinae
rubeotic glaucoma
Rubin-Holth punch
Rubinstein
    R. cryoextractor
    R. cryophake
    R. cryoprobe
    R. irrigation cannula
Rubinstein-Taybi syndrome
ruby
    r. diamond knife
    r. laser
Rucker body
rudimentary eye
rudiment lens
Ruedemann
    R. eye implant
    R. lacrimal dilator
    R. operation
    R. tonometer
Ruedemann-Todd tendon tucker
ruff
    papillary r.
ruffed canal
Ruggeri reflex
Ruiz
    R. fundus contact lens
    R. fundus laser lens
    R. microkeratome
    R. plano fundus lens implant
    R. procedure
    R. trapezoidal keratotomy
Ruiz-Nordan trapezoidal marker

R

NOTES

445

rule
    accommodation r.
    astigmatism with the r.
    Behren r.
    Javal r.
    Kestenbaum r.
    Knapp r.
    Kollner r.
    Krimsky-Prince accommodation r.
    Luedde transparent r.
    Pischel scleral r.
    Prentice r.
    Prince r.
ruler
    biometric r.
    Bio-Pen biometric r.
    BVI AXIS biometric r.
    Helveston scleral marking r.
    Hyde astigmatism r.
    Hyde-Osher keratometric r.
    Scott No. 2 curved r.
    Thornton double corneal r.
    Thornton limbal incision r.
    Weck astigmatism r.
Rumex titanium instrument
Rumison side port fixation occluder
running nylon penetrating keratoplasty
    suture
rupture
    choroidal r.
    indirect choroidal r.
    scleral r.
    traumatic choroidal r.

ruptured globe
Rushton ocular measurement
Russell
    R. body
    R. syndrome
    R. viper venom time
Russian
    R. forceps
    R. four-pronged fixation hook
rust
    r. ring
    r. ring of cornea
    r. spot
ruthenium
    r. plaque
    r. red
ruthenium-106 ophthalmic plaque
Rutherford syndrome
Ruysch
    R. membrane
    R. tunic
ruyschiana
    membrana r.
ruyschian membrane
RV275
    Tracoustic R.
Rycroft
    R. cannula
    R. needle
    R. operation
    R. tying forceps

S

S cone excitation
S potential

S3

VISX Star S3

S-100 protein antibody
S5-1804-HUMER lens-folding forceps
Sabin-Feldman dye test
Sabouraud

S. dextrose agar
S. medium

Sabreloc needle
Sabril
saburral

s. amaurosis
s. amaurosis fugax

sac

conjunctival s.
drainage of lacrimal s.
Förster lacrimal s.
lacrimal s.
nasolacrimal s.
tear s.
Tenon s.

saccade

down-gaze s.
foveating s.
hypometric s.
normal upward corrective s.
ocular s.
s. palsy
scanning s.
slow-to-no s.

saccadic

s. abnormality
s. contrapulsion
s. dysmetria
s. eccentric target
s. eye movement
s. fixation
s. intrusion
s. movements of eye
s. pulse
s. pursuit
s. velocity

saccadomania
sacci (*pl. of* saccus)
saccular aneurysm
sacculiform
sacculus lacrimalis
saccus, pl. **sacci**

s. conjunctivae
s. conjunctivalis
s. lacrimalis

Sachs tissue forceps
saddle

s. bridge
Turkish s.

Saemisch

S. operation
S. section
S. ulcer

Saenger

S. pupil
S. sign

Safar operation
SAFE

Structure And Function Evaluation
SAFE study

safety

s. of cyclosporine
S. and Efficacy of a Heparin-
Coated Intraocular Lens in
Uveitis
s. glasses
s. lens
s. spectacles

Safil synthetic absorbable surgical
suture
Safir Ophthalmetron
SAGE

Statpac-like Analysis for Glaucoma
Evaluation

sagittal

s. axis
s. axis of eye
s. axis of Fick
s. depth
s. height

SAI

surface asymmetry index

Sainton sign
Sakler erysiphake
Salagen
saline

Blairex sterile s.
CIBA Vision S.
Hydrocare preserved s.
hypertonic s.
Lens Plus s.
Murine sterile s.
phosphate-buffered s.
Soft Mate s.
SoftWear S.
s. solution
sorbic acid Sorbi-Care s.
Sterile Preserved S.

saline-saturated wool dressing

S

salivary
s. gland
s. nucleus
Salleras procedure
salmon
s. patch
s. patch hue
salmon-patch hemorrhage
salt-and-pepper
s.-a.-p. appearance
s.-a.-p. chorioretinitis
s.-a.-p. fundus
s.-a.-p. retinopathy
salts
gold s.
Salus
S. arch
S. sign
Salzmann
S. nodular corneal degeneration
S. nodular corneal dystrophy
S. nodule
Salz nucleus splitter
Samoan conjunctivitis
Sampaoelesi line
sampling error
Sanchez-Bulnes lacrimal sac retractor
Sanchez-Salorio syndrome
sand
S. process
s.'s of Sahara keratitis
Sanders
S. disease
S. disorder
S. operation
Sanders-Castroviejo suturing forceps
Sanders-Retzlaff-Kraff (SRK)
Sanders-Retzlaff-Kraff formula
Sandimmune
SANDO
sensory ataxic neuropathy with dysarthria and ophthalmoplegia
Sandt forceps
sanguineous cataract
Sanson image
Sanyal conjunctivitis
SAP
standard automated perimetry
Sappey fiber
sapphire knife
saprophytic bacteria
saprophyticus
Staphylococcus s.
saquinavir sulfate
sarcoid
Boeck s.
s. uveitis

sarcoidosis
s. infiltration
pediatric ocular s.
sarcoidosis-associated uveitis
sarcoma, pl. **sarcomata**
Ewing s.
granulocytic s.
hemorrhagic s.
Kaposi s.
melanotic s.
multifocal hemorrhagic s.
reticulum cell s.
sarcomatosum
ectropion s.
glioma s.
s. senilis
s. spasticum
s. uveae
Sartorius SM 111
satellite
s. ganglionic cell
s. lesion
SatinCrescent
S. implant knife
S. tunneler
SatinShortCut implant knife
SatinSlit
S. implant knife
S. keratome
Sato
S. cataract needle
S. corneal knife
S. keratoconus
S. lid retractor
S. operation
S. procedure
Satoyoshis syndrome
Sattler
S. advancement forceps
S. layer
S. veil
saturated color
saturation
color s.
SaturEyes contact lens
Saturn
S. II contact lenses
S. ring
saturninus
halo s.
saucering of rim
saucerization
saucer-shaped cataract
Sauer
S. corneal débrider
S. infant speculum
S. suture forceps
Sauflon PW lens
Saupe cilia forceps

Sauvineau ophthalmoplegia
Saverburger irrigation/aspiration tip
Savin
>S. operation
>S. procedure

saw
>Stryker s.

Sayoc
>S. operation
>S. procedure

Sayre elevator
SB
>scleral buckle

SBS
>shaken baby syndrome

SBV
>single binocular vision

SC
>scleral cautery
>stem cell
>subconjunctival

s̄c
>without correction

scaffolding
>capillary s.

scale
>Activities of Daily Vision S. (ADVS)
>disk damage likelihood s. (DDLS)
>Esterman s.
>Expanded Disability Status S. (EDSS)
>Fitzpatrick sun-sensitivity s.
>Griffith s.
>Klyce/Wilson s.
>Kuppuswamy s.
>Kurtzke Expanded Disability Status S.
>Resource-Based Relative Value S. (RBRVS)
>Snell-Sterling visual efficiency s.
>visual analogue s. (VAS)

scalloped
>s. border
>s. contour
>s. pupil

scalloping
scalpel
>Feather incision s.
>s. guard
>Guyton-Lundsgaard s.

Microcap s.
Myocure blade s.

ScalpelTec
>S. phaco keratome slit blade
>S. wound-enlargement blade

scalp flap
scaly plaque
scan
>axial CT s.
>choroidal s.
>computed tomography s.
>computerized tomography s.
>coronal CT s.
>cross-vector A-s.
>duplex s.
>gallium s.
>isotope s.
>limited gallium s.
>magnetic resonance imaging s.
>MRI s.
>Opthascan Mini-A s.
>orbital CT s.
>OTI ultrasound B & A s.
>radioisotope s.
>technetium s.
>US-2000 echo s.

ScanMaker 4 flatbed scanner
scanner
>Dine digital s.
>Heidelberg laser tomographic s.
>laser tomography s. (LTS)
>ScanMaker 4 flatbed s.
>Zeiss-Humphrey 840 UBM s.

scanning
>s. excimer laser
>gallium s.
>s. laser glaucoma test
>s. laser ophthalmoscope (SLO)
>S. Laser Ophthalmoscope perimetry
>s. laser polarimeter
>s. laser polarimetry (SLP)
>s. prism
>s. saccade
>s. slit confocal microscope

scar
>chorioretinal s.
>corneal s.
>disciform macular s.
>facetted corneal s.
>gray-white corneal s.
>herpes simplex s.
>linear s.

NOTES

scar *(continued)*
    peripapillary s.
    s. plate
    punched-out chorioretinal s.
    vascularized s.
scarification
scarifier
    Desmarres s.
    s. knife
    Kuhnt corneal s.
Scarpa staphyloma
scarring
    bulbar conjunctival s.
    conjunctival s.
    corneal s.
    episcleral s.
    ghost s.
    gossamer s.
    linear s.
    quiescent stromal s.
    stromal ghost s.
    subretinal s.
scatter
    beam s.
    forward light s.
    light s.
    s. pattern
    peripheral light s.
    s. photocoagulation
    sclerotic s.
scattergram
scattering
    light s.
    Rayleigh s.
    reflective s.
scatterplot
SCE
    serous choroidal effusion
Scedosporium apiospermum
SCH
    suprachoroidal hemorrhage
Schaaf foreign body forceps
Schachar lens
Schacher ganglion
Schachne-Desmarres lid everter
Schaedel cross-action towel clamp
Schaefer
    S. fixation forceps
    S. sponge holder
Schaffer sign
Schaumann inclusion body
Scheie
    S. akinesia
    S. anterior chamber cannula
    S. blade
    S. cataract-aspirating cannula
    S. cataract-aspirating needle
    S. classification
    S. electrocautery

    S. goniopuncture knife
    S. goniotomy knife
    S. operation
    S. ophthalmic cautery
    S. syndrome
    S. technique
    S. thermal sclerostomy
    S. trephine
Scheie-Graefe fixation forceps
Scheie-Westcott corneal section scissors
Scheimpflug
    S. photography
    S. principle
    S. slit image
    S. videophotography system
Scheiner
    S. experiment
    S. principle
    S. theory
schematic eye
schenckii
    Sporothrix s.
Schepens
    S. binocular indirect
    ophthalmoscope
    S. electrode
    S. forceps
    S. Gelfilm
    S. hollow hemisphere implant
    S. operation
    S. orbital retractor
    S. refractor
    S. retinal detachment unit
    S. scleral depressor
    S. spoon
    S. technique
    S. thimble depressor
Schepens-Pomerantzeff ophthalmoscope
scheroma
Schilder
    S. disease
    S. encephalitis
Schillinger suture support
Schimek operation
Schiötz
    S. tonofilm
    S. tonometer
    S. tonometry
Schirmer
    S. filter paper
    S. operation
    S. syndrome
    S. tear quality test
    S. tear test strip
    S. 1 test
    S. test I, II
schisis cavity
schisis-related detachment

schistosa
> *Enhydrina s.*

Schlegel lens
schleiferi
> *Staphylococcus s.*

Schlemm
> S. canal

Schlichting dystrophy
Schlieren phenomenon
Schmalz operation
Schmid-Fraccaro syndrome
Schmidt keratitis
Schmincke tumor
Schnabel
> S. cavern
> S. optic atrophy

Schnaitmann bifocal
Schnidt clamp
Schnyder
> central crystalline dystrophy of S.
> S. crystalline corneal dystrophy

Schöbl scleritis
Schocket
> S. anterior chamber tube shunt
> S. scleral depressor
> S. tube implant

Schöler treatment
Schön theory
school myopia
Schott lid speculum
Schubert-Bornschein congenital stationary night blindness
Schultz
> S. fiber basket
> S. iris retractor

Schumann giant type eye magnet
Schwalbe
> S. anterior border ring
> S. line (SL)
> S. space

Schwann
> S. cell
> cords of S.

schwannoma
> malignant s.
> melanotic s.
> oculomotor nerve s.
> orbital s.

Schwartz-Jampel syndrome
Schwartz syndrome
Schweigger
> S. capsule forceps

> S. extracapsular forceps
> S. hand perimeter

Schweninger-Buzzi macular atrophy
science
> vision s.

scientific investigation
scieropia
scimitar scotoma
scintigraphy
scintillans
> synchesis s.

scintillating
> s. granule
> s. scotoma
> s. vision loss

scintillation
scintillography
> lacrimal s.

scirrhencanthis
scirrhophthalmia
scissors
> Aebli corneal section s.
> alligator s.
> anterior chamber synechia s.
> Atkinson corneal s.
> bandage s.
> Barraquer corneoscleral s.
> Barraquer-de Wecker iris s.
> Barraquer vitreous strand s.
> Becker corneal section spatulated s.
> Berens corneal transplant s.
> Berens iridocapsulotomy s.
> Berkeley Bioengineering mechanized s.
> Birks Mark II Instruments micro trabeculectomy s.
> Bonn iris s.
> canalicular s.
> capsulotomy s.
> Castroviejo anterior synechia s.
> Castroviejo corneal section s.
> Castroviejo corneal transplant s.
> Castroviejo iridocapsulotomy s.
> Castroviejo keratoplasty s.
> Castroviejo synechia s.
> Castroviejo-Vannas capsulotomy s.
> Cohan-Vannas iris s.
> Cohan-Westcott s.
> conjunctival s.
> corneal section spatulated s.
> corneoscleral right/left hand s.
> curved iris s.

S

NOTES

scissors *(continued)*
    curved tenotomy s.
    de Wecker iris s.
    dissecting s.
    enucleation s.
    eye suture s.
    Fine suture s.
    Frost s.
    Giardet corneal transplant s.
    Gill s.
    Gill-Hess s.
    Gills-Welsh s.
    Gills-Welsh-Vannas angled micro s.
    Girard corneoscleral s.
    Glasscock s.
    Grieshaber vertical cutting s.
    Grieshaber vitreous s.
    Guist enucleation s.
    Haenig irrigating s.
    Halsted strabismus s.
    Harrison s.
    Hoskins-Castroviejo corneal s.
    Hoskins-Westcott tenotomy s.
    House-Bellucci alligator s.
    Huey s.
    Hunt chalazion s.
    iridectomy s.
    iridocapsulotomy s.
    iridotomy s.
    iris s.
    Irvine probe-pointed s.
    Karakashian-Barraquer s.
    Katzin s.
    Keeler intravitreal s.
    keratectomy s.
    keratoplasty s.
    Kirby s.
    Knapp iris s.
    Knapp strabismus s.
    Kramp s.
    Kreiger-Spitznas vibrating s.
    Lagrange sclerectomy s.
    Lambert-Heiman s.
    Lawton corneal s.
    left-handed cornea s.
    Lister s.
    Littauer dissecting s.
    Littler dissecting s.
    Manson-Aebli corneal section s.
    Mattis corneal s.
    Maunoir iris s.
    Max Fine s.
    Mayo s.
    McClure iris s.
    McGuire corneal s.
    McLean capsulotomy s.
    McPherson-Castroviejo corneal
      section s.
    McPherson corneal section s.

    McPherson-Vannas microiris s.
    McPherson-Westcott conjunctival s.
    McPherson-Westcott stitch s.
    McReynolds pterygium s.
    mechanized s.
    micro Westcott s.
    mini-keratoplasty stitch s.
    Moore-Troutman corneal s.
    Morris vertical s.
    s. movement
    MPC automated intravitreal s.
    Nadler superior radial s.
    Noyes iridectomy s.
    Noyes iris s.
    Nugent-Gradle s.
    O'Brien stitch s.
    Ong capsulotomy s.
    pterygium s.
    ptosis s.
    radial iridotomy s.
    Reeh s.
    Reichling corneal s.
    right-handed cornea s.
    right/left corneoscleral s.
    Rizzuti-McGuire corneal section s.
    Rosenblatt s.
    Scheie-Westcott corneal section s.
    Shield iridotomy s.
    Smart s.
    Spencer eye suture s.
    Spring iris s.
    Stevens eye s.
    Stevens tenotomy s.
    Storz-Westcott conjunctival s.
    strabismus s.
    straight tenotomy s.
    superior radial tenotomy s.
    Sutherland s.
    Sutherland-Grieshaber s.
    Thomas s.
    Thorpe s.
    Thorpe-Castroviejo s.
    Thorpe-Westcott s.
    Troutman-Castroviejo corneal
      section s.
    Troutman conjunctival s.
    Troutman-Katzin corneal
      transplant s.
    Troutman microsurgical s.
    Troutman suture s.
    Vannas capsulotomy s.
    Vannas iridocapsulotomy s.
    Verhoeff s.
    vibrating s.
    s. vitrectomy
    vitreous strand s.
    Walker s.
    Walker-Apple s.
    Walker-Atkinson s.

Wecker iris s.
Werb s.
Westcott conjunctival s.
Westcott stitch s.
Westcott tenotomy s.
Westcott utility s.
Wilmer conjunctival s.
Wincor enucleation s.
Witherspoon vertical s.
Zaldivar iridectomy s.

scissors-shadow

SCL

soft contact lens

sclera, pl. **scleras, sclerae**
bared s.
baring of s.
blanching of s.
blue s.
buckling s.
ectasia of s.
foramen of s.
lamina cribrosa sclerae
lamina fusca sclerae
limbus of s.
massive granuloma of s.
melanosis sclerae
retroequatorial s.
sinus venosus s.
substantia propria sclerae
sulcus s.
white s.

scleral
s. blade
s. buckle (SB)
s. buckling
s. buckling operation
s. buckling procedure
s. canal
s. cautery (SC)
s. channel
s. conjunctiva
s. contact lens
s. crescent
s. cyst
s. deformity
s. degeneration
s. depression
s. depressor
s. ectasia
s. exoplant
s. expander
s. expander ring

s. expansion band
s. expansion band procedure
s. explant
s. explant surgery
s. fistula
s. fistulectomy operation
s. flap
s. flap suture
s. framework
s. furrow
s. grip
s. hook
s. icterus
s. implant
s. indentation
s. infolding
s. lamina cribrosa
s. lip
s. marker
s. melting
s. miniflap
s. necrosis
s. outfolding
s. patch graft
s. pick
s. plexus
s. punch
s. reinforcement
s. resection
s. resection knife
s. rigidity
s. roll
s. rupture
s. search coil
s. search coil technique
s. shell
s. shell glaucoma
s. shortening clip
s. shortening operation
s. show
s. sponge rod
s. spur (SS)
s. staphyloma
s. substance
s. sulcus
s. supporter
s. tissue
s. trabecula
s. tunnel
s. tunnel abscess
s. tunnel incision
s. twist

S

NOTES

scleral *(continued)*
    s. twist-grip forceps
    s. venous sinus
    s. window
scleral-limbal-corneal incision
scleras (*pl. of* sclera)
scleratitis
sclerectasia
    partial s.
    total s.
sclerectasis
sclerectoiridectomy
sclerectoiridodialysis
sclerectome
sclerectomy
    holmium YAG laser s.
    Holth s.
    Iliff-House s.
    nonpenetrating deep s.
    s. punch
    thermal s.
scleriasis
scleriritomy
scleritis
    anterior s.
    anular s.
    brawny s.
    deep s.
    diffuse anterior s.
    gelatinous s.
    herpes simplex s.
    idiopathic s.
    malignant s.
    s. necroticans
    necrotizing nocardial s.
    necrotizing nodular s.
    posterior s.
    Schöbl s.
    syphilitic s.
sclerocataracta
sclerochoroidal
    s. calcification
    s. thickening
sclerochoroiditis
    anterior s.
    posterior s.
scleroconjunctival
scleroconjunctivitis
sclerocornea
sclerocorneal
    s. junction
    s. phacoemulsification
    s. sulcus
scleroiritis
sclerokeratectomy
sclerokeratitis
sclerokeratoiritis
sclerokeratoplasty
sclerokeratosis

sclerolimbus
scleromalacia perforans
scleronyxis
sclerophthalmia
scleroplasty operation
sclerosing
    s. keratitis
    s. orbital granuloma
    s. panencephalitis chorioretinitis
sclerosis, pl. **scleroses**
    arteriolar s.
    central areolar choroidal s.
    choroidal primary s.
    diffuse choroidal s.
    multiple s.
    nuclear s. (NS)
    peripapillary s.
    progressive systemic s.
    relapsing/remitting multiple s. (RR-MS)
    secondary progressive multiple s. (SP-MS)
    systemic s.
    tuberous s.
sclerostomy
    enzymatic s.
    Holmium laser s.
    s. needle
    posterior thermal s.
    Scheie thermal s.
    thermal s.
    trabecuphine laser s.
sclerotic
    s. cataract
    s. coat
    nuclear s. (NS)
    s. scatter
    s. scatter illumination
    s. stroma
sclerotica
    tunica s.
scleroticectomy
scleroticochoroidal canal
scleroticochoroiditis
scleroticonyxis
scleroticopuncture
scleroticotomy
sclerotitis
sclerotome
    Alvis-Lancaster s.
    Atkinson s.
    Castroviejo s.
    Curdy s.
    Guyton-Lundsgaard s.
    Lundsgaard s.
    Lundsgaard-Burch s.
    Walker-Lee s.
sclerotomy
    anterior s.

deep s.
de Wecker anterior s.
foreign body s.
Lindner s.
s. operation
s. port
posterior s.
s. punch
rectangular two-thirds-thickness s.
s. removal of foreign body
s. with drainage
s. with exploration
sclerouveitis
rheumatoid s.
sclopetaria
chorioretinitis s.
retinitis s.
SCMD microkeratome
SCN
suprachiasmatic nucleus
Scobee oblique muscle hook
scolex, pl. **scoleces, scolices**
scoop
Arlt s.
Daviel s.
enucleation s.
Kirby intraocular lens s.
Knapp s.
Lewis s.
Mules s.
Wilder s.
scope
Bjerrum s.
tangent s.
Welch-Allyn Pocket s.
scopolamine hyoscine
scoria
scotodinia
scotograph
scotoma, pl. **scotomata**
absolute s.
altitudinal s.
anular s.
arc s.
arcuate Bjerrum s.
aural s.
bitemporal hemianopic s.
Bjerrum s.
cecocentral s.
central s.
centrocecal s.
color s.

comet s.
congruous homonymous
hemianopic s.
cuneate-shaped s.
double arcuate s.
eclipse s.
equatorial ring s.
false s.
flittering s.
focal s.
frame s.
glaucomatous nerve-fiber bundle s.
hemianopic s.
homonymous hemianopic s.
insular s.
ipsilateral centrocecal s.
junction s.
s. junction
junctional s.
Mariotte s.
motile s.
s. for motion
negative s.
paracentral ring s.
pericecal s.
pericentral s.
peripapillary s.
peripheral s.
physiologic s.
position s.
positive s.
quadrantic s.
relative s.
s. ring
ring s.
scimitar s.
scintillating s.
Seidel s.
sickle s.
superior arcuate s.
suppression s.
thin-rim s.
s. of Traquair
unilateral altitudinal s.
zonular s.
scotomagraph
scotomatous
scotometer
Bjerrum s.
scotometry
scotomization
scotopia

NOTES

scotopic
  s. adaptation
  s. eye
  s. perimetry
  s. sensitivity
  s. sensitivity loss
  s. stimulus
  s. vision
scotopsin
scotoscope
scotoscopy
Scott
  S. lens-insertion forceps
  S. No. 2 curved ruler
scout
  Optikon 2000 placido-based corneal
  topography system Keratron S.
scrape
  corneal epithelial s.
  epithelial s.
  post s.
scraper
  diamond dusted membrane s.
  (DDMS)
  epithelial s.
  Knolle capsule s.
  Kratz capsule s.
  Tano membrane s.
scraping
  conjunctival s.
  corneal epithelial s.
  epithelial s.
scratched contact lens
scratcher
  Jensen capsule s.
  Knolle capsule s.
  Kratz capsule s.
  Kratz-Jensen s.
scratch-resistant spectacle lens
screen
  Bernell tangent s.
  Bjerrum s.
  Grey-Hess s.
  Hess diplopia s.
  Hess-Lee s.
  Mitsubishi HL7955 CRT s.
  tangent s.
screener
  Rosenbaum pocket vision s.
screening
  Modified Clinical Technique
  vision s.
  photo s.
scrofulous
  s. conjunctivitis
  s. keratitis
  s. ophthalmia
  s. rhinitis

scrub
  lid s.
  OCuSoft s.
  s. typhus
scrubber
  Amoils epithelial s.
  Simcoe anterior chamber capsule s.
scurf
  lid s.
scutum region
SD
  standard deviation
SDI-BIOM wide angle viewing system
sea
  s. fan sign
  s. frond
seam
  pigment s.
search
  modified binary s. (MOBS)
Searcy
  S. anchor/fixation
  S. chalazion trephine
  S. oval cup erysiphake
seasonal
  s. allergic conjunctivitis
  s. rhinoconjunctivitis
sebaceous
  s. adenoma
  s. cell
  s. cell carcinoma
  s. gland carcinoma
  s. gland of conjunctiva
  s. glands of conjunctiva gland
  s. inclusion cyst
sebaceum
  adenoma s.
seborrhea
seborrheic
  s. blepharitis
  s. debris
  s. keratosis
SEBR
  spontaneous eye blink rate
sebum palpebrale
Seckel syndrome
seclusion of pupil
secobarbital sodium
second
  s. cranial nerve
  s. sight
secondary
  s. action
  s. amyloidosis
  s. angle-closure glaucoma
  s. anophthalmia
  s. axis
  s. cataract
  s. curve on contact lens

s. deviation
s. dye test
s. exotropia
s. eye
s. focal length
s. focal point
s. intraocular lens
s. keratitis
s. lens implant
s. malignant neoplasm
s. mechanism
s. membrane
s. neovascular glaucoma
s. neovascularization
s. optic atrophy
s. position
s. progressive multiple sclerosis (SP-MS)
s. retinitis
s. strabismus
s. vitreous

second-degree relative
second-grade fusion
secretion
basal tear s.
meibomian s.
oily s.
reflex tear s.
tear s.

secretomotor nerve
secretory epithelial cell
section
nerve cross s.
orbital s.
Saemisch s.
trigeminal nerve root s.

sectioning
noninvasively s.

sector
s. cortical cataract
s. cut
s. defect
s. iridectomy
s. iridectomy operation
s. pallor
s. palsy
s. retinitis pigmentosa

sectoral
s. iris paralysis
s. redness

sectoranopia
congruous homonymous horizontal s.
congruous homonymous quadruple s.

sector-shaped defect
sedimentary cataract
SEE
Surgical Eye Expeditions

seeberi
Rhinosporidium s.

seeding
vitreous s.

Seeligmüller sign
see-saw
s.-s. anisocoria
s.-s. nystagmus

segment
anterior ocular s.
bifocal s.
compensated s.
dissimilar s.
extramedullary s.
Fenhoff external and anterior s.
s. height
inner s.
Intacs corneal ring s.
intramedullary s.
intrastromal corneal ring s. (ICRS)
intratemporal s.
outer s.
posterior s.
prism s.

segmental
s. explant
s. hypoplasia
s. implant
s. iris atrophy
s. lens

segmentation
neodymium:yttrium-lithium-fluoride laser s.

Seibel
S. double-ended LASIK flap lifter and spatula
S. 3-D speculum
S. LASIK flap irrigator and squeegee cannula
S. nucleus chopper
S. paracentesis valve adjuster
S. vertical safety quick chopper

NOTES

S

457

Seidel
    S. scotoma
    S. sign
    S. test
Seiff frontalis suspension set
seizure
    visual s.
Seldane
Selecta II Glaucoma Laser System
selection
    data s.
    stepwise variable s.
selective
    s. facial myectomy
    s. laser trabeculoplasty (SLT)
    s. purinergic
self-adhering lid retractor
self-adjusted glasses
self-centering micromanipulator
self-fixating sideport diamond knife
self-retaining
    s.-r. infusion cannula
    s.-r. irrigating cannula
    s.-r. retractor
self-sealing
    s.-s. scleral puncture
    s.-s. side port
self-stabilizing vitrectomy lens
Selinger operation
sella, pl. **sellae**
    diaphragma sellae
    empty s.
    J-shaped s.
    tilt of s.
    s. turcica
sellar calcification
semicircular canal
semiconductor GaAIAs infrared diode laser photocoagulator
semifinished
    s. blank
    s. contact lens
    s. glass
semilunar
    s. fold
    s. folds of conjunctiva
semilunaris
    plica s.
    raphe plica s.
semiscleral contact lens
semishell implant
senescent
    s. cortical degenerative cataract
    s. disciform macular degeneration
    s. ectropion
    s. elastosis
    s. enophthalmos
    s. entropion
    s. halo

    s. keratosis
    s. macular exudative choroiditis
    s. macular hole
    s. miosis
    s. nuclear degenerative cataract
    s. ptosis
    s. retinoschisis
senile
    s. atrophy
    s. chorioretinitis
    s. choroidal change
    s. disciform macular degeneration
    s. ectropion
    s. elastosis
    s. entropion
    s. exudative macular degeneration
    s. furrow degeneration
    s. guttate choroidopathy
    s. halo
    s. keratosis
    s. lenticular myopia
    s. macular exudative choroiditis
    s. miosis
    s. nuclear sclerotic cataract
    s. reflex
    s. retinoschisis
    s. vitritis
senilis
    arcus s.
    cataract s.
    choroiditis guttata s.
    circus s.
    ectropion s.
    linea corneae s.
    sarcomatosum s.
Senior-Loken syndrome
Senn retractor
senopia
Sensar
    S. acrylic intraocular lens
    S. OptiEdge foldable acrylic IOL
    S. OptiEdge intraocular lens
sensation
    corneal s.
    decreased corneal s.
    s. disturbance
    foreign-body s.
    s. impairment
    light s.
    nociceptive s.
    threshold of visual s.
    s. time
sense
    color s.
    form s.
    light s.
    stereognostic s.
Sensitive
    S. Eyes

S. Eyes daily cleaner
S. Eyes drops
S. Eyes Enzymatic Cleaner
S. Eyes Plus Saline Solution
S. Eyes saline/cleaning solution
S. Eyes Sterile Saline Spray

sensitivity
contrast s.
cornea s.
corneal s.
increment threshold spectral s.
light s.
periocular drug s.
scotopic s.
spatial-contrast s.
spectral s.
s. threshold

sensor
Ocular Vergence and
Accommodation S. (OVAS)
oximetry s.
reliable wave front s.
Shell s.

Sensorcaine with epinephrine
sensorimotor disorder
sensory
s. amblyopia
s. ataxic neuropathy with dysarthria
and ophthalmoplegia (SANDO)
s. correspondence
s. deprivation esotropia
s. deprivation exotropia
s. deprivation nystagmus
s. detachment
s. elevation
s. fiber
s. fusion
s. nerve
s. retina
s. root
s. root of ciliary ganglion
s. system
s. visual pathway

separable acuity
separate image test
separation
centrifugal s.
fluidic ILM s.
s. of retina
vitreofoveal s.
vitreomacular s.
vitreous s.

separator
Allen stereo s.
diamond wound s.
Kirby cylindrical zonal s.
Kirby flat zonal s.
Remy s.

sepsis
hematogenous s.

septa (*pl. of* septum)
septic
s. chorioretinitis
s. retinitis
s. thrombosis

septica
iridocyclitis s.

Septicon
septooptic
s. dysplasia
s. dysplasia syndrome

septum, pl. septa
s. cavum pellucidum
inferior orbital s.
intermuscular s.
orbital s.
s. orbitale
s. sequela
superior orbital s.
tarsus orbital s.

sequela, pl. sequelae
septum s.

Sequels
Diamox S.

sequence
linear sebaceous nevus s.

sequestered space
sera (*pl. of* serum)
Serdarevic
S. Circle of Light
S. speculum
S. suture adjuster

Sereine
S. Cleaner
S. Soaking and Cleaning Solution
S. Wetting and Soaking Solution

serena
gutta s.

series
s. five forceps
Kurova Shursite lens s.
Stanford Achievement Test S.
Zeiss slit-lamp s.

serine protease

NOTES

serious corneal complication
seropositivity rate
serosa
> choroiditis s.
> s. choroiditis
> retinitis centralis s.

serous
> s. chorioretinopathy
> s. choroidal detachment
> s. choroidal effusion (SCE)
> s. cyclitis
> s. cyst
> s. detachment maculopathy
> s. iritis
> s. macular detachment
> s. membrane
> s. pigment epithelial detachment
> s. pigment epithelium
> s. retinal pigment epithelium detachment
> s. retinitis
> s. retinopathy

Serpasil
serpent ulcer of cornea
serpiginous
> s. choroiditis
> s. choroidopathy
> s. corneal ulcer
> s. keratitis
> s. ulceration

serrated conjunctival forceps
Serratia
> *S. liquefaciens*
> *S. marcescens*
> *S. marcescens* infection

serrefine
> ASSI s.
> s. clamp
> Dieffenbach s.
> Lemoine s.

serum, pl. **sera**
> s. laminin-P1
> s. lysozyme

service
> Lighthouse Low Vision S.
> sterilizer monitoring s.

sessile papilloma
set
> Bloomberg trabeculotome s.
> British Standards Institution optotype s.
> Carriazo-Barraquer instrument s.
> Catalano intubation s.
> Crawford lacrimal intubation s.
> diagnostic fitting s.
> DORC subretinal instrument s.
> Fine bimanual handpiece s.
> Impex/Lerner foldable lens removing s.

> Jackson lacrimal intubation s.
> Jaffe laser blepharoplasty and facial resurfacing s.
> Jaffe lid retractor s.
> McIntyre infusion s.
> Mentanium vitreoretinal instrument s.
> pediatric vitrectomy lens s.
> Pettigrove LASIK s.
> Price Donor Cornea Punch s.
> Seiff frontalis suspension s.
> Simcoe lens positioning s.
> Steinert LASIK s.
> STENTube lacrimal intubation s.
> Thomas subretinal instrument s. II
> Tolentino vitrectomy lens s.
> variable power cross-cylinder lens s.
> Volk SuperField multi-adapter transformer lens s.

seton
> Ahmed drainage s.
> S. drainage device
> s. operation

setting
> field diaphragm s.
> luminance s.
> lux s.

setting-sun
> s.-s. phenomenon
> s.-s. sign

Set-Up
> AMO S.-U.

seventh
> s. cranial nerve (CN VII)
> s. cranial nerve palsy

severe visual impairment and blindness (SVI/BL)
Severin
> S. implant
> S. lens

Sewall
> S. forceps
> S. retractor

sew-on lens
sex-linked recessive optic atrophy
SF6
> sulfur hexafluoride
> SF6 gas

SFP
> simultaneous foveal perception

SH
> suprachoroidal hemorrhage

Shaaf cilia foreign body forceps
Shack-Hartmann aberrometer
shadow
> Barrow color s.
> Goethe color s.
> s. graph

Purkinje s.
s. test

shadowing
acoustical s.
hollowing and s.

Shafer sign

Shaffer
S. anterior angle classification
S. operation

Shaffer-Weiss classification

shaft
irrigating grasping forceps with
curved s.
irrigating scissors with straight s.
s. vision

shagreen
anterior capsule s.
anterior mosaic crocodile s.
crocodile s.
s. pattern

shaken baby syndrome (SBS)

shallow
s. chamber
s. detachment

shallowing
anterior chamber s.
s. of chamber

sham-movement vertigo

shaped cataract

shape perception

shaper
Automated Corneal S. (ACS)
Chiron automated corneal s.

sharp
s. hook
s. and pink (S&P)

Sharplan argon laser

Sharpoint
S. microsurgical knife
S. ophthalmic microsurgical suture
S. slit knife
S. spoon blade
S. Ultra-Glide corneal transplant
suture
S. Ultra-Glide ophthalmic transplant
suture
S. Ultra-Guide ophthalmic needle
S. UltraPlug punctum plug
V-lance S.
S. V-lance blade

Sharvelle
S. side-port nucleus manipulator
S. side-port splitter

shaver
USC scleral s.

Shea
S. forceps
S. syndrome

shear force

shearing
S. cortex suction kit
s. injury
S. planar posterior chamber
intraocular lens
S. posterior chamber intraocular
lens implant

sheath
arachnoid s.
bulbar s.
dural s.
eyeball s.
fetal fibrovascular s.
fibrovascular s.
muscle s.
nerve s.
optic nerve s.
pial s.
s. syndrome

sheathing
arteriolar s.
halo s.
peripheral retinal vascular s.
perivascular s.
retinal vein s.
s. of retinal vessel
vascular s.
venous s.
vessel s.

sheathotomy

Sheehy-Urban sliding lens adapter

sheen dystrophy

sheet
Barrier s.
Eye-Pak II s.
foil s.
glassy s.
ground-glass s.
S.'s irrigating vectis
S.'s lens
S.'s lens glide
S.'s lens-inserting forceps
S.'s lens spatula

S

NOTES

sheet *(continued)*
    S.'s microiris hook
    Silastic s.
    Supramid s.
    Teflon s.
sheeting
    micromesh s.
Sheets-McPherson tying forceps
shelf-type implant
shell
    s. implant
    plaster s.
    s. prosthesis
    scleral s.
Shell sensor
Shepard
    S. incision depth gauge
    S. incision irrigating cannula
    S. intraocular lens forceps
    S. intraocular lens-holding forceps
    S. intraocular utility forceps
    S. lens-inserting forceps
    S. microiris hook
    S. optical center marker
    S. radial keratotomy irrigating
      cannula
    S. reversed iris hook
    S. tying forceps
Shepard-Reinstein forceps
Shepherd tomahawk chopper
**Sheridan-Gardiner isolated letter-
  matching test**
Sherman card
Sherrington
    S. law
    S. law of reciprocal innervation
shield
    aluminum eye s.
    Barraquer eye s.
    Buller eye s.
    Cartella eye s.
    cataract mask s.
    Clear View hydrophilic s.
    collagen s.
    corneal light s.
    Cox II ocular laser s.
    Durette external laser s.
    Expo Bubble eye s.
    eye s.
    face s.
    S.'s forceps
    Fox aluminum s.
    Fox eye s.
    Grafco eye s.
    Green eye s.
    Guibor s.
    Hessburg corneal s.
    Hessburg eye s.
    S. iridotomy scissors

    Jardon eye s.
    Mueller eye s.
    Paton eye s.
    plastic eye s.
    pressure s.
    PROSHIELD collagen corneal s.
    ring cataract mask eye s.
    Soft Shield collagen corneal s.
    trigeminal s.
    s. ulcer
    Universal eye s.
    Visitec corneal s.
    Weck eye s.
    wrap-a-round eye s.
shield-shaped
shift
    criterion s.
    eye-head s.
    hyperopic s.
    Purkinje s.
Shigella
    S. flexneri
    S. sonnei
shiny cellophane reflection
shipyard
    s. conjunctivitis
    s. disease
    s. eye
    s. keratoconjunctivitis
Shirmer basal secretion test
Shoch
    S. foreign body pickup
    S. suture
shock
    anaphylactic s.
    s. optic neuropathy
shoelace stitch
Shoemaker intraocular lens forceps
short
    s. ciliary nerve
    s. C-loop lens
    s. posterior ciliary artery
    s. root of ciliary ganglion
    s. sight
    s. wavelength automated perimetry
      (SWAP)
    s. wavelength autoperimetry
ShortCut A-OK small-incision knife
shortening
    cicatricial s.
Shorti LRI diamond knife
short-scale contrast
shortsightedness
shot-silk
    s.-s. phenomenon
    s.-s. reflex
    s.-s. retina
show
    scleral s.

Shprintzen syndrome
shredded iris
Shugrue operation
shunt
    aqueous tube s.
    Baerveldt s.
    dural s.
    opticociliary s.
    Schocket anterior chamber tube s.
    s. vessel
    White glaucoma pump s.
shunting
    left-to-right s.
sialylated chain
sicca
    blepharitis s.
    keratitis s.
    keratoconjunctivitis s. (KCS)
    non-Sjögren keratoconjunctivitis s.
    rhinitis s.
    s. syndrome
    transplantation of submandibular
      gland for keratoconjunctivitis s.
siccus
    pannus s.
Sichel
    S. blade
    S. disease
    S. knife
Sichi
    S. operation
    S. orbital implant
sickle
    s. cell anemia
    s. cell retinopathy
    s. scotoma
sickness
    simulator s.
side-biting spatula
side-cutting spatulated needle
side-port
    s.-p. cannula
    s.-p. fixation knife
side port
siderophone
sideroscope
siderosis
    s. bulbi
    s. cataract
    s. conjunctivae
    s. lentis
    ocular s.

siderotic cataract
sidewall infusion cannula
Sidler-Huguenin endothelioma
Sieger streak
Siegrist
    S. spot
    S. streak
Siegrist-Hutchinson syndrome
Siemens Quantum 2000 Color Doppler
Siepser endocapsular controller
sight
    day s.
    far s.
    line of s.
    long s.
    near s.
    night s.
    old s.
    primary line of s.
    second s.
    short s.
    s. specific
sighted
    partially s.
sign
    Abadie s.
    Argyll Robertson pupil s.
    Arroyo s.
    Baillarger s.
    Ballet s.
    Bárány s.
    Bard s.
    Barré s.
    Battle s.
    Becker s.
    Bekhterev s.
    Bell s.
    Benson s.
    Berger s.
    Bianchi s.
    Bielschowsky s.
    Bjerrum s.
    black dot s.
    black sunburst s.
    Bonnet s.
    Bordier-Fränkel s.
    Boston s.
    Brickner s.
    Brown-Kelly s.
    Brunati s.
    Cantelli s.
    cerebellar eye s.

S

NOTES

sign *(continued)*
Cestan s.
Charcot s.
Charleaux oil droplet s.
Chvostek s.
Cogan lid-twitch s.
Collier tucked lid s.
Cowen s.
Dalrymple s.
digitoocular s.
Dixon Mann s.
doll's eye s.
s. of edema of lower eyelid
Elliot s.
Enroth s.
Gianelli s.
Gifford s.
Goppert s.
Gower s.
Graefe s.
Griffith s.
Grocco s.
Gunn s.
Hennebert s.
Hoaglund s.
Hutchinson s.
Jellinek s.
Jendrassik s.
Joffroy s.
Kestenbaum s.
Knies s.
Kocher s.
Larcher s.
Loewi s.
Lotze local s.
Macewen s.
Magendie s.
Magendie-Hertwig s.
Mann s.
Marcus Gunn pupillary s.
Marfan s.
Maxwell-Lyons s.
May s.
Means s.
Metenier s.
Möbius s.
Möbius-von Graefe-Stellway s.
Munson s.
Nikolsky s.
ocular s.
orbicularis s.
Parrot s.
peek s.
Pick s.
Piltz s.
Prevost s.
pseudo-Graefe s.
Reisman s.
Revilliod s.

Rifkind s.
Ripault s.
Robertson s.
Romaña s.
Romberg s.
Rosenbach s.
Saenger s.
Sainton s.
Salus s.
Schaffer s.
sea fan s.
Seeligmüller s.
Seidel s.
setting-sun s.
Shafer s.
Skeer s.
Stellwag s.
Stimson s.
Sugiura s.
Suker s.
Summerskill s.
swinging flashlight s.
Tay s.
Tellais s.
Theimich lip s.
Topolanski s.
Tournay s.
Trousseau s.
Uhthoff s.
von Graefe s.
Watzke-Allen s.
Weber s.
Weber-Rinne s.
Wernicke s.
white pupil s.
Widowitz s.
Wilder s.
Woods s.
signal
laser Doppler s.
pseudo-CSF s.
Signet Optical lens
signet-ring
s.-r. carcinoma
s.-r. lymphoma
significance
monoclonal gammopathy of
undetermined s. (MGUS)
SilaClean
Siladryl Oral
Silastic
S. intubation
S. plate
S. scleral buckler implant
S. sheet
S. T-tube
Sildenafil
silent
s. central retinal vein obstruction

s. dacryocystitis
s. sinus syndrome
silica gel
silicone
s. acrylate
s. acrylate contact lens
s. band
s. button
s. conformer
s. elastomer lens
s. eye sphere
s. hemisphere
s. intraocular lens
s. introducer
s. lubricant
s. mesh implant
s. nasolacrimal intubation
s. oil
s. oil injection
s. oil tamponade
s. plug
s. punctal plug therapy
s. rod
s. rod and sleeve forceps
s. sponge explant
s. sponge forceps
s. strip
s. tire
s. toric IOL
s. tube
s. tubing
Silicon Graphics Crimson Reality Engine
siliculose, siliquose
s. cataract
Silikon 1000 retinal tamponade
silk traction suture
sillonneur
Silsoft contact lens
Silva-Costa operation
silver
s. compound
Gomori methenamine s. (GMS)
s. nitrate
s. nitrate solution
s. protein
s. tattoo pigment
s. wire effect
Silver-Hildreth operation
silver-wire
s.-w. arteriole

s.-w. reflex
s.-w. vessel
Simcoe
S. anterior chamber capsule scrubber
S. corneal marker
S. cortex extractor aspiration cannula
S. double-barreled irrigating/aspirating unit
S. double-end lens loupe
S. I&A system
S. II PC aspirating needle
S. II PC double cannula
S. II PC lens
S. II PC nucleus delivery loupe
S. interchangeable tip
S. irrigation/aspiration system
S. lens implant forceps
S. lens-inserting forceps
S. lens positioning set
S. notched spatula
S. nucleus erysiphake
S. nucleus forceps
S. nucleus lens loupe
S. posterior chamber lens forceps
S. reverse aperture cannula
S. reverse irrigating/aspirating cannula
S. scleral depressor
S. suture needle
S. upeop
S. wire speculum
Similasan eye drops
Simmons
occult temporal arteritis of S.
simple
s. acute conjunctivitis
s. anisocoria
s. color
s. diplopia
s. episcleritis
s. glaucoma
s. heterochromia
s. hyperopic astigmatism
s. myopia
s. myopic astigmatism
s. optic atrophy
s. plus lens
s. retinitis
simplex
epidermolysis bullosa s.

S

NOTES

simplex *(continued)*
    glaucoma s.
    s. glaucoma
Simpson
    S. lacrimal probe
    S. test
simulans
    Staphylococcus s.
Simulantest
simulator
    s. sickness
    video display terminal s. (VDTS)
simultanagnosia
simultaneous
    s. color contrast
    s. foveal perception (SFP)
    s. macular perception (SMP)
    s. prism cover test (SPC)
Sinarest 12 Hour nasal solution
sine-wave grating
Singapore epidemic conjunctivitis
single
    s. binocular vision (SBV)
    s. cover test
    s. lid eversion
single-action rongeur
single-armed suture
single-cut contact lens
single/double occluder
single-incision system
single-mirror goniolens
single-quadrant testing
single-running suture
single-stitch
    s.-s. aponeurotic tuck technique
    S.-s. PhacoFlex
Single-Vision Thin & Lite 1.67 Semi-Finished Lens with hard coating
sinister
    oculus s. (left eye)
    tension oculus s. (tension of left eye) (TOS)
    visio oculus s. (vision of left eye) (VOS)
sinistrality
sinistrocular
sinistrocularity
sinistrogyration
sinistrotorsion
Sinskey
    S. intraocular lens
    S. IOL manipulator
    S. lens-holding forceps
    S. lens hook
    S. lens-manipulating hook
    S. microiris hook
    S. microlens hook
    S. micro-tying forceps
    S. pick

Sinskey-Wilson foreign body forceps
sinus, pl. **sinus, sinuses**
    anterior chamber s.
    Arlt s.
    Arlt-Jaesche s.
    s. catarrh
    cavernous s.
    s. circularis iridis
    ethmoid s.
    ethmoidal s.
    frontal s.
    s. headache
    s. of Maier
    Maier s.
    s. mucocele
    paranasal s.
    scleral venous s.
    sphenoid s.
    s. venosus sclera
    venous s.
sinusitis
    frontal s.
    maxillary s.
    paranasal s.
sinusoidal grating
Sipple-Gorlin syndrome
Sipple syndrome
SITA
    Swedish interactive thresholding algorithm
SITE
    SITE irrigating/aspirating needle
    SITE irrigation/aspiration machine
    SITE macrobore plus needle
    SITE Phaco I/A needle
    SITE Phaco II handpiece
    SITE TXR diaphragmatic microsurgical system
    SITE TXR 2200 microsurgical unit
    SITE TXR peristaltic microsurgical system
    SITE TXR phacoemulsification system
site
    retinal impact s.
situ keratomileusis procedure
situs inversus
sixth
    s. cranial nerve (CN VI)
    s. cranial nerve palsy
size
    burn spot s.
    dark-adapted pupil s. (DAPS)
    eye s.
    lens s.
    object s.
    pupil s.
    relative s.
    retinal image s.

spot s.
    Thornton guide for optical zone s.

Sjögren
    S. disease
    S. reticular dystrophy
    S. syndrome

Sjögren-Larsson syndrome

SKBM
    Summit Krumeich-Barraquer
    microkeratome
    SKBM microkeratome

Skeele curette

Skeer sign

skein
    Holmgren s.
    test s.
    s. test

skeletal abnormality

Skeleton fine forceps

skew
    s. deviation
    s. motion
    s. pupil

skiameter

skiametry

skiascope

skiascopy bar

skiascotometry

SKILL Card Test

skin
    s. autograft
    s. cancer compound
    s. change
    s. diabetes
    s. flap
    s. graft
    s. hook
    s. marking pen
    s. pupillary reflex

ski needle

skirt
    vitreous s.

Sklar-Schiötz tonometer

skull
    exophthalmos due to tower s.
    s. temple

sky-blue spot

SL
    Schwalbe line

slab-off
    s.-o. grinding
    s.-o. lens

Slade formed irrigation cannula

Slade-type adjustable aspirating LASIK speculum

slant
    antimongoloid s.
    S. haptic
    S. haptic single-piece intraocular lens
    mongoloid s.
    s. muscle operation
    palpebral s.

SLE
    slit-lamp examination

sleeve
    anterior segment s.
    Charles anterior segment s.
    Charles infusion s.
    Charles vitrector with s.
    clear keratin s.
    implant s.
    s. implant
    Labtician oval s.
    phaco s.
    retinal probe s.
    s. spreading forceps
    Stevens-Charles s.
    SupraSLEEVES nylon s.
    Watzke s.

slide
    AO Vectographic Project-O-Chart s.
    epithelial s.
    Polaroid vectograph s.

sliding flap

slimcut blade

SlimFit
    S. ovoid intraocular lens
    S. small-incision ovoid lens

sling
    Arion s.
    fascia lata frontalis s.
    frontalis muscle s.
    s. for implant
    s. procedure
    Supramid s.
    suture s.
    tarsoligamentous s.

slippage

slit
    s. blade knife
    s. illumination
    s. lamp biomicroscope
    S. Lamp 900 BQ

S

NOTES

slit-beam test
slit-lamp
    s.-l. biomicroscopy
    s.-l. cup
    s.-l. examination (SLE)
    s.-l. fluorophotometer
    s.-l. microscope
    s.-l. ophthalmoscopy
SLK
    superior limbic keratoconjunctivitis
SLO
    scanning laser ophthalmoscope
Sloan
    S. letters
    S. M system
    S. optotype
    S. reading card
Sloane
    S. Epi-peeler
    S. flap repositor
    S. micro hoe
    S. trephine
sloping isopter
slough
    conjunctival s.
sloughing base
slow-channel syndrome
slow conjugate roving eye movement
slow-to-no saccade
10 SL/O Zeiss keratometer
SLP
    scanning laser polarimetry
SLT
    selective laser trabeculoplasty
sludging of circulation
sluggish movements of eyes and
  eyelids
SLx
    IRIS Medical OcuLight S.
Sly syndrome
small
    s. aperture Steri-Drape
    s. incision trabeculectomy
small-incision
    s.-i. cataract surgery
    s.-i. phacoemulsification
SmallPort phaco system
Smart
    S. forceps
    S. scissors
smear
    conjunctival s.
    KOH s.
    Tzanck s.
smegmatis
    Mycobacterium s.
Smirmaul
    S. nucleus extractor
    S. technique

Smith
    S. expressor
    S. expressor hook
    S. eyelid operation
    S. intraocular capsular amputator
    S. knife
    S. lid hook
    S. modification
    S. modification of Van Lint lid
      block
    S. orbital floor implant
    S. speculum
    S. trabeculectomy
Smith-Fisher
    S.-F. iris replacer
    S.-F. knife
    S.-F. spatula
Smith-Green cataract knife
Smith-Indian
    S.-I. operation
    S.-I. technique
Smith-Kettlewell Institute Low
  Luminance Card Test
Smith-Kuhnt-Szymanowski operation
Smith-Leiske cross-action intraocular
  lens forceps
Smith-Lemli-Opitz syndrome
Smith-Magenis syndrome
Smith-Riley syndrome
SMON
    subacute myelooptic neuropathy
smooth
    s. cannula
    s. grasping forceps
    s. muscle hamartoma
    s. pursuit
smooth-edged continuous tear
smooth-pursuit movement
SMP
    simultaneous macular perception
SMZ-10A zoom stereo microscope
snail tracks
snake bite-induced ptosis
snake-like
    s.-l. appearance
    s.-l. structure
snare
    Banner enucleation s.
    Castroviejo enucleation s.
    enucleation wire s.
    s. enucleator
    Förster enucleation s.
    Foster enucleation s.
    wire enucleation s.
Sneddon-Wilkinson disease
Snellen
    S. chart
    S. conventional reform implant
    S. entropion forceps

S. fraction
S. lens loupe
S. letter optotype
S. letters
S. line
S. near-vision card
S. notation
S. number
S. ptosis operation
S. reading card
S. reform eye
S. soft contact lens
S. test
S. test type
S. vectis
S. visual acuity
Snell law
Snell-Sterling visual efficiency scale
SnET2
tin ethyl etiopurpurin
Sno-Strips
snow
s. blindness
s. conjunctivitis
s. glasses
snowball opacity
snow-bank exudate
snowflake cataract
snowman graft
snowstorm cataract
Snugfit eye patch
Snyder corneal spring forceps
Soac-Lens
soaking solution
SOCA
Studies of the Ocular Complications in AIDS
Sochlor Solution
society
Canadian Ophthalmology S.
North American Neuro-Ophthalmology S. (NANOS)
Ophthalmic Photographers S. (OPS)
socket
anophthalmic s.
contracted s.
s. contracture
s. discharge
s. prosthesis
s. reconstruction
sodium
s. acetate

s. bicarbonate
s. borate
carboxymethylcellulose s.
cefamandole s.
s. chloride (NaCl)
s. chloride in solution
s. cromoglycate
cromolyn s.
dantrolene s.
diclofenac s.
fluorescein s.
s. fluorescein (NaFl)
flurbiprofen s.
fomivirsen s.
foscarnet s.
ganciclovir s.
s. hexametaphosphate
hyaluronate s.
s. hyaluronate and chondroitin sulfate
s. hyaluronate solution
s. hydroxide
s. lauryl sulfate
naproxen s.
nedocromil s.
pentobarbital s.
s. perborate
phenobarbital s.
s. phosphate
s. propionate
secobarbital s.
sterile acetazolamide s.
stibogluconate s.
S. Sulamyd
S. Sulamyd Ophthalmic
sulfacetamide s.
suramin s.
thiopental s.
valproate s.
warfarin s.
Soemmering
S. crystalline swelling
S. foramen
ring of S.
S. ring
S. ring cataract
S. spot
SOF
superior orbital fissure
Soflens
S. 66
S. contact lens

S

NOTES

Soflens *(continued)*
    S. enzymatic contact lens cleaner
    S. 66 lens
SoFlex series lens
Sof/Pro-Clean
Sofsilk nonabsorbable silk suture
soft
    s. cataract
    s. contact lens (SCL)
    s. contact lens solution
    s. drusen
    s. exudate
    Gonio s.
    s. intraocular lens
    s. IOL cutter
    S. Mate
    S. Mate Comfort Drops for
    Sensitive Eyes
    S. Mate Consept
    S. Mate daily cleaning solution
    S. Mate disinfection and storage
    solution
    S. Mate Enzyme Alternative
    S. Mate Enzyme Plus cleaner
    S. Mate Hands Off daily cleaner
    S. Mate protein remover
    S. Mate saline
    S. Mate Saline for Sensitive Eyes
    S. Plug punctal plug
    S. Shield collagen corneal shield
    s. silicone sponge
    s. tissue swelling
Soft-Cell eye spear
Softcon
SofTec Delivery System
soft-finger tension
SoftGels
    HydroEye S.
SoftPlug
SoftSITE high add aspheric multifocal
  contact lens
soft-tipped
    s.-t. cannula
    s.-t. extrusion handpiece
Soft-Touch A-Probe
software
    IMAGE S.
    PathFinder Corneal Analysis s.
    posterior capsule opacification s.
    Visulas 532 Combi s.
    Visulas InterChange s.
SoftWear
    S. Saline
    S. Saline for Sensitive Eyes
    Solution
solani
    Fusarium s.
Sola Optical USA Spectralite high
  index lens

solar
    s. blindness
    s. burn
    s. damage
    s. keratoma
    s. keratosis
    s. maculopathy
    s. radiation
    s. retinitis
    s. retinopathy
solid
    s. color
    s. silicone with Supramid mesh
    implant
    s. vision
solium
    Taenia s.
Soll suture and incision marker
SOLO-care Multi-Purpose Solution
Solu-Medrol
Solurex L.A.
Solusept
solution
    Adsorbotear Ophthalmic S.
    AK-Dilate Ophthalmic S.
    AK-Nefrin Ophthalmic S.
    AK-Spore S.
    Akwa Tears s.
    Alcon Saline Especially for
    Sensitive Eyes S.
    Alocril ophthalmic s.
    Alomide ophthalmic s.
    AMO Vitrax viscoelastic s.
    Amvisc Plus s.
    apraclonidine ophthalmic s.
    AquaSite Ophthalmic S.
    azelastine hydrochloride
    ophthalmic s.
    balanced saline s.
    balanced salt s. (BSS)
    Barnes-Hind contact lens cleaning
    and soaking s.
    Barnes-Hind wetting s.
    Betadine Sterile Ophthalmic
    Prep S.
    Beta-Ophtiole ophthalmic s.
    Betimol beta-blocker s.
    bimatoprost ophthalmic s.
    BioLon s.
    Bion Tears S.
    Blairex Sterile Preserved Saline S.
    boric acid s.
    Boston Advance Comfort Formula
    Conditioning S.
    Boston Simplicity Multi-Action S.
    brimonidine tartrate ophthalmic s.
    BSS Plus ophthalmic irrigating s.
    BSS sterile irrigating s.
    Claris Cleaning and Soaking S.

ComfortCare GP Wetting and Soaking S.
Comfort Tears S.
Complete Comfort Plus Multi-Purpose S.
ContaClair multi-purpose contact lens s.
CooperVision balanced salt s.
Cosopt ophthalmic s.
Crolom Ophthalmic S.
cromolyn sodium ophthalmic s.
Dakrina Ophthalmic S.
dexamethasone s.
Dey-Drop Ophthalmic S.
disinfecting s.
Domeboro s.
dorzolamide hydrochloride ophthalmic s.
dorzolamide hydrochloride-timolol maleate ophthalmic s.
Dry Eyes s.
Dry Eye Therapy S.
Dwelle Ophthalmic S.
emedastine difurmarate ophthalmic s.
eye irrigating s.
Eye-Lube-A S.
Eye-Sed s.
Eyesine s.
Eye Stream sterile eye irrigating s.
Eye Wash s.
Feldman buffer s.
fluorescein dye and stain s.
Freeman s.
graft preservation s.
Healon s.
hydrolysis of s.
hypertonic s.
HypoTears PF S.
hypotonic s.
Indocin ophthalmic s.
Iocare balanced salt s.
I-Phrine Ophthalmic S.
irrigating s.
Isopto Plain S.
Isopto Tears S.
isotonic s.
Just Tears S.
ketorolac tromethamine ophthalmic s.
ketotifen fumarate ophthalmic s.
K Sol preservation s.

Lacril Ophthalmic S.
latanoprost timolol maleate ophthalmic s.
Lens Plus Sterile Saline S.
levofloxacin ophthalmic s.
Liquifilm Forte S.
Liquifilm Rewetting S.
Liquifilm Tears S.
Lobob Hard Contact Lens Wetting S.
Lobob Rigid Hard Contact Lens Soaking S.
lodoxamide tromethamine ophthalmic s.
loteprednol etabonate ophthalmic s.
LubriTears S.
Lumigan ophthalmic s.
medocromil sodium ophthalmic s.
Miochol s.
Murine s.
Murocel Ophthalmic S.
Mydfrin Ophthalmic S.
Nature's Tears S.
nedocromil sodium ophthalmic s.
Neosporin Ophthalmic S.
Neo-Synephrine Ophthalmic S.
No Rub Opti-Free Express multi-purpose disinfecting s.
Nu-Tears II S.
OcuCoat PF Ophthalmic S.
OcuMax s.
Ocupress Ophthalmic S.
ofloxacin ophthalmic s.
olopatadine hydrochloride ophthalmic s.
ONE s.
ophthalmic s.
Opti-Free Express Multi-Purpose S.
Optimum Cleaning, Disinfecting, and Storage S.
Opti-One Conditioning S.
Opti-One Multi-Purpose S.
Opti-Soak Conditioning S.
Optivar ophthalmic s.
osmium tetroxide s.
oxidation of s.
pemirolast potassium ophthalmic s.
Prefrin Ophthalmic S.
preservatives in s.
ProConcept Wetting and Soaking S.
Puralube Tears S.

S

NOTES

solution *(continued)*
  Pure Eyes Disinfection/Soaking S.
  Pure Eyes soaking s.
  Purilens UV Disinfection S.
  Quixin ophthalmic s.
  Refresh Plus Ophthalmic S.
  Relief Ophthalmic S.
  Ringer lactate s.
  rose bengal red s.
  saline s.
  Sensitive Eyes Plus Saline S.
  Sensitive Eyes saline/cleaning s.
  Sereine Soaking and Cleaning S.
  Sereine Wetting and Soaking S.
  silver nitrate s.
  Sinarest 12 Hour nasal s.
  soaking s.
  Sochlor S.
  sodium chloride in s.
  sodium hyaluronate s.
  soft contact lens s.
  Soft Mate daily cleaning s.
  Soft Mate disinfection and
    storage s.
  SoftWear Saline for Sensitive
    Eyes S.
  SOLO-care Multi-Purpose S.
  solvent s.
  Soquette contact lens soaking s.
  sterility of s.
  Sulster S.
  Tear Drop S.
  TearGard Ophthalmic S.
  Teargen Ophthalmic S.
  Tearisol S.
  Tears Naturale Free S.
  Tears Naturale II S.
  Tears Plus S.
  Tears Renewed S.
  timolol maleate ophthalmic gel-
    forming s.
  Total The All-In-One Hard Contact
    Lens S.
  Travatan ophthalmic s.
  travoprost ophthalmic s.
  Trump s.
  Ultra Tears S.
  Unicare blue and green all-in-one
    cleaning s.
  Unisol 4 Preservative Free
    Saline S.
  Visalens contact lens cleaning and
    soaking s.
  Viscoat s.
  viscoelastic s.
  Viva-Drops S.
  wetting s.
  Zaditor ophthalmic s.
  zinc sulfate s.

solvent solution
somata
  amacrine cell s.
somatic cell
Sondermann canal
sonnei
  Shigella s.
Sonogage
  S. System Corneo-Gage 20 MHz
    center frequency transducer
  S. ultrasound pachometer
sonographer
  Trans-Scan pulsed Doppler s.
sonolucent
  acoustical s.
  s. cleft
  s. lesion
Sonomed
  S. A/B-Scan system
  S. 1500 A-scan instrument
  S. A-Scan system
  S. B-1500 system
Sonometric Ocuscan
SOOF
  suborbicularis oculi fat
    SOOF lift
Soothe eye
SOP
  Bleph-10 S.
  Blephamide S.
  Chloroptic S.
  FML S.
  Lacri-Lube S.
  Pred G S.
Soper
  S. cone contact lens
  S. cone lens
Soquette contact lens soaking solution
sorbic acid Sorbi-Care saline
Sorbi-Care
Sorbinil Retinopathy Trial (SRT)
Soriano operation
Soria operation
Sorsby
  S. maculopathy
  S. pseudoinflammatory macular
    degeneration
  pseudoinflammatory macular
    dystrophy of S.
  S. pseudoinflammatory macular
    dystrophy
  S. syndrome
Sotos syndrome
soul blindness
sound
  lacrimal s.
source
  point s.

Sourdille
>S. forceps
>S. keratoplasty
>S. keratoplasty operation
>S. ptosis operation

southern
>S. blot hybridization assay
>S. blot technique

Sovereign
>S. bifocal lens
>S. SHIELD System

S&P
>sharp and pink

space
>Berger s.
>Blessig s.
>circumlental s.
>episcleral s.
>Fontana s.
>intercellular s.
>interfascial s.
>interlamellar s.
>s. of iridocorneal angle
>Kuhnt s.
>s. myopia
>object s.
>Panum fusional s.
>parafoveal cystic s.
>perichoroidal s.
>perioptic subarachnoid s.
>periscleral s.
>preseptal s.
>prezonular s.
>retrobulbar s.
>retroocular s.
>Schwalbe s.
>sequestered s.
>subarachnoid s.
>subpigment epithelial s.
>subretinal s.
>suprachoroidal s.
>Tenon s.
>zonular s.

space-occupying lesion
spacer
>autogenous hard palate eyelid s.
>eyelid s.
>lower eyelid s.

Spadafora MemoryLens dialer
Spaeth
>S. block
>S. classification
>S. cystic bleb operation
>S. ptosis operation

Spaleck forceps
Spanish silk suture
Spanlang-Tappeiner syndrome
sparganosis
>nodules in s.
>ocular s.

sparing
>foveal s.
>macular s.
>pupillary s.
>recurrent pupillary s.

Sparta microforceps
spasm
>accommodation s.
>s. of accommodation
>accommodative s.
>ciliary s.
>convergence s.
>cyclic ocular motor s.
>facial s.
>hemifacial s.
>near-reflex s.
>s. of the near reflex
>nictitating s.
>oculomotor paresis with cyclic s.
>posttraumatic accommodative s.
>winking s.

spasmodic
>s. mydriasis
>s. strabismus

spasmus nutans
spastic
>s. ectropion
>s. entropion
>s. lagophthalmia
>s. miosis
>s. mydriasis
>s. paretic facial contracture
>s. pseudosclerosis

spasticity of conjugate gaze
spasticum
>ectropion s.
>entropion s.
>sarcomatosum s.

spatia
>s. anguli iridis
>s. anguli iridocornealis
>s. zonularia

spatial
>s. acuity

NOTES

spatial *(continued)*
  s. discrimination
  s. information
  s. interaction
  s. localization
  s. perception disorder
  s. summation
spatial-contrast sensitivity
spatially
  s. resolved value
  s. resolved wavefront aberration
spatiotopic stimulus
spatium
  s. episclerale
  s. interfasciale
  s. intervaginale
  s. perichoroideale
spatula
  AE-2920 Carones LASEK s.
  angled iris s.
  angulated iris s.
  Bangerter iris s.
  Barraquer irrigator s.
  Berens s.
  Birks Mark II micro push/pull s.
  Buratto contact lens spoon and s.
  capsule fragment s.
  Carones LASEK s.
  Castillejos LASIK retreatment s.
  Castroviejo cyclodialysis s.
  Castroviejo double-ended s.
  Castroviejo synechia s.
  Cleasby s.
  corneal fascia lata s.
  corneal graft s.
  Culler iris s.
  cyclodialysis s.
  double s.
  Drews-Sato suture-pickup s.
  Elschnig cyclodialysis s.
  Fisher-Smith s.
  Fox LASIK s.
  French hook s.
  French lacrimal s.
  French pattern s.
  Fukasaku s.
  Gills-Welsh s.
  Green double s.
  Green lens s.
  Green replacer s.
  Guimaraes flap s.
  Guimaraes ophthalmic s.
  Hardten double-ended LASIK flap lifter and s.
  Hersh LASIK retreatment s.
  Hertzog lens s.
  Hirschman s.
  s. hook
  hook s.

iridodialysis s.
iris s.
Jaffe intraocular s.
Jaffe lens s.
Johnston axis marker and s.
Johnston LASIK s.
Katena iris s.
Kimura platinum s.
Kirby angulated iris s.
Knapp iris s.
Knolle lens cortex s.
Knolle lens nucleus s.
Laird s.
LASEK epithelial detaching s.
LASEK epithelial flap repositioning s.
Lindner s.
Lindstrom LASIK s.
MacRae flap flipper/retreatment s.
Maddox LASIK s.
Manhattan Eye & Ear s.
Masket Phaco s.
Maumenee vitreous sweep s.
McIntyre s.
McPherson s.
McReynolds s.
microvitreoretinal s.
needle s.
nucleus s.
Obstbaum lens s.
Obstbaum synechia s.
Olk vitreoretinal s.
Pallin lens s.
Paton double s.
Paton single s.
Paton transplant s.
platinum probe s.
s. probe
probe s.
Rainin clip-bending s.
Rainin lens s.
Rhein LASIK epithelial detaching s.
Rhein LASIK flap elevator and stromal s.
Rhein LASIK flap repositioning s.
Rowen s.
Seibel double-ended LASIK flap lifter and s.
Sheets lens s.
side-biting s.
Simcoe notched s.
Smith-Fisher s.
spoon s.
s. spoon
Steinert double-ended LASIK s.
suture pickup s.
synechia s.
Tan s.

s. temple
Thornton malleable s.
Tooke s.
Vinciguerra-Carones LASEK s.
Vinciguerra PRK/LASEK s.
vitreous sweep s.
Wheeler iris s.
spatula/protector
Arbelaez LASIK s.
spatulated needle
SPC
simultaneous prism cover test
spear
s. developmental cataract
LASIK s.
Merocel surgical s.
PVA s.
Soft-Cell eye s.
Ultracell LASIK s.
Weck-cel surgical s.
Speas operation
special
s. sense vertigo
s. spectacle lens
species
halophilic noncholera *Vibrio* s.
specific
sight s.
speckled corneal dystrophy
spectacle
s. blur
s. correction
s. crown
s. frame
s. frame pad
s. lens
s. magnifier
s. plane
spectacle-borne device
spectacle-induced aniseikonia
spectacles
aphakic s.
Bartel s.
bifocal s.
bridge of s.
cataract s.
clerical s.
compound s.
decentered s.
divers' s.
divided s.
flat top s.

folding s.
Franklin s.
half-eye s.
half-glass s.
Hallauer s.
hemianopic s.
industrial s.
Masselon s.
mica s.
orthoscopic s.
pantoscopic s.
periscopic s.
photochromic s.
prism s.
prismatic s.
protective s.
ptosis crutch s.
pulpit s.
refraction s.
safety s.
stenopeic s.
telescopic s.
temple of s.
tinted s.
wire frame s.
spectacular image
spectra (*pl. of* spectrum)
Spectralite Transitions lens
spectral sensitivity
Spectra-Pritchard 1980-PR photometer
spectrocolorimeter
Spectronic GENESYS 5 spectrophotometer
spectrophotometer
Spectronic GENESYS 5 s.
spectroscopy
H-magnetic resonance s.
magnetic resonance s. (MRS)
noncontact photo-acoustic s. (NC-PAS)
spectrum, pl. **spectra, spectrums**
chromatic s.
color s.
S. color vision meter 712 anomaloscope
electromagnetic s.
facioauriculovertebral s.
fortification s.
S. Lens Analysis System
ocular s.
Raman s.
visible s.

S

NOTES

specula (*pl. of* speculum)
specular
    s. attachment
    s. glare
    s. image
    s. microscope
    s. microscopy
    s. reflection
    s. reflection video-recording system
specularity
Specular reflex slit lamp
speculum, pl. **specula**
    Alfonso pediatric eyelid s.
    aspirating lid s.
    Azar lid s.
    Barraquer-Colibri s.
    Barraquer eye s.
    Barraquer wire s.
    basket-style scleral supporter s.
    Becker-Park s.
    Bercovici wire lid s.
    Berens s.
    Bronson-Park s.
    Brown interchangeable lid s.
    Burch-Lester s.
    Cantera-Olivieri CB s.
    Cantera-Olivieri Hansa s.
    Carpel s.
    Castallo s.
    Castroviejo s.
    Clark s.
    Cook s.
    Culler s.
    Douvas-Barraquer s.
    eye s.
    eyelid s.
    Fanta s.
    fine-wire s.
    Floyd-Barraquer wire s.
    Fox s.
    Gaffee s.
    Ginsberg eye s.
    Grandon eye s.
    Guell type LASIK s.
    Guist s.
    Guist-Bloch s.
    Guyton-Maumenee s.
    Guyton-Park eye s.
    Guyton-Park lid s.
    Hansa s.
    Hirschman s.
    Iliff-Park s.
    Jaffe lid s.
    Kaiser s.
    Kammann adjustable aspirating s.
    Katena s.
    Keeler-Pierse eye s.
    Keizer-Lancaster eye s.
    Kershner reversible eyelid s.

Knapp-Culler s.
Knapp eye s.
Knolle lens s.
Kratz aspirating s.
Kratz-Barraquer wire eye s.
Lancaster eye s.
Lancaster lid s.
Lancaster-O'Connor s.
Lang s.
Lester-Burch s.
lid s.
LidFix s.
Lieberman aspirating s.
Lieberman K-Wire s.
Lindstrom-Chu aspirating s.
Machat adjustable aspirating
  wire s.
Machat-type adjustable aspirating
  LASIK s.
Manche LASIK s.
Maumenee-Park eye s.
McKee s.
McKinney eye s.
McPherson s.
Mellinger s.
Metcher s.
Moria one-piece s.
Mueller s.
Murdock eye s.
Murdock-Wiener eye s.
Murdoon eye s.
nasal s.
Omni-Park s.
Pannu-Kratz-Barraquer s.
Park s.
Park-Guyton s.
Park-Guyton-Callahan s.
Park-Guyton-Maumenee s.
Park-Maumenee s.
Paton single s.
Paton transplant s.
pediatric lid s.
Pierse eye s.
reversible lid s.
Sauer infant s.
Schott lid s.
Seibel 3-D s.
Serdarevic s.
Simcoe wire s.
Slade-type adjustable aspirating
  LASIK s.
Smith s.
stop s.
Sutherland-Grieshaber s.
Weeks s.
Weiss s.
Wiener s.
Williams pediatric eye s.
wire lid s.

Ziegler s.
Zirm LASIK aspiration s.
Speedy-1 Auto refractometer
Spencer
    S. chalazion forceps
    S. eye suture scissors
    S. silicone subimplant
Spencer-Watson
    S.-W. Z-plasty
    S.-W. Z-plasty operation
Spero forceps
sph.
    sphere
    spherical
sphenocavernous syndrome
sphenoccipital fissure
sphenofrontal suture
sphenoid
    s. bone
    s. door jamb
    s. fissure
    greater wing of s.
    lesser wing of s.
    s. sinus
    s. wing meningioma
sphenoidal fissure
sphenoidalis
    ala minor ossis s.
    foramen s.
sphenomaxillary fissure
sphenoorbital suture
sphenopalatine ganglion
sphenorbital
sphere (sph.)
    Carter s.
    diopter s. (DS)
    Doherty s.
    s. end point
    s. implant
    s. introducer
    method of the s.
    Morgagni s.
    Mules vitreous s.
    porous hydroxyapatite s.
    Pyrex eye s.
    silicone eye s.
spherical (sph.)
    s. cornea
    s. equivalent (Deq)
    s. equivalent lens
    s. implant
    s. lens aberration

    s. refraction
    s. refractive error
    S. Twirl
spherocylinder
spherocylindrical lens
spherocylindric lens
spheroidal keratopathy
spheroid degeneration
spherometer
spherophakia
spherophakia-brachymorphia syndrome
spheroprism
sphincter
    s. erosion
    s. fiber
    s. iridis
    iris s.
    s. muscle
    s. muscle of pupil
    s. oculi
    s. oris
    s. pupillae
    s. tear
sphincteric
sphincterismus
sphincteritis
sphincterolysis
sphincterotomy
spider
    s. angioma
    s. telangiectasia
    s. vasculature
Spielmeyer-Sjögren disease
Spielmeyer-Stock disease
Spielmeyer-Vogt
    S.-V. disease
    S.-V. syndrome
spike
    blue s.
    intraocular pressure s.
    retinal s.
spillover cell
spinal
    s. canal tumor
    s. miosis
    s. mydriasis
spina trochlearis
spin-cast
    s.-c. lens
    s.-c. process
spindle
    s. A, B melanoma

S

NOTES

spindle *(continued)*
    Axenfeld-Krukenberg s.
    cataract s.
    s. cataract
    s. cell
    s. cell melanoma
    Krukenberg corneal s.
    Krukenberg pigment s.
spindle-cell tumor
spindle-shaped
    s.-s. area
    s.-s. cell
spinocerebellar
    s. ataxia
    s. degeneration
spiral
    s. field
    Tillaux s.
    s. of Tillaux
spiralis
    Trichinella s.
spiramycin
Spitz nevus
Spivack axis marker
Spizziri cannula knife
SPK
    superficial punctate keratitis
SPKT
    superficial punctate keratitis of Thygeson
splaytooth forceps
splenic retinitis
splenium of corpus callosum
splinter disk hemorrhage
split-beam photographic technique
split-calvarial bone graft
split fixation
splitter
    beam s.
    Brierley nucleus s.
    Goldberg side-port s.
    Koch-Salz nucleus s.
    Kraff nucleus s.
    Rosen phaco s.
    Salz nucleus s.
    Sharvelle side-port s.
    Wan side-port nucleus s.
split-thickness autograft
splitting
    foveal s.
    s. of lacrimal papilla
    s. lacrimal papilla operation
    macular s.
    Minsky intramarginal s.
    stromal s.
SP-MS
    secondary progressive multiple sclerosis
spoke-like sutural cataract
spondylitis
    ankylosing s.

sponge
    cellulose surgical s.
    Custodis s.
    s. explant
    Fuller silicone s.
    grooved silicone s.
    s. implant
    implant s.
    Krukenberg s.
    lens s.
    Lincoff lens s.
    lint-free s.
    Masciuli silicone s.
    Merocel lint-free s.
    Microsponge Teardrop s.
    ophthalmic s.
    Packer tunnel silicone s.
    Pro-Ophtha s.
    radial s.
    soft silicone s.
    Vaiser s.
    VersaTool eye s.
    Visi-Spear eye s.
    vitrectomy s.
    Weck s.
    Weck-cel s.
spongy
    s. appearance
    s. iritis
spontaneous
    s. congenital iris cyst
    s. ectopia lentis
    s. extrusion of lens
    s. extrusion of vitreous
    s. eye blink rate (SEBR)
    s. eyelid retraction
    s. hyphema
    s. intracranial hypotension
    s. peeling
    s. resorption
    s. retinal venous pulsation
    s. retrobulbar hemorrhage
spoon
    Alfonso-McIntyre nucleus s.
    s. blade
    Bunge evisceration s.
    Castroviejo lens s.
    cataract s.
    Culler lens s.
    Cutler lens s.
    Daviel lens s.
    Elschnig s.
    enucleation s.
    evisceration s.
    Fisher s.
    graft carrier s.
    Hess s.
    Kalt s.
    Kirby intracapsular lens s.

Knapp lens s.
s. knife
LASIK aspiration s.
lens s.
needle s.
s. needle
Rizzuti graft carrier s.
Schepens s.
spatula s.
s. spatula
Wehner s.
Wells enucleation s.
sporadic aniridia
sporangium, pl. **sporangia**
Sporanox
Sporothrix schenckii
sporotrichosis
conjunctival s.
spot
acoustic s.
ash leaf s.
baring of blind s.
bear track s.'s
birdshot s.
Bitot s.
blank s.
blind s.
blue s.
blur s.
Brushfield s.
cherry-red s.
chorioretinal atrophic s.
cluster of pigmented s.'s
corneal s.
cotton-wool s. (CWS)
cribriform s.
depigmented s.
dry s.
Elschnig s.
eye s.
flame s.
Förster-Fuchs black s.
Fuchs black s.
Gaule s.
histo s.
Horner-Trantas s.
hot s.
iridescent s.
Lisch s.
Mariotte blind s.
Maurer s.
Maxwell s.

mongolian s.
opacification cherry-red s.
peripheral chorioretinal atrophic s.
physiologic blind s.
retinal blur s.
s. retinoscope
Roth s.
rust s.
Siegrist s.
s. size
sky-blue s.
Soemmering s.
Tay cherry-red s.
white s.
Wies s.
Wölfflin-Krückmann s.
yellow s. (YS)
spotty corneal opacity
SPP
standard pseudoisochromatic plate
SPP color deficiency testing
product
Spratt mastoid curette
spray
Sensitive Eyes Sterile Saline S.
spread
s. function
illusory visual s.
pagetoid s.
visual s.
spreader
Athens suture s.
conjunctiva s.
Costenbader incision s.
Frederick sleeve s.
Gill incision s.
incision s.
Kwitko conjunctival s.
Suarez s.
Wilder band s.
spring
s. catarrh
S. Clip Opticaid
s. conjunctivitis
S. iris scissors
s. ophthalmia
s. pupil
spring-hinge temple
springing mydriasis
springtime conjunctivitis
spud
Alvis foreign body s.

S

NOTES

spud *(continued)*
    Bahn s.
    Corbett s.
    curved needle eye s.
    Davis s.
    Dix foreign body s.
    Ellis foreign body s.
    eye s.
    Fisher s.
    flat eye s.
    foreign body s.
    Francis s.
    Goldstein golf-club s.
    golf-club eye s.
    s. and gouge
    gouge s.
    Hosford s.
    LaForce knife s.
    Levine s.
    needle s.
    s. needle
    O'Brien s.
    Plange s.
    Storz folding-handle eye s.
    s. tool
    Walter s.
    Walton s.

spur
    corneoscleral s.
    Fuchs s.
    Grunert s.
    Michel s.
    scleral s. (SS)

spuria
    polycoria s.

spurious cataract

Sputnik Russian razor blade

Squalamine lactate

squamosa
    blepharitis s.

squamous
    s. cell
    s. cell carcinoma
    s. cell carcinoma of eyelid
    s. metaplasia
    s. papilloma
    s. seborrheic blepharitis

square
    s. prism
    s. pupil

square-wave
    s.-w. jerks
    s.-w. pulse

squashed-tomato appearance

squeegee capsule polisher

Squid instrument/apparatus

squint
    accommodative s.
    s. angle
    angle of s.
    comitant s.
    convergent s.
    s. deviation
    divergent s.
    downward s.
    Duane classification of s.
    external s.
    s. hook
    internal s.
    latent s.
    noncomitant s.
    upward s.

squinting eye

squirrel plague conjunctivitis

SR
    superior rectus
        Ocufit SR

SRF
    subretinal fluid

SRI
    surface regularity index

SR-IV Programmed Subjective refractor

SRK
    Sanders-Retzlaff-Kraff
        SRK formula

SRM
    subretinal membrane

SRNV
    subretinal neovascularization

SRNVM
    subretinal neovascular membrane

SRP
    surgical reversal of presbyopia

^{90}Sr-plaque irradiation

SRT
    Sorbinil Retinopathy Trial
    stereotactic radiation therapy

SS
    scleral spur

SSDLP
    subthreshold subfoveal diode laser
      photocoagulation

S-shaped deformity

SST
    Submacular Surgery Trials

ST
    esotropia

Staar
    S. AA 4207 lens
    S. Aquaflow technique
    S. implantable contact lens
    S. intraocular lens
    S. toric IOL
    S. toric lens
    S. 4203VF lens
    S. 4207VF lens

stab
    s. incision
    s. incision angled blade
stability
    tear film s.
stabilization
    dynamic s.
stabilizer
    mast cell s.
    Stamler corneal transplant s.
    Steinert suction globe s.
Stableflex anterior chamber lens
stable vision
Stahl
    S. caliper block
    S. caliper plate
    S. calipers
    S. lens gauge
    S. nucleus expressor
Stähli pigment line
stain
    acid-fast s.
    calcein-AM s.
    calcofluor white s.
    Diff-Quick s.
    direct fluorescent antibody s.
    ethidium homodimer s.
    fluorescein s.
    Giemsa s.
    Gomori methenamine silver s.
    lissamine green s.
    Live/Dead Kit s.
    Masson trichrome s.
    PAS s.
    rose bengal s.
    VisionBlue trypan blue 0.06% s.
staining
    arc s.
    arcuate s.
    blood s.
    blotchy positive s.
    bright s.
    coarse punctate s.
    conjunctival s.
    corneal stromal blood s.
    fluorescein s.
    focal s.
    immunofluorescent s.
    immunoperoxidase s.
    s. pattern
    punctate s.
    in situ DNA nick end-labeling s.

    stippling and s.
    three o'clock s.
    TUNEL s.
stalk
    optic s.
Stallard
    S. eyelid operation
    S. flap operation
Stallard-Liegard
    S.-L. operation
    S.-L. suture
Stamler
    S. corneal transplant stabilizer
    S. side-port fixation hook
stand
    s. magnifier
    Mayo s.
standard
    American National Standards
      Institute s.
    ANSI s.
    s. automated perimetry (SAP)
    s. deviation (SD)
    s. near card
    s. notation
    s. pseudoisochromatic plate (SPP)
    s. pseudoisochromatic plates color
      deficiency testing product
    s. pseudoisochromatic plates part 2
    s. thickness
stand-off
    edge s.-o.
Stanford Achievement Test Series
Stangel modified Barraquer
  microsurgical needle holder
staphylococcal
    s. allergic keratoconjunctivitis
    s. blepharitis
    s. blepharoconjunctivitis
    s. conjunctivitis
    s. hypersensitivity
Staphylococcus
    S. aureus
    S. epidermidis
    S. epidermis
    S. haemolyticus
    S. hominis
    S. hyicus
    S. intermedius
    S. lugdunensis
    S. saprophyticus
    S. schleiferi

NOTES

Staphylococcus (continued)
    S. simulans
    S. warneri
staphyloma
    anterior corneal s.
    anular s.
    ciliary s.
    congenital anterior s. (CAS)
    s. corneae racemosum
    corneal s.
    equatorial s.
    intercalary s.
    peripapillary s.
    posterior s.
    s. posticum
    projecting s.
    retinal s.
    Scarpa s.
    scleral s.
    uveal s.
staphylomatous
staphylotomy
STAR
    S. S4 ActiveTrak 3-D eye tracking system
    S. S3 ActiveTrak excimer laser system
    S. S4 excimer laser system
    S. S2 SmoothScan excimer laser system
star
    epicapsular lens s.
    S. excimer laser
    s. fold
    s. lens
    lens s.
    Lindstrom S.
    macular s.
    VISX S.
    Winslow s.
stare
    hyperthyroid s.
    postbasic s.
    thyroid s.
Stargardt
    S. and Best disease
    S. dystrophy
    S. maculopathy
    S. syndrome
Star-Optic eye wash
Starr fixation forceps
star-shaped field
starter
    Brown pocket s.
startle myoclonus
stasis, pl. **stases**
    axoplasmic s.
    papillary s.
    venous s.

Stat
    S. aspirator
    S. Scrub handwasher machine
state
    deturgescent s.
    refractive s.
state-of-the-art aberrometer
static
    s. accommodation insufficiency
    s. countertorsion
    s. perimeter
    s. perimetry
    s. refraction
    s. retinoscopy
stationary
    s. cataract
    s. night blindness
statometer
Statpac-like Analysis for Glaucoma Evaluation (SAGE)
Statpac test
Statrol
Stay-Brite
Stay-Wet 3
steady-state accommodation
steal syndrome
Stealth
    S. DBO diamond blade
    S. DBO free-hand diamond knife
Steclin
steel
    Newsom cracker model 8-07116 in stainless s.
Steele-Richardson-Olszewski
    S.-R.-O. disease
    S.-R.-O. syndrome
steep
    s. axis
    s. contact lens
steepening
    corneal s.
    inferior s.
    videokeratographic corneal s.
steepest meridian
steerable I/A
Stefan law
Steiger curve
Steinbrinck anomaly
Steinert
    S. disease
    S. double-ended claw chopper
    S. double-ended LASIK spatula
    S. II claw chopper
    S. LASIK set
    S. suction globe stabilizer
Steinert-Deacon incision gauge
Steinhauser electromucotome

stella
  s. lentis hyaloidea
  s. lentis iridica
stellata
  retinitis s.
stellate
  s. cataract
  s. keratitis
  s. retinopathy
Stellwag
  S. brawny edema
  S. sign
  S. symptom
stem
  brain s.
  s. cell (SC)
  s. palsy
stenochoria
stenocoriasis
stenon duct
stenopeic, stenopaic
  s. disk
  s. iridectomy
  s. spectacles
stenosis
  aqueductal s.
  s. canaliculus
  carotid artery s.
  hemodynamically significant carotid
    artery s. (HSCAS)
  involutional s.
  lacrimal punctal s.
  punctal s.
  punctum s.
Stenotrophomonas maltophilia
Stenstrom ocular measurement
stent
  lacrimal s.
  Supramid occluding s.
STENTube lacrimal intubation set
step
  ComfortCare GP One S.
  corneal graft s.
  s. graft operation
  nasal s.
  Ronne nasal s.
Stephenson needle holder
Stephens soft IOL-inserting forceps
Step-Knife diamond blade knife
stepwise
  s. fashion
  s. variable selection

Sterane
stereo
  s. optic disc photograph
  s. reindeer test
  s. x-ray
stereoacuity
  variable distance s. (VDS)
stereocampimeter
  Lloyd s.
stereognostic sense
stereogram
  random-dot s. (RDS)
stereo-identical point
stereometric parameter
stereo ophthalmoscope
stereooptic disk diapositive
stereo orthopter
stereophantoscope
stereophorometer
stereophoroscope
stereophotography
stereopsis
  coarse s.
  Gross s.
  macular s.
  s. test
stereoscope
stereoscopic
  s. acuity
  s. diplopia
  s. fundus photograph
  s. imaging
  s. parallax
  s. vision
stereoscopy
stereotactic radiation therapy (SRT)
stereotest
  Lang s.
stereoviewer
  Donaldson s.
Steri-Drape
  S.-D. drape
  3M small aperture S.-D.
  small aperture S.-D.
sterile
  s. acetazolamide sodium
  s. adhesive bubble dressing
  s. calcium alginate swab
  s. corneal ulcer
  s. endophthalmitis
  s. hypopyon
  s. indocyanine green kit

S

NOTES

sterile *(continued)*
    s. melt
    S. Preserved Daily Cleaner
    S. Preserved Saline
sterility of solution
sterilizer
    Cox rapid dry heat transfer s.
    s. monitoring service
Steriseal disposable cannula
Steritome microkeratome system
Stern-Castroviejo
    S.-C. locking forceps
    S.-C. suturing forceps
Sterofrin
    Isopto S.
steroid
    s. concentration
    s. diabetes
    s. glaucoma
    s. therapy
steroid-induced
    s.-i. cataract
    s.-i. glaucoma
steroidogenic diabetes
Stevens
    S. eye scissors
    S. iris forceps
    S. muscle hook retractor
    S. needle holder
    S. tenotomy hook
    S. tenotomy scissors
Stevens-Charles sleeve
Stevens-Johnson syndrome
Stevenson
    S. lacrimal sac retractor
    S. refractor
stibogluconate sodium
stick
    fluorescein s.
    needle s.
    Pro-Ophtha s.
Stickler syndrome
sties (*pl. of* sty)
Stifel figure
stiff
    s. pupil
    s. retina
    s. retinal fold
stigma
    Koplik s.
stigmatic
    s. image
    s. lens
stigmatometer
stigmatometric test card
stigmatoscope
stigmatoscopy
Stiles-Crawford effect

stiletto
    Berkeley Bioengineering s.
    Blair s.
    s. knife
stillicidium lacrimarum
Stilling
    canal of S.
    S. color table
    S. color test
    S. plate
Stilling-Turk-Duane syndrome
Stimson sign
stimulator
    CAM vision s.
    optokinetic s.
stimulatory antibody
stimulus, pl. **stimuli**
    accommodative s.
    auditory s.
    blue flash s.
    body-referenced s.
    bright-white flash s.
    s. deprivation
    eye-referenced s.
    flash s.
    flicker fusion s.
    light s.
    optokinetic s.
    proprioceptive s.
    red flash s.
    retinotopic s.
    scotopic s.
    spatiotopic s.
    Vernier s.
stippled
    s. hyperfluorescence
    s. pattern
stippling and staining
stitch
    bow-tie s.
    cuticular s.
    shoelace s.
    triple-throw square knot s.
    s. with twists
    zipper s.
stitch-removal forceps
stitch-removing knife
St. Martin-Franceschetti cataract hook
Stocker
    S. line
    S. needle
    S. operation
Stocker-Holt dystrophy
Stocker-Holt-Schneider dystrophy
Stock operation
Stock-Spielmeyer-Vogt syndrome
Stokes lens
Stolte
    S. capsulorrhexis forceps

S. prechopper, angled handle
S. prechopper, straight handle
stone
S. implant
tear s.
Stone-Jordan implant
stony-hard eye
stop
Bowman needle s.
Castroviejo corneal scissors with inside s.
s. speculum
stop-and-chop phacoemulsification technique
storage
Opti-Free Rinsing Disinfecting and S.
Storz
S. band
S. calipers
S. capsule forceps
S. CAPSULORBLUE intraocular lens
S. cataract knife
S. cilia forceps
S. corneal bur
S. corneal forceps
S. corneal trephine
S. corneoscleral punch
S. DiaPhine trephine
S. folding-handle eye spud
S. handle
S. handpiece
S. keratome
S. keratometer
S. lid plate
S. microscope
S. MicroSeal
S. Microvit magnet
S. Microvit vitrector
S. Millennium microsurgical system
S. Premiere Microvit
S. radial incision marker
S. tonometer
Storz-Atlas hand eye magnet
Storz-Bell erysiphake
Storz-Bonn suturing forceps
Storz-Duredge steel cataract knife
Storzine
Storz-Utrata forceps
Storz-Walker retinal detachment unit
Storz-Westcott conjunctival scissors

Stoxil
strabismal
s. amblyopia
s. deviation
s. nystagmus
strabismic amblyopia
strabismometer
strabismus
absolute s.
accommodative s.
alternate day s.
alternating s.
American Association of Pediatric Ophthalmology and S. (AAPOS)
anatomic s.
A-pattern s.
Bielschowsky s.
bilateral s.
binocular s.
Braid s.
cicatricial s.
comitant s.
concomitant s.
constant s.
convergent s.
cyclic s.
s. deorsum vergens
s. divergence
divergent s.
dynamic s.
external s.
s. fixus
s. forceps
Graves s.
s. hook
horizontal s.
incomitant vertical s.
intermittent s.
internal s.
kinetic s.
latent s.
manifest s.
mechanical s.
mixed s.
monocular s.
monolateral s.
muscular s.
noncomitant s.
nonconcomitant s.
nonparalytic s.
paralytic s.
periodic s.

NOTES

S

strabismus *(continued)*
    relative s.
    s. scissors
    secondary s.
    spasmodic s.
    suppressed s.
    s. surgery
    s. sursum vergens
    unilateral s.
    uniocular s.
    variable s.
    vertical s.
strabometer
strabometry
strabotome
strabotomy
Strachan
    S. disease
    S. syndrome
Strachan-Scott syndrome
straight
    s. mosquito clamp
    s. retinal probe
    s. temple
    s. tenotomy scissors
    s. tying forceps
straight-eyed patient
straight-line bifocal
straight-tip bipolar forceps
strain
    eye s.
Straith eyelid operation
Strampelli
    S. lens
    S. lens implant
Strampelli-Valvo operation
strand
    fibrin s.
    glassine s.
    iris s.
    lysis of restricting s.
    mucin s.
    mucous-like s.
    mucus s.
    restricting s.
    stromal s.
    vitreous s.
strap
    Velcro head s.
stratified squamous epithelium
stratum cerebrale retinae
Straus curved retrobulbar needle
strawberry
    s. hemangioma
    s. nevus
straylight meter
streak
    angioid retinal s.
    angiosis s.

    hypofluorescent s.
    Knapp s.
    lightning s.
    Moore lightning s.
    s. retinoscope
    s. retinoscopy
    Sieger s.
    Siegrist s.
    Verhoeff s.
stream
    Eye S.
Streatfield-Fox operation
Streatfield operation
Streatfield-Snellen operation
strength
    orbicularis s.
strephosymbolia
streptococcal
    s. bacillus
    s. blepharitis
Streptococcus
    S. faecalis
    group B *S.*
    S. pneumococcus
    S. pneumoniae
    S. pyogenes
    S. viridans
streptokinase
Streptomyces
    S. caespitosus
    S. tsukubaensis
stress
    hypoxic corneal s.
stretching
    pupil s.
stretch reflex
stria, pl. **striae**
    striae ciliaris
    concentric s.
    corneal s.
    Haab s.
    Knapp s.
    striae retinae
    vertical s.
    Vogt s.
striascope
striatal nigral degeneration
striate
    s. keratitis
    s. keratopathy
    s. melanokeratosis
    s. opacity
    s. retinitis
    s. visual cortex
striated glasses
striation
    retinal s.
stringy mucus

strip
  Color Bar Schirmer s.
  DET fluorescein s.
  EyeClose Adhesive s.
  Fluorets fluorescein sodium s.'s
  Ful-Glo fluorescein s.
  gliotic s.
  Lacrytest s.'s
  marginal tear s.
  s. procedure
  reagent s.
  Schirmer tear test s.
  silicone s.
  tear test s.
stripe
  central reflex s.
stripper
  Crawford fascial s.
  fascia lata s.
  zonular s.
  zonule s.
stripping
  cortical s.
  s. membrane
stroboscopic disk
stroke-like episode
stroma, pl. **stromata**
  avascular corneal s.
  corneal s.
  iris s.
  s. of iris
  limbal s.
  perilimbal s.
  pigmented s.
  s. plexus
  sclerotic s.
  vitreous s.
  s. vitreum
stromal
  s. anular infiltrate
  s. bed
  s. blood vessel
  s. corneal dystrophy
  s. derma
  s. disease
  s. downgrowth
  s. ectasia
  s. edema
  s. ghost scarring
  s. haze
  s. hydration
  s. ingrowth

  s. keratitis
  s. keratouveitis
  s. line
  s. matrix
  s. melt
  s. melting
  s. necrosis
  s. neovascularization
  s. opacity
  s. photoablation
  s. pocket
  s. ring infiltrate
  s. splitting
  s. strand
  s. thickness
  s. thinning
  s. ulcer
  s. vascularization
  s. wound healing
Stromberg curve
Strow corneal forceps
Struble lid everter
structure
  S. And Function Evaluation
    (SAFE)
  angle s.
  Kolmer crystalloid s.
  snake-like s.
strumous ophthalmia
strut
  optic s.
Stryker
  S. frame
  S. saw
STTOdx ophthalmic surgery system
Student unpaired *t*-test
study
  Advanced Glaucoma Intervention S.
    (AGIS)
  Age-Related Eye Disease S.
    (AREDS)
  Amblyopia Treatment S.
  Beaver Dam Eye S.
  Blue Mountain Eye S.
  Branch Vein Occlusion S.
  case-control s.
  Central Vein Occlusion S. (CVOS)
  CLAMP S.
  CLEERE S.
  CLEK S.
  cohort s.

NOTES

study *(continued)*
    Collaborative Corneal
      Transplantation S.'s (CCTS)
    Collaborative Initial Glaucoma
      Treatment S. (CIGTS)
    Collaborative Longitudinal
      Evaluation of Keratoconus S.
    Collaborative Normal Tension
      Glaucoma S. (CNTGS)
    Collaborative Ocular Melanoma S.
      (COMS)
    Congenital Esotropia
      Observational S. (CEOS)
    Contact Lens and Myopia
      Progression S.
    Controlled High Risk Subjects
      Avonex Multiple Sclerosis
      Prevention S. (CHAMPS)
    Cooperative Ocular Melanoma S.
      (COMS)
    Cornea Donor S. (CDS)
    Cytomegalovirus Retinitis and Viral
      Resistance S. (CRVRS)
    Diabetic Retinopathy Vitrectomy S.
      (DRVS)
    double-blind s.
    Early Treatment Diabetic
      Retinopathy S. (ETDRS)
    Early Treatment for Retinopathy of
      Prematurity S. (ETROP)
    Egna-Neumarkt S.
    Endophthalmitis Vitrectomy S.
      (EVS)
    Fluorouracil Filtering Surgery S.
      (FFSS)
    Glaucoma Laser Trial Followup S.
      (GLTFS)
    Herpetic Eye Disease S.
    Herpetic Eye Disease S. I
      (HEDS1)
    Herpetic Eye Disease S. II
      (HEDS2)
    Infant Aphakia Treatment S.
    Krypton-Argon Regression of
      Neovascularization S. (KARNS)
    Lens Opacities Case-Control S.
    Longitudinal Optic Neuritis S.
      (LONS)
    long-term comparative s.
    Macular Photocoagulation S. (MPS)
    NEI Visual Acuity Impairment
      Survey s.
    S.'s of the Ocular Complications
      in AIDS (SOCA)
    Ocular Hypertension Treatment S.
      (OHTS)
    PERK S.
    Prism Adaptation S. (PAS)
    prospective s.

    Prospective Evaluation of Radial
      Keratotomy S.
    retrospective s.
    SAFE s.
    Temba glaucoma s.
    The Berkeley Orthokeratology S.
    The Silicone S.
    vectographic s.
    VIP S.
    Vision in Preschoolers S.
    Vitrectomy for Macular Hole S.
      (VMHS)
Sturge-Weber
    S.-W. disease
    S.-W. encephalotrigeminal
      angiomatosis
    S.-W. Syndrome
    S.-W. syndrome
Sturge-Weber-Dimitri syndrome
Sturm
    conoid of S.
    interval of S.
    S. interval
stutzeri
    Pseudomonas s.
sty, stye, pl. **sties, styes**
    meibomian s.
    S. Ophthalmic Ointment
    zeisian s.
Style S2 clear-loop lens
styrene contact lens
Suarez spreader
Suarez-Villafranca operation
sub-2 incision
subacute
    s. myelooptic neuropathy (SMON)
    s. necrotizing encephalomyelopathy
    s. sclerosing panencephalitis
subarachnoid
    s. bleed
    s. fluid
    s. hemorrhage
    s. oculomotor nerve lesion
    s. oculomotor nerve palsy
    s. space
subcapsular
    s. cataract
    s. epithelium
    s. plaque
subchoroidal hemorrhage
subciliary incision
subclinical
    s. diabetes
    s. optic neuritis
Subco needle
subconjunctival (SC)
    s. antibiotic
    s. cyst
    s. edema

s. emphysema
s. foreign body
s. hemorrhage
s. injection
s. needle
subconjunctivitis
subcontinent
laryngeal and ocular granulation tissue in children from the Indian s. (LOGIC)
subcortical alexia
subcutaneous
s. amyloid
s. fat atrophy
subduction
subdural hematoma
subepidermal calcified nodule
subepithelial
s. corneal haze
s. corneal opacity
s. fibrosis
s. keratitis
s. nevus
s. opacification
s. plaque
s. plexus
s. punctate corneal infiltrate
subepithelialis
keratitis punctata s.
subfoveal
s. choroidal neovascularization
s. mass
s. neovascular membrane
subhyaloid
s. blood
s. hemorrhage
subimplant
Spencer silicone s.
subinternal limiting membrane hemorrhage
subject
healthy s.
subjective
S. Autorefractor-7
s. device
s. prism-neutralized cover test
s. refraction test
s. refractor
s. testing
s. vertigo
s. vision
subjectoscope

sublatio retinae
subluxated lens
subluxation of lens
subluxed lens
submacular
s. surgery
S. Surgery Trials (SST)
submembrane fluid
subnormal
s. accommodation
s. vision
suboccipital craniectomy
suboptimal vision
suborbicularis
s. oculi fat (SOOF)
s. oculi fat lift
suborbital
subperiosteal
s. abscess
s. implant
subpigment epithelial space
subretinal
s. aspiration cannula
s. fluid (SRF)
s. fluid cuff
s. fluid drainage
s. hemorrhage
s. mass
s. membrane (SRM)
s. neovascularization (SRNV)
s. neovascular membrane (SRNVM)
s. pigment ring
s. scarring
s. space
subscleral
subsclerotic
substance
corneal s.
s. exophthalmos
exophthalmos-producing s. (EPS)
s. of lens
s. P
scleral s.
toxic s.
substantia
s. corticalis lentis
s. propria
s. propria corneae
s. propria sclerae
sub-Tenon
s.-T. anesthesia cannula
s.-T. corticosteroid injection

S

NOTES

sub-Tenon *(continued)*
s.-T. depot
s.-T. parabulbar anesthesia
subterminale
Clostridium s.
subthreshold subfoveal diode laser photocoagulation (SSDLP)
subtilis
Bacillus s.
subtotal thyroidectomy
subtraction topography
subvolution
success
anatomic s.
successive contrast
succulent vessel
succus cineraria Maritima
suction
s. ophthalmodynamometer
perilimbal s.
s. ring
s. trephine
Vactro perilimbal s.
sudden visual loss
sudoriferous cyst
sugar cataract
sugar-induced cataract
sugar-loaf cornea
Sugiura sign
suis
Brucella s.
Suker sign
Sulamyd
Sodium S.
sulbactam
sulcus, pl. **sulci**
chiasmal s.
ciliary s.
corneoscleral s.
s. fixated position
s. fixation
s. infraorbitalis maxillae
infrapalpebral s.
s. infrapalpebralis
intramarginal s.
iridociliary s.
lacrimal s.
optic s.
orbital s.
s. orbitales lobi frontalis
s. sclera
scleral s.
sclerocorneal s.
superior tarsal s.
s. support
supraorbital s.
Sulfacel 15
sulfacetamide
s. phenylephrine

s. and prednisolone
s. sodium
s. sodium and fluorometholone
sulfadiazine
sulfa drug
Sulfair
S. 10
S. Forte
sulfamethoxazole
Sulfamide
sulfanilamide
Sulfasuxidine
sulfate
alkyl ether s.
atropine s.
chondroitin s.
dermatan s.
dimethyl s.
eserine s.
ferrous s.
gentamicin s.
hydroxychloroquine s.
indinavir s.
keratan s.
neomycin s.
phenelzine s.
physostigmine s.
polymyxin B s.
quinine s.
saquinavir s.
sodium hyaluronate and chondroitin s.
sodium lauryl s.
tranylcypromine s.
zinc s.
sulfisoxazole diolamine
sulfonamide
Sulf-10 Ophthalmic
sulfur
s. gas
s. hexafluoride (SF6)
sulfurhexafluoride gas
Sulphrin
Sulpred
Sulster Solution
Sulten-10
summation
spatial s.
Summerskill
S. operation
S. sign
Summit
S. Apex Plus excimer laser
S. Krumeich-Barraquer microkeratome (SKBM)
S. OmniMed excimer laser
S. SVS Apex laser
S. UV 200 Excimed laser
Sumycin

sunburst
  black s.
  s. dial
  s. dial chart
  s. effect
sunburst-type lesion
sunflower cataract
sunglasses
  Costa Del Mar MP2 s.
Sung reverse nucleus chopper
sunrise
  S. LTK system
  s. syndrome
sunset
  s. fundus
  s. syndrome
Super
  S. Field NC slit lamp lens
  S. Pinky ball
  S. punctum plug
Superblade
  Bishop-Harman S.
  S. No. 75 blade
supercilia (*pl. of* supercilium)
superciliaris
  arcus s.
superciliary
  s. arch
  s. muscle
supercilii
  musculus corrugator s.
  musculus depressor s.
supercilium, pl. **supercilia**
superduction
superficial
  s. congestion
  s. corneal line
  s. lamellar keratectomy
  s. lamellar limbo keratoplasty
  s. linear keratitis
  s. line of cornea
  s. punctate keratitis (SPK)
  s. punctate keratitis of Thygeson
  (SPKT)
  s. punctate keratopathy
  s. reticular degeneration of Koby
  s. retinal refractile deposit
superficialis
  keratitis ramificata s.
  xerosis s.

superimposed
  s. amblyopia
  s. ellipse
superinfection
  bacterial s.
  corneal s.
superior
  s. arcuate bundle
  s. arcuate scotoma
  arcus palpebralis s.
  arteriola macularis s.
  arteriola nasalis retinae s.
  arteriola temporalis retinae s.
  s. canaliculus
  s. cervical ganglion
  s. colliculus
  s. commissura of Meynert
  s. conjunctival fornix
  s. cornea
  s. corneal shield ulcer
  s. division palsy
  s. eyelid crease
  fissura orbitalis s.
  s. gaze
  glandula lacrimalis s.
  s. homonymous quadrantic defect
  s. lacrimal gland
  s. limbic keratoconjunctivitis (SLK)
  s. macular arteriole
  musculus tarsalis s.
  s. nasal artery
  s. nasal vein
  s. oblique extraocular muscle
  s. oblique microtremor
  s. oblique muscle and trochlear
  luxation
  s. oblique myokymia
  s. oblique palsy
  s. oblique tack surgery
  s. oblique tendon
  s. oblique tendon sheath syndrome
  s. oblique transposition
  s. ophthalmic vein
  s. orbital fissure (SOF)
  s. orbital fissure syndrome
  s. orbital septum
  s. palpebral furrow
  s. palpebral vein
  s. pole
  s. polioencephalitis
  s. punctum
  s. quadrantanopsia

NOTES

superior *(continued)*
s. radial tenotomy scissors
s. rectus (SR)
s. rectus bridle suture
s. rectus extraocular muscle
s. rectus forceps
s. rim
s. salivary nucleus
s. sector iridectomy
s. tarsal muscle
s. tarsal papillary conjunctivitis
s. tarsal sulcus
s. tarsus
s. tarsus palpebrae
s. temporal artery
s. temporal vein
temporal venulae retina s.
s. tendon of Lockwood
s. vascular arcade
vena ophthalmica s.
venula macularis s.
venula nasalis retinae s.
venula temporalis retinae s.
s. zone of retina
superiores
venae palpebrales s.
superioris
levator palpebrae s.
musculus levator palpebrae s.
superoccipital
superonasal
s. macula
s. paracentral visual field
supertemporal bulbar conjunctiva
supertraction
conus s.
s. conus
supplement
antioxidant s.
ICaps TR dietary s.
MaculaRx Plus nutritional s.
MaxiVision dietary s.
Ocuvite Lutein Antioxidant S.
Supplemental Therapeutic Oxygen for Prethreshold Retinopathy of Prematurity
support
capsular s.
iris s.
Schillinger suture s.
sulcus s.
supporter
scleral s.
suppressant
aqueous s.
suppressed
s. amblyopia
s. strabismus

suppression
s. amblyopia
central s.
facultative s.
macular s.
obligatory s.
orbital fat s.
s. scotoma
suppressor T cell
suppurativa
hyalitis s.
suppurative
s. choroiditis
s. hyalitis
s. keratitis
s. retinitis
s. ulcer
SupraCAPS quarter-globe cap
suprachiasmatic nucleus (SCN)
suprachoroid
s. lamina
s. layer
suprachoroidal
s. hemorrhage (SCH, SH)
s. space
suprachoroidea
lamina s.
supraciliaris
epicanthus s.
supraciliary canal
Supraclens
Opti-Free S.
supraduction
SupraFOIL implant
Supramid
S. bridle collagen suture
S. lens implant
S. lens implant suture
S. occluding stent
S. sheet
S. sling
Supramid-Allen implant
supranuclear
s. cataract
s. control
s. deficiency
s. deviation
s. disorder
s. gaze center
s. input
s. lesion
s. ocular palsy
s. ophthalmoplegia
s. paresis of vertical gaze
s. pathway
supraocular
supraoptic
s. canal
s. commissure

supraorbital
  s. akinesia
  s. arch
  s. arch of frontal bone
  s. artery
  s. canal
  s. foramen
  s. incisure
  s. margin of frontal bone
  s. margin of orbit
  s. nerve
  s. neuralgia
  s. notch
  s. point
  s. reflex
  s. ridge
  s. sulcus
  s. vein
supraorbitale
  foramen s.
supraorbitalis
  incisura s.
  nervus s.
suprapineal recess
suprascleral
suprasellar
  s. aneurysm
  s. lesion
  s. meningioma
  s. tumor
8000 Supra Series auto refractometer
SupraSLEEVES nylon sleeve
supratemporally
supratentorial arteriovenous malformation
suprathreshold static perimetry
Supratome microkeratome
supratrochlear nerve
supravergence
supraversion
Suprax
suprofen
suramin sodium
Surefit AC 85J lens
SureSight autorefractor
Surevue contact lens
surface
  s. analgesia
  anterior corneal s.
  s. asymmetry index (SAI)
  s. breakdown
  concave reflecting s.

  convex reflecting s.
  curved reflecting s.
  s. dyslexia
  ellipsoidal back s.
  s. implant
  s. irregularity
  s. lamellar keratoplasty
  s. lubrication
  ocular s.
  Petzval s.
  s. photorefractive keratectomy
  reflecting s.
  s. regularity index (SRI)
  s. tension
  toric s.
  s. wrinkling retinopathy
Surgamid
surgeon
  American Board of Eye S.'s (ABES)
  American College of Eye S.'s (ACES)
  Fellow of the American College of S.'s (FACS)
  Fellow of the Royal College of S.'s (FRCS)
  vitreoretinal s.
surgery
  American Society of Cataract and Refractive S. (ASCRS)
  American Society of Ophthalmic Plastic and Reconstruction S.
  antiglaucoma s.
  artificial divergency s.
  asymmetric s.
  cataract s.
  ciliodestructive s.
  closed-eye s.
  corneal s.
  cranioorbital s.
  cyclophotocoagulation vitreoretinal s.
  decompression s.
  decompressive s.
  eyelid s.
  eye muscle s.
  eye plaque s.
  failed ptosis s.
  filtration s.
  fistulizing s.
  foldable intraocular lens s.
  glaucoma filtering s.
  glaucoma filtration s.

NOTES

surgery *(continued)*
    intraoperative adjustable suture s.
    keratorefractive s.
    lacrimal s.
    laser s.
    laser-filtering s.
    macular hole s.
    no-stitch phacoemulsification s.
    open globe s.
    orbital decompression s.
    periocular s.
    photorefractive s.
    refractive s.
    retinal s.
    scleral explant s.
    small-incision cataract s.
    strabismus s.
    submacular s.
    superior oblique tack s.
    sutureless cataract s.
    symmetric s.
    vitreous s.
Surg-E-Trol
    S.-E.-T. I/A System
    S.-E.-T. System irrigating/aspirating
      unit
surgical
    s. calipers
    s. caniculotomy
    s. decompression procedure
    S. Eye Expeditions (SEE)
    s. gut suture
    s. keratometry
    s. marking pen
    s. patch grafting
    s. reversal of presbyopia (SRP)
    s. treatment
surgically
    s. induced astigmatism
    s. induced refractive change
Surgicraft suture needle
Surgidev
    S. PC BUV 20-24 intraocular lens
    S. suture
Surgikos disposable drape
SurgiMed suture
SurgiScope
    Marco S.
Surgisol
Surgistar
    S. corneal trephine
    S. ophthalmic blade
Surodex
surplus field
sursumduction
    alternating s.
sursumvergence
    left s.
    right s.

sursumversion
survey
    Baltimore Eye S.
    Health and Activity Limitations S.
      (HALS)
    population-based cross-sectional s.
Susac syndrome
susceptibility kill rate
suspect
    glaucoma s.
suspension
    AK-Cide S.
    AK-Spore H.C. Ophthalmic S.
    AK-Trol S.
    Alrex ophthalmic s.
    brinzolamide ophthalmic s.
    Cortisporin Ophthalmic S.
    fluorometholone ophthalmic s.
    FML-S Ophthalmic S.
    frontalis fascia lata s.
    hydrocortisone s.
    Lotemax ophthalmic s.
    loteprednol etabonate ophthalmic s.
    Poly-Dex S.
    Poly-Pred Ophthalmic S.
    rimexolone ophthalmic s.
    Terra-Cortril Ophthalmic S.
    transconjunctival frontalis s.
    Vexol Ophthalmic S.
suspensory
    s. ligament
    s. ligament of eye
Sussman
    S. four-mirror gonioscope
    S. lens
sustained-release system
sustainer
    Akahoshi nucleus s.
sustentacular
    s. fiber
    s. tissue
Sutcliffe laser shield and retracting
  instrument
Sutherland
    S. lens
    S. rotatable microsurgery instrument
    S. scissors
Sutherland-Grieshaber
    S.-G. scissors
    S.-G. speculum
sutura
    s. ethmoidolacrimalis
    s. ethmoidomaxillaris
    s. frontolacrimalis
    s. infraorbitalis
    s. lacrimoconchalis
    s. lacrimomaxillaris
    s. palatoethmoidalis
    s. palatomaxillaris

sutural developmental cataract
suture
    absorbable s.
    adjustable s.
    s. adjustment
    Alcon s.
    anchor s.
    anchoring s.
    antitorque s.
    Arroyo encircling s.
    Arruga encircling s.
    Atraloc s.
    Axenfeld s.
    16-bite nylon s.
    black braided nylon s.
    black braided silk s.
    black silk bridle s.
    black silk sling s.
    Bondek s.
    braided silk s.
    braided Vicryl s.
    bridge s.
    bridle s.
    buried s.
    canaliculus rod and s.
    cardinal s.
    catgut s.
    cheesewiring of s.'s
    chromic catgut s.
    chromic collagen s.
    chromic gut s.
    clove-hitch s.
    coated Vicryl s.
    compression s.
    s. of cornea operation
    Custodis s.
    Dacron s.
    Davis-Geck s.
    Deknatel silk s.
    Dermalon s.
    Dexon s.
    double-armed s.
    double-running penetrating
      keratoplasty s.
    Ethicon-Atraloc s.
    Ethicon micropoint s.
    Ethicon Sabreloc s.
    s. of eyeball operation
    Faden s.
    fetal Y s.
    figure-of-eight s.
    fixation s.

    Foster s.
    frontolacrimal s.
    frontosphenoid s.
    frontozygomatic s.
    Frost s.
    Gaillard-Arlt s.
    groove s.
    guy s.
    Guyton-Friedenwald s.
    horizontal mattress s.
    infraorbital s.
    interrupted nylon s.
    intracameral s.
    intraluminal s.
    iris s.
    s. of iris operation
    juxtalimbal s.
    lacrimoconchal s.
    lacrimoethmoidal s.
    lacrimomaxillary s.
    lacrimoturbinal s.
    s. lancet
    lancet s.
    s. of lens
    Look s.
    Mannis s.
    mattress s.
    McCannel s.
    McLean s.
    Mersilene s.
    Micro-Glide corneal s.
    micropoint s.
    mild chromic s.
    monofilament nylon s.
    s. of muscle operation
    nonabsorbable s.
    Nurolon s.
    nylon 66 s.
    Ophthalon s.
    palatomaxillary s.
    s. pickup hook
    pickup spatula s.
    s. pickup spatula
    plain catgut s.
    plain collagen s.
    plain gut s.
    Polydek s.
    polyester s.
    polyglactin 910 s.
    polyglycolate s.
    polyglycolic acid s.
    polypropylene s.

NOTES

S

suture *(continued)*
    posterior fixation s.
    postplaced s.
    preplaced s.
    Prolene s.
    Quickert s.
    releasable s.
    rip-cord s.
    s. rotation
    s. rotation technique
    running nylon penetrating
      keratoplasty s.
    Safil synthetic absorbable
      surgical s.
    scleral flap s.
    s. of sclera operation
    Sharpoint ophthalmic
      microsurgical s.
    Sharpoint Ultra-Glide corneal
      transplant s.
    Sharpoint Ultra-Glide ophthalmic
      transplant s.
    Shoch s.
    silk traction s.
    single-armed s.
    single-running s.
    s. sling
    Sofsilk nonabsorbable silk s.
    Spanish silk s.
    sphenofrontal s.
    sphenoorbital s.
    Stallard-Liegard s.
    superior rectus bridle s.
    Supramid bridle collagen s.
    Supramid lens implant s.
    surgical gut s.
    Surgidev s.
    SurgiMed s.
    Swiss silk s.
    Tevdek s.
    traction s.
    transscleral s.
    twisted virgin silk s.
    Verhoeff s.
    Vicryl s.
    virgin silk s.
    white braided silk s.
    Worst s.
    Y s.
    zygomatic s.
    zygomaticofrontal s.
    zygomaticomaxillary s.
    zygomaticosphenoid s.
    zygomaticotemporal s.
SutureGroove gold eyelid weight
sutureless
    s. cataract surgery
    s. transconjunctival pars plana
      vitrectomy

"suture-out" astigmatism
suturing
    s. of eyelid
    s. forceps
    s. needle
    temporary keratoprosthesis s.
suturolysis
Svedberg unit
SVI/BL
    severe visual impairment and blindness
swab
    calcium alginate s.
    sterile calcium alginate s.
    wooden s.
Swan
    S. discission knife
    S. incision
    S. lancet
    S. needle
    S. syndrome
Swan-Jacob gonioprism
SWAP
    short wavelength automated perimetry
Swedish interactive thresholding
  algorithm (SITA)
sweep
    Barraquer s.
    eye s.
    iris s.
    s. view
sweeper
    Tiko zonule s.
Sweet
    S. locator
    S. method
    S. original magnet
swelling
    chronic optic disk s.
    corneal s.
    s. of disk
    optical disk s.
    optic disk s.
    Soemmering crystalline s.
    soft tissue s.
Swets goniotomy knife cannula
swift-cut phaco incision knife
swimmer's goggles
swimming pool conjunctivitis
swinging
    s. flashlight sign
    s. flashlight test
    s. lid flap
    s. light test
Swiss
    S. bladebreaker
    S. silk suture
Swiss-cheese visual field
sycosiform
sycosis tarsi

syllabic blindness
Sylva
    S. anterior chamber irrigator
    S. irrigating/aspirating unit
Sylvian aqueduct syndrome
symblephara
symblepharon
    anterior s.
    inferior s.
    s. lysis
    posterior s.
    s. ring
    total s.
symblepharopterygium
symbol
    test s.
symmetrical astigmatism
symmetric surgery
sympathetic
    s. amaurosis
    s. carotid plexus
    s. heterochromia
    s. hyperactivity
    s. innervation failure
    s. iridoplegia
    s. iritis
    s. nervous system
    s. neuron
    s. ophthalmia
    s. pathway
    s. uveitis
sympathetica
    ptosis s.
sympathizing eye
sympatholytic drug
sympathomimetic eye drops
sympathoparesis
symptom
    afferent visual s.
    Anton s.
    Berger s.
    Epstein s.
    Haenel s.
    halo s.
    Liebreich s.
    Magendie s.
    rainbow s.
    Stellwag s.
    Uhthoff s.
    Wernicke s.
symptomatic blepharospasm
synaphymenitis

synapse
    photoreceptor-bipolar s.
synaptic
    s. body
    s. connection
    s. ridge
synaptophysin antibody
synathroisis
syncanthus
synchesis
    s. corporis vitrei
    s. scintillans
syndectomy
syndermatotic cataract
syndermotica
    cataracta s.
syndesmitis
syndrome
    A s.
    Aarskog s.
    Aase s.
    accommodative effort s.
    acquired Horner s.
    acquired immunodeficiency s.
    (AIDS)
    acute idiopathic blind spot
    enlargement s.
    acute retinal necrosis s.
    adherence s.
    adhesive s.
    Adie s.
    Ahlström s.
    AICA s.
    Aicardi s.
    Alezzandrini s.
    Alport s.
    Alström s.
    Alström-Hallgren s.
    Alström-Olsen s.
    alternating Horner s.
    amniotic band s.
    Andersen s.
    Angelman s.
    Angelucci s.
    Angosky s.
    anterior chamber cleavage s.
    anterior optic chiasmal s.
    antielevation s. (AES)
    anti-Hu s.
    antiphospholipid s.
    Antley-Bixler s.
    Anton s.

S

NOTES

syndrome *(continued)*

Anton-Babinski s.
Apert s.
aqueous misdirection s.
ARN s.
ARRON s.
arteriovenous strabismus s.
Ascher s.
ataxia-telangiectasia s.
AV strabismus s.
Axenfeld s.
Axenfeld-Fieger s.
Axenfeld-Reiger s.
Backhaus s.
Balint s.
Baller-Gerold s.
Bamatter s.
Bannayan s.
Bardet-Biedl s.
bare lymphocyte s.
Barlow s.
Baron-Bietti s.
Bartholin s.
Bartter s.
basal cell nevus s.
Bassen-Kornzweig s.
Batten s.
Batten-Mayou s.
battered-baby s.
battered-child s.
Béal s.
Behçet s.
Behr s.
Benedikt s.
Bernard s.
Bernard-Horner s.
Bielschowsky-Jansky s.
Bielschowsky-Lutz-Cogan s.
Biemond s.
Bietti s.
big blind spot s.
bilateral uveal effusion s.
blepharophimosis ptosis s.
blepharospasm-oromandibular
  dystonia s.
blind spot s.
Bloch-Stauffer s.
Bloch-Sulzberger s.
blue rubber bleb nevus s.
Bonnet-DeChaume-Blanc s.
Bonnier s.
brachial arch s.
brittle cornea s.
Brown-McLean s.
Brown tendon sheath s.
Brown vertical retraction s.
Brueghel s.
Brushfield-Wyatt s.
capsular bag distention s.

capsular exfoliation s.
capsule contraction s.
CAR s.
Carpenter s.
cataract with Down s.
cat's eye s.
cavernous sinus s.
cavernous sinus/superior orbital
  fissure s.
central scotoma s.
Centurion s.
cerebrohepatorenal s.
cervicooculoacoustic s.
Cestan s.
Cestan-Chenais s.
Cestan-Raymond s.
Chandler s.
CHARGE s.
Charles Bonnet s. (CBS)
Charlin s.
Chédiak-Higashi s.
cherry-red spot myoclonus s.
chiasma s.
chiasmal s.
chiasmatic s.
Churg-Strauss s.
Claude Bernard s.
Claude Bernard-Horner s.
Claude-Lhermitte s.
cleavage s.
cleft s.
Coats s.
Cockayne s.
co-contraction s.
Coffin-Lowry s.
Cogan s.
Cogan-Reese s.
Cohen s.
Collins s.
competition swimmer's eyelid s.
computer vision s. (CVS)
congenital adherence s.
congenital fibrosis s.
congenital Horner s.
congenital juxtafoveolar s.
congenital rubella s.
congenital tilted disk s.
Conn s.
conotruncal anomalies face s.
Conradi s.
contact lens overwear s.
contact lens overwearing s.
Cornelia de Lange s.
CPD s.
cranial stenosis s.
craniofacial s.
CREST s.
cri du chat s.
Crouzon s.

Cushing s.
cutaneomucouveal s.
DAF s.
D chromosome ring s.
Degos s.
DeGrouchy s.
Dejean s.
de Lange s.
de Morsier s.
de Morsier-Gauthier s.
DIDMOAD s.
diencephalic s.
DiGeorge s.
dispersion s.
distal optic nerve s.
dorsal midbrain s.
Down s.
Doyne s.
Drews s.
dry eye s. (DES)
D trisomy s.
Duane retraction s.
dural shunt s.
dyscephalic s.
E s.
Eaton-Lambert s.
Edwards s.
Ehlers-Danlos s.
Ehlers-Danlos s. VI, VII
Eisenmenger s.
Ellingson s.
Elschnig s.
embryonic fixation s.
empty sella s.
exfoliation s. (XFS)
extrapyramidal s.
Fabry s.
Falls-Kertesz s.
Fanconi s.
fat adherence s.
fetal hydantoin s.
fetal trimethadione s.
fetal warfarin s.
fibrosis s.
Fiessinger-Leroy-Reiter s.
Fisher s.
Fitz-Hugh-Curtis s.
flaccid canaliculus s.
flecked retina s.
flocculus s.
floppy eyelid s.
Foix s.

Forsius-Eriksson s.
Forssman carotid s.
Foster Kennedy s.
foveomacular cone dysfunction s.
Foville s.
Foville-Wilson s.
Franceschetti s.
Franceschetti-Klein s.
François s.
Fraser s.
Freeman-Sheldon s.
Frenkel anterior ocular traumatic s.
Frey s.
Friedenwald s.
Friedreich s.
Fuchs s.
Fuchs-Kraupa s.
GAPO s.
Gardner s.
Gass s.
Gerstmann s.
Gilbert-Behçet s.
Gitelman s.
Goldberg s.
Goldenhar s.
Goldenhar-Gorlin s.
Goldmann-Favre s.
Goltz s.
Goltz-Gorlin s.
Gorham-Stout s.
Gradenigo s.
Graefe s.
Gregg s.
Greig s.
Greither s.
Grönblad-Strandberg s.
Gruber s.
Guillain-Barré s.
Gunn s.
Hagberg-Santavuori s.
half-moon s.
Hallermann-Streiff s.
Hallermann-Streiff-Francois s.
Hallervorden-Spatz s.
Hallgren s.
Haltia-Santavuori type of Batten s.
Hand-Schüller-Christian s.
Harada s.
Hawes-Pallister-Landor s.
Hay-Wells s.
Heerfordt s.
Heidenhain s.

NOTES

syndrome *(continued)*

hereditary benign intraepithelial dyskeratosis s.
hereditary hyperferritinemia-cataract s.
hereditary optic atrophy s.
heredodegenerative neurologic s.
Hermansky-Pudlak s.
Hertwig-Magendie s.
HHH s.
Hippel-Lindau s.
histoplasmosis s.
HLA-B27 s.
Holmes-Adie tonic pupil s.
Holt-Oram s.
Homén s.
Homer s.
Horner s.
Horner-Bernard s.
Horton s.
Hunter s.
Hunter-Hurler s.
Hurler s.
Hurler-Scheie s.
Hutchinson s.
hyperophthalmopathic s.
hyperviscosity s.
hypotony s.
hypoxic eyeball s.
ICE s.
idiopathic orbital inflammatory s. (IOIS)
idiopathic vitreomacular traction s.
immune recovery vitritis s.
infantile strabismus s.
inflammatory s.
innominate steal s.
internal capsule s.
iridocorneal endothelial s.
iridocyclitis masquerade s.
iridoendothelial s.
iris-nevus s.
iris retraction s. of Campbell
IRVAN s.
Irvine-Gass s.
ischemic chiasmal s.
ischemic ocular s.
Jacod s.
Jacod-Negri s.
Jadassohn-Lewandowsky s.
Jahnke s.
Jansky-Bielschowsky s.
jaw-winking s.
Jeune s.
Johnson s.
Joubert s.
Kasabach-Merritt s.
Kearns-Sayre s. (KSS)
Kehrer-Adie s.

Kennedy s.
KID s.
Kiloh-Nevin s.
Kimmelstiel-Wilson s.
Kloepfer s.
Koeppe s.
Koerber-Salus-Elschnig s.
Krause s.
Kufs s.
lacrimo-auriculo-dento-digital s.
Lambert-Eaton myasthenic s.
Langer-Giedion trichorhinophalangeal s.
Larsen s.
lateral medullary s.
Laurence-Biedl s.
Laurence-Moon s.
Laurence-Moon-Bardet-Biedl s.
Laurence-Moon-Biedl s.
Lawford s.
Leber plus s.
lens-induced UGH s.
Lenz s.
LEOPARD s.
Letterer-Siwe s.
lid imbrication s.
Li-Fraumeni s.
Löfgren s.
LOGIC s.
Lowe oculocerebrorenal s.
Lowe-Terrey-MacLachlan s.
Lyle s.
Lytico-Bodig s.
macular ocular histoplasmosis s.
Magendie-Hertwig s.
MAR s.
Marcus Gunn jaw-winking s.
Marfan s.
Marinesco-Sjögren s.
Marinesco-Sjögren-Garland s.
Marshall s.
masquerade s.
McCune-Albright s.
Meige s.
melanoma-associated retinopathy s.
Melkersson s.
Melkersson-Rosenthal s.
Meretoja s.
microtropic s.
Mietens s.
Mikulicz-Radecki s.
Mikulicz-Sjögren s.
milk-alkali s.
Millard-Gubler s.
Miller s.
Miller-Fisher s.
Milles s.
Möbius s.
Monakow s.

monofixation s.
morning glory s.
Morquio s.
Morquio-Brailsford s.
Mount-Reback s.
mucocutaneous lymph node s.
multifocal choroidopathy s.
multiple evanescent white-dot s.
  (MEWDS)
multiple lentigines s.
myasthenia s.
myasthenia-like s.
Naegeli s.
Nager s.
neurodegenerative s.
neuroleptic malignant s.
Nieden s.
nodulus s.
Nonne s.
Noonan s.
Norman-Wood s.
Nothnagel s.
nystagmus blockage s. (NBS)
ocular histoplasmosis s. (OHS)
ocular ischemic s. (OIS)
ocular motor s.
ocular pseudoexfoliation s.
oculoauditory s.
oculobuccogenital s.
oculocerebral s.
oculocerebrorenal s.
oculocutaneous s.
oculoglandular s.
oculomucous membrane s.
oculopalatal myoclonus s.
oculopharyngeal s.
oculorenal s.
OMM s.
one-and-a-half s.
optic chiasmal s.
opticocerebral s.
opticopyramidal s.
optic tract s.
orbital apex s.
orbital infarction s.
osteoporosis-pseudoglioma s.
Ota nevus s.
outer retinal necrosis s.
overwear s. (OWS)
9p- s.
4p- s.
Pallister-Hall s.

Pancoast superior sulcus s.
paraflocculus s.
paraneoplastic s.
parasellar s.
Parinaud oculoglandular s.
Parinaud-plus s.
Paterson-Brown-Kelly s.
PEHO s.
periaqueductal s.
Petzetakis-Takos s.
pigmentary dispersion s.
pigment dispersion s. (PDS)
plateau iris s.
plus-minus s.
Posner-Schlossman s.
posterior inferior cerebellar
  artery s.
postganglionic Horner s.
Potter s.
prechiasmal optic nerve
  compression s.
preganglionic Horner s.
presumed ocular histoplasmosis s.
  (POHS)
pretectal s.
progressive outer retinal necrosis s.
Proteus s.
pseudoexfoliation s.
pseudo-Foster Kennedy s.
pseudopresumed ocular
  histoplasmosis s. (pseudo POHS)
13q- s.
rainbow s.
Raymond s.
Raymond-Cestan s.
Recklinghausen s.
recurrent corneal erosion s.
red-eyed shunt s.
Reese s.
Refsum s.
Reiter s.
renal coloboma s.
restrictive s.
retinal necrosis s.
retraction s.
rheumatoid hyperviscosity s.
Richner-Hanhart s.
Riddoch s.
Rieger s.
Riley-Day s.
Riley-Smith s.
Ring D chromosome s.

S

NOTES

501

syndrome *(continued)*

Roaf s.
Robinow s.
Rollet s.
Romberg s.
Roth-Bielschowsky s.
Rothmund s.
Rothmund-Thomson s.
Roth spot s.
Rubinstein-Taybi s.
Russell s.
Rutherford s.
Sanchez-Salorio s.
Satoyoshis s.
Scheie s.
Schirmer s.
Schmid-Fraccaro s.
Schwartz s.
Schwartz-Jampel s.
Seckel s.
Senior-Loken s.
septooptic dysplasia s.
shaken baby s. (SBS)
Shea s.
sheath s.
Shprintzen s.
sicca s.
Siegrist-Hutchinson s.
silent sinus s.
Sipple s.
Sipple-Gorlin s.
Sjögren s.
Sjögren-Larsson s.
slow-channel s.
Sly s.
Smith-Lemli-Opitz s.
Smith-Magenis s.
Smith-Riley s.
Sorsby s.
Sotos s.
Spanlang-Tappeiner s.
sphenocavernous s.
spherophakia-brachymorphia s.
Spielmeyer-Vogt s.
Stargardt s.
steal s.
Steele-Richardson-Olszewski s.
Stevens-Johnson s.
Stickler s.
Stilling-Turk-Duane s.
Stock-Spielmeyer-Vogt s.
Strachan s.
Strachan-Scott s.
Sturge-Weber s.
Sturge-Weber-Dimitri s.
sunrise s.
sunset s.
superior oblique tendon sheath s.
superior orbital fissure s.

Susac s.
Swan s.
Sylvian aqueduct s.
tectal midbrain s.
tegmental s.
temporal crescent s.
tendon sheath s.
Terry s.
Terson s.
Thompson s.
tight lens s. (TLS)
tilted disc s. (TDS)
tilted disk s.
Tolosa-Hunt s.
tonic pupil s.
top-of-the-basilar s.
Touraine s.
toxic Strep s.
Treacher Collins s.
Treacher Collins-Franceschetti s.
tubulointerstitial nephritis and
   uveitis s.
UGH s.
UGH+ s.
Uhthoff s.
Ullrich s.
Ullrich-Feichtiger s.
uncal s.
Usher s.
uveal effusion s.
uveitis-vitiligo-alopecia-poliosis s.
uveocutaneous s.
uveoencephalitic s.
uveomeningeal s.
uveomeningitis s.
Uyemura s.
V s.
velocardiofacial s.
vertical retraction s.
visceral larva migrans s.
visual deprivation s.
visual paraneoplastic s.
vitreomacular traction s.
vitreoretinal choroidopathy s.
vitreoretinal traction s.
vitreous wick s.
V-K-H s.
Vogt s.
Vogt-Koyanagi s.
Vogt-Koyanagi-Harada s.
Vogt-Spielmeyer s.
von Graefe s.
von Hippel-Lindau s.
von Recklinghausen s.
Waardenburg s.
Waardenburg-Klein s.
Wagner s.
Wagner-Stickler s.
Walker-Warburg s.

Wallenberg lateral medullary s.
Warburg s.
Weber s.
Weber-Gubler s.
Weill-Marchesani s.
Weill-Reys s.
Weill-Reys-Adie s.
Werner s.
Wernicke s.
Wernicke-Korsakoff s.
Weyers-Thier s.
white dot s.
Wildervanck s.
Wilson s.
windshield wiper s.
wipe-out s.
Wolf s.
Wolfram s.
Wyburn-Mason s.
Zellweger s.

synechia, pl. **synechiae**
anterior s.
anular s.
Castroviejo anterior s.
circular s.
congenital anterior s.
iridocorneal s.
iris s.
peripheral anterior s. (PAS)
posterior s.
s. spatula
total anterior s.
total posterior s.

synechial closure
synechialysis
synechiotomy
Paufique s.
synechotome
synechotomy
synephris
syneresis of vitreous
syneretic vitreous
Synergetics
S. Awh serrated pick
S. DDMS
S. directional laser probe
S. endo illuminator
synergistic divergence
syngeneic epithelium
synizesis pupillae

synkinesia
congenital oculopalpebral s.
lid-triggered s.
synkinesis
external pterygoid levator s.
facial s.
oculocephalic s.
oculomotor nerve s.
pterygoid levator s.
s. pupilla
trigemino oculomotor s.
synkinetic
s. movement
s. near reflex
s. near response
synophrys
synophthalmia, synophthalmos, synophthalmus
synoptophore
synoptoscope
syntenic gene
synthesis
genome s.
synthetic
S. Optics random dot butterfly test
s. penicillin
Synvisc
syphilis
acquired s.
congenital s.
ocular s.
syphilitic
s. cataract
s. chorioretinitis
s. choroiditis
s. dacryocystitis
s. episcleritis
s. iritis
s. keratitis
s. ocular disease
s. optic perineuritis
s. retinitis
s. retinopathy
s. rhinitis
s. scleritis
syphilitica
retinitis s.
syringe
Anel s.
Fink-Weinstein two-way s.
Fragmatome flute s.
Fuchs retinal detachment s.

S

NOTES

syringe *(continued)*
  Fuchs two-way s.
  Goldstein anterior chamber s.
  Goldstein lacrimal s.
  lacrimal s.
  Luer-Lok s.
  Parker-Heath anterior chamber s.
  probe s.
  retinal detachment s.
  tuberculin s.
  two-way s.
  Yale Luer-Lok s.
syringoma
  eyelid s.
  s. tumor
syrup
  Carbodec S.
  Cardec-S S.
  Rondec S.
system
  Accurus vitreoretinal surgical s.
  Aesculap-Meditec MEL60 s.
  afocal optical s.
  Alcon Closure S. (ACS)
  Alcon EyeMap EH-290 corneal
    topography s.
  AMO Prestige advanced cataract
    extraction s.
  AMO Prestige Phaco S.
  Anterior Eye Segment Analysis S.
  AquaLase cataract removal s.
  ArF excimer laser s.
  Automated Quantification of After-
    Cataract automated analysis s.
  autonomic nervous s.
  Autoswitch S.
  Badal stimulus s.
  Beaver clear cornea incision s.
  BIOM noncontact panoramic
    viewing s.
  BIOM noncontact wide-angle
    viewing s.
  Bio-Optics Bambi Cell Analysis S.
  Bio-Optics Bambi image analysis s.
  Bio-Optics telescope s.
  bioptic amorphic lens s.
  Blairex S.
  boxing s.
  British N s.
  Buzard Diamond Barraqueratome
    Microkeratome S.
  Cambridge Research S.'s (CRS)
  Candela videoimaging s.
  Catarex cataract removal s.
  Cavitron irrigation/aspiration s.
  Cavitron-Kelman
    irrigation/aspiration s.
  central nervous s. (CNS)
  Chromos imager s.

  CIBA TearSaver punctual
    gauging s.
  closed-circuit television vision
    enhancement s. (CCTV)
  closed-loop s.
  CMS AccuProbe 450 s.
  Coburn irrigation/aspiration s.
  Combiline S.
  complement s.
  Complete Ophthalmic Analysis S.
    (COAS)
  Computed Anatomy Corneal
    Modeling S.
  Corneal Modeling S.
  corneal topography s. (CTS)
  CorneaSparing LTK s.
  CryoSeal FS S.
  C-Scan corneal topography s.
  delivery s.
  Digital B S.
  dioptric s.
  Dodick photolysis s.
  DORC fast freeze cryosurgical s.
  DORC Hexon Illumination S. 1266
    XII
  dual aspiration pump s.
  DuoVisc viscoelastic s.
  EAS-1000 anterior eye segment
    analysis s.
  EMI digital imaging s.
  ErgoTec vitreoretinal instrument s.
  Evaluation of Posterior Capsular
    Opacification s.
  extrapyramidal s.
  Eye Cap Ophthalmic Image
    Capture S.
  eyeFix speculum s.
  EyeMap EH-290 corneal
    topography s.
  Eye Quip Keratron Scout
    topography s.
  EyeSys S. 2000
  EyeSys corneal analysis s.
  EyeSys 2000 corneal topographic
    mapping s.
  EyeSys corneal topography s.
  EyeSys surface topography s.
  EZE-FIT IOL s.
  FlapMaker microkeratome s.
  full-field s.
  gaussian optical s.
  Grieshaber power injector s.
  Grolman photographic s.
  Guided Trephine S. (GTS)
  Hartmann-Shack wavefront sensor s.
  Hessburg subpalpebral lavage s.
  Hexon illumination s.
  Hodapp-Parrish-Anderson visual
    field staging s.

HPA visual field staging s.
Humphrey ATLAS Eclipse corneal topography s.
Humphrey Instruments vision analyzer overrefraction s.
Humphrey Mastervue corneal topography s.
hyaloid s.
Hybriwix probe s.
IMAGEnet image digitizing s.
IMAGEnet 2000 series digital imaging s.
immune s.
INNOVA S. 920
Integre 532 delivery s.
Inverter vitrectomy s.
IRIS Medical OcuLight green laser s.
IRIS Medical OcuLight infrared laser s.
IRIS OcuLight SLx indirect ophthalmoscope delivery s.
irrigation/aspiration s.
IVEX s.
Jaeger grading s.
Kappa SP lens finishing s.
Katena quick switch I/A s.
Kellan capsular sparing s.
Keratograph corneal topography s.
Keratome excimer laser s.
Keratron Scout topography s.
Koeller illumination s.
Kornmehl LASIK s.
Kowa fluorescein s.
lacrimal s.
LADARTracker Closed-Loop Tracking S.
LADARVision excimer laser s.
LADARWave CustomCornea Wavefront S.
Langerman diamond knife s.
LaserScan LSX excimer laser s.
Legacy cataract surgical s.
Lens Comfort Ultrasound Cleaning and Disinfecting S.
Lens Opacification Classification S. (LOCS)
Lens Opacity Classification S. II
Lens Opacity Classification S. III
lens-plus-eye s.
Lens Plus Oxysept S.
low-vision enhancement s. (LVES)

Mackool s.
Malis bipolar coagulating/cutting s.
Marlin Salt S. II
Massachusetts XII vitrectomy s. (MVS)
Mastel compass-guided arcuate keratotomy s.
Materials Testing S.
McGuire I/A s.
McIntyre coaxial irrigating/aspirating s.
McIntyre I/A s.
McIntyre III nucleus removal s.
McIntyre irrigation/aspiration s.
Medi-Duct ocular fluid management s.
micropigmentation s.
MicroProbe integrated laser and endoscope s.
MicroShape Keratome S.
Microvit probe s.
midget s.
Millennium CX, LX microsurgical s.
Millennium Transconjunctival Standard Vitrectomy 25 S.
Millennium TVS25 S.
Milli-Q water purification s.
MiraSept S.
M.I.S. multi-port illumination s.
MK-2000 keratome s.
Monarch II intraocular lens delivery s.
Monarch II IOL delivery s.
Mot-R-Pak vitrectomy s.
Mport lens insertion s.
M-TEC 2000 Surgical S.
nasolacrimal drainage s.
Nd:YAG Photon LaserPhaco S.
Nelson grading s.
Niamtu video imaging s.
Nidek EC-5000 refractive laser s.
Nidek MK-2000 Keratome S.
nomogram s.
ocular motor s.
Oculex drug delivery s.
oculomotor s.
Oculus BIOM noncontact lens s.
Ocutome II fragmentation s.
OCVM s.
Odyssey phacoemulsification s.
OIS image digitizing s.

NOTES

system (*continued*)

OIS WinStation 5000 Ophthalmic Imaging S.
Olson calibrated cornea trephine s.
OPD-Scan diagnostic s.
optical s.
Opti-Pure S.
optokinetic s.
Orbscan II multidimensional diagnostic s.
Orbscan II topography s.
Orbscan topography analysis s.
osseous s.
parasympathetic nerve s.
parasympathetic nervous s.
PAR CTS corneal topography s.
Passport disposable injection s.
PE-400 ERG/VEP s.
peripapillary choroidal arterial s.
Phacojack Phaco S.
Photon cataract removal s.
Photon Ocular Surgery S.
Phototome S. 2700
pial s.
Placido-disk videokeratoscopy s.
postcanalicular s.
PreClean soak s.
Premiere SmallPort phaco s.
Price corneal transplant s.
printers' point s.
pump-leak s.
pyramidal s.
Quick Care S.
QuickRinse automated instrument rinse s.
Quickswitch irrigation/aspiration ophthalmic s.
Reese Ellsworth classification s.
Refractec ViewPoint CK S.
Reinverting Operating Lens S. (ROLS)
renin-angiotensin s.
RetinaLyze S.
Rhein blade cleaning s.
Rodenstock s.
Scheimpflug videophotography s.
SDI-BIOM wide angle viewing s.
Selecta II Glaucoma Laser S.
sensory s.
Simcoe irrigation/aspiration s.
single-incision s.
SITE TXR diaphragmatic microsurgical s.
SITE TXR peristaltic microsurgical s.
SITE TXR phacoemulsification s.
Sloan M s.
SmallPort phaco s.
SofTec Delivery S.

Sonomed A/B-Scan s.
Sonomed A-Scan s.
Sonomed B-1500 s.
Sovereign SHIELD S.
Spectrum Lens Analysis S.
specular reflection video-recording s.
STAR S4 ActiveTrak 3-D eye tracking s.
STAR S3 ActiveTrak excimer laser s.
STAR S4 excimer laser s.
STAR S2 SmoothScan excimer laser s.
Steritome microkeratome s.
Storz Millennium microsurgical s.
STTOdx ophthalmic surgery s.
Sunrise LTK s.
Surg-E-Trol I/A S.
sustained-release s.
sympathetic nervous s.
T s.
tear drainage s.
tear duct s.
The Wave phacoemulsion s.
TMS corneal topography s.
Tomey topographic modeling s.
Tomey topography s.
Topcon CM-1000 corneal mapping s.
Topcon IMAGEnet digital imaging s.
Topographic Modeling S.-1 (TMS-1)
Topographic Modeling S.-2 (TMS-2)
Topographic Scanning S. (TopSS)
TopSS/AngioScan s.
TopSS topographic scanning s.
trocar-cannula s.
Ultrascan Digital B s.
Ultrasound Biomicroscope S.
Unfolder implantation s.
UniPulse 1040 Surgical CO_2 laser s.
United Sonics J shock phaco fragmentor s.
Veatch ophthalmic ReSeeVit s.
Venturi-Flo valve s.
VERIS III s.
vertebrobasilar s.
vestibular s.
Vision Analyzer/Overrefraction S.
Vision Master excimer laser s.
Visitec surgical vitrectomy s.
visual-evoked response imaging s. (VERIS)
visual sensory s.
Visulab S.

VISUPAC digital imaging s.
VISX Star II stromal photoablation s.
VISX Star S2 excimer laser s.
VISX Twenty/Twenty s.
VISX 20/20 version 4.01 vision keycard s.
Vit Commander S.
vortex s.
Wallach Ophthalmic Cryosurgery S.
water-based tinting s.
Wavefront S.
WaveScan Wavefront s.
Wheeler cyclodialysis s.
Wilmer Cataract Photo-grading S.
Wisconsin age-related maculopathy grading s.
YC 1400 Ophthalmic YAG laser s.

Zaldivar limbal-relaxing incision s.
Zeiss DAS-1 hydrophobic s.
Zeiss fiberoptic illumination s.
zoom s.

systemic
s. amyloidosis
s. bacterial endophthalmitis
s. corticosteroid therapy
s. drug
s. glucocorticoid
s. hyperosmolar agent
s. lupus erythematosus choroidopathy
s. myopathy
s. myositis
s. pathology
s. sclerosis

Szymanowski-Kuhnt operation
Szymanowski operation

S

NOTES

T

    tension
        T lens
        T system

T+

    increased tension

TA

    temporal arteritis

tab

    vitrectomy prism lens t.

tabes dorsalis
tabetic optic atrophy
table

    Reuss color t.
    Stilling color t.

tablet

    Carbiset T.
    Carbiset-TR T.
    Carbodec TR T.
    Ocuvite Lutein t.
    PBZ t.
    PBZ-SR t.

Tac-40
tachistesthesia
tachistoscope
tack

    retinal t.

taco test
tacrolimus
tactile tension
tadpole pupil
Taenia solium
tag

    vitreoretinal t.

tagged image file format (TIFF)
Taillefer valve
Takahashi iris retractor forceps
Takata laser
Takayasu

    idiopathic arteritis of T.

talantropia
Talbot

    T. law
    T. unit

tamoxifen retinopathy
tamponade

    gas t.
    intraocular silicone oil t.
    silicone oil t.
    Silikon 1000 retinal t.

tandem scanning confocal microscope
tangent

    t. perimetry
    t. scope

    t. screen
    t. screen testing

tangential illumination
Tangier disease
Tanne

    T. corneal cutting block
    T. corneal punch
    T. guillotine-style punch

Tano

    T. device
    T. double mirror peripheral
      vitrectomy lens
    T. eraser
    T. membrane scraper
    T. ring

Tansley operation
Tan spatula
tantalum

    t. clip
    t. mesh
    t. mesh implant
    t. "O" ring

TAO

    thyroid-associated ophthalmopathy

TAP

    tension by applanation

tap

    anterior chamber t.
    aqueous t.
    choroidal t.
    vitreous t.

tap-biopsy
tape

    Blenderm t.
    brow t.
    optokinetic t.
    Transpore eye t.

taper-cut needle
tapered-shaft punctum plug
taper-point needle
tapetal light reflex
tapetochoroidal

    t. degeneration
    t. dystrophy

tapetoretinal

    t. degeneration
    t. retinopathy

tapetoretinopathy
tapetum

    t. choroideae
    t. lucidum
    t. nigrum
    t. oculi

taping

    eyelid t.

T

tapioca iris melanoma
tapir
    bouche de t.
target
    accommodative t.
    Air Force test grid t.
    background-presented test t.
    fixation t.
    saccadic eccentric t.
    von Graefe t.
tarsadenitis
tarsal
    t. angle
    t. artery
    t. asthenopia
    t. canal
    t. cartilage
    t. conjunctiva
    t. cyst
    t. ectropion
    t. gland
    t. laceration
    t. membrane
    t. muscle
    t. plate
    t. portion of eyelid
    t. sandwich technique
    t. strip procedure
tarsales
    glandulae t.
tarsalis
    epicanthus t.
tarsectomy
    Blaskovics t.
    Kuhnt t.
tarsi (*pl. of* tarsus)
tarsitis
    tuberculous t.
tarsocheiloplasty
tarsoconjunctival
    t. composite graft
    t. flap
    t. gland
    t. pedicle
tarsoligamentous sling
tarsomalacia
tarsoorbital
tarsophyma
tarsoplasia
tarsoplasty
tarsorrhaphy
tarsotomy
    transverse t.
tarsus, pl. **tarsi**
    inferior t.
    t. orbital septum
    t. osseus
    superior t.

    sycosis tarsi
    tinea tarsi
Tasia operation
tattoo
    t. of cornea operation
    t. pigment
tattooing
    corneal t.
    medical t.
    t. needle
Tauranol
Tavist
Tavist-1
tax double needle
Tay
    T. cherry-red spot
    T. choroiditis
    T. disease
    T. sign
Tay-Sachs disease
Tazarotene
Tazorac
TBUT
    tear breakup test
TCD
    transcranial Doppler
T-cell lymphoma
TCF
    total conjunctival flap
TDME
    tractional diabetic macular edema
TDS
    tilted disc syndrome
TdT
    terminal deoxynucleotidyl transferase
Teale-Knapp operation
tear
    Akwa T.'s
    Androgen T.
    artificial t.'s (AT)
    Bion T.'s
    bloody t.'s
    t. breakup test (TBUT)
    breakup time of t.
    t. clearance rate
    Comfort T.'s
    conjunctival t.
    crocodile t.'s
    t. drainage
    t. drainage system
    T. Drop Solution
    t. duct
    t. duct patency
    t. duct system
    t. film
    t. film breakup time
    t. film debris
    t. film disorder
    t. film instability

t. film stability
t. film test
fishmouth t.
flap t.
t. flow
t. function test
t. gas
giant retinal t. (GRT)
t. gland
horseshoe t.
iatrogenic retinal t.
I-Liqui T.'s
iris sphincter t.
Isopto T.'s
Just T.'s
t. lake
t. layer
Liquifilm T.'s
t. of meniscus
Milroy Artificial T.'s
mucin of t.
t. mucus ferning
Murine T.'s
Muro T.'s
Natural T.'s
nonpreserved artificial t.
operculated t.
operculated retinal t.
t. osmolarity
T.'s Plus
t. pool
t. protein deposit
t. pump
Puralube T.'s
t. quality
t. quantity
reflux of t.
t. of retina
retinal horseshoe t.
t. sac
t. secretion
t. secretion classification
smooth-edged continuous t.
sphincter t.
t. stone
t. test strip
traction-related t.
t. turnover
Ultra T.'s
Visine T.'s

vitreous cells as indicator of
   retinal t.
   t. volume
teardrop pupil
Tear-Efrin
Tearfair
tear-film disturbance
TearGard Ophthalmic Solution
Teargen Ophthalmic Solution
tear-induced retinal detachment
tearing
   nonreflex t.
Tearisol
Tearisol Solution
TearSaver punctum plug
Tearscope
   Keeler T.
   T. Plus photographer
   T. Plus tear film kit
technetium scan
technician
   Certified Paraoptometric T. (CPOT)
technique
   Armaly-Drance t.
   Atkinson t.
   automated tissue delamination t.
   bare scleral t.
   blue field stimulation t.
   Boyden chamber t.
   Brockhurst t.
   Brown-Beard t.
   capsule forceps t.
   chip-and-flip phacoemulsification t.
   closed-dissection t.
   conjunctival advancement t.
   cost-ineffective current screening t.
   crack-and-flip phacoemulsification t.
   Crawford t.
   divide-and-conquer t.
   erysiphake t.
   feeder-frond t.
   flicher-fusion frequency t.
   Fraunfelder "no touch" t.
   frequency doubling t.
   frontalis sling t.
   Goldmann kinetic t.
   Goldmann static t.
   high-tension suturing t.
   Hughes modification of Burch t.
   immunohistochemical t.
   iris-fixation t.
   Kaplan-Meier estimation t.

T

NOTES

technique (*continued*)
  Kaufman-Capella cryopreservation t.
  Knoll refraction t.
  Lambda phacoemulsification t.
  laser-scrape t.
  letterbox t.
  masquerade t.
  Maurice corneal depot t.
  McCannel suture t.
  McLean t.
  McReynolds t.
  microlymphocytotoxicity t.
  Miyake t.
  mustache t.
  O'Brien akinesia t.
  Okamura t.
  open-sky t.
  ophthalmic vitreous surgical t.
  phaco-chop t.
  Phakonit nucleus division t.
  piezoelectric transducer t.
  preferential-looking t.
  push-plus refraction t.
  Quickert three-suture t.
  radioimmunoassay t.
  Scheie t.
  Schepens t.
  scleral search coil t.
  single-stitch aponeurotic tuck t.
  Smirmaul t.
  Smith-Indian t.
  Southern blot t.
  split-beam photographic t.
  Staar Aquaflow t.
  stop-and-chop phacoemulsification t.
  suture rotation t.
  tarsal sandwich t.
  transillumination t.
  transocular t.
  transpupillary t.
  transscleral suture fixation t.
  tumbling t.
  Tzanck t.
  Van Lint modified t.
  Van Milligen eyelid repair t.
  von Graefe t.
Technolas 217 excimer laser
technologist
  Certified Ophthalmic T. (COT)
  Certified Ophthalmic Medical T.
    (COMT)
technology
  Catarex t.
  frequency doubling t. (FDT)
  imaging t.
  in-lab lens casting t.
  nerve fiber t.
  objective noninvasive t.
  WhiteStar power modulation t.

TechnoMed
  T. C-Scan
  T. C-Scan videokeratoscope
Tecnis
  T. foldable intraocular lens
  T. foldable IOL
tectal midbrain syndrome
tectonic
  t. corneal graft
  t. epikeratoplasty
  t. keratoplasty
Teflon
  T. block
  T. implant
  T. injection catheter
  T. iris retractor
  T. plate
  T. plug
  T. sheet
tegmental syndrome
teichopsia
Tektronix digital phonometer
tela, pl. **telae**
  t. cellulosa
  t. conjunctiva
Telachlor
telangiectasia
  calcinosis cutis, Raynaud
    phenomenon, esophageal motility
    disorder, sclerodactyly, and t.
    (CREST)
  essential t.
  generalized essential t. (GET)
  hereditary hemorrhagic t.
  idiopathic acquired retinal t.
  macular t.
  retinal t.
  spider t.
telangiectasis
  bilateral juxtafoveal t. (BJT)
  idiopathic juxtafoveal retinal t.
  idiopathic perifoveal t. (IPT)
  retinal t.
telangiectatic glioma
Teldrin
telebinocular
telecanthus
telecentric fundus camera
telemedical evaluation
telemedicine
teleopsia
telephoto effect
telepresence environment
telescope
  afocal t.
  Eschenbach monocular t.
  Galilean t.
  Hopkins rod lens t.

implantable miniaturized t. (IMT)
monocular t.

telescopic
t. lens
t. spectacles

Telfa
T. pad
T. plastic film dressing

Tellais sign

Teller
T. acuity card
T. visual acuity

Temba glaucoma study

TEMOO mode beam laser

template

temple
cable t.
curl t.
hockey-end t.
t. length
library t.
loafer t.
paddle t.
riding bow t.
skull t.
spatula t.
t. of spectacles
spring-hinge t.
straight t.
Venturi adjusted t.

temporal
t. arteriole of retina
t. arteritis (TA)
t. artery
t. artery biopsy
t. artery pallor
t. bone
t. bulbar conjunctiva
t. canthus
t. crescent
t. crescent syndrome
t. hemianopsia
t. island of visual field
t. lobe
t. lobe field defect
t. lobe unilateral cerebral
  hemisphere lesion
t. loop
t. macula
medial superior t. (MST)
t. modulation perimetry
t. optic disk pallor

t. peaking
t. pit
t. raphe
t. self-sealing clear corneal incision
t. vascular arcade
t. venulae retina superior
t. venule of retina
t. wedge
t. zone
t. zone of retina

temporalis
commissura palpebrarum t.
t. muscle

temporary
t. balloon buckle
t. diabetes
t. intracanalicular collagen implant
t. keratoprosthesis (TKP)
t. keratoprosthesis suturing
t. prism

temporooccipital artery

temporoparietal lobe

tenacious
t. distance fusion
t. proximal fusion

Tendency-Oriented Perimetry (TOP)

tendinous insertion

tendo
t. oculi
t. palpebrarum

tendon
t. advancement
Brown t.
canthal t.
lateral canthal t.
levator t.
Lockwood t.
medial canthal t.
t. recession
t. sheath syndrome
superior oblique t.
tenotomy of ocular t.
t. tucker
Zinn t.

tendotome

tendotomy

tenectomy

Tennant
T. Anchorflex AC lens
T. anchor lens-insertion hook
T. implant
T. lens-inserting forceps

T

NOTES

513

Tennant *(continued)*
    T. lens-manipulating hook
    T. titanium suturing forceps
    T. tying forceps
Tennant-Colibri corneal forceps
Tennant-Troutman superior rectus
  forceps
Tenner
    T. lacrimal cannula
    T. titanium suturing forceps
Tenon
    T. capsule
    T. fascia bulbi
    T. fascia lata
    T. fibroblast
    T. flap
    T. membrane
    T. patch graft
    T. sac
    T. space
tenonectomy
tenonitis
    brawny t.
tenonometer
tenontotomy
tenoplasty
    cyanoacrylate tissue adhesive
      augmented t.
Tenormin
tenosynovitis
tenotome
tenotomist
tenotomize
tenotomy
    Arroyo t.
    Arruga t.
    curb t.
    free t.
    graduated t.
    t. hook
    intrasheath t.
    t. of ocular tendon
    t. operation
    Z marginal t.
tensile strength of vessel
Tensilon
    T. implant
    T. test
tension (T)
    applanation t. (AT)
    t. by applanation (TAP)
    t. of eye
    finger t.
    hard-finger t.
    increased t. (T+)
    intraocular t.
    normal t. (TN)
    normal-finger t.
    ocular t. (Tn)

    t. oculus dextra (tension of right
      eye) (TOD)
    t. oculus sinister (tension of left
      eye) (TOS)
    soft-finger t.
    surface t.
    tactile t.
    t. test
    zonular t.
tensor insertion
tented-up retina
tentorial nerve
tentorii ramus
tenuis
    pannus t.
Tenzel
    T. elevator
    T. forceps
    T. rotational cheek flap
Terak Ophthalmic Ointment
teratogenic association
terfenadine
Terg-A-Zyme
terminal
    t. bulb
    t. deoxynucleotidyl transferase
      (TdT)
    t. deoxynucleotidyl transferase-
      mediated dUTP-digoxigenin nick-
      end labeling (TUNEL)
terminaux
    boutons t.
termini
    carboxy t.
terminus
    incision t.
Terra-Cortril Ophthalmic Suspension
Terramycin
    polymyxin B and T.
    T. w/polymyxin B Ophthalmic
      Ointment
terreus
    Aspergillus t.
Terrien
    T. marginal degeneration
    T. ulcer
Terry
    T. astigmatome
    T. keratometer
    T. silicone capsule polisher
    T. syndrome
Terson
    T. capsule forceps
    T. extracapsular forceps
    T. operation
    T. syndrome
tertiary
    t. position
    t. vitreous

tertius palpebra
tessellated fundus
Tessier
- T. classification
- T. clefting
- T. operation

test
- afterimage t.
- alternate cover t. (ACT)
- alternate cover-uncover t.
- alternating light t.
- Ames t.
- Amsler grid t.
- anaglyph t.
- anomaloscope plate t. (APT)
- Arabic eye t.
- a-wave t.
- Bagolini striated glasses t.
- Bailey-Lovie Near T.
- Bárány caloric t.
- Barraquer-Krumeich t.
- basic secretion t.
- Behçet skin puncture t.
- Bence Jones t.
- Benton Facial Recognition T.
- Berens pinhole and dominance t.
- Berens three-character t.
- Bielschowsky-Parks head-tilt three-step t.
- Bielschowsky three-step head-tilt t.
- Binocular Visual Acuity T.
- biochrome t.
- biometry t.
- biopter t.
- blindness t.
- Bonferroni t.
- breakup time t.
- Brightness Acuity T. (BAT)
- Bruchner t.
- butterfly t.
- caloric irrigation t.
- t. card
- cardinal field t.
- Catford visual acuity t.
- child-friendly VDS t.
- chi-squared test
- cocaine t.
- Color Bar Schirmer Tear T.
- color comparison t.
- color vision t.
- Color Vision Testing Made Easy t. (CVTMET)

- complement fixation t.
- t. condition
- confrontation visual field t.
- contour stereo t.
- contrast sensitivity t. (CST)
- corneal impression t. (CIT)
- corneal staining t.
- cotton thread tear t.
- cover t.
- cover-uncover t.
- critical flicker fusion t.
- cross cover t.
- CRS Color Vision T.
- Cuignet t.
- D-15 t.
- dark-room t.
- DEM t.
- denervation supersensitivity t.
- Developmental Eye Movement t.
- D-15 Hue Desaturated Panel t.
- direct chlamydial immunofluorescence t.
- dissimilar image t.
- dissimilar target t.
- t. distance
- Dix-Hallpike t.
- double Maddox rod t.
- dry eye t. (DET)
- duction t.
- duochrome t.
- Dupuy-Dutemps dacryocystorhinostomy dye t.
- dye disappearance t. (DDT)
- E t.
- edrophonium chloride t.
- Ehrmann t.
- t. eye
- Farnsworth-Munsell 100-hue color vision t.
- Farnsworth Panel D-15 t.
- FastPac 24-2 t.
- F2 Color Vision t.
- Fisher exact t.
- fistula t.
- flashlight t.
- flicker fusion t.
- flicker fusion frequency t. (FFF)
- flicker perimetry t.
- fluorescein angiogram t.
- fluorescein clearance t. (FCT)
- fluorescein dilution t.
- fluorescein dye disappearance t.

NOTES

test *(continued)*

fluorescein instillation t.
fluorescein strip t.
fluorescent antibody t.
fly t.
FM-100 hue t.
fog t.
forced-duction t.
forced generation t.
forward traction t.
Foucault knife edge t.
four-dot t.
Frequency Doubling Perimeter t.
Fridenberg stigmatometric t.
Friedman t.
Frisby stereoacuity t.
Functional Acuity Contrast T.
  (FACT)
Getman-Henderson-Marcus visual
  manipulation t.
glare t.
Glaucoma Hemifield T. (GHT)
Goldmann visual field t.
Graefe t.
Haidinger brush t.
hair bulb incubation t.
hand-motion visual acuity t.
hand-movement visual acuity t.
haploscopic t.
Hardy-Rand-Ritter t.
Harrington-Flocks t.
head-tilt t.
Hemifield glaucoma t.
Hering t.
Hering-Bielschowsky after-image t.
Hess screen t.
higher visual function t.
Hirschberg t.
Holladay contrast acuity t.
Holmgren color t.
Holmgren wool skein t.
Hooper Visual Organization T.
  (HVOT)
HOTV t.
28 Hue de Roth t.
90 hue discrimination t.
100 hue t.
Humphrey 24-2 glaucoma
  hemifield t.
ice pack t.
interference visual acuity t.
intravenous thyrotropin-releasing
  hormone t.
Ishihara t.
Jaeger visual t.
Jenning t.
Jones dye t.
Jones I, II t.
Keystone view stereopsis t.

Kirby-Bauer disk sensitivity t.
Kirsch t.
Kodak Surecell Chlamydia t.
Kolmogorov-Smirnov t.
Krimsky prism t.
Kruskal-Wallis t.
Kveim t.
lacrimal irrigation t.
lactoferrin t.
Lagrange t.
Lancaster red-green t.
Lancaster-Regan t.
Lancaster screen t.
Landolt broken-ring t.
Landolt-C t.
Lang stereo t.
lantern t.
letter t.
t. letter
Lighthouse Distance Visual
  Acuity T.
light projection t.
light-stress t.
line t.
linear visual acuity t.
lupus erythematosus cell t.
macular computerized
  psychophysical t. (MCPT)
Maddox rod t.
Maddox wing t.
magnetic field-search coil t.
major amblyoscope t.
Mann-Whitney U t.
Mantoux t.
Marcus Gunn t.
Marlow t.
Mauthner t.
McNemar t.
Mecholyl t.
Mentor B-VAT II BVS contour
  circles distance stereoacuity t.
Mentor B-VAT II BVS random
  dot E distance stereoacuity t.
microhemagglutination t.
Micro-Reflux T. (MRT)
MicroTrac Direct Specimen T.
mirror rocking t.
Modified Clinical Technique t.
Mollon-Reffin minimal t.
monocular confrontation visual
  field t.
Mr. Color t.
mydriatic provocative t.
Nagel t.
near vision t.
neostigmine t.
neutral density filter t.
nudge t.
nystagmus t.

t. object
objective prism-neutralized cover t.
Octopus 201 perimeter t.
Ocugene glaucoma genetic t.
ocular motility t.
oculocephalic t.
ophthalmic t.
Optec 3000 contrast sensitivity t.
optokinetic t.
ornithine tolerance t.
Otis-Lennon School Ability T.
parallax t.
Parks-Bielschowsky three-step head-
tilt t.
Park three-step t.
passive forced duction t.
P&C t.
Pearson chi-square t.
Pease-Allen Color t.
Pepper Visual Skills for
Reading T.
perimeter corneal reflex t.
peripheral detection t.
photostress t.
pilocarpine t.
pinhole and dominance t.
Polaroid 3D Vectograph t.
primary dye t.
prism adaptation t. (PAT)
prism and alternate cover t.
(PACT)
4 prism diopter base-out t.
prism dissociation t.
prism-neutralized cover t.
prism shift t.
prism vergence t.
Prostigmin t.
provocative t.
pseudoisochromatic color t.
pupil cycle induction t.
Rabinowitz-McDonnell t.
Randot Dot E stereo t.
Randot Stereo Smile t.
Raven Progressive Matrices t.
Rayleigh color matching t.
red-filter t.
red glare t.
red glass t.
rest t.
Rochat t.
rotational t.
Sabin-Feldman dye t.

scanning laser glaucoma t.
Schirmer 1 t.
Schirmer t. I, II
Schirmer tear quality t.
secondary dye t.
Seidel t.
separate image t.
shadow t.
Sheridan-Gardiner isolated letter-
matching t.
Shirmer basal secretion t.
Simpson t.
simultaneous prism cover t. (SPC)
single cover t.
skein t.
t. skein
SKILL Card T.
slit-beam t.
Smith-Kettlewell Institute Low
Luminance Card T.
Snellen t.
Statpac t.
stereopsis t.
stereo reindeer t.
Stilling color t.
subjective prism-neutralized cover t.
subjective refraction t.
swinging flashlight t.
swinging light t.
t. symbol
Synthetic Optics random dot
butterfly t.
taco t.
tear breakup t. (TBUT)
tear film t.
tear function t.
Tensilon t.
tension t.
three-character t.
three-step t.
thyroid function t. (TFT)
thyrotropin-releasing hormone t.
(TRH)
Titmus stereo t.
Titmus stereoacuity t.
Titmus vision t.
TNO stereo t.
traction t.
transillumination t.
TRH t.
triiodothyronine suppression t.
Tumblin-E t.

T

NOTES

test *(continued)*
    tumbling E t.
    tyrosinase t.
    University of Waterloo Colored
      Dot T. (UWCDot)
    VDS t.
    vertical prism t.
    Vistech 6500 contrast t.
    visual manipulation t.
    Visuscope motor t.
    Visuscope sensory t.
    water-drinking t.
    water provocative t.
    Watzke-Allen t.
    W4D t.
    Welland t.
    Werner t.
    Wernicke t.
    Westcott t.
    Wilbrand prism t.
    Wilcoxon matched pairs t.
    Wilcoxon signed rank t.
    Wirt stereo t.
    Wirt stereopsis t.
    Wirt vision t.
    Wolff-Eisner t.
    Worth 4-dot near flashlight t.
    χ^2 t.

tester
    APT-5 Color Vision T.
    Baylor-Video Acuity T. (BVAT)
    Mentor B-VAT II video acuity t.
    Miller-Nadler glare t.
    Phoroptor vision t.
    Prio video display terminal
      vision t.
    Topcon vision t.
    Vistech Multivision Contrast T.
      8000

testing
    antenatal t.
    Bruchner reflex t.
    confrontation visual field t.
    cranial nerve t.
    dark-room t.
    double-quadrant t.
    extraocular muscle t.
    filter glasses for color t.
    forced-duction t.
    four base-out prism t.
    hypothesis t.
    kinetic visual field t.
    lacrimal t.
    levator function t.
    near acuity t.
    near vision t.
    provocative t.
    pursuit t.

    quick estimation by sequential t.
      (QUEST)
    rapid antibiotic susceptibility t.
      (RAST)
    single-quadrant t.
    subjective t.
    tangent screen t.
    visual acuity t.
    visual field t.
    zippy estimating by sequential t.
      (ZEST)
    Zone Quick tear volume t.

tetani
    Clostridium t.

tetany
    t. cataract
    zonular t.

tetartanope
tetartanopia
tetartanopic
tetartanopsia
Tetcaine
tetracaine hydrochloride
Tetracon
tetracycline
tetrad
    Konoto t.
tetraethylammonium chloride
tetrahydrozoline hydrochloride
tetranopsia
Tetrasine Extra Ophthalmic
tetrastichiasis
tetroxide
    osmium t.
Tevdek suture
texaphyrin
    lutetium t. (lu-tex)
text blindness
TFT
    thyroid function test
TG-140 needle
thalamolenticular
thalamopeduncular
thalamus
    optic t.
Thalidomide
Thalomid
Thal procedure
thaw-freeze
Thayer-Martin plate
THC:YAG laser
the
    T. Berkeley Orthokeratology Study
    T. Pointing Game
    T. Safety and Efficacy of a
      Tumor Necrosis Factor Receptor
      Fusion Protein on Uveitis
    T. Silicone Study
    T. Wave phacoemulsion system

Theimich lip sign
Thelazia callipaeda
thelaziasis
Theobald probe
theobromae
    Lasiodiplodia t.
Theodore keratoconjunctivitis
theory
    Alhazen t.
    Barkan t.
    color t.
    Hering t.
    Ladd-Franklin t.
    migration t.
    molecular dissociation t.
    opponent colors t.
    retinex t.
    Scheiner t.
    Schön t.
    trichromatic color t.
    Unna abtropfung t.
    von Frisch t.
    Wollaston t.
    Young-Helmholtz t. of color vision
therapeutic
    t. contact lens
    t. dacryocystorhinostomy
    t. equivalence
    t. iridectomy
therapy
    cidofovir t.
    cobalt t.
    corticosteroid t.
    cytokine t.
    Dry T.
    external beam radiation t.
    fluorescein-potentiated argon laser t. (FPAL)
    ganciclovir t.
    highly active antiretroviral t. (HAART)
    hyperbaric oxygen t. (HBO)
    immunoadsorption t.
    immunomodulatory t.
    laser t.
    maximum tolerated medical t.
    Mini-Drops eye t.
    miotic t.
    mydriatic-cycloplegic t.
    occlusion t.
    photodynamic t. (PDT)
    PhotoPoint laser t.

    radiation t.
    red-filter t.
    silicone punctal plug t.
    stereotactic radiation t. (SRT)
    steroid t.
    systemic corticosteroid t.
    transcorneal oxygen t.
TheraTears lubricant eye drops
thermal
    t. adhesion
    t. burn
    t. cataract
    t. cautery
    t. keratoplasty (TKP)
    t. sclerectomy
    t. sclerostomy
thermocautery
Thermocycler
    Touchdown T.
thermokeratoplasty
    laser t.
thermoluminescence detector (TLD)
thermosclerectomy
thermosclerostomy
thermosclerotomy
thermotherapy
    adjuvant microwave t.
    microwave plaque t.
    transpupillary t. (TT, TTT)
thickening
    sclerochoroidal t.
thick lens
thickness
    central corneal t. (CCT)
    contact lens t.
    t. of contact lens
    standard t.
    stromal t.
Thiel-Behnke corneal dystrophy
Thill Aniseikonia Worksheet
thimerosal
thin lens
thinning
    choroidal t.
    corneal t.
    stromal t.
thin-rim scotoma
thioglycate broth
thiomalate
    gold sodium t.
thiopental sodium

NOTES

thioridazine
 t. hydrochloride
 t. retinal toxicity
 t. retinopathy
third
 t. cranial nerve (CN III)
 t. cranial nerve palsy
 t. framework region (FR3)
 t. order neuron
third-grade fusion
Thomas
 T. brush
 T. calipers
 T. cryoextractor
 T. cryoprobe
 T. cryoptor
 T. cryoretractor
 T. fixation forceps
 T. irrigating-aspirating cannula
 T. Kapsule instrument
 T. operation
 T. retractor
 T. scissors
 T. subretinal instrument set II
Thompson syndrome
Thorazine
Thornton
 T. arcuate blade
 T. double corneal ruler
 T. fixating ring
 T. fixation forceps
 T. guide for optical zone size
 T. limbal fixation ring
 T. limbal incision ruler
 T. malleable spatula
 T. needle
 T. optical center marker
 T. triple micrometer knife
 T. tri-square blade
Thornton-Fine ring
Thorpe
 T. calipers
 T. conjunctival forceps
 T. corneal forceps
 T. foreign body forceps
 T. four-mirror goniolaser
 T. four-mirror goniolaser lens
 T. four-mirror goniolens
 T. four-mirror vitreous fundus laser
  lens
 T. scissors
 T. slit lamp
 T. surgical gonioscope
Thorpe-Castroviejo
 T.-C. calipers
 T.-C. corneal forceps
 T.-C. fixation forceps
 T.-C. goniolens

 T.-C. scissors
 T.-C. vitreous foreign body forceps
Thorpe-Westcott scissors
Thorton
 T. globe fixation ring
 T. optic zone marker
Thrasher lens implant forceps
thread
 mucous t.
threat reflex
three
 t. dimensional
 t. o'clock staining
three-character test
three-mirror
 t.-m. contact lens
 t.-m. prism
three-piece
 t.-p. acrylic intraocular lens
 t.-p. silicone intraocular lens
three-point touch
three-snip
 t.-s. punctum
 t.-s. punctum operation
three-step test
three-toothed forceps
three-wall decompression
threshold
 achromatic t.
 brightness difference t.
 chromatic contrast t.
 color-contrast t.
 t. disease
 displacement t.
 t. effect
 final t.
 light differential t.
 t. limit value (TLV)
 minimum light t.
 prebleached dark-adapted t.
 quantitative static t.
 sensitivity t.
 t. stage III of retinopathy of
  prematurity (TS III ROP)
 tolerance t.
 visual t.
 t. of visual sensation
thromboangiitis obliterans
thrombosed artery
thrombosis
 carotid artery t.
 cavernous sinus t.
 orbital vein t.
 t. in retina
 retinal t.
 septic t.
thromboxane receptor antagonist
thrombus
 fibrin t.

through-the-lid contact ultrasound
thrush
    lid t.
thumb occluder
Thurmond
    T. nucleus-irrigating cannula
    T. pachymetry marker
Thygeson
    T. chronic follicular conjunctivitis
    T. disease
    punctate keratitis of T.
    superficial punctate keratitis of T.
     (SPKT)
    T. superficial punctate keratitis
    T. superficial punctate keratopathy
thymic hypoplasia
thymidine analog
thymoxamine hydrochloride
Thymoxid
thyroid
    t. exophthalmos
    t. eye disease
    t. function test (TFT)
    t. gland disorder
    t. lid retraction
    t. ophthalmopathy
    t. orbitopathy
    t. stare
thyroid-associated ophthalmopathy
  (TAO)
thyroidectomy
    subtotal t.
thyroiditis
    Hashimoto t.
    Riedel t.
thyroid-releasing hormone (TRH)
thyrotoxic exophthalmos
thyrotoxicosis ophthalmoplegia
thyrotropic exophthalmos
thyrotropin-releasing hormone test
  (TRH)
thyroxine, thyroxin
TIA
    transient ischemic attack
tiapride
Tiapridex
tic
    t. douloureux
    local t.
    motor t.
ticarcillin
ticrynafen ointment

tie-over Sellotape dressing
TIFF
    tagged image file format
tight
    t. contact lens
    t. lens syndrome (TLS)
TIGR
    trabecular meshwork-inducible
    glucocorticoid response
tigré
    fundus t.
TIGR **gene**
tigroid
    t. background
    t. fundus
    t. retina
Tiko
    T. pliable iris retractor
    T. zonule sweeper
Tilavist
Tilderquist needle holder
Tillaux
    extraocular muscles of T.
    spiral of T.
    T. spiral
Tillett operation
Tillyer bifocal lens
tilt
    pantoscopic t.
    t. of sella
    visual t.
tilted
    t. disc syndrome (TDS)
    t. disk
    t. disk syndrome
    t. vision
tilting
    t. lens
    t. lens atresia
time
    breakup t. (BUT)
    death-to-preservation t.
    edge-light pupil cycle t.
    fading t.
    implicit t.
    lacrimal transit t.
    noninvasive break-up t. (NIBOT)
    noninvasive tear film breakup t.
     (NITFBUT)
    not invasive break-up t.
    photostress recovery t. (PRT)
    Russell viper venom t.

T

NOTES

time *(continued)*
    sensation t.
    tear film breakup t.
    tumor doubling t.
Timentin
Timex TMX optical eyewear
timolol
    t. gellan
    t. hemihydrate
    t. maleate
    t. maleate ophthalmic gel-forming
     solution
    t. and pilocarpine
Timoptic
    T. Ocudose
    T. Ophthalmic
Timoptic-XE
    T.-X. Ophthalmic
Timpilo
T-incision
tinea tarsi
tin ethyl etiopurpurin (SnET2)
tinnitus
    gaze-evoked t.
tinted
    t. contact lens
    t. spectacles
tinting of spectacle lens
tip
    Binkhorst t.
    diathermy t.
    endolaser probe t.
    flared ABS t.
    Girard irrigating t.
    guillotine cutting t.
    Keeler lancet t.
    Keeler micro round t.
    Keeler micro spear t.
    Keeler puncture t.
    Keeler razor t.
    Keeler triple facet t.
    Kelman t.
    Kelman-Mackool flare t.
    Luer syringe t.
    MicroTip phaco t.
    Mitchell viscoelastic removal I/A t.
    nonaspirating ultrasonic phaco
     chopper t.
    Quad cutting t.
    rotary cutting t.
    Saverburger irrigation/aspiration t.
    Simcoe interchangeable t.
    TurboSonic t.
    Welsh flat olive-t.
tire
    276 t.
    implant t.
    t. implant

    silicone t.
    Watzke t.
tisiris
tissue
    t. adhesive
    adipose t.
    conjunctiva-associated lymphoid t.
    connective t.
    cutaneous t.
    donor t.
    ectopic t.
    epibulbar t.
    epiciliary proliferative t.
    episcleral t.
    t. forceps
    frozen t.
    human allograft t.
    hypergranulation t.
    hyperreflective t.
    limbal t.
    McCarey-Kaufman preserved
     donor t.
    mesoblastic t.
    mucosa-associated lymphoid t.
     (MALT)
    mucosal associated lymphoid t.
    nonfixed t.
    nuclear t.
    orbital adipose t.
    pericanalicular connective t.
    t. plasminogen
    t. plasminogen activator (TPA,
     tPA)
    posterior corneal t.
    pterygial t.
    scleral t.
    sustentacular t.
    transplantation of posterior
     corneal t.
    uveal t.
tissue-specific pericyte
Titan
titanium
    He hook chopper in t.
    t. miniplate
    t. needle
    Newsom cracker model 05-4063
     in t.
    t. suturing forceps
Titmus
    T. stereoacuity test
    T. stereo fly
    T. stereo test
    T. vision test
    T. Washer storage case
TKP
    temporary keratoprosthesis
    thermal keratoplasty

TL-1
>Minolta illuminance meter T.

TLD
>thermoluminescence detector

TLS
>tight lens syndrome

TLV
>threshold limit value

TM
>trabecular meshwork

TMS-1
>Topographic Modeling System-1
>TMS-1 videokeratoscope

TMS-2
>Topographic Modeling System-2
>TMS-2 computer-assisted
>videokeratoscope
>TMS-2 computerized corneal
>topographer

TMS corneal topography system

TN
>normal tension

Tn
>ocular tension

TNO stereo test
tobacco/alcohol amblyopia
tobacco amblyopia
TobraDex Ophthalmic
Tobralcon
tobramycin and dexamethasone
Tobrasol
Tobrex Ophthalmic
Toctron EA-290
TOD
>tension oculus dextra (tension of right
>eye)

Todd
>T. cautery
>T. electrocautery
>T. gouge
>T. paralysis

tolazoline
Tolentino
>T. prism lens
>T. ring
>T. vitrectomy lens
>T. vitrectomy lens set
>T. vitreous cutter

tolerance threshold
Tolman micrometer
Tolosa-Hunt syndrome

Tomas
>T. iris hook
>T. suture hook

tomato-ketchup fundus
tome
>Laschal precision suture t.
>precision suture t.

Tomey
>T. autorefractor
>T. autotopographer
>T. ConfoScan confocal microscope
>T. refractive workstation
>T. retinal function analyzer
>T. TMS-1 photokeratoscope
>T. topographic modeling system
>T. topography system
>T. Trooper AutoLensmeter

tomodensitometry
tomograph
>Heidelberg retina t. (HRT)
>Heidelberg retina t. II (HRT-II)

tomography
>axial t.
>carbonic anhydrase t.
>complex motion t.
>computed t. (CT)
>confocal scanning laser t.
>CSL t.
>3D i-Scan ultrasound t.
>Heidelberg retinal t.
>helical computed t.
>Humphrey model 2000 optical
>coherence t.
>ocular coherence t.
>optical coherence t. (OCT)
>orbital t.
>Retinal Detachment Using Optical
>Coherence T.

Tomycine
TON
>traumatic optic neuropathy

tonic
>t. accommodation
>t. convergence
>t. downward deviation
>t. lid
>t. pupil
>t. pupil syndrome
>t. upward deviation
>t. vergence

tonicity

NOTES

tonofilm
 crescent t.
 Schiötz t.
tonogram
tonograph
tonography
Tonomat applanation tonometer
tonometer
 air-puff contact t.
 air-puff noncontact t.
 Alcon t.
 Allen-Schiötz t.
 AO Reichert Instruments
  applanation t.
 applanation t.
 Barraquer applanation t.
 Barraquer operating room t.
 Berens t.
 Bigliano t.
 biprism applanation t.
 Carl Zeiss t.
 Challenger digital applanation t.
 Coburn t.
 Digilab t.
 Draeger t.
 Durham t.
 electronic t.
 Gartner t.
 Goldmann applanation t. (GAT)
 Harrington t.
 impression t.
 indentation t.
 Intermedics intraocular t.
 Keeler Pulsair t.
 Krakau t.
 Lombart t.
 Mackay-Marg electronic t.
 Maklakoff t.
 McLean t.
 Mueller electronic t.
 noncontact t. (NCT)
 OBF t.
 Pach-Pen XL t.
 Perkins applanation t.
 pneumatic t.
 portable PT100 noncontact t.
 pressure phosphene t.
 ProTon portable t.
 Pulsair t.
 Reichert noncontact t.
 Rosner t.
 Ruedemann t.
 Schiötz t.
 Sklar-Schiötz t.
 Storz t.
 Tonomat applanation t.
 Tono-Pen XL t.
tonometry
 applanation t. (AT)

 automatic t.
 digital t.
 indentation t.
 Schiötz t.
Tono-Pen
 Oculab T.-P.
 T.-P. XL tonometer
tonsil
 cerebellar t.
Tooke
 T. corneal knife
 T. cornea-splitting knife
 T. spatula
Tooke-Johnson corneal knife
tool
 lens simulation sales t.
 spud t.
toothed forceps
TOP
 Tendency-Oriented Perimetry
Topcon
 T. aspheric lens
 T. chart projector
 T. CM-1000 corneal mapping
  system
 T. eye refractometer
 T. 50IA camera
 T. IMAGEnet digital imaging
  system
 T. keratometer
 T. LM P5 digital lensometer
 T. noncontact morphometric
  analysis
 T. perimeter
 T. refractor
 T. RM-A2300 auto refractometer
 T. SL-7E photo slip lamp
 T. SL-E Series slit lamp
 T. SL-1E slit lamp
 T. SP-1000 noncontact specular
  microscope
 T. TRC-501A fundus camera
 T. TRC-50VT retinal camera
 T. TRC-50X retinal camera
 T. TRV-50VT fundus camera
 T. vision tester
topical
 t. anesthesia
 t. anesthetic
 t. cycloplegic
 t. drug
 t. 5-fluorouracil
 t. glucocorticoid
 t. hyperosmolar agent
 NeoDecadron T.
 t. treatment
topiramate

TOPO
topographic simulated keratometric power
top-of-the-basilar syndrome
topogometer
topographer
ASTRAmax stereo t.
Atlas corneal t.
CT 200 corneal t.
Dicon CT 200 corneal t.
Keratron corneal t.
TMS-2 computerized corneal t.
topographic
t. agnosia
t. anatomy
t. astigmatism
t. disorientation
t. echography
t. electroretinography
T. Modeling System-1 (TMS-1)
T. Modeling System-2 (TMS-2)
t. scanning/indocyanine green angiography combination instrument
T. Scanning System (TopSS)
t. simulated keratometric power (TOPO)
topographical electroretinogram
topographically
t. guided therapeutic laser in situ keratomileusis
t. guided therapeutic LASIK
topography
computer-assisted corneal t. (CACT)
computerized corneal t.
confocal laser scanning t.
corneal t.
elevation t.
EyeSys Technologies corneal t.
Holladay Diagnostic Summary t.
optic disc t.
Orbscan corneal t.
subtraction t.
TopSS scanning laser retinal t.
Topolanski sign
topometer
C-Scan color-ellipsoid t.
ToPreSite
TopSS
Topographic Scanning System
TopSS scanning laser ophthalmoscope

TopSS scanning laser retinal topography
TopSS topographic scanning system
TopSS/AngioScan system
TopSS/ICG
Toradol
T. Injection
T. Oral
torcula
toric
t. ablation
back surface t.
t. contact lens
t. intraocular lens
t. intraocular lens axis rotation
posterior t.
t. spectacle lens
t. surface
toricity
Toric-Optima series lens
torn iris
toroidal contact lens
torpor retinae
torque
muscle t.
torsion
Listing t.
torsional
t. deviation
t. diplopia
t. movement
t. nystagmus
t. oscillopsia
torticollis
ocular t.
tortuosity
familial arteriolar t.
t. of retinal vessel
vascularized t.
venous t.
Torulopsis glabrata
TOS
tension oculus sinister (tension of left eye)
total
t. anterior synechia
t. astigmatism
t. blindness
t. cataract
t. conjunctival flap (TCF)
t. hydrophthalmia
t. hyperopia (Ht)

T

NOTES

total *(continued)*
t. hyphema
t. iridectomy
t. keratoplasty
t. ophthalmoplegia
t. posterior synechia
t. sclerectasia
t. steady-state tear flow
t. symblepharon
T. The All-In-One Hard Contact Lens Solution
t. vitrectomy

totale
ankyloblepharon t.

totalis
ophthalmoplegia t.

Toti
T. operation
T. procedure

Toti-Mosher operation

toto
eye removed in t.

touch
corneal endothelial t.
iridocorneal t.
three-point t.
vitreous t.

Touchdown Thermocycler
Touchlite zoom lens
Touraine syndrome
Tournay
T. phenomenon
T. sign

Touton giant cell
towelettes
DisCide disinfecting t.

Townley-Paton operation
toxemic retinopathy of pregnancy
toxic
t. amaurosis
t. amblyopia
t. cataract
t. diabetes
t. follicular conjunctivitis
t. maculopathy
t. optic neuropathy
t. reaction
t. retinal metallosis
t. retinopathy
t. Strep syndrome
t. substance

toxicity
chloroquine t.
hydroxychloroquine t.
light t.
ocular t.
phenothiazine t.
photic retinal t.

retinal t.
thioridazine retinal t.

toxic-nutritional disease
toxicodendron
Rhus t.

toxicogenic conjunctivitis
toxin
botulinum t. A (BTA)
botulinum A t.

toxin-induced myopathy
Toxocara canis
toxocariasis
t. endophthalmitis
ocular t.

Toxoplasma
T. chorioretinitis
T. gondii

toxoplasmic
t. choroiditis
t. retinitis
t. retinochoroiditis
t. uveitis

toxoplasmosis
t. chorioretinitis
congenital t.
fulminant ocular t.
ocular t.
punctate outer retinal t.

Toynbee corpuscle
TPA, tPA
tissue plasminogen activator
intravitreal TPA

T-PRK
tracker-assisted photorefractive keratectomy
T-PRK laser

trabecula, pl. **trabeculae**
anterior chamber t.
scleral t.

trabecular
t. aspiration
t. fiber
t. membrane
t. membrane pigment
t. meshwork (TM)
t. meshwork-inducible glucocorticoid response (TIGR)
t. network
t. outflow

trabeculectomy
ab externo t.
Cairns t.
t. flap
initial t.
t. operation
Pearce t.
phaco t.
small incision t.
Smith t.

trabeculitis glaucoma
trabeculodialysis
trabeculodysgenesis
trabeculopexy
    argon laser t. (ALT)
trabeculoplasty
    argon laser t. (ALTP)
    diode laser t. (DLT)
    laser t.
    pneumatic t.
    selective laser t. (SLT)
trabeculopuncture
trabeculotome
    Allen-Burian t.
    Harms t.
    McPherson t.
trabeculotomy probe
trabeculotomy-trabeculectomy
    combined t.-t.
trabeculum
    corneoscleral t.
trabecuphine laser sclerostomy
trachoma, pl. **trachomata**
    Arlt t.
    Arlt-Jaesche t.
    t. body
    brawny t.
    cicatrizing t.
    follicular t.
    t. gland
    gland t.
    granular t.
    inactive t.
    MacCallan classification of t.
    prosthesis-induced t.
    Türck t.
    World Health Organization
        classification of t.
trachoma-inclusion conjunctivitis (TRIC)
trachomatis
    Chlamydia t.
trachomatosus
    pannus t.
trachomatous
    t. conjunctivitis
    t. dacryocystitis
    t. keratitis
    t. pannus
tracing
    optical ray t.
    ray t.

track
    bear t.'s
    corneal paracentesis t.
    polar bear t.'s
    snail t.'s
tracker
    Purkinje image t.
tracker-assisted
    t.-a. photorefractive keratectomy (T-PRK)
    t.-a. PRK laser
tracking
    pursuit t.
Tracor Northern
Tracoustic RV275
tract
    geniculocalcarine t.
    leiomyoma of uveal t.
    optic t.
    uveal t.
traction
    anterior loop t.
    t. band
    diabetic t.
    epiretinal membrane t.
    foveal t.
    macular t.
    t. macular detachment
    Moss t.
    peripheral vitreoretinal t.
    t. suture
    t. test
    vessel t.
    vitreomacular t.
    vitreopapillary t.
    vitreoretinal t.
    vitreous t.
tractional
    t. diabetic macular edema (TDME)
    t. retinal degeneration
    t. retinal detachment (TRD)
traction-related tear
trained retinal locus
training
    vision t.
Trainor-Nida operation
Trainor operation
Tramacort
Tramadol
tranexamic acid
transantral decompression

NOTES

transcaruncular-transconjunctival approach
transconjunctival
  t. aqueous oozing
  t. cryopexy
  t. frontalis suspension
  t. lower eyelid blepharoplasty
  t. route
transcorneal oxygen therapy
transcranial Doppler (TCD)
transcript
  latency associated t. (LAT)
transducer
  Accuscan T. 400
  Neuroguard pulsed wave t.
  Ocuscan 400 t.
  Sonogage System Corneo-Gage 20
    MHz center frequency t.
  UBM t.
  vector array t.
transducin
transepithelial photoablation
transferase
  terminal deoxynucleotidyl t. (TdT)
transfer function
transferred ophthalmia
transfixion
  t. of iris
  t. of iris operation
transformed migraine
transient
  t. ametropia
  t. blindness
  t. congestion
  t. early exophthalmos
  t. ischemic attack (TIA)
  t. layer of Chievitz
  t. myopia
  t. obscuration of vision
  t. photopsia
  t. unilateral dilation
  t. unilateral mydriasis
  t. vertebrobasilar ischemia
  t. visual loss
  t. visual obscuration
transillumination
  t. technique
  t. test
transilluminator
  Finnoff t.
  halogen Finoff t.
transitional zone
transition zone
translimbal
translocation
  foveal t.
  macular t.
  t. needle
  retinal t.

translucent
transmissibility
  oxygen t. (Dk/L)
transmission
  t. electron microscope
  t. electron microscopy
  ephaptic t.
  light t.
transmitted light
transneuronal degeneration
transocular technique
transorbital leukotomy
transparency
  corneal t.
transparent ulcer of the cornea
trans pars plana
transplant
  corneal t.
  lamellar corneal t.
  McReynolds pterygium t.
  ocular muscle t.
  penetrating corneal t.
transplantation
  amniotic membrane t.
  t. antigen
  autologous chondrocyte t.
  t. of cornea
  corneal t.
  epithelial t.
  limbal autograft t. (LAT)
  limbal-conjunctival autograft t.
    (LCAT)
  limbal stem-cell t.
  t. of muscle operation
  organ t.
  photoreceptor t.
  t. of posterior corneal tissue
  t. of submandibular gland for
    keratoconjunctivitis sicca
Transpore eye tape
transposition
  medial rectus t.
  muscle t.
  superior oblique t.
transpunctal endocanalicular approach
transpupillary
  t. cyclophotocoagulation
  t. laser
  t. retinopexy
  t. technique
  t. thermotherapy (TT, TTT)
Trans-Scan pulsed Doppler sonographer
transscleral
  t. cryopexy
  t. cryotherapy
  t. diathermy
  t. laser cyclophotocoagulation

t. neodymium:yttrium-aluminum-garnet cyclophotocoagulation for glaucoma
t. retinal photocoagulation
t. retinopexy
t. suture
t. suture fixation
t. suture fixation technique
transsclerally sutured posterior chamber lens (TS-SPCL)
transsphenoidal encephalocele
transsynaptic degeneration
transverse
t. axis of Fick
t. suture of Krause
t. tarsotomy
transvitreal
Trantas
T. dot
T. operation
tranylcypromine sulfate
TranZgraft
trap-door
t.-d. fracture
t.-d. scleral buckle operation
trapezoid
t. angled CVD diamond knife
t. single-plane clear corneal incision
trapezoidal keratotomy
trap incision
Traquair
T. island
junctional scotoma of T.
scotoma of T.
trauma, pl. traumas, traumata
air bag-associated t.
blunt t.
corneal t.
intraocular foreign body t.
ocular t.
orbital t.
orbitocranial t.
prevalence of ocular t.
traumatic
t. amblyopia
t. angle recession
t. aniridia
t. atrophy
t. choroidal rupture
t. choroiditis
t. corneal abrasion

t. corneal cyst
t. degenerative cataract
t. endophthalmitis
t. glaucoma
t. gliosis
t. hyphema
t. microhyphema
t. mydriasis
t. myopathy
t. optic neuropathy (TON)
t. ptosis
t. pupillary miosis
t. rent
t. retinopathy
t. scleral cyst
t. wound dehiscence
Travatan ophthalmic solution
travoprost ophthalmic solution
tray
I-tech cannula t.
Trbinger detachment
TRC-50IX ICG-capable fundus camera
TRC-SS2 stereoscopic fundus camera
TRD
tractional retinal detachment
Treacher
T. Collins-Franceschetti syndrome
T. Collins syndrome
treating herpetic anterior uveitis
treatment
An Observation Study on Recurrence of Amblyopia After Discontinuation of T.
antimicrobial t.
argon laser retinal t.
corticosteroid t.
external beam radiation t.
focal laser t.
Imre t.
Ocular Microcirculation View Analysis T. (OMVAT)
PhotoPoint t.
Refresh Liquigel dry eye t.
Schöler t.
surgical t.
topical t.
t. zone laser ablation
tree
vascular t.
trematode infection
trematodiasis

T

NOTES

529

tremor
> head t.
> immunosuppressant-induced head t.
> oculopalatal t.

tremulous
> t. cataract
> t. iris

trepanation
> t. of cornea
> corneal t.

trephination
> elliptical t.
> excimer laser t.
> host t.
> nonmechanical t.
> open-sky t.
> partial-thickness t.

trephine
> Arroyo t.
> Arruga lacrimal t.
> automated t.
> automatic t.
> Bard-Parker t.
> Barraquer t.
> Barron epikeratophakia t.
> Barron-Hessburg corneal t.
> Barron radial vacuum t.
> t. blade
> Bonaccolto t.
> bone t.
> bone-biting t.
> Boston t.
> Brown-Pusey corneal t.
> Caldwell Suction T.
> Cardona corneal prosthesis t.
> Castroviejo corneal transplant t.
> Castroviejo improved t.
> chalazion t.
> corneal prosthesis t.
> Davis t.
> DiaPhine t.
> Dimitry chalazion t.
> disposable t.
> Elliot corneal t.
> Elschnig t.
> epithelial t.
> Gradle corneal t.
> Green t.
> Grieshaber calibrated t.
> Grieshaber corneal t.
> Guyton corneal transplant t.
> hand-held t.
> Hanna t.
> Hessburg-Barron disposable vacuum t.
> Hessburg-Barron suction t.
> Huang LASEK t.
> Iliff lacrimal t.
> Katena t.

> Katzin t.
> King corneal t.
> lacrimal t.
> LASEK alcohol well and epithelial t.
> Lichtenberg corneal t.
> lid t.
> Londermann corneal t.
> Lopez-Enriquez scleral t.
> Martinez disposable corneal t.
> M-brace corneal t.
> Moria t.
> Mueller electric corneal t.
> Ophtec 9.0 mm t.
> Paton corneal t.
> Paufique t.
> Pharmacia corneal t.
> punch t.
> razor-blade t.
> Scheie t.
> Searcy chalazion t.
> Sloane t.
> Storz corneal t.
> Storz DiaPhine t.
> suction t.
> Surgistar corneal t.
> Troutman tenotomy t.
> Walker t.
> Weck t.

Treponema
> *T. pallidum*
> *T. pallidum* hemagglutination

treponemal antibody
Tretinoin
TRH
> thyroid-releasing hormone
> thyrotropin-releasing hormone test
> TRH test

triad
> Charcot t.
> Hoyt-Spencer t.
> Hutchinson t.
> near t.
> t. of retinal cone

trial
> A T. of Bifocals in Myopic Children with Esophoria
> t. case
> t. case and lens
> t. clip
> Complications of Age-Related Macular Degeneration Prevention T. (CAPT)
> t. contact lens
> Correction of Myopia Evaluation T. (COMET)
> Cytomegalovirus Retinitis Retreatment T. (CRRT)

Diabetes Control and
    Complications T.
Early Manifest Glaucoma T.
    (EMGT)
Foscarnet-Ganciclovir CMV
    Retinitis T. (FGCRT)
t. frame
Ganciclovir-Cidofovir CMV
    Retinitis T. (GCCRT)
Glaucoma Laser T. (GLT)
HPMPC Peripheral CMV
    Retinitis T. (HPCRT)
Monoclonal Antibody CMV
    Retinitis T. (MACRT)
Sorbinil Retinopathy T. (SRT)
Submacular Surgery T.'s (SST)
triamcinolone acetonide
Triamond
Fine Finesse T.
triangle
Arlt t.
color t.
fitting t.
frontal t.
Wernicke t.
triangular capsulotomy
Tri-Beeled trapezoidal keratome
tributary vein occlusion
TRIC
trachoma-inclusion conjunctivitis
tricarbocyanine dye
trichiasis repair
trichilemmoma
Trichinella spiralis
trichodysplasia
trichofolliculoma tumor
trichoma
trichomatosis
trichomatous
trichophytosis
trichosis carunculae
trichroic
trichroism
trichromasy
trichromatic, trichromic
t. color theory
trichromatism
anomalous t.
trichromatopsia
anomalous t.
trichromic (*var. of* trichromatic)
tricurve contact lenses

trifacial neuralgia
trifluoperazine hydrochloride
trifluorothymidine
trifluperidol hydrochloride
trifluridine eye drops
trifocal
executive t.
t. glasses
t. lens
trigeminal
t. denervation
t. herpes zoster dermatitis
t. nerve (NV)
t. nerve root section
t. neuralgia
t. neuropathic keratopathy
t. pain
t. reflex
t. sensory ganglion
t. shield
trigemino oculomotor synkinesis
trigeminus
nervus t.
reflex t.
t. reflex
trigger mechanism
trigone
Mueller t.
triiodothyronine suppression test
trilamellar
trilateral retinoblastoma
trimethidium methosulfate
trimethoprim and polymyxin B
triopathy
Tri-Ophtho
triparanol
tripelennamine
Tripier
T. operation
T. operation throw square knot
T. operation triple
T. operation vision
triple
T. Antibiotic
t. facet-tip needle
t. procedure
t. symptom complex
Tripier operation t.
t. vision
Triple-Gen
triple-throw square knot stitch
triplokoria, triptokoria

NOTES

T

triplopia
tripod fracture
Tri-Port sub-Tenon anesthesia cannula
triptokoria (*var. of* triplokoria)
TripTone Caplets
triradiate line
Tris-borate buffer
trisector
    Alfonso nucleus t.
trisodium phosphonoformate hexahydrate
Trisol
tristichia
tritan axis
tritanomal
tritanomalous
tritanomaly
tritanope
tritanopia
tritanopic
tritanopsia
Tri-Thalmic HC
Triton
trocar
    Veirs t.
trocar-cannula system
trochlea
    t. musculi obliqui superioris bulbi
    t. musculi obliqui superioris oculi
    t. of superior oblique muscle
trochlear
    t. fossa
    t. fovea
    t. hamulus
    t. muscle
    t. nerve (CR IV, N.IV)
    t. nerve lesion
    t. nerve nucleus
    t. nerve palsy
    t. tubercle
trochlearis
    fossa t.
    fovea t.
    nervus t.
    spina t.
Trokel
    T. hyperopia conformer
    T. lens
Trokel-Peyman laser lens
troland
tromethamine
    ketorolac t.
    lodoxamide t.
Troncoso
    T. gonioscope
    T. gonioscopic lens implant
Tropheryma whippelii
trophic
    t. change
    t. defect

    t. keratitis
    t. keratopathy
    t. retinal degeneration
    t. ulceration of the cornea
tropia
    alternating t.
    constant monocular t.
    t. deviation
    horizontal t.
    intermittent t.
    vertical t.
tropica
    Leishmania t.
Tropicacyl
tropical
    t. optic neuropathy
    t. polyhexamethylene biguanide
tropicalis
    Candida t.
tropicamide
    hydroxyamphetamine and t.
tropic deviation
tropometer
troposcope
Trousseau sign
Troutman
    T. bladebreaker
    T. blade holder
    T. cannula
    T. conjunctival scissors
    T. corneal dissector
    T. corneal knife
    T. implant
    T. lens loupe
    T. microsurgical scissors
    T. needle holder
    T. nonincisional lamellar dissector
    T. operation
    T. punch
    T. rectus forceps
    T. suture scissors
    T. tenotomy trephine
    T. tying forceps
Troutman-Barraquer
    T.-B. corneal fixation forceps
    T.-B. corneal utility forceps
Troutman-Castroviejo
    T.-C. corneal fixation forceps
    T.-C. corneal section scissors
Troutman-Katzin corneal transplant
    scissors
Troutman-Llobera fixation forceps
Troutman-Tooke corneal knife
Trovert
Truc
    T. flap
    T. operation
true
    t. exfoliation

t. hemianopsia
t. image
t. visual acuity (TVA)
Trujillo
T. LASIK enhancement hook
T. LASIK enhancement rake
T. LASIK enhancement wedge
Trump solution
truncated contact lens
truncation
trunk
facial nerve t.
Trupower aspherical lens
TruPro lacrimal cannula
Trusopt
TruVision lens
Trypanosoma
trypanosomiasis
trypsin-digested explant
trypticase soy broth
TSC
tuberous sclerosis complex
T-sign
TS III ROP
threshold stage III of retinopathy of
prematurity
TS-SPCL
transsclerally sutured posterior chamber
lens
tsukubaensis
Streptomyces t.
Tsuneoka irrigating hook
TT
transpupillary thermotherapy
t-**test**
Student unpaired *t*-t.
TTT
transpupillary thermotherapy
T-tube
cul-de-sac irrigation T.-t.
Houser cul-de-sac irrigator T.-t.
lacrimal duct T.-t.
polyethylene T.-t.
Pyrex T.-t.
Silastic T.-t.
vinyl T.-t.
tube
Ahmed glaucoma drainage t.
Ahmed shunt t.
angled suction t.
anterior chamber t.
Baerveldt glaucoma implant t.

Baerveldt shunt t.
Bowman t.
corneal t.
Crawford t.
encircling polyethylene t.
endotracheal t.
Eppendorf t.
Frazier suction t.
fusion t.
Guibor duct t.
Guibor Silastic t.
Houser cul-de-sac irrigator t.
Jones Pyrex t.
Jones tear duct t.
laser t.
Lester Jones t.
L.T. Jones tear duct t.
Luer t.
Microfuge t.
Molteno shunt t.
Moulton lacrimal duct t.
neural t.
polyethylene t.
Pyrex t.
Questek laser t.
Quickert-Dryden t.
Reinecke-Carroll lacrimal t.
silicone t.
vinyl t.
tuber
frontal t.
tubercle
t. bacillus
caseating t.
lacrimal t.
lateral orbit t.
lateral orbital t.
lateral palpebral t.
optic disk t.
trochlear t.
Whitnall t.
tubercular retinal vasculitis
tuberculin syringe
tuberculoma
optochiasmatic t.
tuberculosis
t. conjunctivitis
intraocular t.
Mycobacterium t.
tuberculous
t. dacryocystitis
t. iritis

NOTES

tuberculous *(continued)*
   t. keratitis
   t. phlyctenulosis
   t. rhinitis
   t. tarsitis
   t. uveitis
tuberous
   t. sclerosis
   t. sclerosis complex (TSC)
tube-shunt procedure
tubing
   bicanalicular t.
   t. introducer forceps
   silicone t.
   viscodissector t.
Tübinger
   T. perimeter
   T. perimetry
tubular
   t. vision
   t. visual field
tubulointerstitial nephritis and uveitis syndrome
tuck
   iris t.
   left superior oblique t.
   t. procedure
tucked lid of Collier
tucker
   Bishop-Peter tendon t.
   Bishop tendon t.
   Burch-Greenwood tendon t.
   Fink tendon t.
   Green muscle t.
   Green strabismus t.
   Ruedemann-Todd tendon t.
   tendon t.
Tudor-Thomas
   T.-T. graft
   T.-T. operation
tuft
   cystic retinal t.
   neovascular t.
   retinal t.
   vitreoretinal t.
   zonular-traction retinal t.
tularemia
   oculoglandular t.
tularemic conjunctivitis
tularensis
   conjunctivitis t.
   Francisella t.
Tulevech cannula
Tulio phenomenon
tulle gras dressing
Tumblin-E test
tumbling
   t. E cube
   t. E test

   t. procedure
   t. technique
   t. technique operation
tumor
   anemone cell t.
   t. apex
   apical t.
   benign t.
   brain t.
   Brooke t.
   carcinoid t.
   cerebellar astrocytoma t.
   cerebellopontine angle t.
   chiasmal t.
   choristoma t.
   choroidal melanocytic t.
   Coerens t.
   collision t.
   congenital limbal corneal dermoid t.
   conjunctival lymphoid t.
   craniofacial fibro-osseous t.
   cystic hydrocystoma t.
   dermoid t.
   t. doubling time
   ependymoma t.
   epithelial t.
   eyelid t.
   t. of eyelid
   fibroosseous t.
   fossa t.
   Grawitz t.
   hair follicle t.
   histiocytic t.
   t. of interior of eye
   interior eye t.
   intrasellar t.
   Koenen t.
   lacrimal gland epithelial t.
   lymphoid t.
   lymphoproliferative t.
   malignant epithelial t.
   medulloblastoma t.
   melanocytic iris t.
   mesenchymal t.
   metastasis of t.
   t. metastasis
   metastatic choroidal t.
   mixed t.
   mucinous adenocarcinoma t.
   neurogenic t.
   nonepithelial t.
   ocular adnexal t.
   optic nerve t.
   t. of optic nerve
   orbital t.
   Pancoast t.
   papilliform t.
   phakomatous choristoma t.

pilomatrixoma t.
pituitary t.
plasma cell t.
pleomorphic spindle cell t.
primitive neuroectodermal t.
 (PNET)
Rathke pouch t.
retinal anlage t.
rhabdoid t.
Schmincke t.
spinal canal t.
spindle-cell t.
suprasellar t.
syringoma t.
trichofolliculoma t.
vascular t.
Warthin t.
waxy t.
Wilms t.
Zimmerman t.
tunable dye laser
TUNEL
 terminal deoxynucleotidyl transferase-
 mediated dUTP-digoxigenin nick-end
 labeling
 TUNEL assay
 TUNEL staining
tungsten-halogen lamp
tunic
 Brücke t.
 fibrous t.
 fibrovascular t.
 Ruysch t.
 vascular t.
tunica
 t. adnata oculi
 t. albuginea oculi
 t. conjunctiva
 t. conjunctiva bulbi oculi
 t. conjunctiva palpebra
 t. fibrosa bulbi
 t. fibrosa oculi
 t. interna bulbi
 t. nervea
 t. nervosa oculi
 t. sclerotica
 t. sensoria bulbi
 t. uvea
 t. vasculosa bulbi
 t. vasculosa lentis
 t. vasculosa oculi

tunnel
 t. field
 scleral t.
 t. vision
tunneled implant
tunneler
 crescent scleral t.
 SatinCrescent t.
turbidity-reducing unit
TurboSonic tip
TurboStaltic pump
turbo-tip of phacoemulsification unit
turcica
 sella t.
Türck trachoma
Turkish saddle
Turk line
turnover
 epithelial t.
 tear t.
Turtle chart
tutamina oculi
Tutoplast
TVA
 true visual acuity
Tween
tweezers
 jeweler's t.
twelfth nerve palsy
twenty/twenty
 t. argon-fluoride excimer laser
 T. drops
twice daily (b.i.d.)
twilight
 t. blindness
 t. vision
twin cone
Twirl
 Spherical T.
twirling method
Twisk microscissors
twist
 t. fixation hook
 scleral t.
 stitch with t.'s
twisted virgin silk suture
twitch
 Cogan lid t.
two-angled polypropylene loop
two-handed phacoemulsification
two-light discrimination
two-plane lens

NOTES

535

two-staged Baerveldt glaucoma implant
two-way
  t.-w. cataract-aspirating cannula
  t.-w. syringe
  t.-w. towel clip
Tycos manometer
tying forceps
tying/stitch removal forceps
tyloma conjunctivae
tylosis ciliaris
tyloxapol
Tyndall
  T. effect
  T. phenomenon
type
  t. 1, 2 diabetes
  Jaeger test t.
  t. 1 herpes simplex virus
  point system test t.
  Snellen test t.

typhlology
typhlosis
typhus
  epidemic t.
  scrub t.
typical
  t. achromatopsia
  t. coloboma
typoscope
tyramine hydrochloride
Tyrell iris hook
tyrosinase-negative type oculocutaneous albinism
tyrosinase-positive type oculocutaneous albinism
tyrosinase test
tyrosinemia type I, II, III
Tzanck
  T. smear
  T. technique

UBM
 ultrasound biomicroscopy
  UBM transducer
UCVA
 uncorrected visual acuity
UEA-1
 Ulex europaeus agglutinin 1
UGH
 uveitis glaucoma hyphema
  UGH syndrome
UGH+ syndrome
Uhthoff
 U. phenomenon
 U. sign
 U. symptom
 U. syndrome
UL
 upper lid
Ulanday double cannula
ulcer
 acne rosacea corneal u.
 ameboid u.
 anular u.
 bacterial infectious corneal u.
 catarrhal corneal u.
 central corneal u.
 chronic serpiginous u.
 community-acquired corneal u.
 conjunctival u.
 contact lens-induced peripheral u.
  (CLPU)
 corneal u.
 dendriform u.
 dendritic herpes simplex corneal u.
 descemetocele u.
 fascicular u.
 fungal corneal u.
 geographic herpes simplex
  corneal u.
 herpes simplex corneal u.
 herpetic u.
 hypopyon u.
 infectious corneal u.
 Jacob u.
 marginal catarrhal u.
 marginal corneal u.
 metaherpetic u.
 Mooren corneal u.
 noncentral u.
 oval-shaped vernal u.
 peripheral corneal u.
 pneumococcal u.
 pneumococcus u.
 ring u.
 rodent u.

 Saemisch u.
 serpiginous corneal u.
 shield u.
 sterile corneal u.
 stromal u.
 superior corneal shield u.
 suppurative u.
 Terrien u.
 visually insignificant infectious
  corneal u.
 von Hippel internal corneal u.
 xerophthalmic u.
ulceration
 catarrhal marginal u.
 u. of cornea
 frank corneal u.
 geographic u.
 herpes epithelial tropic u.
 indolent u.
 Mooren u.
 necrotizing sclerocorneal u. (NSU)
 perilimbal u.
 rheumatoid related u.
 serpiginous u.
ulcerative keratitis
ulcerogranuloma
ulceromembranous
ulcerosa
 blepharitis u.
ulcus serpens corneae
ulectomy
ulerythema ophryogene
Ulex europaeus agglutinin 1 (UEA-1)
Ulloa operation
Ullrich-Feichtiger syndrome
Ullrich syndrome
Ultex
 U. bifocal
 U. lens
 U. lens implant
Ultima
 Dioptron U.
 U. 2000 photocoagulator
Ultra
 U. mag lens
 U. Tears
 U. Tears Solution
 U. view SP slit lamp lens
Ultracaine
UltraCare Disinfecting
 Solution/Neutralizer with Color
Ultracell LASIK spear
Ultra-Image A-scan
Ultra-Lase
ultra-late phase

U

Ultram
Ultramatic
 U. Project-O-Chart (UPOC)
 U. Project-O-Chart projector
 U. Rx Master Phoroptor
 U. Rx Master phoroptor retractor
ultramicrotome
 Reichert-Jung Ultracut u.
Ultrapred
UltraPulse laser
ultrascan
 Digital B System u.
 U. Digital B system
 U. Digital 2000 contact ultrasound
 A-scan
Ultra-select nitinol guide wire
UltraShaper Keratome
Ultrasharp round blade microKnife AU
 681-21-3
ultrasonic
 u. cataract-removal lancet
 u. cataract-removal lancet needle
 u. insonification
 u. micrometer
 U. pachymeter
 u. pachymetry
ultrasonogram
 A-scan u.
 B-scan u.
 Doppler u.
 gray-scale u.
ultrasonography
 A-scan u.
 B-scan u.
 Contact B-scan u.
 CooperVision u.
 Doppler u.
 water-bath u.
ultrasound
 Acuson u.
 Alcon Digital B 2000 u.
 Axisonic II u.
 U. Biomicroscope System
 u. biomicroscopy (UBM)
 CooperVision u.
 3D i-Scan ophthalmic u.
 Doppler u.
 high-gain digital u.
 kinetic u.
 ocular u.
 Ocuscan A-scan biometric u.
 u. pachometer
 u. pachymeter-KMI RK-5000
 renal u.
 through-the-lid contact u.
UltraTears
UltraThin surgical blade
ultraviolet
 u. A (UVA)

 u. B (UVB)
 u. blocker
 u. burn
 u. filter
 u. keratoconjunctivitis
 u. keratopathy
 u. light
 u. radiation
 u. ray ophthalmia
ultraviolet-induced injury
Ultravue lens
Ultrazyme enzymatic cleaner
umbilicated cataract
umbra
umbrella
 u. iris
 U. punctum plug
umbrella-like pattern
unaberrated chart
Unasyn
uncal syndrome
uncinate
 u. procedure
 u. process of lacrimal bone
unconventional outflow
uncorrected visual acuity (UCVA)
uncrossed diplopia
uncut spectacle lens
underaction
 congenital superior oblique u.
undercorrection
underlying
 u. conus
 u. cornea
underpigmentation
underwater diathermy unit
undine dropper
undissociated alkaloid
undulatory nystagmus
unequal retinal image
Unfolder implantation system
ung
 ointment
unguis
 os u.
 pterygium u.
unharmonious ARC
Unicare blue and green all-in-one
 cleaning solution
Unicat diamond knife
unifocal
 u. helioid choroiditis
 u. optic nerve lesion
unilateral
 u. acute idiopathic maculopathy
 u. altitudinal scotoma
 u. arcus
 u. conjunctivitis
 u. corneal lattice dystrophy

u. hearing loss
u. hemianopsia
u. lesion
u. microtremor
u. papilledema
u. proptosis
u. ptosis of eyelid
u. sporadic retinoblastoma
u. strabismus
uniocular
u. hemianopsia
u. strabismus
Uniplanar style PC II lens
UniPulse 1040 Surgical CO_2 laser system
UniShaper Keratome
Unisol
U. Plus
U. 4 Preservative Free Saline Solution
unit
Alcon cryosurgical u.
Alcon irrigating/aspirating u.
Alcon 20,000 Legacy u.
Alcon 10,000 Master u.
Alcon phacoemulsification u.
Aloe reading u.
Amoils cryosurgical u.
Angström u.
AO Ful-Vue diagnostic u.
AO Reichert Instruments Ful-Vue diagnostic u.
Bishop-Harman irrigating/aspirating u.
Bovie electrocautery u.
Bovie electrosurgical u.
Bovie retinal detachment u.
Bracken irrigating/aspirating u.
Charles irrigating/aspirating u.
Cilco Ultrasound u.
Coburn irrigation/aspiration u.
Cooper I&A u.
Cooper irrigating/aspirating u.
CooperVision irrigating/aspirating u.
CooperVision irrigation/aspiration u.
cryosurgical u.
DeVilbiss irrigating/aspirating u.
diathermy u.
Dougherty irrigating/aspirating u.
Drews irrigating/aspirating u.
Drews-Rosenbaum irrigating/aspirating u.

Fink irrigating/aspirating u.
Fox irrigating/aspirating u.
Frigitronics cryosurgical u.
Gass irrigating/aspirating u.
Gibson irrigating/aspirating u.
Girard ultrasonic u.
Hartstein irrigating/aspirating u.
Holzknecht u.
Hyde irrigating/aspirating u.
Hyde irrigator/aspirator u.
Intermedics Phaco I/A u.
IOLAB irrigating/aspirating u.
irrigation/aspiration u.
Irvine irrigating/aspirating u.
Keeler cryophake u.
Keeler cryosurgical u.
Kelman-Cavitron I/A u.
Kelman-Cavitron irrigating/aspirating u.
Kelman cryosurgical u.
Kelman irrigating/aspirating u.
Kelman phacoemulsification u.
Krymed Cryopexy u.
u. of light
log u.
u. of luminous flux
u. of luminous intensity
McIntyre irrigating/aspirating u.
microcautery u.
Mira diathermy u.
N_2O cryosurgical u.
u. of ocular convergence
Ocutome vitrectomy u.
OMS Empac Irrigation/Aspiration u.
Peczon I/A u.
Peyman vitrectomy u.
Peyman vitreophage u.
Phaco Cavitron irrigating/aspirating u.
Phaco Emulsifier Cavitron u.
Pierce I/A u.
Premiere irrigation/aspiration u.
Rollet irrigating/aspirating u.
Schepens retinal detachment u.
Simcoe double-barreled irrigating/aspirating u.
SITE TXR 2200 microsurgical u.
Storz-Walker retinal detachment u.
Surg-E-Trol System irrigating/aspirating u.
Svedberg u.
Sylva irrigating/aspirating u.

U

NOTES

unit *(continued)*
  Talbot u.
  turbidity-reducing u.
  turbo-tip of phacoemulsification u.
  underwater diathermy u.
  Visitec aspiration u.
  Visitec irrigating/aspirating u.
  Visitec vitrectomy u.
  Vitrophage-Peyman u.
unitas
  oculi u. (both eyes)
United Sonics J shock phaco fragmentor system
unity conjugacy planes
univariate
  u. linear regression
  u. polytomous logistic regression
Universal
  U. conformer
  U. eye shield
  U. II forceps
  U. implant
  U. Pathfinder knife
  U. phaco chopper/manipulator
  U. slit lamp
  U. soft tip cannulated sliding extrusion needle
universale
  angiokeratoma corporis diffusum u.
University
  U. of Waterloo chart
  U. of Waterloo Colored Dot Test (UWCDot)
Univis
  U. bifocal
  U. lens
UniVisc
Univision low-vision microscopic lens
Unna abtropfung theory
unoprostone
  u. isopropyl
  u. isopropyl ester
unpegged hydroxyapatite implant
unrefined refraction
unstained wet mount
unwanted migration of pigment
unzipper
  Katzen flap u.
up
  base u. (BU)
UPA
  urokinase-type plasminogen activator
up-and-down staircases procedure
upbeat nystagmus
updrawn pupil
upgaze
UPOC
  Ultramatic Project-O-Chart
  UPOC projector

upper
  u. canaliculus
  u. eyelid
  u. hemianopsia
  u. lid (UL)
  u. palpebral conjunctiva
  u. punctum
  u. retina
  u. tarsal conjunctiva
upside-down
  u.-d. ptosis
  u.-d. reversal of vision
uptake
  lacrimal gland gallium u.
upward
  u. gaze
  u. squint
URAM E2 compact MicroProbe laser
urate band keratopathy
uratic
  u. conjunctivitis
  u. iritis
Ureaphil Injection
uremic
  u. amaurosis
  u. amblyopia
  u. optic neuropathy
  u. retinitis
Uribe orbital implant
urica
  cornea u.
  keratitis u.
urinary
  u. GAG assay
  u. glycosaminoglycan measurement assay
urine refractometry
Urokinase
urokinase-type plasminogen activator (UPA)
Urrets-Zavalia retinal surgical lens
US-2000 echo scan
USA
  Dutch Ophthalmic U.
USC
  U. marker
  U. scleral planer
  U. scleral shaver
Usher syndrome
UTAS 2000 electroretinography instrument
uterque
  oculi u. (each eye) (OU)
  visio oculus u. (vision of both eyes) (VOU)
Utrata
  U. capsulorrhexis forceps
  U. foldable lens cutter
  U. retriever

Utrata-Kershner capsulorrhexis cystitome forceps
utricular reflex
UV
    U. blocking filter
    U. Nova Curve lens
UVA
    ultraviolet A
UVB
    ultraviolet B
uvea
    tunica u.
uveae
    ectropion u.
    entropion u.
    sarcomatosum u.
uveal
    u. atrophy
    u. coat
    u. effusion
    u. effusion syndrome
    u. entropion
    u. framework
    u. juvenile xanthogranuloma
    u. melanocyte
    u. melanoma
    u. metastasis
    u. neurofibroma
    u. nevus
    u. osteoma
    u. staphyloma
    u. tissue
    u. tract
    u. tract hamartoma
    u. tract hemangioma
uvealis
    pars u.
uveitic
    u. band keratopathy
    u. glaucoma
uveitides
uveitis, uveitides, pl. **uveitides**
    anterior u.
    aspergillosis u.
    bacterial u.
    Behçet u.
    bilateral u.
    candidal u.
    chronic anterior u. (CAU)
    endogenous u.
    excessive rebound u.
    Förster u.

    Fuchs u.
    fungal u.
    u. glaucoma hyphema (UGH)
    granulomatous anterior u.
    herpes simplex u.
    heterochromic u.
    HLA-B27-associated u.
    immune recovery u.
    u. intermedia
    intermediate u.
    Kirisawa u.
    lens-induced u.
    leptospiral u.
    nongranulomatous anterior u.
    parasitic u.
    peripheral u.
    phacoanaphylactic u.
    phacogenic u.
    phacolytic u.
    phacotoxic u.
    posterior u.
    protozoan u.
    Safety and Efficacy of a Heparin-Coated Intraocular Lens in U.
    sarcoid u.
    sarcoidosis-associated u.
    sympathetic u.
    The Safety and Efficacy of a Tumor Necrosis Factor Receptor Fusion Protein on U.
    toxoplasmic u.
    treating herpetic anterior u.
    tuberculous u.
    viral u.
    vitiligo u.
    Vogt-Koyanagi bilateral u.
    zoster u.
uveitis-vitiligo-alopecia-poliosis syndrome
uveocutaneous syndrome
uveoencephalitic syndrome
uveoencephalitis
uveolabyrinthitis
uveomeningeal syndrome
uveomeningitis syndrome
uveomeningoencephalitis
uveoneuraxitis
uveoparotitis
uveoplasty
uveoretinitis
uveoscleral outflow
uveoscleritis
uveovertex drainage

U

NOTES

Uvex lens
uviban
UWCDot
   University of Waterloo Colored Dot Test

Uyemura
   U. operation
   U. syndrome

V
    volume
       V pattern
       V syndrome
VA
    VA magnetic orbital implant
Va$_{cc}$
    corrected visual acuity
Vac
    Vaper V. II
vaccinia
    blepharoconjunctivitis v.
    v. gangrenosa
    generalized v.
    v. infection
    keratitis v.
    progressive v.
vaccinial keratitis
vacciniforme
    hydroa v.
vaccinulosa
    keratitis post v.
Vac-Down
Vactro
    V. perilimbal suction
    V. perilimbal suction apparatus
vacuolar configuration
vacuole
    autophagic v.
    cortical v.
    nonmembrane-bound v.'s
Vac-Up
vacuum-centering guide
vaginae
    v. externa nervi optici
    v. interna nervi optici
    v. oculi
vagus nerve paralysis
Vahlkampfia **cyst**
Vaiser-Cibis muscle retractor
Vaiser sponge
valacyclovir
valganciclovir
Valilab electrocautery
ValleyLab cautery
valproate sodium
Valsalva
    V. maneuver
    V. retinopathy
Valtrex
value
    Abbe v.
    C v.
    Dk v.
    equivalent oxygen percentage v.

    ocular hemodynamic v.
    p v.
    predictive v.
    prismatic dioptric v.
    spatially resolved v.
    threshold limit v. (TLV)
valve
    Ahmed glaucoma v. (AGV)
    Ahmed glaucoma biplate v.
    Béraud v.
    Bianchi v.
    Bochdalek v.
    filtering v.
    Foltz v.
    v. of Hasner
    Hasner v.
    Huschke v.
    Krause v.
    Krupin v.
    Krupin-Denver v.
    v. of Rosenmüller
    Rosenmüller v.
    Taillefer v.
    Van Herick v.
van
    v. den Berg stray-light meter
    v. der Hoeve disease
    V. Herick filtration
    V. Herick modification
    V. Herick valve
    v. Heuven anatomical classification
      of diabetic retinopathy
    V. Lint akinesia
    V. Lint anesthesia
    V. Lint-Atkinson lid akinetic block
    V. Lint block
    V. Lint flap
    V. Lint injection
    V. Lint modified technique
    V. Milligen eyelid repair technique
    V. Milligen operation
Vancocin
vancomycin
Vander vitreoretinal injection cannula
vanillism
vanishing bone disease
Vannas
    V. capsulotomy
    V. capsulotomy scissors
    V. iridocapsulotomy scissors
Vantage ophthalmoscope
Vaper Vac II
variabilis
    erythrokeratodermia v. (EKV)

V

variable
- v. distance stereoacuity (VDS)
- v. power cross-cylinder lens set
- v. strabismus

variance
- analysis of v. (ANOVA)

varians
- metamorphopsia v.

variant
- Heidenhain v.
- Miller-Fisher v.

variation
- coefficient of v.
- diurnal v.

Vari bladebreaker

varicella
- v. iridocyclitis
- v. keratitis
- v. zoster ophthalmicus
- v. zoster virus (VZV)

varicella-zoster retinitis

varices (*pl. of* varix)

varicoblepharon

varicose ophthalmia

Varigray
- V. implant
- V. lens

Varilux
- V. lens implant
- V. Pangamic thin plastic lens

varix, pl. varices
- conjunctival v.
- orbital v.
- vortex vein v.

VAS
- visual analogue scale

vasa sanguinea retinae

Vasco-Posada orbital retractor

vascular
- v. abnormality
- v. arcade
- v. cataract
- v. cerebellar disease
- v. circle of optic nerve
- v. coat of eyeball
- v. congestion
- v. disorder
- v. endothelial cell
- v. endothelial growth factor (VEGF)
- v. filling defect
- v. frond
- v. funnel
- v. hamartoma
- v. keratitis
- v. lamina of choroid
- v. loop
- v. network
- v. occlusion

- v. occlusive disease
- v. optical disk swelling without visual loss
- v. plexus
- v. retinopathy
- v. sheathing
- v. tree
- v. tumor
- v. tunic

vascularization
- conjunctival v.
- corneal v.
- v. elsewhere in the retina (VNE)
- stromal v.

vascularized
- v. scar
- v. tortuosity

vasculature
- choroidal v.
- disk v.
- perimacular v.
- retinal v.
- spider v.

vasculitis
- benign retinal v.
- granulomatous v.
- hypocomplementemic urticarial v. (HUV)
- idiopathic retinal v.
- leukocytoclastic v.
- limbal v.
- necrotizing v.
- obstructive retinal v.
- orbital v.
- v. retinae
- retinal v.
- tubercular retinal v.

vasculonebulous keratitis

vasculopathic downbeat nystagmus

vasculopathy
- exudative idiopathic polypoidal choroidal v.
- idiopathic polypoidal choroidal v. (IPCV)
- polypoidal choroidal v.
- radiogenic v.
- retinal v.

vasoactive amine

Vasocidin Ophthalmic

Vasocine

VasoClear
- V. A
- V. Ophthalmic

Vasocon
- V. Regular
- V. Regular Ophthalmic

Vasocon-A Ophthalmic

vasodilator

Vasosulf Ophthalmic

vault
    lens v.
vaulting of contact lens
VBIO
    Video Binocular indirect ophthalmoscope
VC
    acuity of color vision
VDA
    visual discriminatory acuity
VDS
    variable distance stereoacuity
      VDS test
VDTS
    video display terminal simulator
VE
    visual efficiency
Veatch ophthalmic ReSeeVit system
VECP
    visual-evoked cortical potential
vectis
    Anis irrigating v.
    anterior chamber irrigating v.
    aspirating/irrigating v.
    cul-de-sac irrigating v.
    Drews-Knolle reverse irrigating v.
    irrigating anterior chamber v.
    irrigating/aspirating v.
    Look irrigating v.
    Peczon I/A v.
    Pierce I/A irrigating v.
    Pierce irrigating v.
    plastic disposable irrigating v.
    Sheets irrigating v.
    Snellen v.
vectograph chart
vectographic study
vector
    v. analysis
    v. array transducer
vegetable ophthalmia
VEGF
    vascular endothelial growth factor
veil
    dimple v.
    pigmented v.
    Sattler v.
    vitreal v.
    vitreous v.
veiling glare
vein
    angular v.
    anterior ciliary v.

anterior conjunctival v.
aqueous v.
Ascher v.
branch retinal v. (BRV)
central retinal v. (CRV)
choroid v.
ciliary v.
cilioretinal v.
conjunctival v.
endophlebitis of retinal v.
episcleral v.
facial v.
frontal diploic v.
Galen v.
inferior nasal v.
inferior ophthalmic v.
inferior palpebral v.
inferior temporal v.
Kuhnt postcentral v.
lacrimal v.
muscular v.
nasofrontal v.
nicking of retinal v.
occlusion of branch v.
occlusion of retinal v.
ophthalmic v.
ophthalmomeningeal v.
opticociliary shunt v.
palpebral v.
posterior ciliary v.
posterior conjunctival v.
retinal v.
superior nasal v.
superior ophthalmic v.
superior palpebral v.
superior temporal v.
supraorbital v.
vortex v.
Veinlaser Captured-Pulse laser
Veirs
    V. cannula
    V. trocar
Velcro head strap
velocardiofacial syndrome
velocimeter
    Doppler v.
    laser Doppler v.
velocimetry
    laser Doppler v.
velocity
    v. error

NOTES

velocity *(continued)*
    retinal-slip v.
    saccadic v.
velonoskiascopy, belonoskiascopy
velum
    corneal v.
Velva Kleen
VEM
    vergence eye movement
vena, pl. **venae**
    v. angularis
    venae anteriores conjunctivales
    v. centralis retinae
    v. choroideae oculi
    v. ciliares anteriores
    v. diploica frontalis
    venae episclerale
    v. facialis
    v. lacrimalis
    v. nasofrontalis
    v. ophthalmica inferior
    v. ophthalmica superior
    v. ophthalmomeningea
    venae palpebrales
    venae palpebrales inferiores
    venae palpebrales superiores
    v. vorticosae
venography
    orbital v.
venomanometer
    Zeimer v.
venomanometry
venous
    v. beading
    v. congestion
    v. engorgement
    v. hemangioma
    v. loop
    v. occlusive disease
    v. pulsation
    v. sheathing
    v. sheath patch
    v. sinus
    v. stasis
    v. stasis retinopathy (VSR)
    v. stenosis retinopathy
    v. tortuosity
Vented Gas Forced Infusion (VGFI)
venter frontalis musculi occipitofrontalis
ventricle
    cerebral v.
ventriculography
venturi
    V. adjusted temple
    V. aspiration vitrectomy device
    v. effect
Venturi-Flo valve system
venula, pl. **venulae**
    v. macularis inferior

    v. macularis superior
    v. medialis retinae
    v. nasalis retinae inferior
    v. nasalis retinae superior
    v. retinae medialis
    v. temporalis retinae inferior
    v. temporalis retinae superior
venule
    v. banking
    macular v.
    retinal v.
    right-angle deflected v.
VEP
    visual-evoked potential
VER
    visual-evoked response
vera
    polycoria v.
Verga lacrimal groove
vergence
    ability v.
    v. eye movement (VEM)
    v. facility
    fusional v.
    v. of lens
    negative vertical v.
    power v.
    reduced v.
    reflux v.
    tonic v.
    vertical v.
    zero v.
vergens
    strabismus deorsum v.
    strabismus sursum v.
Vergés phaco chopper
Verhoeff
    V. capsule forceps
    V. lens expressor
    V. operation
    V. scissors
    V. streak
    V. suture
Verhoeff-Chandler
    V.-C. capsulotomy
    V.-C. operation
verification
    prescription v.
VERIS
    visual-evoked response imaging system
    VERIS III system
vermiform
    v. contraction
    v. movement
vermis
    cerebellar v.
    dorsal v.
Vernacel

vernal
    v. catarrh
    v. conjunctivitis
    v. keratoconjunctivitis (VKC)
    v. keratoconjunctivitis refractory
Vernier
    V. optometer
    V. stimulus
    V. visual acuity
verruca vulgaris papilloma
VersaTool eye sponge
version
    ductions and v.'s (D&V)
    v. movement
vertebral angiography
vertebrobasilar
    v. artery
    v. artery insufficiency
    v. system
    v. vascular abnormality
verteporfin
vertex, pl. **vertices**
    v. of distance
    front v.
    v. of power
    v. refractionometer
vertexmeter
vertical
    v. axis
    v. axis of eye
    v. axis of Fick
    v. comitant deviation
    v. diplopia
    v. divergence
    v. divergence position
    v. duction
    v. forceps
    v. fusional vergence amplitude
    v. fusion range
    v. gaze
    v. gaze center
    v. gaze paresis
    v. hemianopsia
    v. illumination
    v. meridian
    v. movement
    v. muscle
    v. myoclonus
    v. nystagmus
    v. parallax
    v. phoria
    v. plane

    v. prism bar
    v. prism test
    v. retraction syndrome
    right gaze v.'s
    v. strabismus
    v. strabismus fixus
    v. stria
    v. tropia
    v. vergence
    v. vertigo
vertices (*pl. of* vertex)
verticillata
    cornea v.
    corneal v.
vertigo
    benign paroxysmal positional v.
     (BPPV)
    objective v.
    ocular v.
    sham-movement v.
    special sense v.
    subjective v.
    vertical v.
vertometer
Verwey eyelid operation
vesicle
    chorionic v.
    clear lid v.
    compound v.
    cornea v.
    corneal v.
    lens v.
    lenticular v.
    lid v.
    multilocular v.
    ocular v.
    ophthalmic v.
    optic v.
    pinocytotic v.
vesicula ophthalmica
vesicular
    v. keratitis
    v. keratopathy
vesiculation
    eyelid v.
vesiculosus linear endothelial
V-esotropia
vessel
    v. abnormality of retina
    anomalous v.
    beaded telangiectatic bulbar
     conjunctival v.

V

NOTES

vessel *(continued)*
    choroidal v.
    ciliary v.
    collateral v.
    congested v.
    conjunctival v.
    disk neurovascular v.
    disk new v.
    episcleral blood v.
    feeder v.
    frond of v.
    ghost v.
    neovascularization of new v.'s
      elsewhere (NVE)
    opticociliary shunt v.
    optociliary shunt v.
    orbital v.
    perilimbal conjunctival v.
    retinal v.
    v. sheathing
    sheathing of retinal v.
    shunt v.
    silver-wire v.
    stromal blood v.
    succulent v.
    tensile strength of v.
    tortuosity of retinal v.
    v. traction
vestibular
    v. cortex
    v. nerve
    v. nucleus
    v. nystagmus
    v. organ
    v. pupillary reaction
    v. system
vestibulocerebellar ataxia
vestibulocochlear
vestibuloocular
    v. reflex
    v. response (VOR)
vestibulotoxicity
    gentamicin-induced v.
Vexol
    V. 1%
    V. Ophthalmic Suspension
V-exotropia
VF
    visual field
VF-14 questionnaire
VFC
    viscous fluid controller
VFQ
    Visual Function Questionnaire
VFQ-25
    25-Item Visual Function Questionnaire
VGFI
    Vented Gas Forced Infusion
V-groove gauge

VG slit lamp
VH
    vitreous hemorrhage
VHF
    visual half-field
VI
    visual impairment
Vibramycin
vibrating scissors
Vibratome
vibratory nystagmus
Vibrio vulnificus
Vickerall round ringed forceps
Vickers
    V. forceps
    V. needle holder
vicrosurgery
Vicryl suture
VID
    visible iris diameter
vidarabine
Vidaurri
    V. double irrigation cannula
    V. irrigator
video
    V. Binocular indirect
      ophthalmoscope (VBIO)
    v. display terminal simulator
      (VDTS)
    v. keratography
    v. specular microscope
videoendoscope
    fiberoptic v.
videokeratograph
    EyeSys v.
videokeratographer
    Humphrey 992 v.
videokeratographic corneal steepening
videokeratography
    computer-assisted v.
    computerized corneal v.
videokeratoscope
    computer-assisted v.
    EyeSys v.
    Keratron v.
    PAR-C-Scan v.
    TechnoMed C-Scan v.
    TMS-1 v.
    TMS-2 computer-assisted v.
videometer
videooculographic image
videooculography
vidian
    v. nerve
    v. neuralgia
    v. neurectomy
Viers
    V. erysiphake
    V. needle

V. operation
V. rod
Vieth-Mueller
V.-M. circle
V.-M. horopter
view
axial v.
Caldwell v.
Caldwell-Waters v.
coronal v.
field of v.
Miyake v.
sweep v.
Waters v.
vigabatrin
Villasenor-Navarro fixation ring
Villasensor ultrasonic pachymeter
villus, pl. **villi**
pectinate villi
Vinciguerra
V. LASEK protector
V. PRK/LASEK spatula
Vinciguerra-Carones LASEK spatula
vinyl
v. T-tube
v. tube
violet
v. haptic
v. vision
visual v.
VIP
Vision in Preschoolers
VIP Study
Vira-A Ophthalmic
viral
v. blepharitis
v. capsid antigen
v. conjunctivitis
v. keratitis
v. keratoconjunctivitis
v. ocular disease
v. uveitis
Virchow corpuscle
virgin silk suture
viridans
Streptococcus v.
VIRIDIS-LITE photocoagulator
VIRIDIS photocoagulator
Viroptic Ophthalmic
virtual
v. focus
v. image

v. point
v. reality head-mounted display
(VR-HMD)
V. Retinal Display (VRD)
virus
alpha herpes v.
BK v.
cytomegalic inclusion v.
Epstein-Barr v. (EBV)
herpes simplex v. (HSV)
herpes simplex v. type I
herpes zoster v.
human immunodeficiency v. (HIV)
human T-lymphotropic v.
influenza v.
JC v.
lymphocytic choriomeningitis v.
molluscum v.
Newcastle disease v.
type 1 herpes simplex v.
varicella zoster v. (VZV)
virustatics
Visalens
V. contact lens cleaning and
soaking solution
V. Wetting
VISC
vitreous infusion suction cutter
visceral
v. larva migrans (VLM)
v. larva migrans syndrome
v. myopathy
Viscoat solution
viscocanalostomy
viscodelamination
visco dissection
viscodissector
v. tubing
vitreoretinal v.
viscoelastic
CoEase v.
v. material
Optimize v.
v. solution
Visco expression cannula
Viscoflow cannula
Viscolens lens
viscosimeter
capillary tube plasma v.
viscosity
high v.
viscotechnique

V

NOTES

viscous
 v. fluid controller (VFC)
 v. ochre fluid
 v. xanthochromic fluid
Visculose
visibility
 v. acuity
 v. curve
visible
 v. drusen
 v. iris diameter (VID)
 v. spectrum
Visi-Drape
 V.-D. Elite ophthalmic drape
 V.-D. mini aperture drape
 V.-D. mini incise drape
Visiflex drape
visile
Visine
 V. AC
 Advanced Relief V.
 V. Extra Ophthalmic
 V. L.R.
 V. L.R. ophthalmic
 V. Original
 V. Tears
 V. Tears PF
Visine-A
visio
 v. oculus
 v. oculus dextra (vision of right eye) (VOD)
 v. oculus sinister (vision of left eye) (VOS)
 v. oculus uterque (vision of both eyes) (VOU)
vision
 6/6 v.
 20/20 v.
 achromatic v.
 acuity of color v. (VC)
 ambulatory v.
 V. analyzer
 V. Analyzer/Overrefraction System
 artificial v.
 best-corrected v.
 binocular single v. (BSV)
 blue v.
 blurred v.
 blurring of v.
 botulism-induced blurred v.
 V. Care enzymatic cleaner
 central island of v.
 central keyhole of v.
 cerebral tunnel v.
 chromatic v.
 color v. (CV)
 cone v.
 counting fingers v.

 crystal clear v.
 day v.
 decreasing v.
 v. deprivation myopia
 dichromatic v.
 dimness of v.
 direct v.
 distance v.
 distortion of v.
 double v. (DV)
 duplicity theory of v.
 eccentric v.
 extramacular binocular v.
 facial v.
 false v.
 field of v.
 finger v.
 finger-counting v.
 form v.
 foveal v.
 glare v.
 green v.
 half v.
 halo v.
 hand-motion v. (HMV)
 haploscopic v.
 Helmholtz theory of color v.
 Hering theory of color v.
 indirect v.
 iridescent v.
 keyhole v.
 line of v.
 linear v.
 loss of v.
 v. loss
 low v.
 macular binocular v.
 V. Master excimer laser system
 misty v.
 monocular v.
 motion v.
 multiple v.
 naked v. (Nv)
 NAS-NRC Committee on V.
 near v.
 night v.
 no-light-perception v.
 obscure v.
 organ of v.
 oscillating v.
 peripheral v.
 persistence of v.
 phantom · v.
 photopic v.
 Pick v.
 pinhole v.
 V. in Preschoolers (VIP)
 V. in Preschoolers Study
 pseudoscopic v.

rainbow v.
reading v.
red v.
residual v.
v. rod
rod v.
v. science
scotopic v.
shaft v.
single binocular v. (SBV)
solid v.
stable v.
stereoscopic v.
subjective v.
subnormal v.
suboptimal v.
V. Tech lens
tilted v.
v. training
transient obscuration of v.
Tripier operation v.
triple v.
tubular v.
tunnel v.
twilight v.
upside-down reversal of v.
violet v.
word v.
yellow v.
VisionBlue trypan blue 0.06% stain
VisionLAB
Visi-Spear eye sponge
Visitec
    V. angled lens hook
    V. aspiration unit
    V. capsule polisher curette
    V. Company lens
    V. corneal shield
    V. corneal suture manipulating
    hook
    V. cortex extractor
    V. double-cutting cystitome
    V. intraocular lens dialer
    V. iris retractor
    V. irrigating/aspirating cannula
    V. irrigating/aspirating unit
    V. lens pusher
    V. manipulator
    V. micro double-iris hook
    V. microhook
    V. microiris hook
    V. nucleus removal loupe

    V. RK zone marker
    V. straight lens hook
    V. surgical vitrectomy system
    V. vitrectomy unit
Visolett
Visometer
    Lotman V.
Vista
    Blue V.
Vistacon
Vistaject-25, -50
Vistaquel
Vistaril
Vistazine
Vistech
    V. 6500 contrast test
    V. Multivision Contrast Tester
    8000
    V. wall chart
Vistide
visual
    v. aberration
    V. Activities Questionnaire
    v. acuity decrease
    v. acuity testing
    v. agnosia
    v. allesthesia
    v. analogue scale (VAS)
    v. angle
    v. aphasia
    v. association area
    v. attentiveness
    v. axis
    v. blackout
    v. cell
    v. cone
    v. confusion
    v. corkscrew defect
    v. cortex
    v. cycle
    v. deprivation syndrome
    v. development
    v. direction
    v. disability
    v. discrimination
    v. discriminatory acuity (VDA)
    v. disturbance
    v. efficiency (VE)
    v. extinction
    v. field (F, VF)
    v. field damage
    v. field defect

NOTES

visual *(continued)*
    v. field index
    v. field testing
    v. function
    v. function evaluation
    V. Function Questionnaire (VFQ)
    v. half-field (VHF)
    v. hallucination
    v. halo
    v. image
    v. impairment (VI)
    v. inattention
    v. line
    v. manipulation test
    v. memory
    v. orbicularis reflex
    v. organ
    v. paraneoplastic syndrome
    v. pathway
    v. pathway disease
    v. perception
    v. performance result
    v. perseveration
    v. pigment
    v. plane
    v. point
    v. preservation
    v. process
    v. prognosis
    v. projection
    v. psychophysics
    v. purple
    v. radiation
    v. seizure
    v. sensory system
    v. spread
    v. threshold
    v. tilt
    v. violet
    v. white
    v. yellow
    v. zone
visuale
    organum v.
visual-evoked
    v.-e. cortical potential (VECP)
    v.-e. potential (VEP)
    v.-e. response (VER)
    v.-e. response imaging system
    (VERIS)
visualization
    contrast v.
    double-contrast v.
visually
    v. evoked potential mapping
    v. insignificant infectious corneal
    ulcer
visual-spatial agnosia
Visual-Tech machine

visual-vestibulo-ocular response
Visudyne
Visulab System
Visulas
    V. argon C laser
    V. argon/YAG laser
    V. 532 Combi software
    V. Combi 532/YAG laser
    V. InterChange software
    V. 532 laser
    V. Nd:YAG laser
    V. 690s PDT laser
    V. YAG C, E, S laser
    V. YAG II plus laser
VisuMed MEL60 laser
visuoauditory
visuognosis
visuolexic
visuometer
visuopsychic
visuosensory
visuospatial disorder
VISUPAC digital imaging system
visus
    linea v.
    organum v.
Visuscope
    Cüppers V.
    V. motor
    V. motor test
    V. ophthalmoscope
    V. sensory test
Visuskop
Visutron
VISX
    V. CAP
    V. contoured ablation method
    V. Contoured Ablation Pattern
    V. 2020 excimer laser
    V. procedure
    V. Refractive Planner
    V. S2, S3 excimer laser
    V. Star
    V. Star II stromal photoablation
    system
    V. Star S3
    V. Star S3 ActiveTrak laser
    V. Star S2 excimer laser system
    V. Star S2 laser
    V. Twenty/Twenty excimer laser
    V. Twenty/Twenty system
    V. 20/20 version 4.01 vision
    keycard system
    V. WaveScan
Vit
    V. Commander foot pedal
    V. Commander handpiece
    V. Commander System
Vit-A-Drops

VitaLase Er:YAG laser
vital dye
VitalEyes
Vitallium
    V. implant
    V. miniplate
vitamin
    v. A deficiency
    ICaps ocular v.
    Ocuvite PreserVision v.'s
vitelliform
    v. degeneration of macula
    v. macular degeneration
    v. macular dystrophy
    v. maculopathy
vitelline macular degeneration
vitelliruptive
    v. degeneration
    v. macular dystrophy
vitellirupture
vitiliginous chorioretinitis
vitiligo, pl. **vitiligines**
    v. iridis
    perilimbal v.
    v. uveitis
Vitrase
Vitrasert intravitreal implant
Vitravene
Vitrax
vitrea
    lamina v.
    membrana v.
vitreal
    v. bleed
    v. cell
    v. detachment
    v. hemorrhage
    v. lamina
    v. liquefaction
    v. membrane
    v. veil
vitrectomy
    anterior v.
    automated v.
    closed-system pars plana v.
    complete v.
    core v.
    v. instrument
    lens-sparing v.
    V. for Macular Hole Study
      (VMHS)
    manual v.

open-sky v.
pars plana Baerveldt tube insertion
  with v.
partial v.
pneumatic v.
port v.
3-port pars plana v.
posterior v.
v. prism lens tab
v. for proliferative retinopathy
scissors v.
v. sponge
sutureless transconjunctival pars
  plana v.
total v.
Weck-cel v.
vitrector
    Alcon v.
    Cilco v.
    CooperVision v.
    Frigitronics v.
    guillotine v.
    Kaufman type II v.
    mechanical v.
    Microvit v.
    Peyman v.
    Storz Microvit v.
vitrectorhexis
vitrei
    synchesis corporis v.
vitrein
vitreitis
    dense v.
    idiopathic v.
vitreocapsulitis
vitreociliary glaucoma
vitreofoveal separation
vitreolysis
    YAG v.
vitreomacular
    v. interface
    v. separation
    v. traction
    v. traction syndrome
Vitreon sterile intraocular fluid
vitreopapillary traction
vitreophage
    Kaufman v.
vitreoretinal (VR)
    v. adhesion
    v. aspirate
    v. attachment

V

NOTES

vitreoretinal *(continued)*
    v. choroidopathy syndrome
    v. condensation
    v. contusion
    v. degeneration
    v. disorder
    v. dysplasia
    v. infusion cutter
    v. interface
    v. micropick
    v. surgeon
    v. tag
    v. traction
    v. traction syndrome
    v. tuft
    v. viscodissector
vitreoretinochoroidopathy
vitreoretinopathy
    anterior proliferative v. (APVR)
    closed-funnel v.
    erosive v.
    exudative v.
    familial exudative v. (FEVR)
    proliferative diabetic v. (PDVR)
    release of traction for hypotony
      and v.
vitreotapetoretinal dystrophy
vitreous
    v. abscess
    v. aspirating needle
    v. aspiration
    v. aspiration biopsy
    v. base
    v. block
    v. block glaucoma
    v. blood
    v. body
    v. breakthrough hemorrhage
    v. bulge
    v. cavity
    v. cell
    v. cells as indicator of retinal
      tears
    v. chamber
    v. clouding
    v. coloboma
    coloboma of v.
    v. contraction
    core v.
    cortical v.
    v. culture
    detached v.
    v. detachment
    v. face
    v. fiber
    v. floater
    v. fluff
    v. fluorophotometry

v. foreign body
v. foreign body forceps
v. gel
v. haze
v. hemorrhage (VH)
v. hernia
v. herniation
v. humor
hyperplastic primary v.
v. inflammation
v. infusion suction cutter (VISC)
knuckle of loose v.
v. lacuna
v. lamina
liquified v.
loss of v.
v. loss
v. membrane
micelles in v.
v. neovascularization
v. opacity
organized v.
v. pencil
persistent anterior hyperplastic
  primary v.
persistent hypertrophic primary v.
  (PHPV)
persistent posterior hyperplastic
  primary v.
persistent primary hyperplastic v.
posterior v.
primary persistent hyperplastic v.
v. prolapse
puff of loose v.
v. retraction
secondary v.
v. seeding
v. separation
v. skirt
spontaneous extrusion of v.
v. strand
v. strand scissors
v. stroma
v. surgery
v. sweep spatula
syneresis of v.
syneretic v.
v. tap
tertiary v.
v. touch
v. traction
v. transplant needle
v. veil
v. wick syndrome
vitreous-aspirating cannula
vitreum
    corpus v.
    stroma v.

vitrina
>   v. ocularis
>   v. oculi

vitritis
>   immune recovery v.
>   senile v.

vitronectin bind
Vitrophage-Peyman unit
vitrosin
ViVa binocular infrared vision analyzer
Viva-Drops
>   V.-D. eye drops
>   V.-D. Solution

Vizor al
VKC
>   vernal keratoconjunctivitis

V-K-H
>   Vogt-Koyanagi-Harada
>   V-K-H syndrome

V-lance
>   V.-l. blade
>   V.-l. blade/knife
>   V.-l. Sharpoint

V-lancet knife
VLM
>   visceral larva migrans

VMHS
>   Vitrectomy for Macular Hole Study

VNE
>   vascularization elsewhere in the retina

VOD
>   visio oculus dextra (vision of right eye)

Vogt
>   V. cataract
>   V. cornea
>   V. degeneration
>   V. disease
>   glaukomflecken of V.
>   limbal girdle of V.
>   limbal palisades of V.
>   V. line
>   V. operation
>   palisades of V.
>   V. stria
>   V. syndrome
>   white limbal girdle of V.
>   V. white limbal girdle

Vogt-Barraquer
>   V.-B. corneal needle
>   V.-B. eye needle

Vogt-Koyanagi
>   V.-K. bilateral uveitis
>   V.-K. syndrome

Vogt-Koyanagi-Harada (V-K-H)
>   V.-K.-H. disease
>   V.-K.-H. syndrome

Vogt-Spielmeyer
>   V.-S. disease
>   V.-S. syndrome

volitantes
>   muscae v.

Volk
>   V. aspheric lens
>   V. conoid lens implant
>   V. coronoid lens
>   V. High Resolution aspherical lens
>   V. Minus noncontact adapter
>   V. 3 Mirror ANF+ lens
>   V. 3 Mirror gonio fundus laser lens
>   V. Plus noncontact adapter cap and equipment
>   V. Quadraspheric lens
>   V. retinal scale adapter
>   V. SuperField aspherical lens
>   V. SuperField multi-adapter transformer lens set
>   V. SuperField NC lens
>   V. SuperMacula 2.2 focal laser lens
>   V. SuperQuad 160 contact lens
>   V. SuperQuad 160 panretinal lens
>   V. Transequator lens
>   V. ultra field aspherical lens adapter
>   V. yellow filter adapter

Volkmann cataract
Volon A
Voltaren Ophthalmic
volume (V)
>   choroidal blood v. (ChBVol)
>   tear v.

voluntary
>   v. convergence
>   v. convergency
>   v. eye movement
>   v. nystagmus
>   v. saccadic oscillation

volvulus
>   *Onchocerca v.*

von
>   v. Ammon operation

NOTES

V

von *(continued)*
- v. Arlt recess
- v. Blaskovics-Doyen operation
- v. Frisch theory
- v. Gierke disease
- v. Graefe cataract knife
- v. Graefe cautery
- v. Graefe cystitome
- v. Graefe electrocautery
- v. Graefe fixation forceps
- v. Graefe iris forceps
- v. Graefe knife needle
- v. Graefe muscle hook
- v. Graefe operation
- v. Graefe prism dissociation method
- v. Graefe sign
- v. Graefe strabismus hook
- v. Graefe syndrome
- v. Graefe target
- v. Graefe technique
- v. Graefe tissue forceps
- v. Helmholtz eye model
- v. Hippel angioma
- v. Hippel disease
- v. Hippel internal corneal ulcer
- v. Hippel-Lindau disease
- v. Hippel-Lindau syndrome
- v. Hippel operation
- v. Mondak capsule fragment-clot forceps
- v. Noorden incision
- v. Recklinghausen disease
- v. Recklinghausen syndrome

VOR
vestibuloocular response

vortex, pl. **vortices**
- v. corneal dystrophy
- Fleischer v.
- v. keratopathy

- v. lentis
- v. pattern
- v. system
- v. vein
- v. vein varix

vortex-like clump

vorticosae
vena v.

VOS
visio oculus sinister (vision of left eye)

Vossius lenticular ring

VOU
visio oculus uterque (vision of both eyes)

V-pattern
- V.-p. esotropia
- V.-p. exotropia

VR
vitreoretinal

VRD
Virtual Retinal Display

VR-HMD
virtual reality head-mounted display
biocular VR-HMD

VS
without glasses

VSG 2/3F graphic card

V-slit lamp

VSR
venous stasis retinopathy

Vuero meter

vulnificus
- v. keratitis
- *Vibrio v.*

V-Y advancement myotarsocutaneous flap for upper eyelid reconstruction

Vygantas-Wilder retinal drainage probe

VZV
varicella zoster virus
- VZV dendrite
- VZV disciform lesion

Waardenburg-Jonkers
    corneal dystrophy of W.-J.
    dystrophy of W.-J.
Waardenburg-Klein syndrome
Waardenburg syndrome
Wachendorf membrane
Wadsworth lid forceps
Wadsworth-Todd
    W.-T. cautery
    W.-T. electrocautery
Wagener-Clay-Gipner classification
Wagner
    W. disease
    W. epiretinal membrane dissector
    W. hereditary vitreoretinal
      degeneration
    W. hyaloid retinal degeneration
    W. retinitis
    W. silicone oil cannula
    W. syndrome
    W. vitreoretinal dystrophy
Wagner-Stickler syndrome
Wainstock suturing forceps
waking ptosis
Waldeau fixation forceps
Waldeyer gland
Waldhauer operation
Walker
    W. coagulator
    W. electrode
    W. lid everter
    W. micro pin
    W. scissors
    W. trephine
Walker-Apple scissors
Walker-Atkinson scissors
Walker-Lee sclerotome
Walker-Warburg syndrome
wall
    eye w.
    w. push maneuver
Wallace-Maloney fixation diamond knife
Wallach
    W. cryosurgery freezer
    W. cryosurgical pencil
    W. Ophthalmic Cryosurgery System
Wallenberg lateral medullary syndrome
wallerian degeneration
wall-eyed bilateral internuclear
    ophthalmoplegia
Walser corneoscleral punch
Walter
    W. Reed implant
    W. Reed operation
    W. spud

Walton
    W. punch
    W. spud
Wan
    W. side-port nucleus manipulator
    W. side-port nucleus splitter
wand
    Connor angled w.
    Connor curved w.
    Connor straight irrigating w.
    Connor straight nonirrigating w.
    Powell w.
Wang lens
Warburg syndrome
warfarin sodium
warm-same
    cold-opposite, w.-s. (COWS)
warneri
    Staphylococcus w.
warpage
    contact lens-induced w.
    corneal w.
wart
    Hassall-Henle w.
    Henle w.
Warthin tumor
wartlike body
wash
    Eye W.
    eye w., eyewash (collyr.)
    Irrigate eye w.
    Lavoptik eye w.
    Star-Optic eye w.
washout
    anterior chamber w.
    color w.
water
    w. cell
    w. content
    w. fissure
    w. provocative test
water-based tinting system
water-bath ultrasonography
water-contact angle
water-drinking test
watered-silk retina
water-silk reflex
Waters view
watery
    w. discharge
    w. eye
Watt stave bender
Watzke
    W. band
    W. cuff

W

Watzke *(continued)*
- W. forceps
- W. operation
- W. sleeve
- W. tire

Watzke-Allen
- W.-A. sign
- W.-A. test

wave
- w. aberration map
- b w.

wave-edge knife

waveform
- blood flow velocity w. (BFVW)
- pendular-jerk w.

wavefront
- w. aberration function
- convergent w.
- w. error
- W. System

wavefront-guided
- w.-g. ablation
- w.-g. LASIK

WaveScan
- VISX W.
- W. Wavefront system

waxy
- w. exudate
- w. lesion
- w. tumor

W4D
- Worth 4-dot
- W4D test

WDSCL
- well-differentiated small-cell lymphoma

wear
- enzymatic cleaner for extended w.
- orthokeratology lens w.
- protective sports eye w.

Weaver
- W. chalazion forceps
- W. trocar introducer

Weber
- W. knife
- W. law
- W. paralysis
- W. sign
- W. syndrome

Weber-Elschnig
- W.-E. lens
- W.-E. lens loupe

Weber-Gubler syndrome

Weber-Rinne sign

web eye

Webster needle holder

Weck
- W. astigmatism ruler
- W. eye shield
- W. knife
- W. microscope
- W. sponge
- W. trephine

Weck-cel
- W.-c. sponge
- W.-c. surgical spear
- W.-c. vitrectomy

Wecker iris scissors

wedge
- Livingston peribulbar w.
- w. resection
- temporal w.
- Trujillo LASIK enhancement w.

Wedl cell

Weeker operation

Weeks
- W. bacillus
- W. needle
- W. operation
- W. speculum

weeping eczematous lesion

Wegener granulomatosus conjunctivitis

WEH/CHOP
- Wills Eye Hospital/Children's Hospital of Philadelphia

Wehner spoon

Weibel-Palade body

Weigert ligament

weight
- EyeClose external eyelid w.
- gold w.
- SutureGroove gold eyelid w.

Weil
- W. disease
- W. lacrimal cannula

Weil-Felix reaction

Weill-Marchesani syndrome

Weill-Reys-Adie syndrome

Weill-Reys syndrome

Weinstein
- W. fixation ring
- W. fixation ring and flap lifter

Weisinger operation

Weiss
- W. gold dilator
- W. reflex
- W. ring
- W. self-retaining cannula
- W. speculum

Welch
- W. Allyn SureSight autorefractor
- W. four-drop device
- W. rubber bulb erysiphake

Welch-Allyn
- W.-A. halogen penlight
- W.-A. ophthalmoscope
- W.-A. Pocket scope

welchii
- *Clostridium* w.

Welcker
    cribra orbitalis of W.
welder's
    w. conjunctivitis
    w. keratoconjunctivitis
well
    alcohol w.
    LASEK alcohol w.
Welland test
well-differentiated small-cell lymphoma (WDSCL)
Wells enucleation spoon
Welsh
    W. cortex extractor
    W. cortex stripper cannula
    W. flat olive-tip
    W. flat olive-tip double cannula
    W. iris retractor
    W. pupil-spreader forceps
    W. silastic erysiphake
Wendell Hughes operation
Werb
    W. operation
    W. right-angle probe
    W. scissors
Werdnig-Hoffmann disease
Wergeland
    W. double cannula
    W. double needle
Werner
    W. syndrome
    W. test
Wernicke
    W. encephalopathy
    W. pupil
    W. reaction
    W. sign
    W. symptom
    W. syndrome
    W. test
    W. triangle
Wernicke-Korsakoff
    W.-K. psychosis
    W.-K. syndrome
WESDR
    Wisconsin Epidemiologic Study of Diabetic Retinopathy
Wesley-Jessen lens
Wessely ring
West
    W. gouge
    W. Indian amblyopia

    W. lacrimal cannula
    W. lacrimal sac chisel
    W. operation
Westcott
    W. conjunctival scissors
    W. stitch scissors
    W. tenotomy scissors
    W. test
    W. utility scissors
Westergren method
Western
    W. blot
    W. immunoblotting analysis
Westphal
    W. phenomenon
    W. pupillary reflex
Westphal-Piltz
    W.-P. phenomenon
    W.-P. reflex
Westphal-Strümpell disease
wet
    w. ARMD
    bedewing to w.
    w. cell
    w. dressing
    w. eye
    Lens W.
    w. macular degeneration
    w. mount
Wet-cote
wet-field
    w.-f. cautery
    w.-f. diathermy
    w.-f. electrocautery
Wet-N-Soak
    W.-N.-S. Plus
wetting
    w. angle
    w. angle of contact lens
    Liquifilm W.
    w. solution
    Visalens W.
Wetting/Rewetting
    Optimum by Lobob Gas Permeable W.
Weve
    W. electrode
    W. operation
Weyers-Thier syndrome
WF
    wide field
Wharton-Jones operation

NOTES

W

Whatman
    W. filter
    W. No. 1 qualitative-type filter
      paper
Wheeler
    W. blade
    W. cyclodialysis system
    W. cystitome
    W. discission knife
    W. eye sphere implant
    W. halving repair
    W. iris spatula
    W. method
    W. operation
    W. procedure
Wheeler-Reese operation
wheel rotation
whippelii
    Tropheryma w.
Whipple
    W. disease
    W. disk
white
    w. braided silk suture
    calcofluor w.
    w. cell
    w. dot
    w. dot syndrome
    w. of eye
    w. fundus reflex
    W. glaucoma pump shunt
    w. laser
    w. laser lesion
    w. light
    w. light tandem-scanning confocal
      microscope
    w. limbal girdle of Vogt
    w. pigment
    w. pupil
    w. pupillary reflex
    w. pupil sign
    w. retinal necrosis
    w. ring
    w. ring of cornea
    w. sclera
    w. spot
    w. stromal infiltrate
    w. tunica fibrosa oculi
    visual w.
    w. without pressure
white-centered hemorrhage
whitening
    ischemic retinal w.
    retinal w.
WhiteStar power modulation technology
white-to-white measurement
Whitnall
    W. ligament

    W. sling operation
    W. tubercle
Whitney superior rectus forceps
Whitten fixation ring
whole-globe enucleation
whorled corneal opacities
whorl lens
whorl-like configuration
Wicherkiewicz eyelid operation
wick
    filtering w.
wicking
    w. glue patch
wide-angle glaucoma
wide field (WF)
wide-field eyepiece
widening
    palpebral fissure w.
Widmark conjunctivitis
Widowitz sign
width
    angle w.
    anterior chamber angle w.
    curve w.
    orbital w.
Wieger ligament
Wiener
    W. corneal hook
    W. keratome
    W. operation
    W. scleral hook
    W. speculum
Wies
    W. chalazion forceps
    W. operation
    W. procedure
    W. spot
Wilbrand
    anterior knee of von W.
    W. prism test
Wilcoxon
    W. matched pairs test
    W. signed rank test
Wild
    W. lens
    W. operating microscope
Wilde forceps
Wilder
    W. band spreader
    W. cystitome
    W. cystitome knife
    W. lacrimal dilator
    W. lens loupe
    W. scleral depressor
    W. scleral retractor
    W. scoop
    W. sign
Wildervanck syndrome
WildEyes costume contact lens

Wildgen-Reck
    W.-R. localizer
    W.-R. locator
Wilkerson intraocular lens-insertion forceps
Willebrandt
Williams
    W. pediatric eye speculum
    W. probe
Willis
    circle of W.
Wills
    W. cautery
    W. Eye Hospital
    W. Eye Hospital/Children's Hospital of Philadelphia (WEH/CHOP)
    W. Hospital utility forceps
    W. spud and bur
    W. utility eye forceps
Wilmer
    W. Cataract Photo-grading System
    W. conjunctival scissors
    W. Eye Institute
    W. operation
    W. Ophthalmological Institute
    W. refractor
    W. retractor
Wilmer-Bagley expressor
Wilms tumor
Wilson
    W. degeneration
    W. disease
    W. recession hook
    W. syndrome
Wiltmoser optical arm
Wincor enucleation scissors
wind-blown contaminant
window
    clear w.
    w. defect
    scleral w.
windshield wiper syndrome
wing cell
winking
    jaw w.
    w. spasm
wink reflex
Winslow star
Winter Helping Hand
Wintersteiner rosette
wipe débridement
wipe-out syndrome

Wipes-SPF
    Lid W.-S.
wire
    cheese w.
    w. enucleation snare
    w. frame spectacles
    Kirschner w.
    w. lid speculum
    w. mesh implant
    Ultra-select nitinol guide w.
wire-loop keratoscope
wiring
    copper w.
    interosseous w.
Wirt
    W. stereopsis test
    W. stereo test
    W. vision test
Wisconsin
    W. age-related maculopathy grading system
    W. Epidemiologic Study of Diabetic Retinopathy (WESDR)
Wise
    W. iridotomy laser lens
    W. iridotomy-sphincterotomy laser lens
with
    w. contact lenses (c̄cl)
    w. correction (cc)
    w. motion
Witherspoon vertical scissors
without
    w. correction (s̄c)
    w. glasses (VS)
with-the-rule (WTR)
    w.-t.-r. astigmatism
W.K. Kellogg Eye Center
wobbly eye
Wolfe
    W. forceps
    W. graft
    W. method
    W. ptosis operation
Wolff-Eisner
    W.-E. prism
    W.-E. test
Wölfflin-Krückmann spot
Wolfram syndrome
Wolfring
    gland of W.
    W. lacrimal gland

NOTES

W

Wolf syndrome
Wollaston
    W. doublet
    W. theory
Wood
    W. lamp
    W. lens
wooden swab
Woods
    W. Concept lens
    W. light examination
    W. sign
wool saturated in saline dressing
Wooten needle
word
    w. blindness
    w. vision
working lens
Worksheet
    Thill Aniseikonia W.
workstation
    Light Blade laser w.
    Tomey refractive w.
World Health Organization classification of trachoma
worse eye
Worst
    W. Claw lens
    W. corneal bur
    W. goniotomy lens
    W. implantation forceps
    W. Medallion lens
    W. needle
    W. operation
    W. pigtail probe

    W. Platina iris-fixated lens
    W. suture
Wort circle
Worth
    W. amblyoscope
    W. concept of fusion
    W. 4-dot (W4D)
    W. 4-dot near flashlight test
    W. ptosis operation
    W. strabismus forceps
wound
    w. closure
    w. dehiscence
    w. gape
    open-sky cataract w.
    puncture w.
wrap-a-round eye shield
Wrattan filter
wreath pattern stromal infiltrate
Wright
    W. fascia needle
    W. operation
    W. ophthalmic needle
wrinkling
    macular surface w.
    w. membrane
    retinal w.
WTR
    with-the-rule
    WTR astigmatism
Wucherer conjunctivitis
Wullstein-House cup forceps
Wundt-Lamansky law
Wyburn-Mason syndrome
Wydase

χ (*var. of* chi)
X
exophoria
X cell
X chrom contact lens
x
axis of cylindric lens
x axis
Xalatan
Xalcom
xanthelasma
x. around eyelid
florid x.
xanthelasmatosis
x. bulbi
x. iridis
xanthism
xanthochromic fluid
xanthocyanopsia
xanthogranuloma
juvenile x. (JXG)
juvenile iris x.
necrobiotic x.
uveal juvenile x.
xanthogranulomatosis
xanthokyanopy
xanthoma
x. elasticum
x. palpebrarum
x. planum
xanthomatosis
x. bulbi
cerebrotendinous x.
x. iridis
xanthophane
xanthophyll pigment
xanthopsia, xanthopia
xanthopsin
Xe
xenon
xenon (Xe)
x. arc
x. arc photocoagulation
x. arc photocoagulator
xenophthalmia
xeroderma
x. of Kaposi
x. pigmentosum
xeroma

xerophthalmia
xerophthalmic ulcer
xerophthalmicus
fundus x.
xerophthalmus
Xeroscope grid distortion
xerosis
x. conjunctivae
conjunctival x.
x. of cornea
corneal x.
Corynebacterium x.
x. superficialis
xerotic
x. degeneration
x. keratitis
X-esotropia
X-exotropia
XFS
exfoliation syndrome
X-linked
X.-l. achromatopsia
X.-l. blue cone monochromatism
X.-l. cone
X.-l. cone dystrophy
X.-l. congenital night blindness
X.-l. fashion
X.-l. juvenile retinopathy
X.-l. juvenile retinoschisis
X.-l. retinitis
X.-l. retinitis pigmentosa (XLRP)
XLRP
X-linked retinitis pigmentosa
Xomed Surgical Products
XP
exophoria
x-ray
orbital x.-r.
polytome x.-r.
stereo x.-r.
x-ray-induced cataract
X-strabismus
XT
exotropia
X(T)
intermittent exotropia
Xylocaine with epinephrine
xylosoxidans
Alcaligenes x.

X

Y

   Y cell
   Y hook
   Y suture

YAG

   yttrium-aluminum-garnet
   YAG cyclocryotherapy
   YAG laser
   YAG laser cyclophotocoagulation
   YAG laser disruption
   YAG vitreolysis

Yaghouti LASIK polisher
Yale

   Y. Luer-Lok
   Y. Luer-Lok needle
   Y. Luer-Lok syringe

Yamagishi viscocanalostomy cannula
Yannuzzi fundus laser lens
Yasuma protocol
Yates correction
y axis
Yazujian bur
YC 1400 Ophthalmic YAG laser system
yellow

   y. blindness
   y. dye laser

indicator y.
y. light reflex
y. point
y. spot (YS)
y. spot of retina
y. vision
visual y.

yellow-mutant oculocutaneous albinism
yellow-ochre hemorrhage
yellow-white choroidal mass
yield

   lens to y.

yoke

   y. movement
   y. muscle

yoked muscle
Yorktown-style designer series display
Youens lens
Young

   Y. operation
   Y. theory of light

Young-Helmholtz theory of color vision
YS

   yellow spot

Y-sutures of crystalline lens
yttrium-aluminum-garnet (YAG)

   y.-a.-g. laser

Y

Z

Z axis of Fick
Z band
Z marginal tenotomy
Z myotomy
Zacril
Zacutex
Zaditen
Zaditor ophthalmic solution
Zaldivar
Z. anterior procedure (ZAP)
Z. degree gauge
Z. iridectomy forceps
Z. iridectomy scissors
Z. knife
Z. limbal-relaxing incision system
Z. LRI marker
Z. micro acrylic lens implantation forceps
Z. reverse capsulorrhexis forceps
ZAP
Zaldivar anterior procedure
ZAP diamond knife
zeaxanthin
Zeeman effect
Zeimer venomanometer
Zeis
gland of Z.
Z. gland
zeisian
z. gland
z. sty
Zeiss
Z. carbon arc slit lamp
Z. cine adapter
Z. DAS-1 hydrophobic system
Z. FF450 fundus camera
Z. fiberoptic illumination system
Z. goniolens
Z. gonioscope
Z. IOL Master laser interferometer
Z. LA 110 projection Lensmeter
Z. lens
Z. OM-3 operating microscope
Z. operating field loupe
Z. ophthalmoscope
Z. OpMi-6 FR microscope
Z. photocoagulator
Z. slit-lamp series
Z. vertex refractionometer
Z. VISULAS 532, 532s laser
Z. VISULAS 532s laser
Z. VISULAS YAG II laser

Zeiss-Barraquer
Z.-B. cine microscope
Z.-B. surgical microscope
Zeiss-Comberg slit lamp
Zeiss-Gullstrand
Z.-G. lens
Z.-G. loupe
Zeiss-Humphrey 840 UBM scanner
Zeiss-Nordenson fundus camera
Zellballen pattern
Zellweger syndrome
Zenapax
Zenarestat
Zentel
Zentmyer line
Zephiran
Zernike
Z. coefficient
Z. decomposition
zero
z. optical power
z. power lenses
z. vergence
ZEST
zippy estimating by sequential testing
Zestril
zidovudine
Ziegler
Z. blade
Z. cautery
Z. cilia forceps
Z. electrocautery
Z. iris knife-needle
Z. knife
Z. lacrimal dilator
Z. operation
Z. probe
Z. puncture
Z. speculum
Zimmerman tumor
Zinacef
zinc
z. acetate
bacitracin z.
z. bacitracin
z. sulfate
z. sulfate solution
Zincfrin
Zinn
anulus of Z.
circle of Z.
Z. circlet
Z. corona
Z. ligament
Z. membrane

Z

Zinn (*continued*)
    Z. ring
    Z. tendon
    zone of Z.
    zonule of Z.
    Z. zonule
Zinn-Haller arterial circle
zinnii
    anulus z.
    circulus z.
zipped angle
zipper stitch
zippy estimating by sequential testing (ZEST)
Zirm LASIK aspiration speculum
Zithromax
zithromycin
Zöllner
    Z. figure
    Z. line
Zolyse
zona, pl. **zonae**
    z. ciliaris
    z. ophthalmica
zonal granuloma
zone
    ablation z.
    anterior optic z.
    apical z.
    z. B-cell lymphoma
    blur z.
    Bowman z.
    Boyd z.
    capillary-free z.
    central steep z.
    choroidal watershed z.
    ciliary z.
    z. of contact lens
    z. of discontinuity
    z. 1 disease
    extravisual z.
    fissure z.
    foveal avascular z. (FAZ)
    interpalpebral z.
    junctional z.
    lens z.
    limbal z.
    markers for z.
    nasal z.
    neutral z.
    nuclear z.
    null z.
    optical z. (OZ)
    posterior optical z. (POZ)
    pupillary z.
    Z. Quick tear volume testing
    retinal z.
    temporal z.
    transition z.

    transitional z.
    visual z.
    z. of Zinn
zonula, pl. **zonulae**
    z. adherens
    z. ciliaris
    z. occludens
zonular
    z. attachment
    z. band
    z. fiber
    z. keratitis
    z. nuclear cataract
    z. pulverulent cataract
    z. scotoma
    z. space
    z. stripper
    z. sutural cataract
    z. tension
    z. tetany
zonulares
    fibrae z.
zonularia
    spatia z.
zonular-traction retinal tuft
zonule
    ciliary z.
    lens z.
    z. stripper
    Zinn z.
    z. of Zinn
zonulitis
zonulolysis, zonulysis
    Barraquer z.
    enzymatic z.
zonulotomy
zoom system
zoster
    z. ophthalmicus
    z. sine eruptio
    z. sine herpete
    z. uveitis
Zostrix
Zovirax
Z-plasty
    Spencer-Watson Z.-p.
Zuckerkandl dehiscence
Zurich suturing forceps
zygoma
zygomatic
    z. bone
    z. foramen
    z. foramen of Arnold
    z. fracture
    z. nerve
    z. suture
zygomatici
    facies orbitalis ossis z.
    processus frontosphenoidalis ossis z.

zygomaticofacial
 z. canal
 z. foramen
 z. nerve
zygomaticofrontal suture
zygomaticomaxillary suture
zygomaticoorbital
 z. artery
 z. foramen
 z. process
 z. process of the maxilla
zygomaticoorbitale
 foramen z.

zygomaticosphenoid suture
zygomaticotemporal
 z. canal
 z. foramen
 z. nerve
 z. suture
zygomaticus
 nervus z.
zygomycosis
Zylik operation
Zyrtec

NOTES

Z

Appendix 1
Anatomical Illustrations

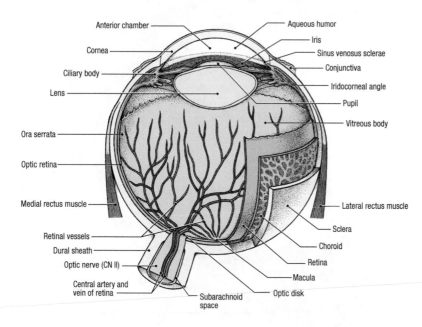

Figure 1. Structure of the eye.

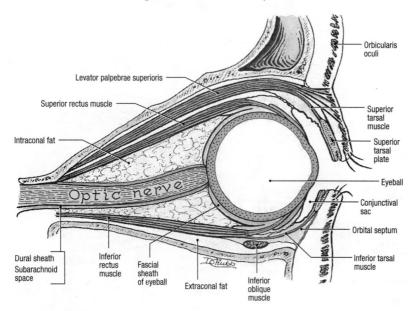

Figure 2. Orbital contents and upper eyelid, sagittal view.

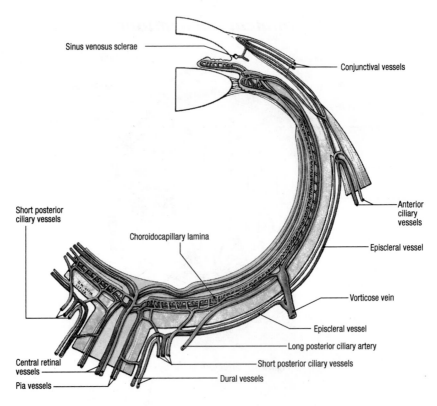

Figure 3. Blood supply to the eyeball.

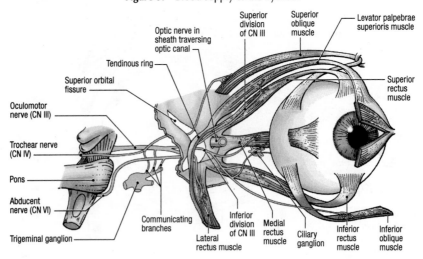

Figure 4. Distribution of ocular cranial nerves.

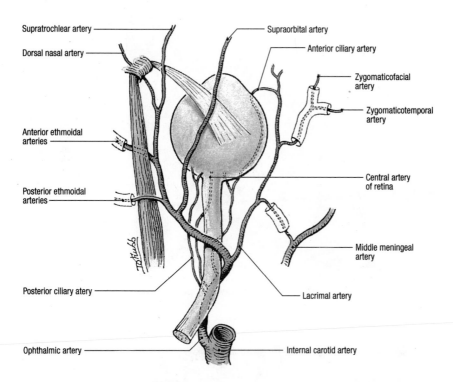

Supratrochlear artery

Dorsal nasal artery

Anterior ethmoidal arteries

Posterior ethmoidal arteries

Posterior ciliary atery

Ophthalmic artery

Supraorbital artery

Anterior ciliary artery

Zygomaticofacial artery

Zygomaticotemporal artery

Central artery of retina

Middle meningeal artery

Lacrimal artery

Internal carotid artery

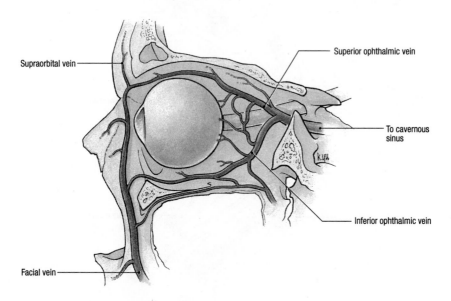

Supraorbital vein

Facial vein

Superior ophthalmic vein

To cavernous sinus

Inferior ophthalmic vein

Figure 5. Ophthalmic arteries (top), ophthalmic veins (bottom).

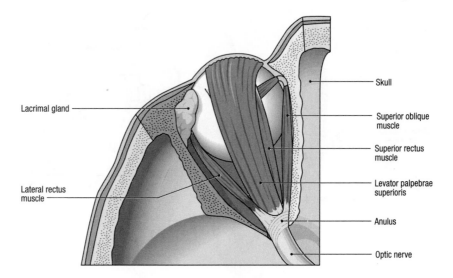

Lacrimal gland

Lateral rectus
muscle

Skull

Superior oblique
muscle

Superior rectus
muscle

Levator palpebrae
superioris

Anulus

Optic nerve

Figure 6. Orbital cavity, superior view.

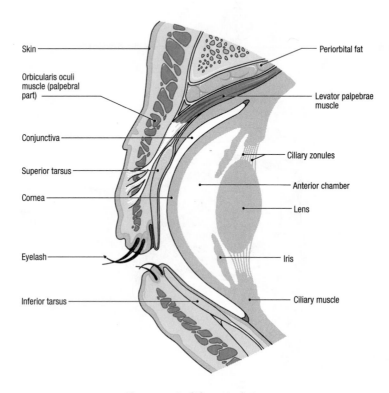

Skin

Orbicularis oculi
muscle (palpebral
part)

Conjunctiva

Superior tarsus

Cornea

Eyelash

Inferior tarsus

Periorbital fat

Levator palpebrae
muscle

Ciliary zonules

Anterior chamber

Lens

Iris

Ciliary muscle

Figure 7. Eyelids, sagittal view.

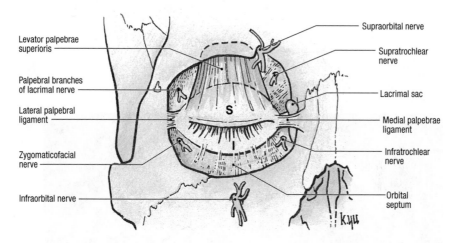

Supraorbital nerve

Levator palpebrae superioris

Supratrochlear nerve

Palpebral branches of lacrimal nerve

Lacrimal sac

Lateral palpebral ligament

Medial palpebrae ligament

Zygomaticofacial nerve

Infratrochlear nerve

Infraorbital nerve

Orbital septum

Figure 8. Orbital septum and eyelid, anterior view. (S) Superior and (I) inferior tarsal plates.

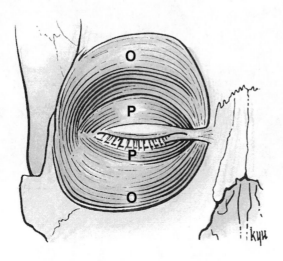

Figure 9. Orbicularis oculi, anterior view. (O) Orbital parts of the orbicularis oculi, (P) palpebral parts of the orbicularis oculi.

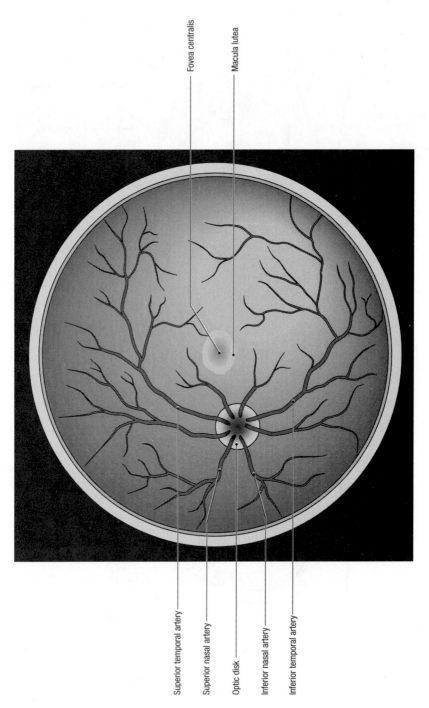

Fovea centralis

Macula lutea

Figure 10. The fundus.

Superior temporal artery

Superior nasal artery

Optic disk

Inferior nasal artery

Inferior temporal artery

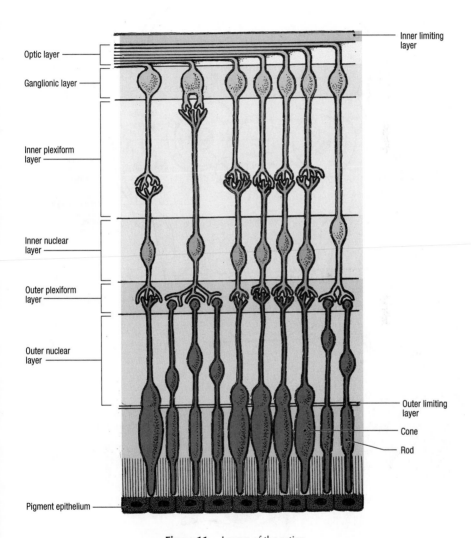

Figure 11. Layers of the retina.

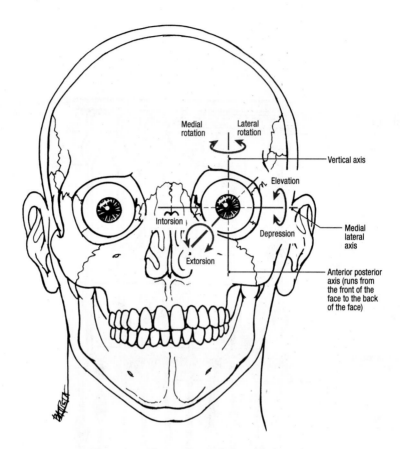

Figure 12. The motions and axes of the eye.

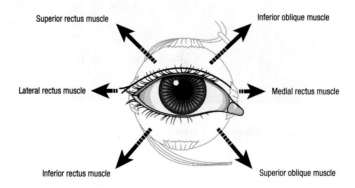

Figure 13. Extraocular eye movements.

Movements of the Eyes and the Muscles Employed

Sideways motion (ab- and adduction)	Vertical motion	Oblique motion		Rolling motion
Dextroversion	**Elevation (lifting)**	**Dextroelevation**	**Levoelevation**	**Extorsion (outward rolling)**
Right eye: lateral rectus	Superior rectus	Right eye: superior rectus	Left eye: superior rectus	Inferior rectus
Left eye: medial rectus	Inferior oblique	Left eye: inferior oblique	Right eye: inferior oblique	Inferior oblique
Levoversion	**Depression (lowering)**	**Dextrodepression**	**Levodepression**	**Intorsion (inward rolling)**
Right eye: medial rectus	Inferior rectus	Right eye: inferior rectus	Left eye: inferior rectus	Superior rectus
Left eye: lateral rectus	Inferior oblique	Left eye: superior oblique	Right eye: superior oblique	Superior oblique

Figure 14. Movements of the eyes and the muscles employed.

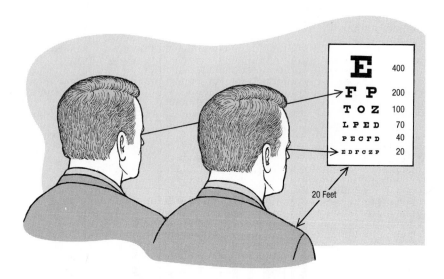

Figure 15. Snellen test of visual acuity.

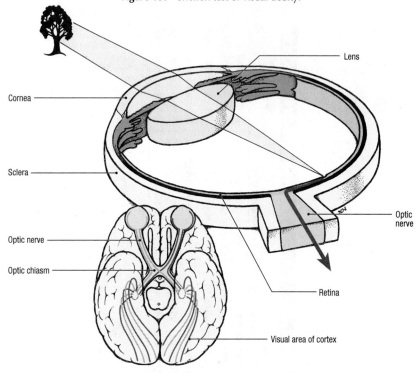

Figure 16. Vision. Light passes through the cornea and is focused onto the retina by the lens. Cells in the retina then transmit this information through the optic nerve to the visual area of the cortex.

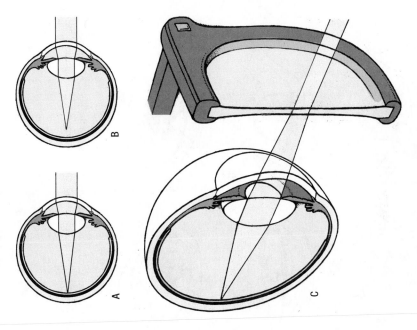

Figure 18. Myopia. (A) Normal (20/20) vision, light rays focus sharply on retina. (B) Myopic (nearsighted) vision, light rays from a distance come to a sharp focus in front of the retina. (C) Myopia corrected by eyeglasses with concave lenses.

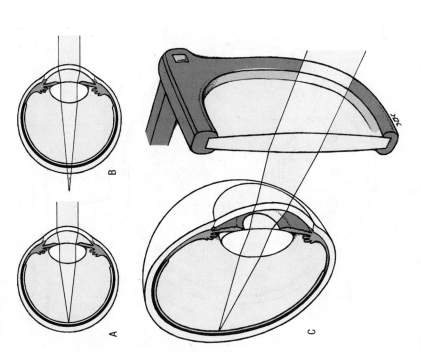

Figure 17. Hyperopia. (A) Normal (20/20) vision, light rays focus sharply on retina. (B) Hyperopic (farsighted) vision, light rays from close objects come to a sharp focus behind the retina. (C) Hyperopia corrected by eyeglasses with convex lenses.

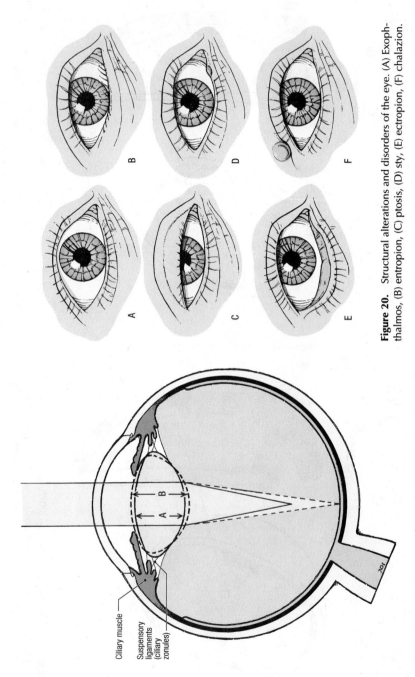

Figure 20. Structural alterations and disorders of the eye. (A) Exophthalmos, (B) entropion, (C) ptosis, (D) sty, (E) ectropion, (F) chalazion.

Figure 19. Lens accommodation. (A) Lens focuses image in front of retina; image is blurred. (B) Lens accommodates to focus on retina; image is sharp.

Ciliary muscle

Suspensory ligaments (ciliary zonules)

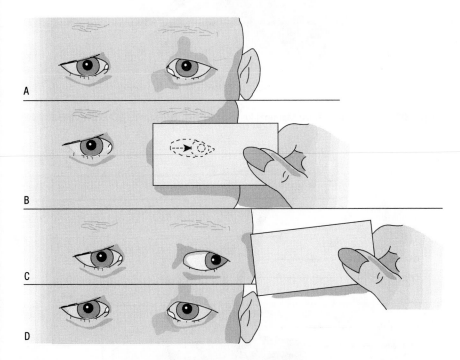

Figure 21. Technique for cover test to test for exophoria (misalignment). (A) Child's eyes appear to be in good alignment. (B) Left eye is then covered for 5 seconds. (C) When card is removed, left eye moves back to alignment. (D) This "drifting" indicates a misalignment.

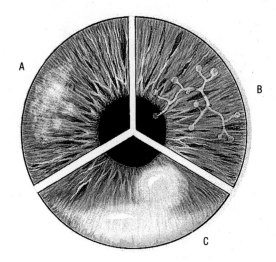

Figure 22. Corneal ulcers. (A) Marginal keratitis, (B) herpes dendrite, (C) hypopyon ulcer.

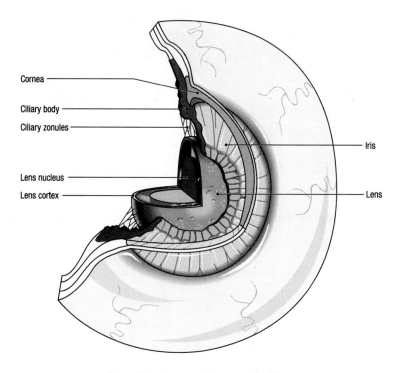

Cornea

Ciliary body

Ciliary zonules

Lens nucleus

Lens cortex

Iris

Lens

Figure 23. Cataract. Note opacity of lens.

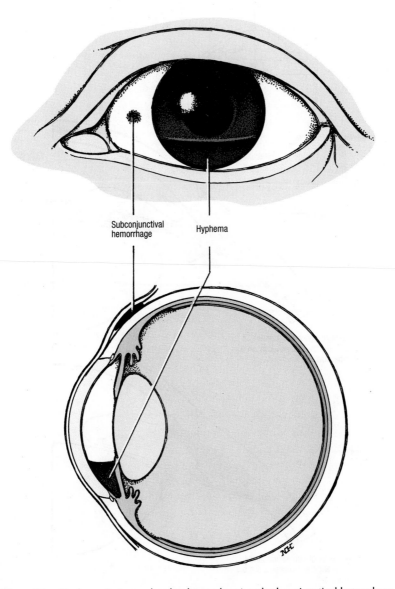

Subconjunctival
hemorrhage

Hyphema

Figure 24. Hyphema (anterior chamber hemorrhage) and subconjunctival hemorrhage.

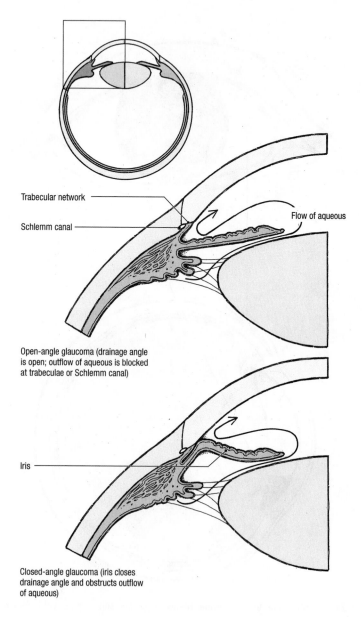

Trabecular network

Schlemm canal

Flow of aqueous

Open-angle glaucoma (drainage angle
is open; outflow of aqueous is blocked
at trabeculae or Schlemm canal)

Iris

Closed-angle glaucoma (iris closes
drainage angle and obstructs outflow
of aqueous)

Figure 25. Glaucoma.

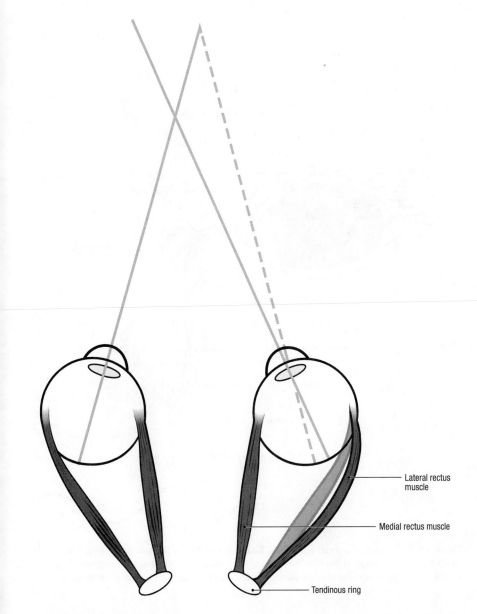

Lateral rectus
muscle

Medial rectus muscle

Tendinous ring

Figure 26. Diagram of the condition of strabismus, where one eye cannot focus with the other. View of eyeballs and their musculature from above with lines of vision indicated. Note that right eye has an elongated muscle which does not allow it to turn the eyeball far enough to focus on a point in the distance.

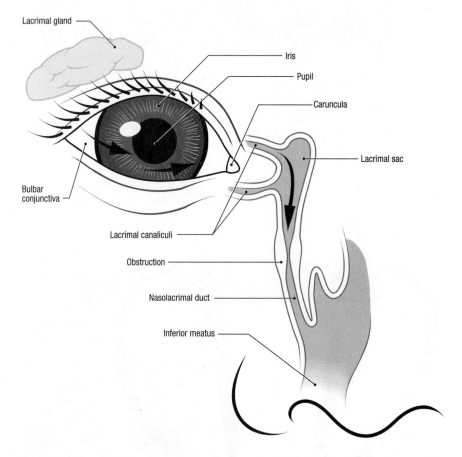

Figure 27. Obstructed lacrimal apparatus. Tears are secreted by the lacrimal gland. Tears, after passing over the eyeball, drain into the lacrimal sac. The nasolacrimal duct is obstructed, preventing tears from emptying into the inferior meatus of the nose and causing inflammation.

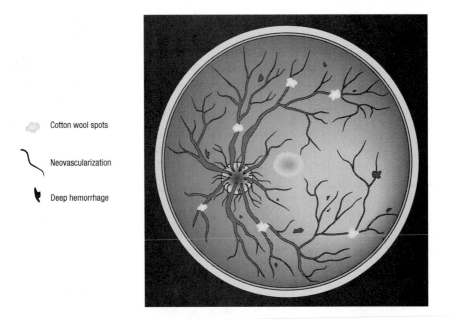

Cotton wool spots

Neovascularization

Deep hemorrhage

Figure 28. Retina afflicted with proliferative diabetic retinopathy as seen through an ophthalmoscope.

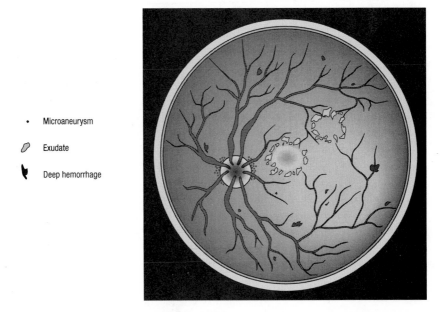

Microaneurysm

Exudate

Deep hemorrhage

Figure 29. The retina as seen through an ophthalmoscope. Retina shows various characteristics associated with background diabetic retinopathy.

A19

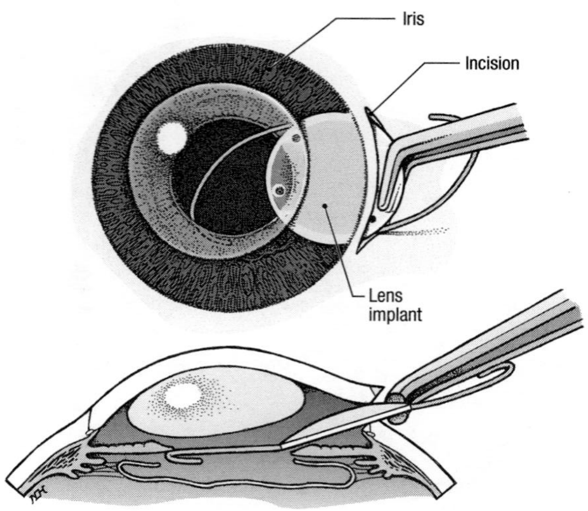

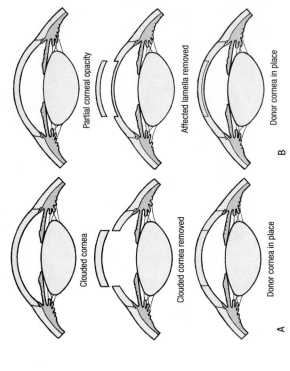

Figure 31. Full and partial corneal transplantation. (A) Penetrating keratoplasty. A full-thickness (7 to 8 mm) disk is removed from the host and replaced with a matching full-thickness button from the donor. (B) Lamellar keratoplasty. A thin layer of corneal tissue is excised from the host eye, sparing the stroma and entire endothelium.

A

Clouded cornea

Clouded cornea removed

Donor cornea in place

B

Partial corneal opacity

Affected lamella removed

Donor cornea in place

Figure 30. Intraocular lens implant insertion into the anterior chamber of the eye.

Iris

Incision

Lens implant

Appendix 2

Cranial Nerves

1. Nerves of the Head and Neck Region

Nerve	Origin	Course	Innervation
Abducent	Pons	Intradural on clivus; traverses cavernous sinus and superior orbital fissure to enter orbit	Lateral rectus
Ansa cervicalis	Hypoglossal	Descends on external surface of carotid sheath	Omohyoid, sternohyoid, and sternothyroid
Deep petrosal	Internal carotid plexus	Traverses cartilages of foramen lacerum, joins greater petrosal nerve at entrance of pterygoid canal	Lacrimal gland, mucosa of nasal cavity, palate, and upper pharynx
Glossopharyngeal	Rostral end of medulla	Exits cranium via jugular foramen, passes between superior and middle constrictors of pharynx to tonsillar fossa, enters posterior third of tongue	Somatic to stylopharyngeus; visceral to parotid gland; sensory of posterior tongue, pharynx, tympanic cavity, auditory tube, carotid body, and sinus
Great auricular	Cervical plexus	Ascends over sterno-cleidomastoid; anterior and parallel to external jugular	Skin of auricle, adjacent scalp, and over angle of jaw
Greater occipital	Medial branch of posterior ramus of spinal nerve C2	Pierces deep muscles of neck and trapezius to ascend posterior scalp to vertex	Posterior scalp
Greater petrosal	Genu of facial nerve	Exits facial canal via hiatus for greater petrosal nerve	Pterygoid ganglion for innervation of lacrimal, nasal, palatine, and upper pharyngeal mucous glands

(continued)

Appendix 2

Nerve	Origin	Course	Innervation
Hypoglossal	Between pyramid and olive of myelencephalon	Hypoglossal canal, medial to angle of mandible, between mylohyoid and hypoglossus to muscles of tongue	Intrinsic and extrinsic muscles of tongue
Intermediate	Facial nerve	Acoustic meatus to distal end of facial nerve	Pterygopalatine and submandibular ganglia via greater petrosal nerve, chorda tympani; tongue and palate
Lesser occipital	Cervical plexus	Parallel to anterosuperior border of sterno-cleidomastoid	Skin of posterior surface of auricle and adjacent scalp
Lesser petrosal	Tympanic plexus	Tympanic cavity to middle cranial fossa; sphenopetrosal fissure or foramen ovale	Otic ganglion for secretomotor innervation of parotid gland
Long thoracic	Anterior rami	Distally on external surface of serratus anterior	Serratus anterior
Nerve to mylohyoid	Inferior alveolar nerve	Inferior alveolar nerve of mandibular foramen to groove on medial aspect of ramus of mandible	Mylohyoid and anterior belly of digastric muscle
Nerve to tensor tympani	Otic ganglion	Cartilaginous portion of pharyngotympanic tube to semicranial of tensor tympani	Tensor tympani
Nerve to tensor veli palatini	Anterior mandibular nerve	Branch of nerve to medial pterygoid	Tensor veli palatini
Olfactory	Olfactory cells in olfactory epithelium of roof of nasal cavity	Foramen of cribriform plate to ethmoid, to olfactory bulbs	Olfactory mucosa; sense of smell
Phrenic	Cervical plexus	Superior thoracic aperture between mediastinal pleura and pericardium	Diaphragm; pericardial sac, mediastinal pleura, diaphragmatic peritoneum

(*continued*)

Nerve	Origin	Course	Innervation
Posterior inferior nasal	Greater palatine	Greater palatine canal through plate of palatine bone	Mucosa of inferior concha and walls of inferior and middle meatuses
Subclavian	Brachial plexus	Posterior to clavicle, anterior to brachial plexus and subclavian artery	Subclavius; sternoclavicular joint
Supraclavicular, lateral, intermediate, and medial	Cervical plexus	Center or posterior border of sternocleido-mastoid; fan out as they descend into lower neck, upper thorax, and shoulder	Skin of lower anterolateral neck, uppermost thorax, and shoulder
Supraorbital	Frontal nerve	Supraorbital foramen, breaks up into small branches	Mucous membrane of frontal sinus, conjunctivae, and skin of forehead
Suprascapular	Brachial plexus	Posterior triangle of neck; under superior transverse scapular ligament	Supraspinatus, infraspinatus muscles; superior and posterior glenohumeral joint
Supratrochlear	Facial nerve	Supraorbital nerve, divides into two or more branches	Skin in middle of forehead to hairline
Transverse cervical	Cervical plexus	Posterior border of sternocleido-mastoid muscle, runs anteriorly across muscle	Skin overlying anterior triangle of neck
Trochlear	Dorsolateral aspect of mesocephalon below inferior colliculus	Passes around brainstem to enter dura in edge of tentorium close to posterior clinoid process; runs in lateral wall of cavernous sinus, entering orbit via superior orbital fissures	Superior oblique muscle
Upper subscapular	Brachial plexus	Posteriorly enters subscapularis	Superior portion of subscapularis

2. Nerves of the Facial Region

Nerve	Origin	Course	Innervation
Auriculotemporal	Mandibular nerve	Passes between neck of mandible and external acoustic meatus to accompany superficial temporal artery	Skin anterior to auricle, posterior temporal region, tragus, helix of auricle, exterior acoustic meatus, upper tympanic membrane
Buccal	Mandibular nerve	Infratemporal fossa, passes anteriorly to reach cheek	Skin and mucosa of cheek, buccal gingiva
Chorda tympani	Facial nerve	Traverses tympanic cavity, passes between incus and malleus; exits temporal bone via petrotympanic fissure; enters infratemporal fossa, merges with lingual nerve	Submandibular and sublingual glands; taste sensation from anterior tongue
Deep temporal	Mandibular nerve	Temporal fossa to temporalis muscle	Temporalis; periosteum of temporal fossa
External nasal	Anterior ethmoidal nerve	Runs in nasal cavity and emerges on face between nasal bone and lateral nasal cartilage	Skin on dorsum of nose including tip of nose
Facial	Posterior border of pons	Runs through internal acoustic meatus and facial canal of petrous part of temporal bone, exiting via stylomastoid foramen; intraparotid plexus	Stapedius, posterior belly of digastric, stylohyoid facial and scalp muscles; skin of external acoustic meatus
Greater palatine	Branch of pterygopalatine ganglion (maxillary nerve)	Passes inferiorly through greater palatine canal and foramen	Palatine glands; mucosa of hard palate

(continued)

Nerve	Origin	Course	Innervation
Inferior alveolar	Terminal branch of posterior mandibular nerve	Lateral and medial pterygoid muscles of infratemporal fossa to enter mandibular canal of mandible	Lower teeth, periodontium, periosteum, and gingiva of lower jaw
Infraorbital	Terminal branch of maxillary nerve	Runs in floor of orbit and emerges at infraorbital foramen	Skin of cheek, lower lid, lateral side of nose and inferior septum and upper lip, upper premolar incisors and canine teeth; mucosa of maxillary sinus and upper lip
Lesser palatine	Pterygopalatine ganglion (maxillary nerve)	Passes inferiorly through palatine canal and lesser palatine foramen	Glands of soft palate; mucosa of soft palate
Lingual	Terminal branch of posterior mandibular nerve	Joins chorda tympani, passes anteroinferiorly between lateral and medial pterygoid muscles, oral cavity	Submandibular ganglion and submandibular and sublingual salivary glands
Mandibular	Trigeminal ganglion	Foramen ovale to infratemporal fossa, divides into anterior and posterior trunks, ramifying into smaller branches, bifurcating into lingual and inferior alveolar nerve	Muscles of mastication, mylohyoid, anterior belly of digastric, tensor tympanic, tensor veli palatini; skin overlying mandible, teeth, gingiva, tongue, and temporo-mandibular joint
Masseteric	Mandibular nerve	Passes laterally through mandibular notch	Masseter; temporo-mandibular joint
Maxillary	Trigeminal nerve	Anteriorly through foramen rotundum, to pterygopalatine fossa, sends roots to pterygoid ganglion (maxillary nerve); continues anteriorly through infraorbital fissures as infraorbital nerve	Pterygopalatine ganglion, lacrimal gland, mucosal glands of nasal cavity, palate, and upper pharynx; skin overlying maxillary mucosa of posteroinferior nasal cavity, maxillary sinus, upper half of mouth (teeth, gingiva and mucosa of palate, vestibule and cheek)

(*continued*)

Nerve	Origin	Course	Innervation
Mental	Terminal branch of inferior alveolar nerve	Mandibular canal at mental foramen	Skin of chin; skin and mucosa of lower lip
Nasopalatine	Pterygopalatine ganglion (maxillary nerve)	Exits pterygopalatine fossa via sphenopalatine foramen; runs anteroinferiorly across nasal septum, to incisive foramen to palate	Mucosal glands of nasal septum; mucosa of nasal septum, anterior-most hard palate
Nerve to lateral and medial pterygoid	Anterior mandibular nerve	Arises in infratemporal fossa, inferior to foramen ovale	Lateral and medial pterygoid muscles
Nerve to pterygoid canal	Formed by merger of greater and deep petrosal nerves	Traverses pterygoid canal, to pterygoid ganglion in pterygoid fossa	Pterygopalatine ganglion
Nerve to stapedius	Facial nerve	Arises as facial nerve, descends posterior to muscle in facial canal	Stapedius
Pharyngeal	Pterygopalatine ganglion	Passes posteriorly through palatovaginal canal	Supplies mucosa of nasopharynx posterior to the pharyngotympanic tubes
Superior alveolar	Maxillary nerve	Posteriorly emerges from pterygomaxillary fissure into infratemporal fossa to posterior aspect of maxilla; Middle and anterior: arises from infraorbital nerve of maxillary sinus, descends walls of sinus	Mucosa of maxillary sinus, maxillary teeth and gingiva

(continued)

Nerve	Origin	Course	Innervation
Trigeminal	Lateral surface of pons by two roots: motor and sensory	Crosses medial part of crest of petrous part of temporal bone, trigeminal cave of dural mater lateral to body of sphenoid and cavernous sinus; motor root passes ganglion to become part of mandibular nerve	Motor: somatic; muscles of mastication, mylohyoid, anterior belly of digastric, tensor tympanic, tensor veli palatini; Sensory: dura of anterior and middle cranial fossa, skin of face, teeth, gingiva, mucosa of nasal cavity, paranasal sinuses, and mouth
Zygomatic	Maxillary nerve	Arises in floor of orbit, divides into two temporal nerves, traverses foramina of same; communicating branch joins lacrimal nerve	Skin over zygomatic arch, anterior temporal region; conveys secretory postsynaptic parasympathetic fibers from pterygopalatine ganglion to lacrimal gland

3. Nerves of the Eye Region

Nerve	Origin	Course	Innervation
Anterior ethmoid	Nasociliary nerve	Arises in orbit, passes via anterior ethmoidal foramen, cranial cavity via cribriform plate of ethmoid to nasal cavity	Dural of anterior cranial fossa; mucous membranes of sphenoidal sinus, ethmoid cells and upper nasal cavity
Ciliary, long and short	Nasociliary nerve; short ciliary ganglion	Passes to posterior aspect of eyeball	Cornea, conjunctiva; ciliary body and iris
Frontal	Ophthalmic nerve	Crosses orbit on superior aspect of levator palpebrae superioris; divides into supraorbital and supratrochlear branches	Skin of forehead, scalp, eyelid, and nose; conjunctiva of upper lid and mucosa of frontal sinus
Infratrochlear	Nasociliary nerve	Follows medial wall of orbit to upper eyelid	Skin, conjunctiva, lining of upper eyelid

(continued)

Nerve	Origin	Course	Innervation
Lacrimal	Ophthalmic nerve	Palpebral fascia of upper eyelid near lateral angle of eye	Small area of skin and conjunctiva of lateral part of upper eyelid
Nasociliary	Ophthalmic nerve	Arises in superior orbital fissure, anteromedially across retrobulbar orbit, providing sensory root to ciliary ganglion; terminates as infratrochlear nerve	Ciliary ganglion (short) coveys postsynaptic sympathetic and parasympathetic to ciliary body and iris; tactile sensation for eyeball; mucous membrane of ethmoid cells, anterosuperior nasal cavity; skin of dorsum and apex of nose
Oculomotor	Interpeduncular fossa of mesencephalon	Dura of posterior clinoid process, lateral wall of cavernous sinus, enters orbit through superior orbital fissure and divides into superior and inferior branches	All extraocular muscles except superior oblique and lateral rectus; presynaptic parasympathetic fibers to ciliary ganglions for ciliary body and sphincter pupillae
Ophthalmic	Trigeminal ganglion	Anteriorly in lateral wall of cavernous sinus to enter orbit through superior orbital fissure, branching into frontal, nasociliary, and lacrimal nerve	General sensation from eyeball; mucous membrane of ethmoid cells, frontal sinus, dura of anterior cranial fossa, falx cerebri, and tentorium cerebelli, anterosuperior nasal cavity; skin of forehead, upper lid, and dorsum and apex of nose
Optic	Ganglion cells of retina	Exits orbit via optic canals; fibers from nasal half of retina cross to contralateral side at chiasm; passes via optic tracts to geniculate bodies, superior colliculus and pretectum	Vision from retina
Posterior ethmoidal	Nasociliary	Leaves orbit via posterior ethmoid foramen	Supplies ethmoid and sphenoid paranasal sinuses

Sample Reports and Dictation

ARGON LASER TRABECULOPLASTY

PREOPERATIVE DIAGNOSIS: Open angle glaucoma, right eye.

POSTOPERATIVE DIAGNOSIS: Open angle glaucoma, right eye.

OPERATION: Argon laser trabeculoplasty, right eye.

ANESTHESIA: Topical.

PROCEDURE: The patient was brought to the laser room in satisfactory condition with appropriate informed consent of the risks, benefits, and alternatives of the procedure having been explained, including pain, glaucoma, decreased vision, need for further surgery, and bleeding. Drops of Iopidine and pilocarpine had been placed while in the holding area. The patient was seated at the slit lamp apparatus and the head positioned and secured. The argon laser aiming beam was focused carefully using a trabeculoplasty lens. Laser shots were placed along the trabecular meshwork approximately every 2 to 3 laser spot widths apart for 180 degrees of the trabecular meshwork. The spot width was 50 microns and the duration of 1 laser shot was 0.1 second. A total of 60 shots were given consisting of 600 to 800 mJ. A satisfactory reaction at the trabecular meshwork was considered to be a blanching or bubble production at the point of laser application. The patient's head was released, and drops of Iopidine were instilled.

Postoperative instructions were reviewed, which included alerting the patient to possible symptoms of elevated intraocular pressure in the operated eye. Followup examination in the office was prescribed to occur 1 to 3 hours after the procedure.

CHALAZION INCISION AND DRAINAGE

OPERATION: Chalazion incision and drainage of the right eye.

PROCEDURE: The patient was brought into the operating room. The right eye was prepped and draped for the procedure. Chalazion forceps were used to grasp the upper eyelid. The pretarsal conjunctival surface of the chalazion was incised. The contents of the chalazion were curetted. Chalazion forceps were removed. Hemostasis was achieved with a modified amount of pressure. Maxitrol ointment was placed in the eye with an overlying eye pad. The patient was reversed from anesthesia and transferred to the recovery area in stable condition.

DACRYOCYSTITIS RHINOSTOMY AND REPAIR OF CANALICULAR ATRESIA

PREOPERATIVE DIAGNOSES:
1. Chronic dacryocystitis, right side.
2. Canalicular atresia, upper and lower canaliculus, right side.

POSTOPERATIVE DIAGNOSES:
1. Chronic dacryocystitis, right side.
2. Canalicular atresia, upper and lower canaliculus, right side.

OPERATION:
1. Dacryocystitis rhinostomy of right side.
2. Repair of canalicular atresia, upper and lower canaliculus, right side, with placement of lacrimal microtube.

ANESTHESIA: Local infiltrative with monitored anesthesia care.

INDICATIONS: The patient is a 36-year-old male who has noted constant epiphora since birth. He is also noted to have a mass of the right lacrimal fossa and episodic discharge.

PROCEDURE: After informed consent was obtained, the patient was taken to the operating room and placed supine on the operating room table. Previously, a gentian violet marking pen had been used to mark the furthest clinical extent of the atretic canaliculi, both upper and lower. In addition, the caruncle was marked out should a conjunctivodacryocystorhinostomy with lacrimal Jones tube placement be necessary. The patient received appropriate preoperative monitoring and sedation, and a solution of 2% lidocaine with 1:100,000 epinephrine in a 50/50 mixture with 0.75% bupivacaine was given subcutaneously in the area of the previously demarcated dacryocystorhinostomy incision. The anterior ethmoidal nerve was also blocked utilizing 2 mL of this same solution by injecting 10 mm superior to the medial canthal tendon on the right side in the medial orbit. The lateral wall of the nose was also infiltrated with this same solution as was the anterior head of the middle turbinate. The head of the middle turbinate was also packed in the area of the middle meatus of the nose with a 4% cocaine-soaked gauze. General endotracheal tube anesthesia had been obtained without incident. The surgeon performed the surgical scrub. Upon his return, the patient was prepped and draped in usual sterile fashion for ophthalmic surgery. A hard corneal shield was placed before the cornea of the right eye after a series of 0.5% topical tetracaine drops had been applied.

The reconstruction of the atretic canaliculi was performed first. Examination of the upper and lower canaliculi revealed distal atresia of the upper and lower canaliculus. A cutdown was performed over the more proximal segment of canaliculi, and a sterile safety pin was used to dilate the atretic segment of canaliculus. A quadruple 0-Bowman probe was then used to cannulate the atretic canaliculus. Care was taken to avoid creating a false track; however, the course of the track marked out the presumed course of the atretic but functional canaliculi, both upper and lower. A similar procedure was performed on the lower after the upper had been completed. Further dilation was performed with a pediatric punctum dilator. After this, a triple 0-Bowman probe was placed and stenosis was noted at the level of the common canaliculus through the inferior punctum. A double 0 and then single 0 Bowman probe was advanced through the remaining portion of the canaliculus to the level of the hard stop of the nasal bone. Irrigation at this point produced reflux. There was no ability to decompress the lacrimal sac. Further dilatation was performed so that a #1 Bowman probe could be admitted through both the superior and inferior atretic canaliculi.

Attention was next directed to the dacryocystorhinostomy portion of the procedure. A #15-Bard-Parker blade was used to incise the previously demarcated dacryocystorhinostomy site. A hemostat was used to spread the fibers of the orbicularis muscle, and the sharp edge of a Freer periosteal elevator was used to strip periosteum down to the level of periorbita. A very enlarged lacrimal sac was noted, and the lacrimal sac was reflected laterally to allow for exposure of the bony nasolacrimal fossa. While retracting the lacrimal sac, a large amount of green to brown mucopurulent debris was expressed through the superior portion of the sac. This was cultured and allowed for further inspection of the nasolacrimal fossa, which was noted to be markedly enlarged from the normal diameter. The medial wall of the lacrimal sac was then sent for biopsy. The rhinostomy began by in-fracturing at the level of the lacrimal maxillary suture. A Kerrison punch was used to enlarge the rhinostomy to a final diameter of 15 mm. Superiorly, the rhinostomy had been enlarged so that no bony edge was closer than 5 mm to the exit of the common canaliculus. Hemostasis was achieved with direct digital pressure, Bovie cautery, and topical thrombin-soaked Gelfoam. The area was then packed with the Gelfoam soaked in topical thrombin.

Attention was directed back to the now reconstructed canaliculi. A 0-Bowman probe was inserted through the superior canaliculus, through the common canaliculus to exit the medial portion of the lacrimal sac. In a similar fashion, a double 0-Bowman probe was passed through the inferior canaliculus. The anterior lacrimal sac flap was fashioned with Westcott scissors, as was the posterior lacrimal sac flap. The nasal mucosa was then incised with cutting cautery, fashioning an anterior and posterior H-flap. The cocaine-soaked gauze was removed from the right naris. Alignment of the rhinostomy through the lacrimal sac and common canaliculus was noted to be adequate. The lacrimal probes were removed, and a Guibor tube was placed through the superior and inferior canaliculus, through the rhinostomy to exit the right naris. The posterior lacrimal sac and posterior nasal mucosal flap were noted to align without tension. The rhinostomy was then packed with Gelfoam soaked in topical thrombin. The anterior flaps were closed with an interrupted 4-0 chromic suture in a horizontal mattress fashion. The deep layers of the orbicularis muscle were closed with a 5-0 Vicryl suture. The skin layers were closed with a series of interrupted mini-vertical mattress sutures. The nose was further packed with a nasal tampon coated with Maxitrol ointment at the tip and soaked in topical thrombin. The Guibor tube had been tied upon itself in the nose. The lacrimal microtube tension was adjusted in the medial canthus. A single dental roll and an eye patch were placed. The patient was extubated without incident and moved to the recovery room in stable condition.

ENUCLEATION OF THE EYE

OPERATION: Enucleation of right eye.

PROCEDURE: The patient was brought to the operating room and prepped and draped in the usual fashion. The left eye was approached, and a 360-degree conjunctival peritomy was performed with Westcott scissors. Wet-field cautery was used for hemostasis during the procedure. Dissection took place in all 4 quadrants to loosen the Tenon capsule from the scleral adhesions.

Next, the rectus muscles were isolated in turn and cut with cautery. Finally, the oblique muscles were isolated and cut with cautery, and then a large curved hemostat was placed on the optic nerve. The optic nerve was then cut with curved scissors, and the eye removed from the socket. There was about a 0.25-cm stump of optic nerve attached to the globe, and the clamp was left on the remaining optic nerve segment for hemostasis. After approximately 5 minutes, this was removed and hemostasis was noted to be excellent. The enucleated eye was sent for pathology.

Finally, the implant ball was placed into the socket, and the Tenon capsule was closed with 4-0 Vicryl suture in an interrupted fashion in 2 different layers. The conjunctiva was closed with 8-0 Vicryl suture in a running fashion with meticulous closure.

A conformer was placed into the conjunctival sac, and Maxitrol ointment placed in the socket. The patient had subconjunctival injections of Decadron and gentamicin, and a pad and Fox shield were placed over the eye.

EXTRACAPSULAR CATARACT EXTRACTION WITH INSERTION OF INTRAOCULAR LENS

OPERATION: Extracapsular cataract extraction with insertion of an intraocular lens, left eye.

PROCEDURE: Prior to surgery, a Honan intraocular pressure reducer balloon was placed over the left eye. The balloon pressure was then inflated to 30 mmHg and allowed to remain in place for 45 minutes prior to surgery. The patient was taken to the operating room where local anesthesia was administered with lidocaine 2% with epinephrine for a Nadbath lid block. Retrobulbar anesthesia and akinesia were achieved with an equal mixture of Marcaine 0.75% with epinephrine and lidocaine 4% along with Wydase. The patient was then prepped and draped in the usual sterile ophthalmic manner, and attention was directed to the left eye.

A lid speculum was inserted between the lids, and the intraocular pressure was measured with a Schiotz tonometer. The remainder of the procedure was conducted through the use of the Weck ophthalmic microscope.

The eye was stabilized with a 4-0 black silk superior rectus traction suture and was subsequently deflected downward. A limbal peritomy was performed with Westcott scissors from 10 o'clock around to 2 o'clock. Eraser bipolar cautery was utilized to effect hemostasis. A scleral incision was made 2 mm superior to the superior limbus with a 6610 Beaver blade to one-half the depth of the sclera for 12 mm in length. The dissection was then carried posteriorly from the base of the incision into clear cornea. A #75-Beaver blade was utilized to create a stab wound into clear cornea at 2 o'clock to provide an access port. A keratome was utilized to enter the anterior chamber through the base of the corneoscleral wound at 10 o'clock.

Healon was injected into the anterior chamber through a cystitome needle. The needle was subsequently used to affect an anterior capsulotomy, and capsule forceps were utilized to affect a circular tear capsulorrhexis capsulotomy. Balanced salt solution was injected underneath the capsule to dissect the nucleus free from the capsule.

The 10 o'clock incision was then enlarged with right and left cutting corneoscleral scissors to 12 mm in length. Through the use of a lens loop and Colibri forceps, the nucleus was expressed through the wound. Two interrupted 10-0 nylon sutures were then inserted through the corneoscleral wound, dividing the wound into equal thirds.

A Cavitron irrigation and aspiration tip was inserted through the wound, and lens cortical material was irrigated and aspirated. Following this, the posterior capsule was noted to be intact, and Healon was injected into the anterior chamber.

An IOLAB posterior chamber intraocular lens, Model G-708G of 22 diopters lens power, had previously been soaked in balanced salt solution. The lens was flushed with fresh balanced salt solution and coated with Healon. Angled McPherson tying forceps were then used to insert the lens through the scleral incision with the inferior foot of the haptic passing beneath the anterior capsule at 6 o'clock. Long-angled McPherson tying forceps were then used to place the superior foot of the haptic through the pupil behind the anterior capsule at 12 o'clock. A Sinskey hook was utilized to rotate the lens and ensure its stability. Miochol was injected into the anterior chamber to constrict the pupil.

Balanced salt solution was then utilized to deepen the chamber and firm up the eye. Additional 10-0 nylon interrupted sutures were utilized to close the corneoscleral wound. At the completion of the maneuver, the wound was watertight. The eye evidenced normal pressure and the pupil was round, central, and lay immediately over the haptic of the posterior chamber lens. The conjunctival wound was coapted with bipolar cautery. Gentamicin and Celestone, 0.5 mL each, were separately injected through the inferior conjunctival cul-de-sac into the sub-Tenon space. The Barraquer lid speculum was removed, Maxitrol ointment instilled, and a patch and Fox shield placed over the eye.

HYPERTROPIA REPAIR

PREOPERATIVE DIAGNOSIS: Right hypertropia secondary to right superior oblique palsy.

POSTOPERATIVE DIAGNOSIS: Right hypertropia secondary to right superior oblique palsy.

OPERATION: A 5-mm resection of right superior rectus muscle and myectomy of the right inferior oblique muscle.

PROCEDURE: The patient was taken to the operating room. After intravenous sedation with Versed and fentanyl, she was given a peribulbar injection of Marcaine and Wydase. A pressure-lowering device was placed in the eye for 10 minutes to achieve hypotony. The area around both eyes were prepared with iodine and water and draped in the usual fashion as a sterile field. The right conjunctival cul-de-sac was irrigated with dilute Betadine solution. A lid speculum was placed in the right palpebral fissure.

An incision was made in the inferotemporal bulbar conjunctiva of the right eye. The right inferior and right lateral rectus muscles were identified through this incision and retracted. A muscle hook was then placed into the inferotemporal orbit, and the inferior oblique muscle was retrieved. This muscle was secured on 2 hemostats. The muscle between the hemostat was excised with the ends of the muscle cauterized. The stumps were then released into the orbit. The conjunctiva was closed with a running 6-0 Vicryl suture.

Attention was then turned to the superior bulbar conjunctiva where an incision was made between the 10 o'clock and the 2 o'clock position at the limbus. Relaxing incisions were made posteriorly at the 2 o'clock and 10 o'clock positions. The superior rectus muscle was isolated with blunt and sharp dissection and secured with a muscle hook. Additional anesthesia was given with a local infiltration on the muscle with 2% Xylocaine. Two 6-0 Vicryl sutures were placed through the temporal and nasal margins of the muscle. These sutures were drawn taut and tied. The muscle was then reinserted and resutured to the globe with the same sutures at a point 5 mm posterior to the original insertion. The stump on the insertion site was cauterized. The conjunctiva was then closed with interrupted 6-0 Vicryl sutures.

At the conclusion of the procedure, TobraDex ointment was instilled, the conjunctiva was closed, and a monocular patch was applied. The patient tolerated the procedure well and left the operating room in good condition.

HYPHEMA IRRIGATION

PREOPERATIVE DIAGNOSIS: Hyphema OS.

POSTOPERATIVE DIAGNOSIS: Hyphema OS.

OPERATION: Irrigation of hyphema OS.

INDICATIONS: Uncontrolled intraocular pressure after hyphema post cataract surgery.

HISTORY: The patient underwent an uneventful trabeculectomy in the left eye 5 years ago. Although the surgery was uneventful, the following day he had an almost total hyphema. No surgical intervention was done, but his intraocular pressure was controlled with medication. Eventually the intraocular pressure became well-controlled by the trabeculectomy, although a fibrous plaque was left on his lens because of the absorbed blood. Ironically, he underwent cataract surgery with posterior chamber intraocular lens implant in this eye to restore the vision and to be able to obtain a fundus view because of his diabetic retinopathy. The procedure was uneventful, and a foldable posterior chamber lens was implanted. At the end of the surgery the eye looked perfect. The following day he presented to the office with an almost total hyphema in the left eye and an intraocular pressure of 73. He stated that morning he had noticed some discomfort in the eye and change in his vision. Because of the fact that it took so long for the eye to attain a functional status, as with his first hyphema, it was elected to irrigate the hyphema immediately.

PROCEDURE: The patient was given some intravenous sedation by the anesthesiologist and then given topical anesthesia with 1% Xylocaine with epinephrine and tetracaine. The previous cataract incision was opened with a 2.5-mm keratome. The IA tip of the Legacy machine was used to irrigate some of the blood from the anterior chamber. Intracameral Xylocaine was also used for anesthesia. Some of the blood could not be aspirated but was actually removed with capsulorrhexis forceps after Viscoat was placed in the anterior chamber. Several attempts were made to irrigate the blood which seemed to be trapped in the superior chamber; whether it had originated in this area or near the trabeculectomy site could not be determined with certainty. At this point, irrigation and forceps removed no additional blood. It was elected to terminate the procedure at this point. Most of the optic of the lens was clean. Whether rebleeding would occur was impossible to say. The incision was closed with 1 interrupted 10-0 nylon suture. The anterior chamber was then reformed with BSS. Then 40 mg of triamcinolone was injected subconjunctivally at the nasal inferior fornix. The speculum was removed, and a light patch and shield were applied. The patient tolerated the procedure well and was returned to the recovery room in good condition.

PARS PLANA VITRECTOMY, MEMBRANE PEELING, SCLERAL BUCKLE, ENDOLASER, AND GAS-FLUID EXCHANGE

OPERATION: Pars plana vitrectomy for complex retinal detachment, membrane peeling, scleral buckle, endolaser, and gas-fluid exchange

PROCEDURE: Following informed consent and the identification of the patient, the patient was brought into the operating room, alert, and in stable condition. Regional anesthesia and akinesia were obtained using a mixture of Marcaine, lidocaine, and Wydase given in a retrobulbar block. The patient was then prepped and draped in the usual sterile fashion for ophthalmic procedure. The lid speculum was placed. A conjunctival peritomy was performed to 360 degrees using Westcott scissors and 0.12 forceps. Stevens scissors were used to dissect in each of the 4 quadrants. A muscle hook was used to grasp the inferior rectus muscle, and the muscle was then bridled using 4-0 black silk suture. Each of the 4 rectus muscles was bridled in a similar fashion.

Once all of the muscles were isolated and each muscle was cleaned using a Q-tip, 4-0 white silk suture bites were placed in each of the 4 quadrants in preparation for placing the scleral buckle. A Ruby blade was used to enter the eye 4 mm posterior to the surgical limbus infratemporally, and a trocar cannula infusion system was put into position. The position was checked with a light pipe prior to turning the infusion on.

Additional sclerotomies were made supratemporally and supranasally using the Ruby blade, also 4 mm posterior to the surgical lumbus. The light pipe and ocutome were then inserted through the sclerotomy sites, and the cortical vitreous was removed from the posterior surface in the lens to the anterior surface of the retina. The retina was noted to be detached, and there was noted to be a large open macular hole present; in addition, there were membranes present on the surface of the retina creating a star-fold infratemporally.

A Michel pick was used to raise membranes from the surface of the retina and peel back the posterior hyaloid to approximately the equator. The ocutome probe was used to remove remaining vitreous from the eye. Subretinal fluid was drained through a macular hole and also through a small retinotomy which was made near the supratemporal arcade. At this time, a 287 scleral buckle element was placed for 360 degrees around the eye, and the 4 pre-placed sutures were then tightened and tied, with the notch rotated posteriorly. The ends of the buckle were tied together using 4-0 white silk suture. Scleral plugs were placed into the sclerotomy sites prior to placing the buckle. An air-fluid exchange was then performed, and the retina was noted to flatten nicely. Additional drainage of fluid was performed through the retinotomy site. Several minutes were allowed to pass for additional fluid to accumulate, and this fluid was removed using active suction. Active suction was also used prior to the gas-fluid exchange to raise portions of the posterior hyaloid.

Once the retina was completely flattened, approximately 500 endolaser spots were placed along the buckle and around the retinotomy site. A gas-gas exchange was then performed using SF-6 gas. The sclerotomy sites were closed using 7-0 Vicryl suture material. The conjunctiva was closed using 6-0 plain suture material. All of the bridle sutures were removed prior to closing of the conjunctiva. Subconjunctival injection of Ancef and dexamethasone was performed. Atropine drops were placed topically on the eye, and the eye was then patched in closed position with an eye shell placed on top. The patient tolerated the procedure well and was transferred to the recovery room in stable condition.

PENETRATING KERATOPLASTY

OPERATION: Penetrating keratoplasty, 7.75 mm in a 7.5-mm bed, right eye.

PROCEDURE: After clearance from the anesthesiologist and topical anesthesia with 0.75% bupivacaine, the right eye was prepped and draped in the usual fashion, and massage was done until the bulb and orbit were soft. The Goldman-McNeill blepharostat was inserted and sutured to the episclera with Vicryl suture. The recipient cornea was measured, and a 7.75-mm trephine was selected for the donor, which was prepared in the usual fashion. A 7.5-mm trephine was then used for the recipient until penetration occurred. Additional deepening of the outer quadrants was done with a Supersharp. Curved corneal scissors to the right and left were used to completely excise the recipient button. The fluid centrally was cleaned up with cellulose sponges.

The pupil was enlarged by first creating snip incisions with Vannas scissors and then extending these, and small amounts of capsule and cortical material were also excised. A very small amount of bleeding occurred, but this stopped spontaneously. The Healon was then placed, as well as Miochol, and the donor corneal button was transferred to the operative field, where it was secured in position using 4 interrupted 10-0 nylon sutures followed by a 10-0 nylon suture in running fashion with the knot superiorly. Prior to tying this, the interrupted sutures were removed, the running suture tension was adjusted, and a permanent knot was created and buried in recipient stroma. The suture tension was adjusted further. The intraocular Healon was evacuated and replaced with balanced salt solution, and the wound was assessed with saline sponges and found to be watertight and in good position with a deep anterior chamber and no evidence of vitreous to the wound. The blepharostat was removed, and subconjunctival injections of gentamicin, Ancef, and Celestone were given and a drop of Betagan 0.5% was instilled. A semi-pressure patch and shield were placed over the operated eye, and the patient was brought to the recovery room in good condition.

PTERYGIA REMOVAL AND PLACEMENT OF CONJUNCTIVAL GRAFT

PREOPERATIVE DIAGNOSIS: Invasive pterygia, right eye.

POSTOPERATIVE DIAGNOSIS: Invasive pterygia, right eye.

OPERATION: Pterygia removal with placement of autologous free-floating conjunctival grafts (nasal and temporal).

ANESTHESIA: Intravenous anesthesia.

INDICATIONS: The patient is a 48-year-old Hispanic male referred for evaluation and treatment of severe invasive pterygia nasally and temporally in both eyes. The diagnosis is confirmed. The patient desires removal of these invasive and destructive lesions and is felt to be an excellent candidate for the same. He was electively admitted through the outpatient unit at this time for the above-indicated desired procedure OD.

PROCEDURE: The patient was taken to the operating room and placed on the operating table in the supine position. An IV was started and separate amounts of fentanyl and pentothal were administered intravenously. After a suitable plane of anesthesia was obtained, 4.5 mL of standard retrobulbar medication was injected in a peribulbar fashion around the right eye, which was then prepped and draped in the usual sterile fashion. Clean sterile drapes were then placed over the patient's right eye. A blepharostat was placed between the lids of the right eye. The operating microscope was then swung in position over the patient's right eye, and the entire procedure was done under direct visualization with the operating microscope.

The pterygia were easily visualized arising from the medial and temporal interpalpebral bulbar conjunctiva and encroaching onto the cornea for approximately 3.0 to 3.5 mm temporally and 2.5 to 3.0 mm nasally. The head of the nasal lesion was grasped with 0.12 corneal forceps, elevated vertically off the plane of the cornea with the plane of dissection obtained at the level of the Bowman membrane, and a superficial keratectomy was performed to peel the lesion back to the level of the limbus. It was then undermined on the bulbar conjunctiva with Westcott scissors, and the base was completely excised. The temporal lesion was removed in an identical fashion. Handheld thermocautery was used to obtain hemostasis in both beds. The edge of the cut conjunctiva was then reapproximated to the underlying episcleral tissues with interrupted 8-0 Vicryl sutures $\times$ 7 in both nasal and temporal beds. This resulted in a bare scleral defect measuring 5 mm horizontally and 7 mm vertically on both sides.

Locking Castroviejo forceps were placed at the 2 o'clock position, and the eye was rotated infratemporally to expose the superior nasal intermuscular quadrant. A 6 $\times$ 9-mm ellipse was drawn in this virgin bulbar conjunctiva. It was undermined with 2% Xylocaine with 1:100,000 epinephrine, and then the conjunctiva was removed, preserving the underlying Tenon capsule. The conjunctival graft was then rotated medially into the nasal site and sutured with interrupted 8-0 Vicryl sutures $\times$ 8. The Castroviejo forceps were then placed at the 10 o'clock position, and the eye was rotated inferonasally, exposing the supratemporal intermuscular quadrant. Again, a 6 $\times$ 9-mm ellipse was drawn in like fashion with thermocautery unit, undermined with Xylocaine, excised with Westcott scissors, rotated into the recipient bed, and sutured into the site with interrupted 8-0 Vicryl sutures $\times$ 8.

At the end of the procedure, sponge and needle counts were correct. The conjunctival grafts were in good order with no blood, air, or fluid under the graft. The edges were approximated well. There was no undue tension in any direction on the grafts and they were in good order. Homatropine ophthalmic drops were placed by instillation in this eye. Maxitrol ophthalmic drops were also placed by instillation, and Steri-Drapes and blepharostat were removed. The eye was dressed with a soft patch and Fox shield. The patient was then placed on a gurney and returned to the outpatient area, discharged in satisfactory postoperative condition.

The patient will have 1 month of convalescence. During that time, his sutures will be dissolving on their own, and he will be tapered off medication. He initially will be restricting activity such that he will not rub, scratch, or itch the eye; in any way get the eye wet or dirty; or be exposed to excessively dirty or dusty environments. He is to use Advil or extra-strength Tylenol for pain relief, but avoid aspirin-containing products for at least 48 hours. He is to leave the Fox shield and patch on the right eye at all times until he is seen in the office 24 hours after the procedure for patch removal and institution of topical medications. He and his family understand these postoperative stipulations well and will be compliant with them. I anticipate he will have dramatic improvement in his ocular motility status with hopeful total prevention of recurrence of the recurrent pterygia and taking of the graft.

PTOSIS REPAIR

OPERATION: Repair of ptosis, right and left eyes.

PROCEDURE: The patient was brought into the operating room. The eyes were prepped and draped for bilateral eyelid surgery. Tetracaine was applied to both eyes. The upper lid crease was demarcated with a marking pen on both upper lids. The excess upper eyelid skin tissue was then demarcated with a marking pen. Intravenous sedation was given. Lidocaine 2% with epinephrine was used to infiltrate both upper eyelids. Adequate anesthesia was achieved.

The right eye was addressed first. Utilizing a #15-Bard-Parker blade, an incision was made along the lid crease. The incision was then carried along through the superior margin of the demarcated upper eyelid excess tissue. Utilizing sharp dissection as well as the unipolar cutting and coagulating Bovie, the eyelid skin and orbicularis were removed. Areas of thinning of the intramuscular septum with prolapsed fat were addressed. The prolapsed fat was excised where indicated. Hemostasis was achieved with unipolar Bovie. A 4 × 4 moistened saline sponge was placed over the right upper eyelid. Attention was then directed to the left upper eyelid. The excess upper lid skin was removed in a similar fashion. Hemostasis was achieved with a Bovie. Closure was then performed of the right upper eyelid. Several supratarsal fixation sutures were placed to address the ptosis. The skin was then closed with a running 6-0 Prolene suture. The left eye was closed in a similar fashion. The patient tolerated the procedure well. The drapes were removed. Maxitrol ointment was placed in each eye. The patient was transferred to the recovery area in stable condition.

TRABECULECTOMY

PREOPERATIVE DIAGNOSIS: Poorly controlled open angle glaucoma left eye.

POSTOPERATIVE DIAGNOSIS: Poorly controlled open angle glaucoma left eye.

OPERATION: Trabeculectomy left eye.

INDICATIONS: Poorly controlled intraocular pressure in a patient who is poorly compliant with medications.

PROCEDURE: The patient was given Versed and fentanyl intravenously. She was given a retrobulbar block OS with 2% Xylocaine with Wydase. She was then prepped and draped for surgery in the usual manner.

The lids OS were retracted with the speculum. Superior rectus suture of 4-0 silk was placed with the operating microscope in position. The Alcon V-lance was used to make an entrance into the anterior chamber at the 11:30 position; the conjunctiva in the supertemporal quadrant was ballooned up using a 30-gauge needle and balanced saline solution. Blunt scissors were used to open the conjunctiva and Tenon capsule in the supertemporal quadrant, and dissection was carried up to the limbus bluntly. The anterior part of the conjunctival flap was retracted with 8-0 silk sutures. The sclera in the supertemporal quadrant was marbleized with the bipolar cautery. The trabeculectomy flap with the base at the limbus was outlined with ophthalmic cautery and then incised along the cautery lines with a #75-Beaver blade. Then the Alcon crescent knife was used to make a lamellar dissection in the eighth section of the triangle in the sclera well into clear cornea. The anterior chamber was entered with a #75-Beaver blade, and a block of clear-colored tissue was excised with the trabeculectomy punch. A peripheral iridectomy was made with the Vannas scissors. There was a small amount of bleeding encountered originally, but this eventually stopped; 1 drop of 10% phenylethyl was used to help stop the bleeding. The apex of the scleral flap was tacked and was sutured down loosely with one 10-0 nylon suture. The run-off from the trabeculectomy site was tested by injecting balanced saline solution into the anterior chamber, and it was seen to be excellent. Prior to the performance of the iridectomy, Miochol was irrigated into the anterior chamber. The conjunctiva was then closed using running interlocking 9-0 Vicryl suture. The superior rectus suture was then removed. The anterior chamber was deepened with balanced saline solution. Then 0.3 mL of 5-fluorouracil was injected subconjunctivally in the inferior fornix. A sterile dressing and atropine were applied at the cornea. The speculum was removed and a light patch applied. The patient tolerated the procedure well and was returned to the outpatient area in good condition.

Appendix 4
Common Terms by Procedure

Argon Laser Trabeculoplasty
argon laser aiming beam
argon laser trabeculoplasty
blanching
bubble production
Iopidine
laser shots
open angle glaucoma
pilocarpine
slit lamp apparatus
spot width
trabecular meshwork
trabeculoplasty lens

Chalazion Incision and Drainage
chalazion
chalazion forceps
hemostasis
Maxitrol ointment
pretarsal conjunctival surface

Dacryocystitis Rhinostomy and Repair of Canalicular Atresia
anterior ethmoidal nerve
atretic canaliculi
Bard-Parker blade
Bovie cautery
Bowman probe
canalicular atresia
canaliculus
chronic dacryocystitis
cocaine-soaked gauze
common canaliculus
conjunctivodacryocystorhinostomy
cutdown
cutting cautery
dacryocystitis rhinostomy
dacryocystorhinostomy incision
epiphora

Freer periosteal elevator
Guibor tube
hard corneal shield
hard stop
H-flap
horizontal mattress fashion
inferior punctum
in-fracturing
Kerrison punch
lacrimal fossa
lacrimal Jones tube
lacrimal maxillary suture
lacrimal microtube
lacrimal sac
Maxitrol ointment
medial canthal tendon
middle meatus
middle turbinate
mini-vertical mattress sutures
mucopurulent debris
nasal tampon
nasolacrimal fossa
orbicularis muscle
pediatric punctum dilator
periorbita
superior canaliculus
thrombin-soaked Gelfoam
topical tetracaine drops
Westcott scissors

Enucleation of the Eye
conformer
conjunctival peritomy
conjunctival sac
curved hemostat
curved scissors
Decadron
enucleation
Fox shield
gentamicin

hemostasis
implant ball
Maxitrol ointment
oblique muscles
optic nerve
rectus muscles
scleral adhesions
subconjunctival injection
Tenon capsule
Westcott scissors
wet-field cautery

Extracapsular Cataract Extraction With Insertion of Intraocular Lens

access port
akinesia
angled McPherson tying forceps
anterior capsulotomy
anterior chamber
balanced salt solution
balloon pressure
Barraquer lid speculum
Beaver blade
bipolar cautery
capsule forceps
Cavitron irrigation and aspiration tip
Celestone
circular tear capsulorrhexis capsulotomy
coapted
Colibri forceps
conjunctival cul-de-sac
corneoscleral wound
cystitome needle
epinephrine
eraser bipolar cautery
extracapsular cataract extraction
Fox shield
gentamicin
haptic
Healon
Honan intraocular pressure reducer
    balloon

inferior foot
intraocular lens
intraocular pressure
IOLAB posterior chamber intraocular
    lens
keratome
lens cortical material
lens loop
lid speculum
lidocaine
limbal peritomy
long-angled McPherson tying forceps
Marcaine
Maxitrol ointment
Miochol
Nadbath lid block
posterior capsule
retrobulbar anesthesia
right and left cutting corneoscleral
    scissors
Schiotz tonometer
scleral incision
Sinskey hook
stab wound
sub-Tenon space
superior limbus
superior rectus traction suture
Weck ophthalmic microscope
Westcott scissors
Wydase

Hypertropia Repair

Betadine solution
conjunctival cul-de-sac
fentanyl
hypertropia
hypotony
inferior oblique muscle
inferior rectus muscle
inferotemporal bulbar conjunctiva
inferotemporal orbit
lateral rectus muscle
lid speculum

Marcaine
monocular patch
muscle hook
myomectomy
palpebral fissure
peribulbar injection
relaxing incisions
superior bulbar conjunctiva
superior oblique palsy
superior rectus muscle
TobraDex ointment
Versed
Wydase
Xylocaine

Hyphema Irrigation
anterior chamber
capsulorrhexis forceps
epinephrine
fibrous plaque
hyphema
IA tip
intracameral
intraocular pressure
keratome
Legacy machine
nasal inferior fornix
subconjunctivally
tetracaine
trabeculectomy
triamcinolone
Viscoat
Xylocaine

Pars Plana Vitrectomy, Membrane Peeling, Scleral Buckle, Endolaser, and Gas-Fluid Exchange
active suction
air-fluid exchange
akinesia
Ancef
atropine drops

black silk suture
bridle sutures
complex retinal detachment
conjunctival peritomy
cortical vitreous
dexamethasone
endolaser spots
eye shell
gas-fluid exchange
gas-gas exchange
inferior rectus muscle
lid speculum
lidocaine
light pipe
macular hole
Marcaine
membrane peeling
Michel pick
muscle hook
ocutome probe
pars plana vitrectomy
posterior hyaloid
retinotomy
retrobulbar block
Ruby blade
scleral buckle
scleral plugs
sclerotomy site
SF-6 gas
Stevens scissors
subconjunctival injection
subretinal fluid
supratemporal arcade
surgical lumbus
trocar cannula infusion system
Westcott scissors
white silk suture bites
Wydase

Penetrating Keratoplasty
Ancef
balanced salt solution
Betagan

blepharostat
bupivacaine
Celestone
cellulose sponges
curved corneal scissors
donor corneal button
episclera
gentamicin
Goldman-McNeill blepharostat
Healon
Miochol
nylon sutures
penetrating keratoplasty
recipient button
recipient cornea
recipient stroma
saline sponges
semi-pressure patch
snip incisions
subconjunctival injections
Supersharp
suture tension
trephine
Vannas scissors
Vicryl suture

Pterygia Removal and Placement of Conjunctival Graft

autologous free-floating conjunctival graft
bare scleral defect
blepharostat
Bowman membrane
bulbar conjunctiva
conjunctival graft
corneal forceps
epinephrine
episcleral tissues
fentanyl
Fox shield
hand-held thermocautery
homatropine ophthalmic drops

interpalpebral bulbar conjunctiva
invasive pterygia
locking Castroviejo forceps
Maxitrol ophthalmic drops
nasal bed
operating microscope
pentothal
peribulbar fashion
recipient bed
retrobulbar medication
Steri-Drapes
superficial keratectomy
temporal bed
Tenon capsule
Vicryl sutures
virgin bulbar conjunctiva
Westcott scissors
Xylocaine

Ptosis Repair

Bard-Parker blade
epinephrine
hemostasis
intramuscular septum
lidocaine
marking pen
Maxitrol ointment
moistened saline sponge
orbicularis
prolapsed fat
Prolene suture
ptosis
sharp dissection
supratarsal fixation sutures
tetracaine
unipolar cutting and coagulating Bovie
upper lid crease

Trabeculectomy

Alcon crescent knife
Alcon V-lance
anterior chamber
atropine

balanced saline solution
Beaver blade
bipolar cautery
blunt scissors
cautery lines
conjunctiva
conjunctival flap
fentanyl
5-fluorouracil
inferior fornix
iridectomy
lamellar dissection
limbus
marbleized
Miochol
open angle glaucoma
operating microscope
ophthalmic cautery

peripheral iridectomy
phenylethyl
retrobulbar block
run-off
scleral flap
silk sutures
speculum
superior rectus suture
supertemporal quadrant
Tenon capsule
trabeculectomy flap
trabeculectomy punch
trabeculectomy site
Vannas scissors
Versed
Vicryl suture
Wydase
Xylocaine

Appendix 5
Drugs by Indication

ALLERGIC DISORDERS (OPHTHALMIC)
Adrenal Corticosteroid
  HMS Liquifilm®
  medrysone

ANESTHESIA (OPHTHALMIC)
Local Anesthetic
  Fluoracaine®
  proparacaine and fluorescein

BLEPHARITIS
Antifungal Agent
  Natacyn® [US/Can]
  natamycin

BLEPHAROSPASM
Ophthalmic Agent, Toxin
  Botox® [US/Can]
  botulinum toxin type A

CATARACT
Adrenergic Agonist Agent
  AK-Dilate® Ophthalmic
  AK-Nefrin® Ophthalmic
  Mydfrin® Ophthalmic [US/Can]
  Neo-Synephrine® Ophthalmic
  phenylephrine

CHORIORETINITIS
Adrenal Corticosteroid
  A-HydroCort® [US/Can]
  Alti-Dexamethasone [Can]
  A-methaPred®
  Apo®-Prednisone [Can]
  Aristocort® Forte Injection
  Aristocort® Intralesional Injection
  Aristocort® Tablet [US/Can]
  Aristospan® Intra-articular Injection
    [US/Can]
  Aristospan® Intralesional Injection
    [US/Can]
  Betaject™ [Can]
  betamethasone (systemic)
  Betnesol® [Can]
  Celestone® Phosphate
  Celestone® Soluspan® [US/Can]
  Celestone®
  Cel-U-Jec®
  Cortef® [US/Can]
  cortisone acetate
  Cortone® [Can]
  Decadron®-LA
  Decadron® [US/Can]
  Decaject®
  Decaject-LA®
  Delta-Cortef®
  Deltasone®
  Depo-Medrol® [US/Can]
  Depopred®
  dexamethasone (systemic)
  Dexasone® [US/Can]
  Dexasone® L.A.
  Dexone®
  Dexone® LA
  Hexadrol® [US/Can]
  hydrocortisone (systemic)
  Hydrocortone® Acetate
  Kenalog® Injection [US/Can]
  Key-Pred®
  Key-Pred-SP®
  Medrol® Tablet [US/Can]
  methylprednisolone
  Meticorten®
  Orapred™
  Pediapred® [US/Can]
  PMS-Dexamethasone [Can]
  Prednicot®
  prednisolone (systemic)
  Prednisol® TBA

prednisone
Prelone®
Solu-Cortef® [US/Can]
Solu-Medrol® [US/Can]
Solurex L.A.®
Sterapred®
Sterapred® DS
Tac™-3 Injection
Triam-A® Injection
triamcinolone (systemic)
Triam Forte® Injection
Winpred™ [Can]

CMV RETINITIS
Antiviral Agent
  Valcyte™
  valganciclovir

CONJUNCTIVITIS (ALLERGIC)
Adrenal Corticosteroid
  HMS Liquifilm®
  medrysone
Antihistamine
  Alertab® [OTC]
  Aller-Chlor® [OTC]
  Aller-Dryl® [OTC]
  Allerdryl® [Can]
  Allermax® [OTC]
  Allernix [Can]
  Altaryl® [OTC]
  Anti-Hist® [OTC]
  ANX®
  Apo®-Dimenhydrinate [Can]
  Apo®-Hydroxyzine [Can]
  Atarax® [US/Can]
  azatadine
  Banophen® [OTC]
  Benadryl® [US/Can]
  brompheniramine
  chlorpheniramine
  Chlor-Trimeton® [OTC]
  Chlor-Tripolon® [Can]

Claritin® [US/Can]
Claritin® RediTabs®
clemastine
cyproheptadine
Dermamycin® [OTC]
Derma-Pax® [OTC]
dexchlorpheniramine
dimenhydrinate
Dimetane® Extentabs® [OTC]
Dimetapp® Allergy [OTC]
Dimetapp® Allergy Children's [OTC]
Diphedryl® [OTC]
Diphenhist® [OTC]
diphenhydramine
Diphen® [OTC]
Diphenyl® [OTC]
Dramamine® Oral [OTC]
Dytuss® [OTC]
Genahist® [OTC]
Geridryl® [OTC]
Gravol® [Can]
Hydramine® [OTC]
Hydrate®
hydroxyzine
Hyrexin® [OTC]
Hyzine-50®
levocabastine
Livostin® [US/Can]
Lodrane® 12 Hour [OTC]
loratadine
Medi-phedryl® [OTC]
Miles® Nervine [OTC]
ND-Stat® Solution [TC]
Nolahist® [US/Can]
Novo-Hydroxyzine [Can]
olopatadine
Optimine® [US/Can]
Patanol® [US/Can]
Periactin® [US/Can]
phenindamine
PMS-Diphenhydramine [Can]
PMS-Hydroxyzine [Can]
Polaramine®

Polydryl® [OTC]
Polytapp® Allergy Dye-Free Medication [OTC]
Q-Dryl® [OTC]
Quenalin® [OTC]
Restall®
Scot-Tussin® Allergy [OTC]
Siladryl® Allergy® [OTC]
Silphen® [OTC]
Tavist®
Tavist®-1 [OTC]
Vistacot®
Vistaril® [US/Can]
Antihistamine/Decongestant Combination
Andehist NR Drops
Carbaxefed RF
carbinoxamine and pseudoephedrine
Hydro-Tussin™-CBX
Palgic®-D
Palgic®-DS
Rondec® Drops
Rondec® Tablets
Rondec-TR®
Antihistamine, H1 Blocker, Ophthalmic
Apo®-Ketotifen [Can]
Emadine®
emedastine
ketotifen
Antihistamine, Ophthalmic
Astelin® [US/Can]
azelastine
Optivar™
Corticosteroid, Ophthalmic
Alrex™ [US/Can]
Lotemax™ [US/Can]
loteprednol
Mast Cell Stabilizer
Alamast™ [US/Can]
Alocril™ [US/Can]
nedocromil (ophthalmic)
pemirolast

Nonsteroidal Antiinflammatory Drug (NSAID)
Acular® [US/Can]
Acular® PF
Apo®-Ketorolac [Can]
ketorolac
Novo-Ketorolac [Can]
Ophthalmic Agent, Miscellaneous
Alamast™ [US/Can]
pemirolast
Phenothiazine Derivative
Anergan®
Phenergan® [US/Can]
promethazine

CONJUNCTIVITIS (BACTERIAL)
Antibiotic, Ophthalmic
levofloxacin
Quixin™ Ophthalmic

CONJUNCTIVITIS (VERNAL)
Adrenal Corticosteroid
HMS Liquifilm®
medrysone
Mast Cell Stabilizer
Alomide® [US/Can]
lodoxamide tromethamine

CORNEAL EDEMA
Lubricant, Ocular
Muro 128® [OTC]
sodium chloride

CYCLOPLEGIA
Anticholinergic Agent
AK-Pentolate®
atropine
Atropine-Care®
Atropisol® [US/Can]
Cyclogyl® [US/Can]
cyclopentolate
Diopentolate® [Can]

Diotrope® [Can]
homatropine
Isopto® Atropine [US/Can]
Isopto® Homatropine
Isopto® Hyoscine
Mydriacyl® [US/Can]
Sal-Tropine™
scopolamine
tropicamide

DRY EYES
Ophthalmic Agent, Miscellaneous
Akwa Tears® [OTC]
AquaSite® [OTC]
artificial tears
balanced salt solution
Bion® Tears [OTC]
BSS® [US/Can]
BSS® Plus [US/Can]
carbopol 940 (Canada only)
carboxymethylcellulose
Cellufresh® [OTC]
Celluvisc® [US/Can]
collagen implants
Eye-Stream® [US/Can]
hydroxypropyl cellulose
HypoTears [OTC]
HypoTears PF [OTC]
Isopto® Tears [US/Can]
Lacrinorm [Can]
Lacrisert® [US/Can]
Liquifilm® Tears [OTC]
Moisture® Eyes [OTC]
Moisture® Eyes PM [OTC]
Murine® Tears [OTC]
Murocel® [OTC]
Nature's Tears® [OTC]
Nu-Tears® [OTC]
Nu-Tears® II [OTC]
OcuCoat® [US/Can]
OcuCoat® PF [OTC]
Puralube® Tears [OTC]

Refresh® [OTC]
Refresh® Plus [US/Can]
Refresh® Tears [US/Can]
Teardrops® [Can]
Teargen® [OTC]
Teargen® II [OTC]
Tearisol® [OTC]
Tears Again® [OTC]
Tears Naturale® [OTC]
Tears Naturale® Free [OTC]
Tears Naturale® II [OTC]
Tears Plus® [OTC]
Tears Renewed® [OTC]
Ultra Tears® [OTC]
Viva-Drops® [OTC]

EPISCLERITIS
Adrenal Corticosteroid
HMS Liquifilm®
medrysone

ESOTROPIA
Cholinesterase Inhibitor
echothiophate iodide
Phospholine Iodide®

EYE INFECTION
Antibiotic/Corticosteroid, Ophthalmic
AK-Cide®
AK-Trol®
bacitracin, neomycin, polymyxin B,
   and hydrocortisone
Blephamide® [US/Can]
Cortimyxin® [Can]
Cortisporin® Ophthalmic [US/Can]
Dexacidin®
Dexacine™
Dioptimyd® [Can]
Dioptrol® [Can]
FML-S®
Maxitrol® [US/Can]
Metimyd®
Neo-Cortef® [Can]

NeoDecadron® Ocumeter®
neomycin and dexamethasone
neomycin and hydrocortisone
neomycin, polymyxin B, and dexa-
    methasone
neomycin, polymyxin B, and hydro-
    cortisone
neomycin, polymyxin B, and pred-
    nisolone
Poly-Pred®
Pred-G®
prednisolone and gentamicin
sulfacetamide and prednisolone
sulfacetamide sodium and fluo-
    rometholone
TobraDex® [US/Can]
tobramycin and dexamethasone
Vasocidin® [US/Can]
Antibiotic, Ophthalmic
  Akne-Mycin®
  AK-Poly-Bac®
  AK-Spore® Ophthalmic Solution
  AK-Sulf®
  AKTob®
  AK-Tracin®
  Alcomicin® [Can]
  Apo®-Oflox [Can]
  Apo®-Tetra [Can]
  A/T/S®
  Baciguent® [US/Can]
  bacitracin
  bacitracin and polymyxin B
  bacitracin, neomycin, and
    polymyxin B
  Bleph®-10
  Brodspec®
  Carmol® Scalp
  Cetamide® [US/Can]
  chloramphenicol
  Chloromycetin® Parenteral [US/Can]
  Chloroptic® Ophthalmic
  Ciloxan™ [US/Can]

ciprofloxacin
Cipro® [US/Can]
Diochloram® [Can]
Diogent® [Can]
Diosulf™ [Can]
Emgel®
EmTet®
Erycette®
EryDerm®
Erygel®
Erythra-Derm™
erythromycin (ophthalmic/topical)
Floxin® [US/Can]
Garamycin® [US/Can]
Garatec [Can]
Genoptic®
Gentacidin®
Gentak®
gentamicin
Klaron®
Levaquin® [US/Can]
levofloxacin
LID-Pack® [Can]
Mycitracin® [OTC]
Nebcin® [US/Can]
neomycin, polymyxin B, and grami-
    cidin
Neosporin® Ophthalmic Ointment
    [US/Can]
Neosporin® Ophthalmic Solution
    [US/Can]
Neosporin® Topical [US/Can]
Neotopic® [Can]
Novo-Tetra [Can]
Nu-Tetra [Can]
Ocu-Chlor® Ophthalmic
Ocuflox® [US/Can]
Ocu-Sul®
ofloxacin
Optimyxin® Ophthalmic [Can]
Optimyxin Plus® [Can]
oxytetracycline and polymyxin B

Pentamycetin® [Can]
PMS-Polytrimethoprim [Can]
PMS-Tobramycin [Can]
Polycidin® Ophthalmic
Polysporin® Ophthalmic
Polysporin® Topical [OTC]
Polytrim® [US/Can]
Quixin™ Ophthalmic
Romycin®
Sebizon®
Sodium Sulamyd® [US/Can]
Staticin®
Sulf-10®
sulfacetamide
Sumycin®
Terramycin® w/Polymyxin B Ophthalmic
tetracycline
Theramycin Z®
TOBI™ [US/Can]
tobramycin
Tobrex® [US/Can]
Tomycine™ [Can]
trimethoprim and polymyxin B
Triple Antibiotic®
T-Stat®
Wesmycin®

EYE IRRITATION
Adrenergic Agonist Agent
AK-Con™
Albalon®
Allersol®
Clear Eyes® [OTC]
Clear Eyes® ACR [OTC]
naphazoline
Naphcon® [OTC]
Naphcon Forte® [Can]
phenylephrine and zinc sulfate
Privine® [OTC]
VasoClear® [OTC]
Vasocon® [Can]

Zincfrin® [US/Can]
Ophthalmic Agent, Miscellaneous
Akwa Tears® [OTC]
AquaSite® [OTC]
artificial tears
Bion® Tears [OTC]
HypoTears [OTC]
HypoTears PF [OTC]
Isopto® Tears [US/Can]
Liquifilm® Tears [OTC]
Moisture® Eyes [OTC]
Moisture® Eyes PM [OTC]
Murine® Tears [OTC]
Murocel® [OTC]
Nature's Tears® [OTC]
Nu-Tears® [OTC]
Nu-Tears® II [OTC]
OcuCoat® [US/Can]
OcuCoat® PF [OTC]
Puralube® Tears [OTC]
Refresh® [OTC]
Refresh® Plus [US/Can]
Refresh® Tears [US/Can]
Teardrops® [Can]
Teargen® [OTC]
Teargen® II [OTC]
Tearisol® [OTC]
Tears Again® [OTC]
Tears Naturale® [OTC]
Tears Naturale® Free [OTC]
Tears Naturale® II [OTC]
Tears Plus® [OTC]
Tears Renewed® [OTC]
Ultra Tears® [OTC]
Viva-Drops® [OTC]

EYELID INFECTION
Antibiotic, Ophthalmic
mercuric oxide
Ocu-Merox®
Pharmaceutical Aid
boric acid

GIANT PAPILLARY CONJUNCTIVITIS
Mast Cell Stabilizer
  Crolom®
  cromolyn sodium

GLAUCOMA
Adrenergic Agonist Agent
  AK-Dilate® Ophthalmic
  AK-Nefrin® Ophthalmic
  Dionephrine® [Can]
  dipivefrin
  Epifrin®
  Epinal®
  epinephrine
  epinephryl borate
  Mydfrin® Ophthalmic [US/Can]
  Neo-Synephrine® Ophthalmic
  Ophtho-Dipivefrin™ [Can]
  phenylephrine
  PMS-Dipivefrin [Can]
  Prefrin™ Ophthalmic
  Primatene® Mist [OTC]
  Propine® [US/Can]
Alpha2-Adrenergic Agonist Agent,
    Ophthalmic
  Alphagan® P [US/Can]
  apraclonidine
  brimonidine
  Iopidine® [US/Can]
Beta-Adrenergic Blocker
  Apo®-Timol [Can]
  Apo®-Timop [Can]
  Betagan® [US/Can]
  betaxolol
  Betimol®
  Betoptic® S [US/Can]
  carteolol
  Cartrol® Oral [US/Can]
  Cosopt® [US/Can]
  dorzolamide and timolol
  Gen-Timolol [Can]

Kerlone®
levobunolol
metipranolol
Novo-Levobunolol [Can]
Nu-Timolol [Can]
Ocupress® Ophthalmic [US/Can]
Optho-Bunolol® [Can]
OptiPranolol® [US/Can]
PMS-Levobunolol [Can]
PMS-Timolol [Can]
Tim-AK [Can]
timolol
Timoptic® [US/Can]
Timoptic® OcuDose®
Timoptic-XE® [US/Can]
Beta-Adrenergic Blocker, Ophthalmic
  Betaxon® [US/Can]
  levobetaxolol
Carbonic Anhydrase Inhibitor
  acetazolamide
  Apo®-Acetazolamide [Can]
  Azopt® [US/Can]
  brinzolamide
  Cosopt® [US/Can]
  Daranide® [US/Can]
  Diamox® [US/Can]
  Diamox Sequels®
  dichlorphenamide
  dorzolamide
  dorzolamide and timolol
  methazolamide
  Neptazane® [US/Can]
  Trusopt® [US/Can]
Cholinergic Agent
  carbachol
  Carbastat® [US/Can]
  Carboptic®
  Diocarpine [Can]
  Isopto® Carbachol [US/Can]
  Isopto® Carpine [US/Can]
  Miocarpine® [Can]
  Miostat® Intraocular [US/Can]

P6E1®
pilocarpine
pilocarpine and epinephrine
Pilocar®
Pilopine HS® [US/Can]
Piloptic®
Salagen® [US/Can]
Cholinesterase Inhibitor
  echothiophate iodide
  Phospholine Iodide®
  physostigmine
Diuretic, Osmotic
  mannitol
  Osmitrol® [US/Can]
  urea
Ophthalmic Agent, Miscellaneous
  Bausch & Lomb® Computer Eye
    Drops [OTC]
  bimatoprost
  glycerin
  Lumigan™
  Osmoglyn®
  unoprostone
Prostaglandin
  latanoprost
  Xalatan® [US/Can]
Prostaglandin, Ophthalmic
  Travatan™
  travoprost

GLIOMA
Antineoplastic Agent
  CeeNU® [US/Can]
  lomustine
Antiviral Agent
  interferon alfa-2b and ribavirin combination pack
  Rebetron™ [US/Can]
Biological Response Modulator
  interferon alfa-2b
  interferon alfa-2b and ribavirin combination pack

Intron® A [US/Can]
Rebetron™ [US/Can]

GONOCOCCAL OPHTHALMIA NEONATORUM
Topical Skin Product
  silver nitrate

HYPERTENSION (OCULAR)
Alpha2-Adrenergic Agonist Agent, Ophthalmic
  Alphagan® P [US/Can]
  brimonidine
Beta-Adrenergic Blocker
  Betagan® [US/Can]
  levobunolol
  Novo-Levobunolol [Can]
  Optho-Bunolol® [Can]
  PMS-Levobunolol [Can]

INTRAOCULAR PRESSURE
Ophthalmic Agent, Miscellaneous
  glycerin
  Osmoglyn®

IRIDOCYCLITIS
Adrenal Corticosteroid
  HMS Liquifilm®
  medrysone
Anticholinergic Agent
  Diotrope® [Can]
  Isopto® Hyoscine
  Mydriacyl® [US/Can]
  scopolamine
  tropicamide

KERATITIS
Adrenal Corticosteroid
  Flarex® [US/Can]
  fluorometholone
  Fluor-Op®
  FML® [US/Can]

FML® Forte [US/Can]
Anticholinergic Agent
   Diotrope® [Can]
   Mydriacyl® [US/Can]
   tropicamide
Mast Cell Stabilizer
   Crolom®
   cromolyn sodium
   Opticrom® [US/Can]

KERATITIS (EXPOSURE)

Ophthalmic Agent, Miscellaneous
   Akwa Tears® [OTC]
   AquaSite® [OTC]
   artificial tears
   Bion® Tears [OTC]
   HypoTears [OTC]
   HypoTears PF [OTC]
   Isopto® Tears [US/Can]
   Liquifilm® Tears [OTC]
   Moisture® Eyes [OTC]
   Moisture® Eyes PM [OTC]
   Murine® Tears [OTC]
   Murocel® [OTC]
   Nature's Tears® [OTC]
   Nu-Tears® [OTC]
   Nu-Tears® II [OTC]
   OcuCoat® [US/Can]
   OcuCoat® PF [OTC]
   Puralube® Tears [OTC]
   Refresh® [OTC]
   Refresh® Plus [US/Can]
   Refresh® Tears [US/Can]
   Teardrops® [Can]
   Teargen® [OTC]
   Teargen® II [OTC]
   Tearisol® [OTC]
   Tears Again® [OTC]
   Tears Naturale® [OTC]
   Tears Naturale® Free [OTC]
   Tears Naturale® II [OTC]
   Tears Plus® [OTC]
   Tears Renewed® [OTC]
   Ultra Tears® [OTC]
   Viva-Drops® [OTC]

KERATITIS (FUNGAL)

Antifungal Agent
   Natacyn® [US/Can]
   natamycin

KERATITIS (HERPES SIMPLEX)

Antiviral Agent
   trifluridine
   vidarabine
   Vira-A®
   Viroptic® [US/Can]

KERATITIS (VERNAL)

Antiviral Agent
   trifluridine
   Viroptic® [US/Can]
Mast Cell Stabilizer
   Alomide® [US/Can]
   lodoxamide tromethamine

KERATOCONJUNCTIVITIS (VERNAL)

Mast Cell Stabilizer
   Alomide® [US/Can]
   lodoxamide tromethamine

MACULAR DEGENERATION

Ophthalmic Agent
   verteporfin
   Visudyne™ [US/Can]

MIOSIS

Alpha-Adrenergic Blocking Agent
   dapiprazole
   Rev-Eyes™
Cholinergic Agent
   acetylcholine

carbachol
Carbastat® [US/Can]
Carboptic®
Diocarpine [Can]
Isopto® Carbachol [US/Can]
Isopto® Carpine [US/Can]
Miocarpine® [Can]
Miochol-E® [US/Can]
Miostat® Intraocular [US/Can]
P_6E_1®
pilocarpine
pilocarpine and epinephrine
Pilocar®
Pilopine HS® [US/Can]
Piloptic®
Nonsteroidal Antiinflammatory Drug
    (NSAID)
Alti-Flurbiprofen [Can]
Ansaid® Oral [US/Can]
Apo®-Flurbiprofen [Can]
flurbiprofen
Froben® [Can]
Froben-SR® [Can]
Novo-Flurprofen [Can]
Nu-Flurprofen [Can]
Ocufen® Ophthalmic [US/Can]

MYDRIASIS

Adrenergic Agonist Agent
AK-Dilate® Ophthalmic
AK-Nefrin® Ophthalmic
Dionephrine® [Can]
Mydfrin® Ophthalmic [US/Can]
Neo-Synephrine® Ophthalmic
phenylephrine
Prefrin™ Ophthalmic
Anticholinergic/Adrenergic Agonist
Cyclomydril® Ophthalmic
cyclopentolate and phenylephrine
Murocoll-2®
phenylephrine and scopolamine
Anticholinergic Agent
AK-Pentolate®

atropine
Atropine-Care®
Atropisol® [US/Can]
Cyclogyl® [US/Can]
cyclopentolate
Diopentolate® [Can]
Diotrope® [Can]
homatropine
Isopto® Atropine [US/Can]
Isopto® Homatropine
Mydriacyl® [US/Can]
Sal-Tropine™
tropicamide

NEURITIS (OPTIC)

Adrenal Corticosteroid
A-HydroCort® [US/Can]
Alti-Dexamethasone [Can]
A-methaPred®
Apo®-Prednisone [Can]
Aristocort® Forte Injection
Aristocort® Intralesional Injection
Aristocort® Tablet [US/Can]
Aristospan® Intra-articular Injection
    [US/Can]
Aristospan® Intralesional Injection
    [US/Can]
Betaject™ [Can]
betamethasone (systemic)
Betnesol® [Can]
Celestone®
Celestone® Phosphate
Celestone® Soluspan® [US/Can]
Cel-U-Jec®
Cortef® [US/Can]
cortisone acetate
Cortone® [Can]
Decadron® [US/Can]
Decadron®-LA
Decaject®
Decaject-LA®
Delta-Cortef®
Deltasone®

Depo-Medrol® [US/Can]
Depopred®
dexamethasone (systemic)
Dexasone® [US/Can]
Dexasone® L.A.
Dexone® LA [US]
Dexone®
Hexadrol® [US/Can]
hydrocortisone (systemic)
Hydrocortone® Acetate
Kenalog® Injection [US/Can]
Key-Pred®
Key-Pred-SP®
Medrol® Tablet [US/Can]
methylprednisolone
Meticorten®
Orapred™
Pediapred® [US/Can]
PMS-Dexamethasone [Can]
Prednicot®
prednisolone (systemic)
Prednisol® TBA
prednisone
Prelone®
Solu-Cortef® [US/Can]
Solu-Medrol® [US/Can]
Solurex L.A.®
Sterapred®
Sterapred® DS
Tac™-3 Injection
Triam-A® Injection
triamcinolone (systemic)
Triam Forte® Injection
Winpred™ [Can]

OCULAR INJURY
Nonsteroidal Antiinflammatory Drug
    (NSAID)
    flurbiprofen
    Ocufen® Ophthalmic [US/Can]

OCULAR REDNESS
Adrenergic Agonist Agent
    AK-Dilate® Ophthalmic

AK-Nefrin® Ophthalmic
Albalon®
Allersol®
Clear Eyes® [OTC]
Clear Eyes® ACR [OTC]
Collyrium Fresh® [OTC]
Dionephrine® [Can]
Eyesine® [OTC]
Geneye® [OTC]
Mallazine® Eye Drops [OTC]
Murine® Plus Ophthalmic [OTC]
Mydfrin® Ophthalmic [US/Can]
Naphazoline
Naphcon® [OTC]
Naphcon Forte® [Can]
OcuClear® [OTC]
Optigene® [OTC]
oxymetazoline
phenylephrine
Prefrin™ Ophthalmic
Privine® [OTC]
tetrahydrozoline
Tetrasine® [OTC]
Tetrasine® Extra [OTC]
Twice-A-Day® [OTC]
VasoClear® [OTC]
Vasocon® [Can]
Visine® Extra [OTC]
Visine® L.R. [OTC]
Antihistamine/Decongestant
    Combination
    Albalon®-A Liquifilm [Can]
    naphazoline and antazoline
    naphazoline and pheniramine
    Naphcon-A® [US/Can]
    Opcon-A® [OTC]
    Vasocon-A® [US/Can]
    Visine-A™ [OTC]

OPHTHALMIC DISORDERS
Adrenal Corticosteroid
    Acthar®
    A-HydroCort® [US/Can]

AK-Dex®
AK-Pred®
A-methaPred®
Apo®-Prednisone [Can]
Aristocort® Forte Injection
Aristocort® Intralesional Injection
Aristocort® Tablet [US/Can]
Aristospan® Intra-articular Injection
   [US/Can]
Aristospan® Intralesional Injection
   [US/Can]
Baldex®
Betaject™ [Can]
betamethasone (systemic)
Betnesol® [Can]
Celestone®
Celestone® Phosphate
Celestone® Soluspan® [US/Can]
Cel-U-Jec®
Cortef® [US/Can]
corticotropin
cortisone acetate
Cortone® [Can]
Decadron® Ocumeter®
Deltasone®
Depo-Medrol® [US/Can]
Depopred®
dexamethasone (ophthalmic)
Diodex® [Can]
Diopred® [Can]
Econopred®
Econopred® Plus
Flarex® [US/Can]
fluorometholone
Fluor-Op®
FML® [US/Can]
FML® Forte [US/Can]
H.P. Acthar® Gel
hydrocortisone (systemic)
Hydrocortone® Acetate
Inflamase® Forte [US/Can]
Inflamase® Mild [US/Can]
Kenalog® Injection [US/Can]

Maxidex® [US/Can]
Medrol® Tablet [US/Can]
methylprednisolone
Meticorten®
Metreton®
Ophtho-Tate® [Can]
Pred Forte® [US/Can]
Pred Mild® [US/Can]
Prednicot®
prednisolone (ophthalmic)
prednisone
Solu-Cortef® [US/Can]
Solu-Medrol® [US/Can]
Sterapred®
Sterapred® DS
Tac™-3 Injection
Triam-A® Injection
triamcinolone (systemic)
Triam Forte® Injection
Winpred™ [Can]

OPHTHALMIC SURGERY
Nonsteroidal Antiinflammatory Drug
   (NSAID)
   diclofenac
   Voltaren® [US/Can]
   Voltaren Ophtha® [Can]

OPHTHALMIC SURGICAL AID
Ophthalmic Agent, Miscellaneous
   GenTeal™ [US/Can]
   Gonak™ [OTC]
   Goniosol® [OTC]
   hydroxypropyl methylcellulose

RETINOBLASTOMA
Antineoplastic Agent
   Cosmegen® [US/Can]
   cyclophosphamide
   Cytoxan® [US/Can]
   dactinomycin
   Neosar®
   Procytox® [Can]

REYE SYNDROME
Ophthalmic Agent, Miscellaneous
  glycerin
  Osmoglyn®

STRABISMUS
Cholinesterase Inhibitor
  echothiophate iodide
  Phospholine Iodide®
Ophthalmic Agent, Toxin
  Botox® [US/Can]
  botulinum toxin type A

SURGICAL AID (OPHTHALMIC)
Ophthalmic Agent, Viscoelastic
  Biolon® [US/Can]
  chondroitin sulfate-sodium
    hyaluronate
  Cystistat® [Can]
  Eyestil [Can]
  Healon® [Can]
  Healon® GV [Can]
  Hyalgan®
  Provisc®
  sodium hyaluronate
  Supartz®
  Suplasyn® [Can]
  Viscoat®
  Vitrax®

UVEITIS
Adrenal Corticosteroid
  rimexolone
  Vexol® [US/Can]
Adrenergic Agonist Agent
  AK-Dilate® Ophthalmic
  AK-Nefrin® Ophthalmic
  Dionephrine® [Can]
  Mydfrin® Ophthalmic [US/Can]
  Neo-Synephrine® Ophthalmic
  phenylephrine
  Prefrin™ Ophthalmic
Anticholinergic Agent
  atropine
  Atropine-Care®
  Atropisol® [US/Can]
  homatropine
  Isopto® Atropine [US/Can]
  Isopto® Homatropine
  Isopto® Hyoscine
  scopolamine

XEROPHTHALMIA
Ophthalmic Agent, Miscellaneous
  Akwa Tears® [OTC]
  AquaSite® [OTC]
  Artificial tears
  Bion® Tears [OTC]
  HypoTears [OTC]
  HypoTears PF [OTC]
  Isopto® Tears [US/Can]
  Liquifilm® Tears [OTC]
  Moisture® Eyes [OTC]
  Moisture® Eyes PM [OTC]
  Murine® Tears [OTC]
  Murocel® [OTC]
  Nature's Tears® [OTC]
  Nu-Tears® [OTC]
  Nu-Tears® II [OTC]
  OcuCoat® [US/Can]
  OcuCoat® PF [OTC]
  Puralube® Tears [OTC]
  Refresh® [OTC]
  Refresh® Plus [US/Can]
  Refresh® Tears [US/Can]
  Teardrops® [Can]
  Teargen® [OTC]
  Teargen® II [OTC]
  Tearisol® [OTC]
  Tears Again® [OTC]
  Tears Naturale® [OTC]
  Tears Naturale® Free [OTC]
  Tears Naturale® II [OTC]
  Tears Plus® [OTC]
  Tears Renewed® [OTC]
  Ultra Tears® [OTC]
  Viva-Drops® [OTC]